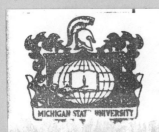

ELECTRONIC FETAL-MATERNAL MONITORING:

Antepartum, Intrapartum

Luis A. Cibils, MD
Mary Campau Ryerson Professor
Department of Obstetrics and Gynecology
The University of Chicago
The Chicago Lying-In Hospital

John Wright • PSG Inc
Boston • Bristol • London

Library of Congress Cataloging in Publication Data

Cibils, Luis A   1927–
    Electronic fetal-maternal monitoring.

    Bibliography: p.
    Includes index.
    1. Fetal heart rate monitoring.   2.   Labor (Obstetrics)
I. Title. [DNLM: 1. Fetal monitoring. 2.   Prenatal
Diagnosis.   3.   Labor. WQ 209 C567e]
RG628.3.H42C52   618.3′207547   80-24362
ISBN 0-88416-192-7

Printed in the United States of America.

International Standard Book Number: 0-88416-192-7

Library of Congress Catalog Card Number: 80-24362

Dedicated with affection to my wife and children
whose encouragement and tolerance during my intermittent isolations
made my work easier

Contents

Foreword

It seems only yesterday that the fetus in utero and the uterine environment were almost completely shrouded in mystery. The gender of the child was principally a matter of sheer speculation. Its size was estimated by abdominal palpation with notorious lack of accuracy. The growth pattern of the fetus was not a subject for serious study inasmuch as antenatal care and observations were not being systematically made. A question of whether the fetus had a severe malformation was dealt with as a matter of fear rather than a subject to be seriously evaluated. The condition of the fetus in utero at a given time and the question of whether the fetus would tolerate labor had not seriously been brought forward. Whether labor could be safely induced and whether the infant would be likely to survive if born were questions yet to be raised.

A small body of useful basic information began to accumulate quietly in the literature. Notable contributions in the last half of the 19th century were the demonstrations of uterine contractility patterns in labor by Friedrich Schatz and the description of uterine contractility during the last two trimesters of pregnancy by John Braxton Hicks. Notable in the first quarter of the 20th century were the contributions of Bell and others concerning the use of oxytocic agents and the relationship of various oxytocic products to physiologic stimulation of uterine contractility. In the second quarter of the 20th century were the contributions of Sir Joseph Barcroft and his *Researches on Prenatal Life* and the work of Theobald who brought the safe use of oxytocin into the arena of clinical obstetrics. Just at mid-century came the work of S.R.M. Reynolds who contributed to and summarized the knowledge of uterine physiology up to mid-century.

In the 1950s there came on the scene Alvarez and Caldeyro-Barcia. Working in Montevideo, Uruguay, these workers laid the foundation for much of the development of what became the field of Maternal and Fetal Medicine. They contributed massively to our ability to measure accurately parameters of uterine activity, and they taught a systematic approach to the clinician's understanding of uterine physiology. Their work spread extremely rapidly beyond the boundaries of their native Uruguay. The last 30 years have seen a quantum leap in our understanding of fetal and uterine physiology. Nearly all of the old questions—diagnostic, therapeutic, and prognostic—have been at least partly answered. The body of new knowledge is now housed largely within the subspecialty of Maternal and Fetal Medicine.

The author of this book arrived on the scene just after the critical mid-century turning point. He was fortunate to come under the influence of Professor Raoul Palmer in France, to work in Spain, then to go from his native Paraguay to join Alvarez and Caldeyro-Barcia at la Sección Fisiología Obstétrica in Montevideo as an active participant in the exciting work being conducted there. Starting from that point he has been ever since in the mainstream of the growing specialty of Maternal and Fetal Medicine. Many of the developments described by Dr. Cibils have a partly autobiographical flavor. The work presented here is a testament to Dr. Cibils' rich knowledge of the currents and countercurrents that have been active in the development of much of this specialty.

This book, 10 years in the dreaming and several years in the writing, is presented as Dr. Cibils' testament to how it all came about. It also represents a progress note as to the current state of the art. Finally, it should serve as a benchmark from which future progress can be measured as we advance further in our understanding of the fetus and the problems it faces in the uterine environment.

Charles H. Hendricks, MD
Department of Obstetrics and Gynecology
The School of Medicine
The University of North Carolina at Chapel Hill
June 1980

Preface

Intrapartum monitoring has become, in the United States, a common procedure to follow spontaneous, enhanced, or induced labor. At some institutions, almost every patient admitted to the labor–delivery suite is attached to a monitoring device and the tracing thus obtained is used in making decisions regarding the management of her case. It is probably safe to state that, in this country, every hospital prepared to give obstetric care is equipped with one or several electronic monitoring apparatuses; it is almost a "status symbol" for any self-respecting institution. The massive availability of this new tool, ostensibly devised and applied to improve fetal and maternal care, has occurred simultaneously with a sharp increase in the proportion of pregnancies terminated by cesarean section. The possible cause-and-effect relationship has been pointed out by many, with such persistence that national authorities—scientific as well as administrative—have decided to investigate the matter carefully. It is possible that part of that increased rate of operations could be ascribed to the rapid introduction of continuous electronic monitoring in clinical practice. More specifically, it is possible that a significant number of those operations are indeed indicated because many physicians were not completely familiar with the methods of precise interpretation of the tracings—a strong probability, since all those undertaking that task have not been systematically and thoroughly prepared. To properly discharge the responsibility, the clinician must dedicate time to specialized training, under competent supervision—a requirement not available to many and thus the explanation for some hasty and not-too-fortunate decisions.

This book was conceived with the awareness of these facts and with the hope that it may contribute to understanding better the pathophysiology of mother and fetus during advanced gestation, labor, and delivery. It should help in minimizing misinterpretations, thereby timing more precisely either active interference by the obstetrician or abstention from it. The general method was the one I learned from my teachers Raoul Palmer and Roberto Caldeyro-Barcia, that is, the review of the physiologic principles governing the functions under study to plan a rational management of their alterations. It was my fortune to have had the opportunity to spend several years with Drs. Hermogenes Alvarez and Roberto Caldeyro-Barcia when the foundations of the subspecialty Fetal Maternal Medicine were being laid by them in Montevideo. Much of the content of this work is the reflection of their teachings: the critical evaluation of carefully recorded laboratory observations and their confrontation with clinical experience are prerequisites to postulate plausible mechanisms as the basis for suggesting therapeutic measures. This philosophy, and the continuing experience of daily learning from my colleagues and collaborators through more than two decades, form the basis for the interpretations and the recommendations made to manage specific clinical conditions.

The book is divided in two sections: monitoring of the mother and monitoring of the fetus. In each, detailed descriptions of instrumentation and techniques are given with discussion of the principles on which the various methods are based. These, as well as all technical steps, are illustrated with pictures and drawings; also, the reasons for the preference of specific methods are given when a choice is available. The first section includes the factors governing the functions of the uterus, the changes brought about by pregnancy, and the systemic repercussions of labor. Special emphasis is given to the various hypotheses that attempt to explain the maintenance of pregnancy and the onset of spontaneous labor. An extensive review of the pharmacologic response of the uterus to drugs commonly used in labor and a special chapter dedicated to anesthetic methods should facilitate understanding some of the concepts.

The second section, monitoring of the fetus, surveys the numerous patterns one may observe during labor, and their clinical significance is described. Electronic monitoring as a means of antepartum surveillance is discussed in detail. To complete, a review is made of the possible advantages and potential problems derived from the use of these relatively new but extensively applied monitoring techniques.

The abundant illustrations constitute a veritable atlas documenting the patterns that could be recorded in the most frequently observed clinical circumstances. At the same time, the discussions of pathophysiologic processes are elaborated with the help of original illustrations. These are taken from work in which I directly participated, or when that was not the case, from publications by others who made original contributions to the points under study. A reasonably complete bibliography of the English language literature closes each chapter.

I want to express special thanks to my friends and colleagues who in Montevideo, Cleveland, and Chicago advised me, shared in many discussions, and/or assisted in planning some of the investigations reported here. I owe much to all of them; however, the concepts included here are strictly my own and thus they may not be made responsible for inacuracies or mistakes. I must also extend my thanks to the numerous authors and publishers who allowed me the use of their illustrations to make some important points or document original contributions. My thanks also to my secretaries Mrs. Doris Compton and Ms. Linda Mary Benjamin for their help and patience during the preparation of the manuscript. Finally, I want to express my appreciation to the publisher, the PSG Publishing Company, for its courtesy and consideration in accepting my requests and for its efforts in maintaining high standards of publication.

Luis A. Cibils
Chicago, Illinois

CHAPTER 1
History of Intrapartum Monitoring

Recording of uterine contractions has been a long sought aim of clinicians and physiologists dedicated to studying the function and controlling factors of the human uterus. The study of muscle strips in vitro and animal uteri in vivo suggested that the uterus was an autonomous organ but with a behavior altogether different from other organs composed primarily of smooth muscle. Lack of proper animal models and the inability to study the human uterus in vivo because of inadequate methods made exploring its physiology difficult.

UTERINE CONTRACTIONS

It was not until 1872, when Friedrich Schatz published his historic work, that the understanding of uterine physiology started to emerge from total empiricism. In fact, the extraordinary quality of his *internal recordings* has remained unsurpassed for more than a century, the present methods being only less cumbersome and more accurate. The elements to study uterine function, however, were all there in tracings obtained with a rotating drum and a pen floating on a mercury column (Figure 1-1). His method involved using a small bag of 70 to 80 ml of volume introduced between the membranes and the lower segment, filled with liquid and connected to a mercury manometer. Schatz obtained excellent tracings of the first stage, second stage, and bearing down efforts (Figure 1-2), varying the turning speed of his recording drum. Tracings obtained today with electronic transducers and recorders are of no better quality. The most important drawback of his method was that it required much manipulation to apply the bag; Semmelweis's concepts of puerperal infection were still being resisted by

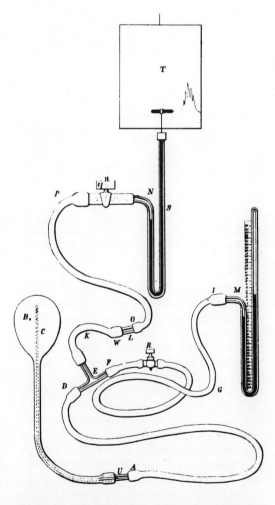

Figure 1-1 Apparatus used by Schatz to record uterine contractions. The intrauterine bag (B, C) is connected to two mercury manometers, one for visual reading (M) and the other (N) for recording on a rotating drum (T) with a floating pen. Reprinted from Schatz (1872).

1

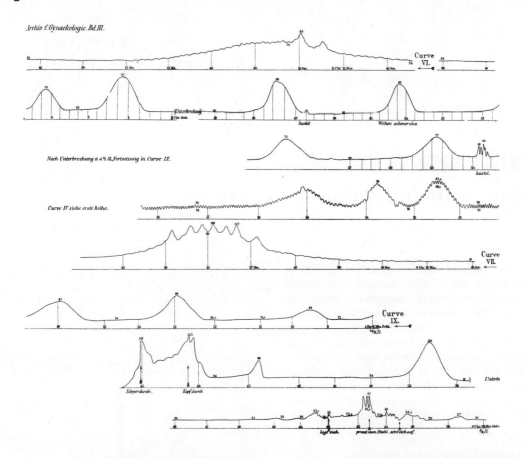

Figure 1-2 Intrauterine pressure tracing obtained at variable speeds of the rotating drum, and running from right to left. On the fourth tracing from the top, note the pressure changes produced by respiratory movements, and on the fifth the pushing efforts superimposed on the contractions. Reprinted from Schatz (1872).

some powerful members of the medical profession, and the principles of antisepsis were being introduced by Lister but not yet widely accepted or practiced. Perhaps because of the inherent danger, Schatz's extraordinary work remained buried for many decades and exercised no influence on understanding the physiology of labor. Another plausible explanation is that Schatz did not belong to the academic establishment of his time, and his work was given the same reception as that of the genial Semmelweis (had it not been for Pasteur and Lister, his ideas would have been ignored for many more years). Be that as it may, Schatz should be acknowledged as the man who devised the first method to explore, and made the first accurate recordings of, the human uterus in labor, a method still used by many with some technical modifications. Evolution toward current techniques was slow, with small steps taken by in-

vestigators such as Poullet (1878), Polaillon (1879), and Westermark (1893) who made a significant improvement by reducing the size of the intrauterine balloon to 2 ml capacity. The German authors at that time were doing original work on uterine physiology and pharmacology.

The dangers of bleeding and particularly infections, inherent in internal methods of recording uterine contractions, deterred these studies and provided incentive to develop *external methods* for recording the contractions that could usually be palpated by the clinicians. But it was not until 1896 that Schaeffer reported on the observations made with an apparatus to be applied on the uterus. This very crude device proved, nevertheless, the possibility of such recordings and the soundness of the concept; thus Schaeffer should be credited as the originator of external recordings. The technical problems involved in developing a reliable and convenient recorder were almost insurmountable, and thus internal methods continued, sporadically, to be used in investigating uterine physiology.

Shortly after World War I, in 1922, Rucker reported his pharmacologic studies made with the Voorhees' bag, thus being the first one in this country to apply a reliable method of observation and setting the stage for others to follow investigations in this area. Later Salerno (1938), with the same technique, *correlated uterine contractions with changes in fetal heart rate* (FHR), thereby establishing the importance of simultaneous recordings of both parameters—the basis of current concepts of fetal monitoring.

However, the need for a reliable external monitor was still much felt because of the always present possibility of infection following the use of internal methods and manipulations required for insertion. Then Dodek (1932) described a relatively primitive and simple apparatus (Figure 1-3) to record the contractions of the uterus at different stages of labor. He studied with it the pharmacology of certain drugs and ascertained the intrinsic irregularity of contractions in spontaneous labor (Figure 1-4). Refinements in design were soon made by others; changes in the pickup system and writing gears resulted in smaller

devices. As a result of the Frey and Lorand reports in 1933, such recorders became very popular. The designers claimed that they could record a number of variables of uterine contractions, proved later to be inaccurate when precise intrauterine tracings were obtained simultaneously. At the time, however, these apparatuses provided the only easy way to make good observations in the manner reported by Moir (1935) for uterine response to a number of drugs used in clinical obstetrics.

Woodbury, Hamilton, and Torpin (1938) made *simultaneous recordings of uterine contractions and vascular pressures* and studied the relationships between them as well as the pharmacologic effects of some drugs commonly used in obstetrics. With this model they were able to estimate changes in blood flow into the intervillous space (IVS), a most critical function repetitively altered by uterine contractions.

In 1934, Adair and Davis described a method to record the *uterine contractions during the puerperium* by inserting an intrauterine bag, fluid-filled and connected to a recorder. This system was used to make a complete pharmacologic study of the puerperal uterus, and the effect of ergot derivatives (Figure 1-5) during the first two weeks postpartum.

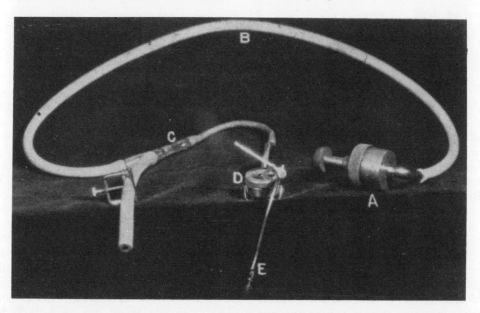

Figure 1-3 Apparatus designed by Dodek to record uterine contractions. The plunger (A) applied over the uterus transmits pressure changes through tubing (B) to writing arm (E). From Dodek SM: A new method for graphically recording the contractions of the parturient human uterus. *Surg Gynecol Obstet* 55:45, 1932. By permission of *Surgery, Gynecology, and Obstetrics.*

4

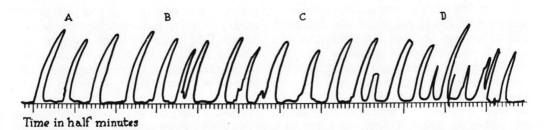

Figure 1-4 Tracing obtained with external recorder documents irregular pattern of contractions in middle first stage of primipara (half-minute intervals). From Dodek SM: A new method for graphically recording the contractions of the parturient human uterus. *Surg Gynecol Obstet* 55:45, 1932. By permission of *Surgery, Gynecology, and Obstetrics.*

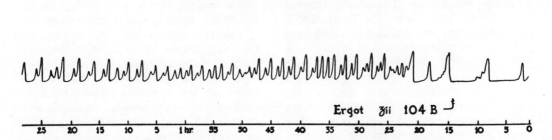

Figure 1-5 Tracing (running right to left) obtained during puerperium with an intrauterine bag was used to carry out pharmacologic studies with ergot derivatives. Reprinted from Adair FL, Davis ME: A study of human uterine motility. *Am J Obstet Gynecol* 27:383, 1934.

To study the *second stage of the second twin,* Moir (1936) very ingeniously used the placenta, a natural intrauterine balloon, by cannulating the umbilical vein of the first twin and connecting it to a recording system. The same setup was used to study the *contractility and pharmacology of the third stage* by Alvarez and Caldeyro-Barcia in the early 1950s.

Fenning (1939) developed the first electronic recorder, in a way similar to the electrocardiogram (ECG), based on the principle of a condenser, and with it he made accurate studies of *uterine contractility in advanced pregnancy* (Figure 1-6). A simplified ink recorder gave him equivalent tracings in 1940, and it helped him to make an exhaustive study of contractions on over 500 patients in labor (Figure 1-7). Wolf (1942) obtained intrauterine records with a transabdominal needle and compared them with tracings obtained by external methods (Figure 1-8). Perhaps because

this work was published during the early stages of World War II, which created marked difficulties in communications, it did not stimulate similar studies, and the author did not follow with further publications.

Because of the relative inaccuracy of external methods and intrauterine bags, Karlson (1944) devised a small strain gauge, which he placed on a flexible, narrow metal tape and introduced between the membranes and myometrium. These gauges were placed in tandem to study the *"motility within the various parts of the uterus"* and its influence upon cervical dilatation and duration of labor. Later on, Lindgren (1960) made exhaustive studies of abnormal labors with this method.

Reynolds, Heard, and Bruns (1947) devised the tokodynamometer (TKD), a multigauged instrument applied abdominally in various regions of the uterus to obtain *simultaneous external recordings of a contraction.* This instrument, in

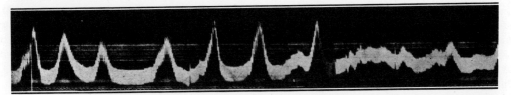

Uterine contractions in false labor.

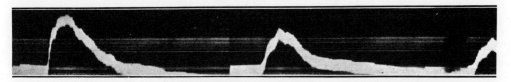

A graph obtained three hours after expulsion of the placenta.

Figure 1-6 Tracings obtained with an external electronic apparatus devised by Fenning. *(Above)* During prelabor. *(Below)* Postpartum. Reprinted from Fenning C, et al: Indirect external hysterography. *Am J Obstet Gynecol* 38:670, 1939.

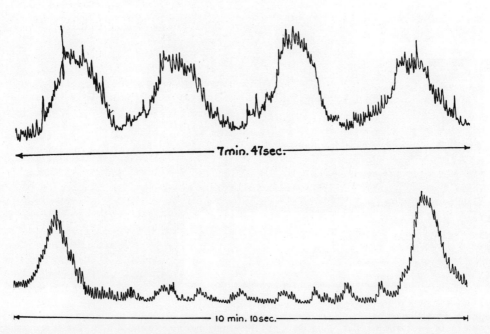

Figure 1-7 External tracings obtained with an ink recorder. *(Above)* Active first stage. *(Below)* Advanced prelabor. Reprinted from Fenning C: A mechanical ink-writing recorder suitable for recording uterine motility during pregnancy and labor. *Am J Obstet Gynecol* 40:330, 1940.

the hands of its designers, did much to help in understanding patterns of normal and abnormal uterine contractions. It supplied the basic material for the first comprehensive book on the physiology of the uterus and its clinical application, by Reynolds, Harris, and Kaiser (1954), which disseminated the concept of "fundal dominance."

The turning point in the modern approach to the study of uterine physiology came in June 1947 when Alvarez and Caldeyro-Barcia in Montevideo, Uruguay, made their first recording of uterine contractions by *transabdominal intra-uterine needle* (Figure 1-9).

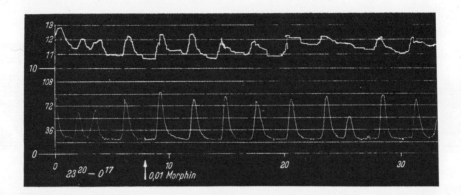

Figure 1-8 Simultaneous tracings obtained by Wolf. *(Above)* External. *(Below)* Internal transabdominal needle. Note difference in quality of recordings. Reprinted from Wolf (1942).

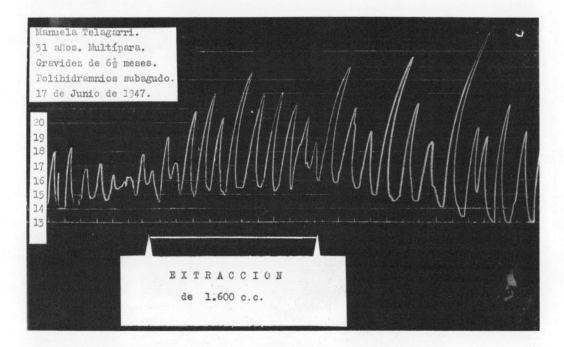

Figure 1-9 First intrauterine contractions recording obtained with a transabdominal needle on a smoked drum. Note the scale cm of water, the irregular contractions, and fluctuating baseline. Reprinted from Alvarez and Caldeyro-Barcia (1948).

7

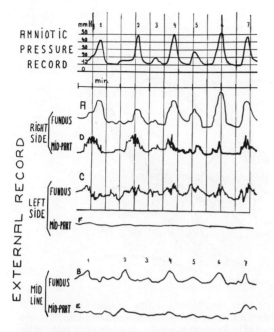

Figure 1-10 Simultaneous recordings using internal and external methods. *(Above)* Intraamniotic pressure. *(Center)* Regional uterine activity obtained with polygraph. *(Below)* Midline region with tokodynamometer. Note higher values from right-side areas and absolute intrauterine pressure values obtained with amniotic catheter. Reprinted from Caldeyro-Barcia R, et al: A better understanding of uterine contractility through simultaneous recording with an internal and seven channel external method. *Surg Gynecol Obstet* 91:641, 1950. By permission of *Surgery, Gynecology, and Obstetrics.*

Their first publications were in Uruguayan journals, but soon their continuing work spilled over to foreign journals with wider readerships. Their original research attracted not only many young workers from various parts of the world but also some established authorities. Then, with Reynolds, they (1950) studied and compared the validity of internal and external recordings by obtaining *simultaneous tracings* with their transabdominal catheter and the TKD (Figure 1-10). Shortly after these publications Alvarez and Caldeyro-Barcia (1952) broadened the study of the pregnant uterus by implanting, within various topographic areas of its wall, microballoons (Figure 1-11) to record the local contractions, thus providing a tracing of *simultaneous pressure changes in distant regions of the uterus and in the*

amniotic activity (Figure 1-12). It enabled them to refine the concept of fundal dominance to the concept of the triple descending gradient and to define better the patterns of coordinated and incoordinated uterine contractions. Their first comprehensive study of uterine contractility and pharmacology was published in 1954.

Because of the potential danger posed by the transabdominal insertion of a needle to guide the passage of the recording catheter, Williams and Stallworthy in 1952 described an apparently more simple method of passing a *catheter through the cervix,* using a Drew-Smythe trocar as guide, between the membranes and lower segment, before piercing the amnion. A varient of this method is currently the most widely used intrauterine recording technique in the United States. (See Chapter 4, Instrumentation.)

Several cardiovascular parameters had been established by Woodbury (1938). Some hypotheses about IVS pressures and their relationship to intraamniotic pressure and contractions were accepted as factual, based on his observations. In 1959 Hendricks and collaborators, by inserting an *open-end catheter in each of these spaces, demonstrated their almost identical values, thus correcting old misunderstandings and establishing the concept of uniform intrauterine pressure* (Figure 1-13). Continuing to simplify the available methods, Hendricks (1959) found that this same system of using an open-end catheter was highly satisfactory in recording the activity of the empty puerperal uterus (Figure 1-14), thus enormously facilitating pharmacologic studies of old and new drugs. This method was also used in 1962 to study simultaneous intramyometrial pressures during labor and postpartum.

Many elements influenced by uterine contractions were not adequately measured or understood as late as 1962. Among them were the changes occurring in *IVS blood flow* during contractions. But in 1964 Borell and co-workers made simultaneous recordings of intrauterine pressures and obtained serial *placentographs* by injecting contrast medium in the abdominal aorta during a uterine contraction and during periods of relaxation. This method, first used in early human gestation, was later applied to nonhuman primates at term. Finally it was used by the same authors and by Bieniarz in human pregnancy at term to evaluate IVS blood flow in normal and pathologic pregnancies.

8

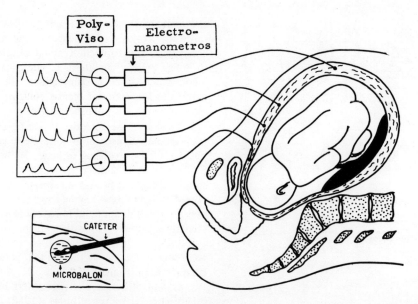

Figure 1-11 Method of recording topographic activity of human myometrium during advanced gestation and puerperium. Fluid-filled microballoons are implanted in different regions of the myometrium and connected to strain gauges and Polyviso recorder. Another catheter is usually inserted in the amniotic cavity. Inset: detail of catheter tip and microballoon anchored in the myometrium. Reprinted from Caldeyro-Barcia R, Alvarez H: Abnormal uterine action in labour. *J Obstet Gynaecol Br Emp* 59:646, 1952.

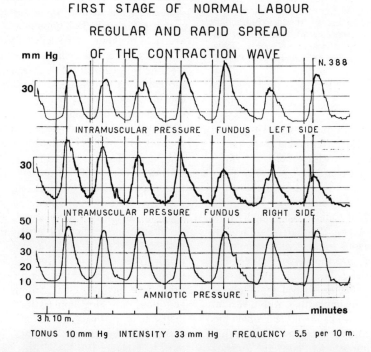

Figure 1-12 Simultaneous intraamniotic and two intramyometrial pressure recordings obtained in normal first stage. Note the differences in pressure between the two fundal regions. Shown at bottom, average values for intraamniotic pressure. After Caldeyro-Barcia and Alvarez (1952).

SIMULTANEOUS AMNIOTIC FLUID AND INTERVILLOUS SPACE PRESSURE RECORDINGS

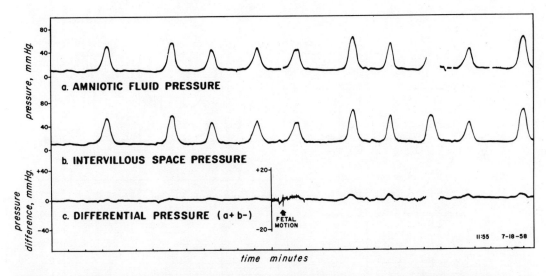

Figure 1-13 Simultaneous pressure tracings recorded during labor with open-end transabdominal catheter. *(A)* Intraamniotic. *(B)* IVS. *(C)* Differential pressure between A and B, almost a straight line with minimal fluctuation around zero. Reprinted from Hendricks CH, et al: Pressure relationships between the intervillous space and the amniotic fluid in human term pregnancy. *Am J Obstet Gynecol* 77:1028, 1959.

FETAL MONITORING

Recording of fetal heart sounds during labor underwent a similar slow process of development. *Auscultation,* first applied to the intrauterine fetus in 1822 by Kergaradec, was the only practical method until very recently. However, more reliable methods of documenting and recording were being tried for many years. The first *fetal ECG* was obtained in 1906 by Cremer shortly after Eintoven had discovered the possibility of recording the adult ECG (Figure 1-15). Because of the technical difficulties encountered at the time, it was not possible to use the ECG to record the FHR, and therefore it remained for many years largely as a curiosity. The development of excellent electrocardiographs and the science of electrocardiography did little to overcome the problem of obtaining good signals through the abdominal and uterine walls. Much later it was used sporadically to establish fetal life or as a clever means to document multiple gestation, but its practical use was not yet apparent. The fetal signal obtained was so small compared to that of the mother that it was impossible to feed a tachometer and record the FHR. It was used in research to obtain tracing strips at high speed and, in these, to count by hand the frequency at variable time sequences. It was while using this method that Swartwout, Campbell, and Williams (1961) first described the rapid oscillations of the fetal heart rate in midpregnancy and advanced gestation.

The need to obtain distinct and large fetal signals was fulfilled in 1958 by Caldeyro-Barcia and collaborators, who implanted transabdominally one electrode into the fetus. It was then possible to obtain *continuous FHR tracings* simultaneously with the intrauterine pressure changes during prelabor and labor (Figure 1-16), but this method was impractical for routine clinical use. Because of this very important limitation, other methods were simultaneously being explored. Thus in 1957 Hon and Hess first obtained fetal ECGs with abdominal electrodes that were good enough to feed the tachometer and record FHR

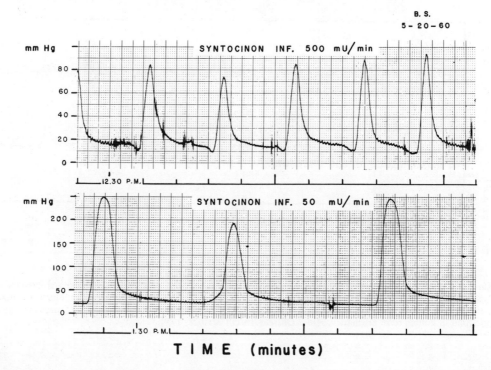

POST PARTUM RECORDS (after 3rd stage)

INTRAUTERINE CATHETER STILL IN SITU

B. S.
5 - 20 - 60

Figure 1-14 One of the first postpartum intrauterine pressure recordings obtained with the transabdominal catheter used to record labor and left untouched after third stage. Note the excellent tracing (respiratory changes in upper recording) and the high pressure readings.

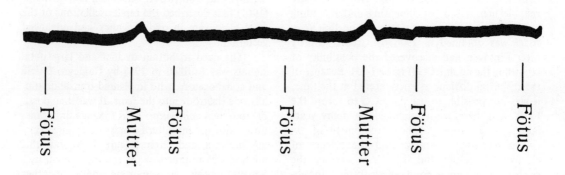

Figure 1-15 First fetal ECG recorded with external electrodes. The small deflections of the baseline are the fetal complexes interrrupting the maternal tracing. Reprinted from Cremer M: Ueber die direkte Ableitung, der Aktionstrome des menschlichen Herzens vom Oesophagus und uber des Elektrocardiogramm des Fotus. *Munch Med Wochenschr* 53:811, 1906.

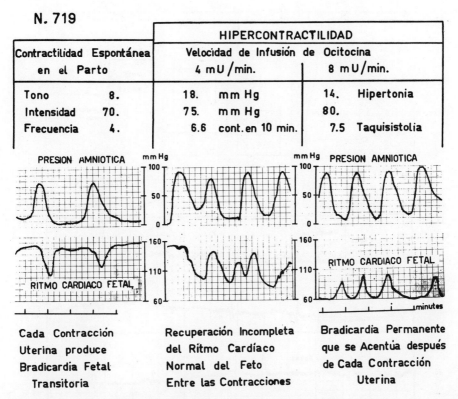

N. 719

Contractilidad Espontánea en el Parto	HIPERCONTRACTILIDAD	
	Velocidad de Infusión de Ocitocina	
	4 mU/min.	8 mU/min.
Tono 8.	18. mm Hg	14. Hipertonia
Intensidad 70.	75. mm Hg	80.
Frecuencia 4.	6.6 cont. en 10 min.	7.5 Taquisistolia

Cada Contracción Uterina produce Bradicardia Fetal Transitoria	Recuperación Incompleta del Ritmo Cardíaco Normal del Feto Entre las Contracciones	Bradicardia Permanente que se Acentúa después de Cada Contracción Uterina

Figure 1-16 First continuous recording of intrauterine pressure changes and FHR obtained by direct methods—intraamniotic catheter and intrafetal electrode. Three different periods of an overstimulated labor leading to severe bradycardia due to polysystoly. Reprinted from Caldeyro-Barcia (1958).

continuously. They did this by simultaneously recording ECGs from two areas with two preamplifiers. The second one was maternal only and was used to cancel the maternal ECG recorded in the same tracing with the fetal ECG obtained by the first preamplifier with the leads on the uterus. Thus they obtained only fetal QRS complexes going through a third preamplifier to feed the tachometer (Figure 1-17). This basic concept was further perfected by Hon and constitutes the basis for the current techniques of continuous monitoring with abdominal electrodes.

Later, in 1963, the *clip electrode* was designed by Hon, to be applied to the fetal scalp, and with this a signal larger than the maternal one was obtained to feed the tachometer directly. This concept, too, is basic to all modern monitors. The prerequisite of rupturing the membranes to apply the scalp electrode precluded the routine application of this technique. And, technical difficulties interfered with obtaining an artifact-free abdominal ECG. Thus out of necessity alternative methods were explored.

For many, phonocardiograms were not clean enough for FHR monitoring, but in 1968 when Bishop applied the *Doppler principle to ultrasound,* the signal generated was good enough to obtain satisfactory continuous tracings—the basis of the most widespread method now used for the so-called external monitoring of FHR. When technically well recorded, it gives an excellent tracing of baseline and accelerations and decelerations, but it does not give a consistently good tracing of baseline oscillations (or beat-to-beat variability). Other parallel investigations culminated in a perfected phonocardiogram with which Hammacher (1967) claims it is possible to obtain tracings comparable to those recorded with the direct intrafetal electrode (Figure 1-18).

Other important functions were later on amenable to continuous monitoring, at least as experimental observations in humans. Thus, Pose

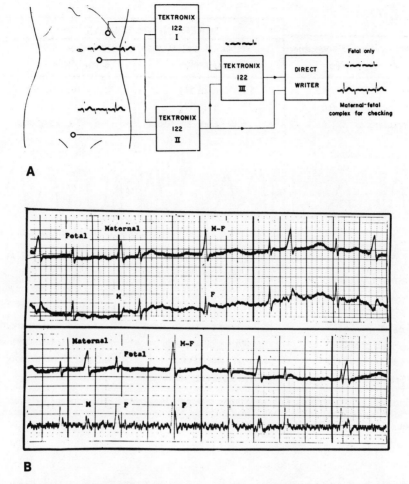

Figure 1-17 *(A)* Schematic of preamplifiers arranged to obtain a good fetal ECG signal to feed cardiotachometer. *(B)* Tracings obtained without and with the cancellation amplifier, the latter showing large fetal R waves to trigger the tachometer. Adapted from Hon EH, Hess OW: Instrumentation of fetal electrocardiography. *Science* 125:553, 1957. Copyright 1957 by the American Association for the Advancement of Science.

et al in 1963 obtained continuous simultaneous tracings of uterine contractions, FHR, blood pressure, contractions, and *either blood or muscular fetal oxygen pressure (pO₂)* (Figure 1-19). *Continuous fetal pH* was successfully recorded in 1976 by Stamm and co-workers, who used an electrode implanted in the scalp.

Fetal respiratory movements (breathing) were successfully recorded in 1971 by Boddy and Robinson using ultrasound signals, a method of observation further developed by Dawes for the study of normal and abnormal fetuses (Figure 1-20). Later Goodlin and associates, in 1972, proposed the evaluation of *systolic time intervals,*

which they recorded as a means to assess fetal well-being. In analyzing their records they also assessed the value of the *pre-ejection period.* These two research methods have not been refined to make their use practical in clinical obstetrics. Intrapartum continuous recording of fetal capillary pO₂ with an electrode applied over the skin was obtained by Huch et al in 1977 (Figure 1-21). This noninvasive method should have useful clinical application when some technical difficulties are resolved.

With all these variables recorded simultaneously it has been possible to begin to understand some of the physiologic and pathophysiologic

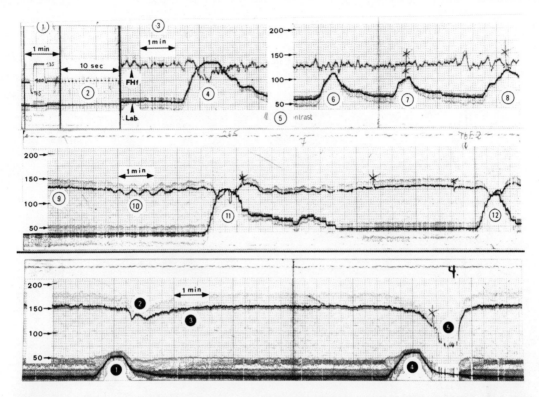

Figure 1-18 Three tracings obtained with external methods, of uterine contractions and FHR, this one with a phonocardiogram. *(Above)* Normal oscillations of the baseline. *(Center)* Some diminution. *(Below)* Absent silent oscillations. The tracings are very similar to those obtained by direct methods. Courtesy K. Hammacher.

phenomena affecting the human fetus during advanced pregnancy, labor, and delivery. Many studies carried out in primates have been useful in facilitating that understanding. However, because other observations seem not to occur in the same way in subhumans or human primates, direct extrapolation of concepts is not warranted. The legal as well as ethical impediments have markedly limited the progress of our understanding of the various processes involved in human labor and

delivery. Research has literally exploded in the past 10 years, to advance our knowledge in a positive way. Nevertheless, although monitoring equipment is available in almost every small and large hospital in the country, the ability to obtain good tracings and interpret them correctly is generally lacking, preventing laboratory advances from being applied successfully to clinical medicine. Closing this gap should be given high priority in the forthcoming years.

14

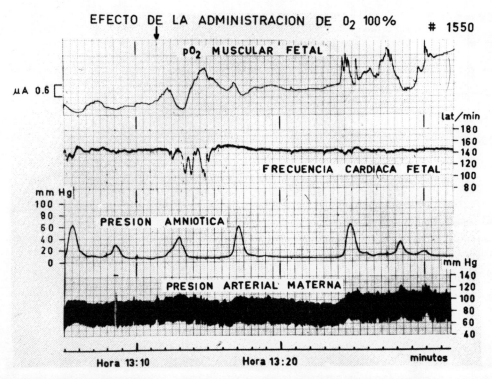

EFECTO DE LA ADMINISTRACION DE O_2 100%   # 1550

pO_2 MUSCULAR FETAL

μA 0.6

lat/min

FRECUENCIA CARDIACA FETAL

mm Hg

PRESION AMNIOTICA

mm Hg

PRESION ARTERIAL MATERNA

Hora 13:10   Hora 13:20   minutos

Figure 1-19   Record obtained at term pregnancy with an anencephalic fetus. *(First)* Tracing obtained with intramuscular electrode inserted transabdominally records relative pO_2 changes. *(Second)* Continuous FHR. *(Third)* Intrauterine pressure. *(Fourth)* Maternal arterial pressure. Note wide fluctuations in the pO_2 tracing and the simultaneous FHR deceleration when it dropped below threshold. Reprinted from Pose (1963).

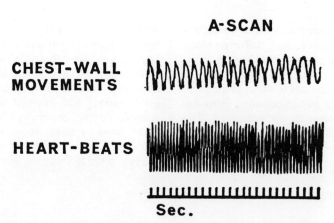

A-SCAN

CHEST-WALL
MOVEMENTS

HEART-BEATS

Sec.

Fig. 4—An A-scan ultrasonic record of chest-wall movements
(fetal breathing) and heart-beat echo from a human fetus in
utero.

Gestational age 38 weeks.

Figure 1-20   Simultaneous tracings by A-scan ultrasonography (sec). *(Above)* Fetal respiratory movements. *(Below)* Heartbeats. Reprinted from Boddy and Robinson (1971).

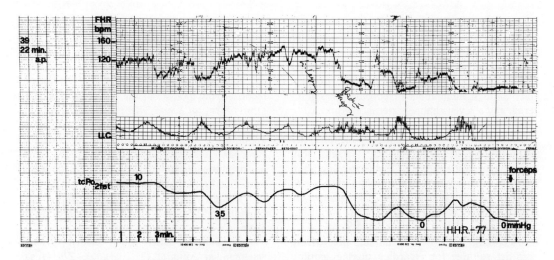

Figure 1-21 Continuous fetal pO₂ level obtained with skin electrode on the scalp, simultaneously recorded with uterine contractions and FHR. Reprinted from Huch A, et al: Continuous transcutaneous monitoring of fetal oxygen tension during labour. *Br J Obstet Gynaecol* 84(suppl 1): 1977.

BIBLIOGRAPHY

Adair FL, Davis ME: A study of human uterine motility. *Am J Obstet Gynecol* 27:383, 1934.

Alvarez H, Caldeyro-Barcia R: Estudios sobre la fisiología de la actividad contractil del útero humano. Primera comunicación: Nueva técnica para registrar la actividad contractil del útero humano grávido. *Arch Ginecol Obstet (Uruguay)* 7:7, 1948.

Alvarez H, Caldeyro-Barcia R: Estudios sobre la fisiología de la actividad contractil del útero humano. Segunda comunicación: La actividad contractil rítmica del útero humano grávido. *Arch Ginecol Obstet (Uruguay)* 7:79, 1948.

Alvarez H, Caldeyro-Barcia R: Estudios sobre la fisiología de la actividad contractil del útero humano. Tercera comunicación: Estudios de los valores absolutos de la presión intrauterina como medida de la actividad contractil del útero. El tono uterino. *Arch Ginecol Obstet (Uruguay)* 7:139, 1948.

Alvarez H, Caldeyro-Barcia R: Estudios sobre la fisiología de la actividad contractil del útero humano. Cuarta comunicación: El parto del segundo gemelo, y el alumbramiento estudiados por medio del registro de la presión intraplacentaria. *Arch Ginecol Obstet (Uruguay)* 8:42, 1949.

Alvarez H, Caldeyro-Barcia R: La actividad contractil uterina en el estado grávido-puerperal. *I Congr Urug Ginec Obstet* 1:507, 1949.

Alvarez H, Caldeyro-Barcia R: Contractility of the human uterus recorded by new methods. *Surg Gynecol Obstet* 91:1, 1950.

Alvarez H, Caldeyro-Barcia R: Studies on the contractility of the pregnant uterus. *Proc I World Cong Fertil Steril* 217, 1953.

Alvarez H, Caldeyro-Barcia R: Fisiopatolgía de la contracción uterina y sus aplicaciones en clínica obstétrica. *II Cong Lat-Am Obstet Ginecol (Brasil)* 1:1, 1954.

Bieniarz J, Crottogini JJ, Curuchet E, et al: Aortocaval compression by the uterus in late human pregnancy. *Am J Obstet Gynecol* 100:203, 1968.

Bishop EH: Ultrasonic fetal monitoring. *Clin Obstet Gynecol* 11:1154, 1968.

Boddy K, Robinson JS: External method for detection of fetal breathing in utero. *Lancet* 2:1231, 1971.

Borell U, Fernstrom I, Ohlson L, et al: Effect of uterine contractions on the human uteroplacental blood circulation. *Am J Obstet Gynecol* 89:881, 1964.

Caldeyro-Barcia R: Estudio de la anoxia fetal intrauterina mediante el ECG fetal y el registro continuo de la frecuencia cardíaca fetal. *III Cong Lat-Am Obstet Ginecol (Mexico)* 2:388, 1958.

Caldeyro-Barcia R, Alvarez H: Abnormal uterine action in labour. *J Obstet Gynaecol Br Emp* 59:646, 1952.

Caldeyro-Barcia R, Alvarez H, Reynolds SRM: A better understanding of uterine contractility through simultaneous recording with an internal and a seven channel external method. *Surg Gynecol Obstet* 91:641, 1950.

Cremer M: Ueber die direkte Ableitung, der Aktionstrome des menschlichen Herzens vom Oesophagus und uber des Elektrocardiogramm des Fotus. *Munch Med Wochenschr* 53:811, 1906.

Dodek SM: A new method for graphically recording the contractions of the parturient human uterus. *Surg Gynecol Obstet* 55:45, 1932.

Fenning C: A mechanical ink-writing recorder suitable for recording uterine motility during pregnancy and labor. *Am J Obstet Gynecol* 40:330, 1940.

Fenning C: Clinical and physiological aspects of uterine motility during pregnancy and labor. *Am J Obstet Gynecol* 43:791, 1942.

Fenning C, David, ME, Adair FL: Indirect external hysterography. *Am J Obstet Gynecol* 38:670, 1939.

Frey E: Der Hysterotonograph. *Zbl Gynak* 57:545, 1933.

Goodlin R, Girard R, Hollmen A: Systolic time intervals in the fetus and neonate. *Obstet Gynecol* 39:295, 1972.

Hammacher K: The diagnosis of fetal distress with an electronic fetal heart monitor, in *Intrauterine Dangers to the Fetus*, Symposium, Prague, 1966. Amsterdam, Excerpta Medica, 1967, pp 228–233.

Hendricks CH, Eskes TKAB, Saameli K: Uterine contractility at delivery and the puerperium. *Am J Obstet Gynecol* 83:890, 1962.

Hendricks CH, Moawad AH: Round ligament motility. In vivo studies in man. *J Obstet Gynaecol Br Comwlth* 72:618, 1965.

Hendricks CH, Quilligan EJ, Tyler CW, et al: Pressure relationships between the intervillous space and the amniotic fluid in human term pregnancy. *Am J Obstet Gynecol* 77:1028, 1959.

Hon EH: Instrumentation of fetal heart rate and fetal electrocardiography. II. A vaginal electrode. *Am J Obstet Gynecol* 86:772, 1963.

Hon EH, Hess OW: Instrumentation of fetal electrocardiography. *Science* 125:553, 1957.

Huch A, Huch R, Schneider N, et al: Continuous transcutaneous monitoring of fetal oxygen tension during labour. *Br J Obstet Gynaecol* 84(suppl 1):1977.

Karlson S: A contribution to the methods of recording the motility of the human uterus. *Acta Obstet Gynecol Scand* 24(suppl 4):1944.

Kergaradec AJ: Memoire sur l'auscultation appliquée à l'etude de la grossesse ou recherches sur deux nouveaux signes propres à faire reconnaître plusieurs circonstances de l'etat de gestation. *Acad Roy Med (Paris)* 1822.

Lindgren L: The causes of fetal head moulding in labour. *Acta Obstet Gynecol Scand* 39:46, 1960.

Lorand S: Uber einen neuen Wehenzeichnenden Apparat (Tokograph). *Zbl Gynak* 57:554, 1933.

Moir JC: The merits and demerits of oxytocic drugs in the postpartum period. *Proc R Soc Med* 28:1654, 1935.

Moir JC: Expulsive force of the uterus during labour. *Lancet* 1:414, 1936.

Polaillon J: Rapport sur l'instrument de M. Poullet. *Bull Soc Chir (Paris)* 5:8, 1879.

Pose SV, Escarcena L, Caldeyro-Barcia R: La presión parcial de oxígeno en el feto durante el parto. *IV Cong Mex Ginecol Obstet* 2:41, 1963.

Poullet J: Présentation d'instruments. *Bull Soc Chir (Paris)* 4:476, 1878.

Rucker MP: The actions of the commoner ecbolics in the first stage of labor. *Am J Obstet Gynecol* 3:134, 1922.

Reynolds SRM, Harris JS, Kaiser IW: *Clinical Measurement of Uterine Forces in Labor.* Springfield, Ill, Thomas, 1954.

Reynolds SRM, Heard OO, Burns P: Recording uterine contraction patterns in pregnant women: Application of the strain gauge in a mutlichannel tokodynamometer. *Science* 106:427, 1947.

Salerno JP: Observations on intrauterine pressure during first stage of labor. *Am J Obstet Gynecol* 36:294, 1938.

Schatz F: Beitrage zur physiologeischen Geburskunde. *Arch Gynak* 3:58, 1872.

Stamm O, Latscha U, Janecek P, et al: Development of a special electrode for continuous subcutaneous pH measurement in the infant scalp. *Am J Obstet Gynecol* 124:193, 1976.

Swartwout JR, Campbell WE, Williams LG: Observations on the fetal heart rate. *Am J Obstet Gynecol* 82:301, 1961.

Westermark F: Experimentelle Untersuchungen uber die Wehentätigkeit des menschlichen Uterus bei der physiologischen Geburt. *Skand Arch Physiol* 4:331, 1893.

Wolf W: Die Wirkung des Morphiums und Atropins auf die Muskulatur des Corpus Uteri. *Arch Gynaekol* 173:614, 1942.

Woodbury RA, Hamilton WF, Torpin R: The relationship between abdominal, uterine and arterial pressures during labor. *Am J Physiol* 121:640, 1938.

CHAPTER 2
Physical Basis of Monitoring Uterine Contractions

The uterus is formed essentially by smooth muscle. Collagen and elastic fibers, in nonhomogeneous distribution, give support to shape this hollow viscus. As a smooth-muscle organ, the uterus functions in a different manner from other organs formed by nonstriated muscle: it does not have intrinsic ganglia known to influence its contractility. However, in recent years nerve endings have been identified very close to muscle cell membranes. Thus, its action does not seem obviously influenced by nerve stimuli; nevertheless it possesses a unique quality of automaticity that allows it to function satisfactorily even when completely denervated. The gross anatomy of the human uterus, either nonpregnant or pregnant, looks simple because it appears as a primitive structure without identifiable layers. It seems to be constituted by a mesh or net involving the uterus in a spiral from the insertion of the fallopian tubes downward. These descriptions tend more to satisfy the imagination of the anatomists and their need to extrapolate findings of well-identified layers of muscle in animal uteri than to be a demonstrable reality. In fact, the uterine corpus appears as a homogeneous structure with the sphincter of the cervix as the only part distinct in arrangement. Even the classic regions of corpus, lower segment, and cervix are arbitrary divisions. Structurally they are somewhat different, but the change in composition, from the fundus to the cervix, is so subtle that a given region is very similar to an adjacent one and not quite like another a little farther down.

The sphincter of the internal os closes the cavity of the uterus, thus making it a single, isolated, hollow viscus, with the physical properties of such an organ. Below the sphincter, the amount of connective tissue increases markedly in the cervix, where its composition at the lowest part is almost exclusively collagen and elastic

fibers, with predominance of the former (Figure 2-1). The so-called resting tone is the minimal pressure recorded in the uterine cavity, assumed to be produced by the muscle fibers in a rested (or tonic) state. However, this state of rest may be exceptional; some part of the uterus is probably always in a state of activity at any given time throughout the life of a woman, the exception possibly being during certain moments of active labor. By means of a thin transcervical catheter it is possible to measure the alterations of intrauterine pressure in the nonpregnant state and

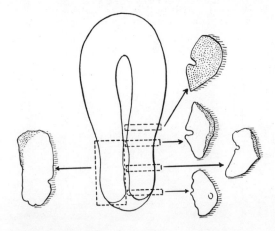

Figure 2-1 Schematic of the composition of the lower uterine segment and cervix. *(Left)* Vertical section of the cervix taken from the area outlined by the dotted rectangle. *(Right)* Four horizontal sections from lower corpus, and upper, middle, and lower cervix. The spotted area represents tissue predominantly muscular while the white areas indicate predominance of collagen tissue. Reprinted from Danforth DN: The distribution and functional activity of the cervical musculature. *Am J Obstet Gynecol* 68:1261, 1954.

thereby observe the changes that occur during the ovarian cycle (Figure 2-2), even though this may seem to constitute a "leaky" system.

This observation indicates that the uterine smooth muscle, unlike the smooth muscle fibers from other organs of the body, is directly and fundamentally influenced by the ovarian hormones estrogen and progesterone.

Estrogens

When injected intraarterially or intravenously, these steroid hormones have a marked influence on the vascular reactivity of the myometrium. They trigger an almost immediate and prolonged vasodilatation, probably by direct action on the arteriolar smooth muscles. On the other hand, a much slower effect takes place on the contractile mechanism involving the synthesis of ac-

tomyosin, the production of high-energy phosphates needed to release the energy required for the contraction, the intracellular and extracellular distribution of sodium, potassium, chloride, and calcium ions involved in the contraction, and the enzymes that participate in the chemical reactions occurring during the contraction. The first objective demonstration of the action of estrogens was obtained by Csapo (1948) after stimulation of the synthesis, extraction of actomyosin from myometrium, and subsequent in vitro study (1950) of its contracting properties (Figures 2-3 and 2-4).

Among the primary important effects of estrogens upon ions is the facilitation of the exchange of calcium, which activates specific enzyme systems. This movement of calcium ions within the cellular compartments appears to be an important controlling mechanism of a number of enzymes. On the other hand, estrogens promote the uptake of several essential and nonessential

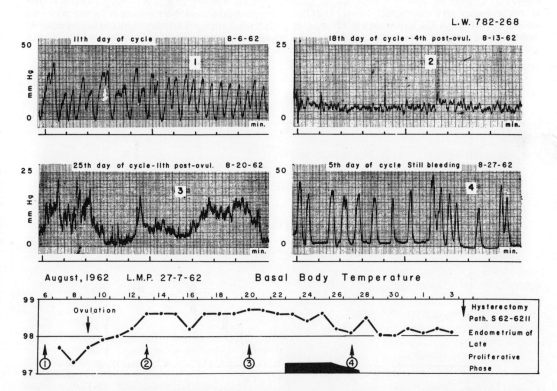

Figure 2-2 Uterine contractility throughout the normal ovarian cycle. Records made at weekly intervals, at dates shown in the lower basal body temperature (BBT) chart matching the records. Note completely different patterns corresponding to the various periods. Hysterectomy at the last arrow in BBT chart revealed an endometrium in the late proliferative phase. Reprinted from Cibils LA: Contracility of the nonpregnant human uterus. *Obstet Gynecol* 30:441, 1967.

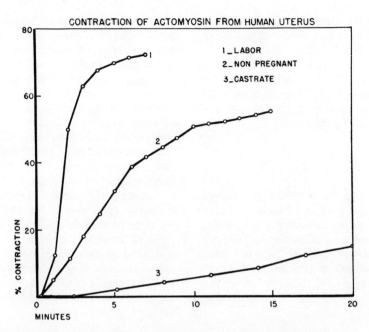

Figure 2-3 Contracting capacity of substance (actomyosin) extracted from uterine muscle from (1) a woman in labor at term pregnancy, (2) a nonpregnant woman, and (3) an ovariectomized patient. Note marked difference in rate and amount of contraction, the highest seen in advanced pregnancy when estrogens are very high, and the lowest in the castrated when estrogens are very low. Reprinted from Csapo A: Actomyosin content of the uterus. *Nature* 162:218, 1948.

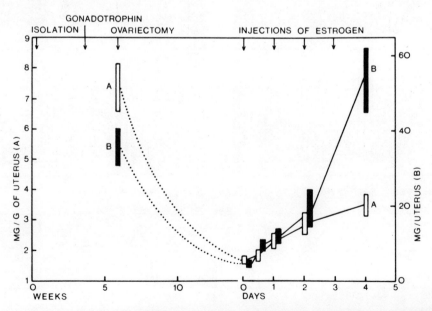

Figure 2-4 The effect of estrogen stimulation and suppression on actomyosin concentration and content in the uterus. *(A)* Open bars, mg/gm of uterus; *(B)* solid bars, mg/uterus. *(Left)* After stimulation with gonadotropin, then the effect of ovariectomy, and the response to daily injections of estrogen. Reprinted from Csapo A: Actomyosin formation by estrogen action. *Am J Physiol* 162:406, 1950.

amino acids and the incorporation of ribonucleoside triphosphates into RNA. As a stimulator of energy sources, it increases muscular glycogen levels. In the past few years specific estrogen receptor sites (binding factors that seem to be formed by proteins) have been identified in the myometrial cells.

Upon uptake by the myometrium, estrogens combine with a cytosol estrogen-binding receptor and remain stable for several hours. Estradiol may be found in the cell nucleus, cytosol, and mitochondria. Estrogens also enhance the affinity of oxytocin receptors, which are located in the cytoplasm, and increase the number of oxytocin and progesterone-binding receptors. The estrogenic effect of increasing the resting membrane potential of the myometrium, may influence the occurrence of rapid rhythmic contractions in the proliferative phase of the cycle. It is not known whether this change is the consequence of water–electrolyte redistribution or another mechanism. Nevertheless, the gross composition of the uterus changes throughout the ovarian cycle, affecting total water content, its distribution, the ionic concentration in the intracellular space

(Figures 2-5 and 2-6), and, with these, the membrane potential of the cells.

Progesterone

Thus, the effect of progesterone and, probably, the ratio of estrogens to progesterone are important in influencing the function of the myometrium. This belief served as the basis for Csapo's hypothesis of progesterone control of pregnancy. He originally reported that progesterone decreases the myometrium membrane potential, but later he showed that, in fact, it significantly increases it to a state of hyperpolarization, thereby interfering with the propagation of the contraction wave because of the effect of progesterone on conduction velocity.

At the molecular level, the influence of various hormones and other substances such as prostaglandins on the mechanism of contraction of the myometrium will be reviewed (see Chapter 8, which includes a discussion of several hypotheses postulated to explaining the onset of spontaneous labor).

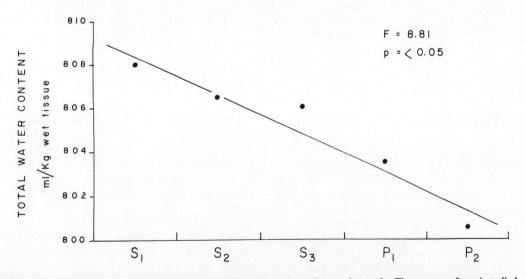

Figure 2-5 Total water content in human myometrium throughout the ovarian cycle. The groups of uteri studied have been arranged in chronologic sequence starting in early secretory phase (S_1) when water content is highest to the preovulatory stage when it is lowest. Reprinted from Cibils LA, Schweid DE: Electrolyte content and distribution in human myometrium. II. Childbearing age group. *Am J Obstet Gynecol* 94:619, 1966.

SODIUM, POTASSIUM and CHLORIDE INTRACELLULAR
CONCENTRATIONS in HUMAN MYOMETRIUM THROUGHOUT the
OVARIAN CYCLE (Estrogen & Progesterone metabolite curves after Loraine
& Bell)

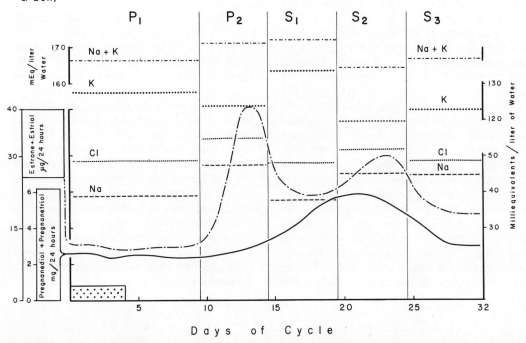

Figure 2-6 *(Scale, right)* Sodium, potassium, and chloride ions. *(Scale, upper left)* Sum of Na⁺ + K⁺ concentrations in human myometrium throughout the ovarian cycle. Cases are grouped according to stage of cycle starting by early proliferative (P₁). *(Scales, left)* These findings are plotted concurrently with normal urinary estrogens and progesterone metabolite excretion curves (after Loraine and Bell, 1963). Reprinted from Cibils LA, Schweid DE: Electrolyte content and distribution in human myometrium. *Am J Obstet Gynecol* 94:619, 1966.

PHYSIOLOGY

The mechanical effect of the growing conceptus (fetus, placenta, and amniotic fluid) influences myometrium and seems to facilitate its adptation to the increasing volume. The physical laws that govern this organ have a changing effect because the shape of the uterus is not the same throughout gestation. From the time the conceptus completely fills the uterine cavity, between the 10th and 12th weeks of gestation, until the 20th week, the uterus has a roughly spherical shape. The radius of the curvature in various areas is approximately of the same order. But at about midpregnancy the uterus grows more rapidly in the longitudinal axis, taking an ovoidal shape. This phenomenon, known as accommodation of the uterus, progresses as pregnancy advances (Figure 2-7), and, with it, important differences are established for the radius of the fundus, midsection, and cervical region of the organ. Laplace's law may be applied to the full-term pregnant uterus: T = pr/2, where T is tension, p the pressure in a given area, and r the radius corresponding to the area corresponding to the uterine wall. This equation indicates that the tension in various areas of the uterus in advanced gestation is not uniform because of the ovoid shape; therefore radii vary at different areas of the walls. The midsection has the greatest radius, followed by the fundus, and then the cervix (the

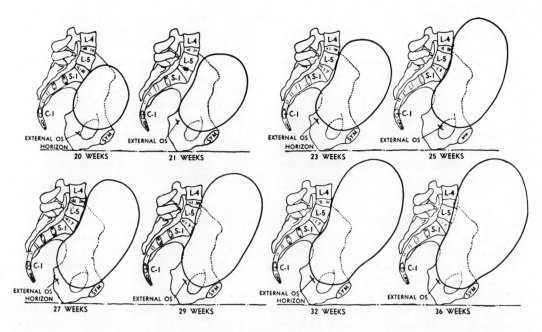

Figure 2-7 Drawings from lateral x-rays to illustrate the change in shape of the uterus from spheroid (at 20 weeks) to progressively more ellipsoid as pregnancy advances. One can appreciate the differences in radius for the upper and lower poles. Reprinted from Gillespie EC: Principles of uterine growth in pregnancy. *Am J Obstet Gynecol* 59:949, 1950.

radius of the fundus is approximately double that of the cervix). Since the resistance to stretching is a direct function of the radius of the curvature in a hollow muscular organ and since the tension of the fundus is about twice that of the cervical region, less resistance is found around the cervical area. In addition, the uterine musculature is thickest at the fundus and diminishes toward the lower part, being thinnest around the cervix. Furthermore, the tension of a muscle, within certain limits, increases its contractile efficiency, hence the more efficient fundal activity. A number of conditions, therefore, converge to favor the preponderance of the fundal area of the uterus over that of the cervix, leading to the ultimate formation of the lower segment and cervical dilatation as a consequence of active labor. Fundamental to this process of cervical dilatation as a consequence of labor is the anatomic constitution of the cervix, which is predominantly formed by collagen tissue in its upper third and almost exclusively by it in the lower third. This contrasts with approximately 30% collagen content per unit of weight in the uterine corpus, the remaining 70% being muscular tissue.

Pressure Measurements

Internal The pressure developed by the contraction of the myometrium in advanced gestation follows Pascal's law of equal distribution in a closed-fluid system and affects the intrauterine contents. Thus, it is possible to record the *intrauterine pressure* with a closed fluid-filled connecting system and obtain the absolute values of those pressures at any given time by means of nonelastic catheters of small caliber introduced transabdominally. The degree of pressure developed will be proportional to the extent of uterine muscle contracting or the intensity of the contraction or both. A strong localized contraction may produce a pressure comparable to that of a weaker contraction propagated to a larger area of myometrium because the elastic properties of the noncontracting area of the uterus, by giving in, dampen the effect of the strong localized contraction. The first studies of absolute intrauterine pressures were carried out with this recording method, but because of the relative risks it was never applied to routine clinical use. Transvaginal and transcervical insertion of a catheter into the uterine cavity is the current technique used to record intrauterine pressures. Theoretical objections to the concept of obtaining true pressure values with this procedure are based on the possible leak of pressure through the ruptured membranes. However a review of the tracings recorded by transabdominal catheters shows that the pressure values are equivalent, for the same patient, before and after rupture of the membranes — suggesting that the lower part of the uterus adapts to the presenting part by closing all areas of potential loss of pressure.

When there is no excess of amniotic fluid or frank polyhydramnios (and this occurs in the majority of labors), the intrauterine volume is not significantly altered during first stage in spite of the important changes going on in the lower segment and corpus, thinning and thickening respectively. As the collagen-rich (or muscle-poor) cervix is "taken up" by the contractions, the muscle-rich (or collagen-poor) fundus gains in thickness (brachystasis), and thus mass, to increase its local tension. At the same time, the lower segment stretches, overtaken by the stronger fundal region, and becomes thinner (mecystasis). However, the intrauterine content, being noncompressible, does not change volume, and therefore the differences in intrauterine pressure readings, which may be recorded as labor progresses, will reflect actual alterations in the intensity of contractions.

Other methods of recording intrauterine pressure have been proposed, to minimize the potential artifacts induced by the ruptured membranes. These are called intrauterine extraovular recording methods. Karlson (1944) used small strain gauges mounted on a steel tape slipped between the membranes and the lower segment. A similar idea led Csapo to propose the insertion of small fluid-filled balloons between the lower segment and membranes. Variations of these methods have been used by investigators for special studies, particularly of the physiology of the lower segment during first and second stages of labor. However, the most reliable and popular technique for recording intrauterine pressures is the transvaginal catheter.

The *internal,* or *intrauterine open catheter,* methods have the important advantage of furnishing the actual pressure values and, hence, accurate information of the strength of contractions and the resting tone. Further, they enable one to make a good estimate of the coordination of contractions by the profile of the tracing — critical when there is suspicion of abnormal contractility. The patient's movements do not affect the actual recording or the patterns, but the value of the resting tone needs to be adjusted if there are changes in the level of the uterine fundus in relationship to the recording transducer.

The most significant drawback of internal methods is the requirement to enter the amniotic cavity, making them invasive techniques. This unavoidable step increases the chances of contamination and clinical infection. Other minor inconveniences of the methods are the patient's discomfort produced by the vaginal manipulations needed to insert the catheter, and the need for local anesthesia when the transabdominal route is used. In addition, the internal extraovular methods do not provide accurate pressure readings, which vary according to the size of the small balloon and the proximity of the strain gauge to a hard fetal part (head or limb) that may directly press on it.

External The *external recording techniques* aim at obtaining tracings of the contractions of the uterus with instruments applied over both uterus and anterior abdominal wall. These techniques record only moments of increased consistency of the uterine wall as the muscle contracts. Thus, local changes are recorded over the area where the recording device is placed. Each recorder has a small piston connected to a strain gauge in the center of a cup-like applicator. Its movements are translated into electric signals that are recorded. This principle is used by the several models available.

Compared to internal methods, the external techniques have advantages and disadvantages. They cannot determine true intrauterine pressure but only relative changes when the device has not been manipulated. Similarly, they do not indicate the true resting tone of the uterine muscle but only the activity of the small area of application. A limitation expected from all indirect methods is their inability to produce information regarding the coordination of the contractions. Only the simultaneous application of several recording devices over a number of areas of the uterus enables one to gain information about coordination of the contractions. The interposition of the abdominal wall adds to the lack of precision of this method. Among the advantages are easy application and absence of the manipulations that would produce patient discomfort or facilitate contamination of amniotic fluid. External recording does not require penetration of the amniotic sac and therefore may be applied repeatedly at any stage of advanced gestation. The external methods are very widely used because they produce a satisfactory tracing for routine cases. They probably are the more frequently used method in this country.

Several ways of analyzing the tracings have been proposed so that recording techniques may be used in research as well as in the clinical management of cases. These applications will be reviewed in Chapter 4, where techniques and instrumentation are discussed.

BIBLIOGRAPHY

Cibils LA: Contractility of the nonpregnant human uterus. *Obstet Gynecol* 30:441, 1967.

Cibils LA, Schweid DE: Electrolyte content and distribution in human myometrium. II. Childbearing age group. *Am J Obstet Gynecol* 94:619, 1966.

Csapo A: Actomyosin content of the uterus. *Nature* 162:218, 1948.

Csapo A: Actomyosin formation by estrogen action. *Am J Physiol* 162:406, 1950.

Danforth DN: The fibrous nature of the human cervix, and its relation to the isthmic segment in gravid and nongravid uteri. *Am J Obstet Gynecol* 53:541, 1947.

Danforth DN: The distribution and functional activity of the cervical musculature. *Am J Obstet Gynecol* 68:1261, 1954.

Gillespie EC: Principles of uterine growth in pregnancy. *Am J Obstet Gynecol* 59:949, 1950.

Greiss FC, Anderson SG: Effect of ovarian hormones on the uterine vascular bed. *Am J Obstet Gynecol* 107:829, 1970.

Karlson S: A contribution to the methods of recording the motility of the human uterus. *Acta Obstet Gynecol Scand* 24(suppl 4): 1944.

Killian AP, Rosenfield CR, Battaglia FC, et al: Effect of estrogens on the uterine blood flow of oophorectomized ewes. *Am J Obstet Gynecol* 115:1045, 1973.

Loraine JA, Bell ET: Hormone excretion during the normal menstrual cycle. *Lancet* 1:1340, 1963.

Moawad AH: The sympathetic nervous system and the uterus, in Josimovich JB (ed): *Uterine Contraction.* New York, Wiley, 1973, pp 65–82.

Resnik R, Killian AP, Battaglia FC, et al: The stimulation of uterine blood flow by various estrogens. *Endocrinology* 94:1192, 1974.

Rorie DC, Newton M: Histologic and chemical studies of the smooth muscle in the human cervix and uterus. *Am J Obstet Gynecol* 99:466, 1967.

Segal SJ, Scher W, Koide SS: Estrogens, nucleic acids, and protein synthesis in uterine metabolism, in Wynn R (ed): *Biology of the Uterus.* New York, Plenum, 1977, pp 139–201.

Schwalm H, Dubrauszky V: The structure of the musculature of the human uterus—muscles and connective tissue. *Am J Obstet Gynecol* 94:391, 1966.

CHAPTER 3
Physical Basis of Monitoring Fetal Heart Rate, Oxygenation, and Acid–Base Status

Fetal well-being may be assessed by recording and analyzing either the mechanical activity of the heart and its consequences, or the electric current produced by the cardiac contraction. In addition, alterations of fetal blood homeostasis, pO_2, and pH have recently been successfully observed. All have been investigated as possible sources of information for following the progress of the fetus through early gestation, advanced pregnancy, and labor.

It seems that the fetal heart initiates its activity as early as the fifth week of gestation, when rhythmic contractions start in a still incompletely developed organ. By the eighth or ninth week the electrical activity of the human fetal heart has already the profile of the adult ECG. At about this time the blood-forming tissues and vessels have developed so well that blood pumping by the heart can be ascertained with adequate means of observation. Sounds produced by the heart valves may be heard if sensitive microphones are used. Likewise, the movements of these valves as well as that of the circulating blood are amenable to recording by appropriate instruments. Both of these phenomena are intermittent but occur with predictable regularity.

The fetus requires as much oxygen as the adult, and oxygen pressure (or concentration) may undergo wide variations that reflect oscillations in the maternal oxygen supply available in the IVS. The normal oxygen concentration in the fetus is instrumental in the maintenance of an overall homeostasis reflected in an acid–base status, with a pH in the range of that of the mother. During normal active labor the repetitive interruptions of blood supply to the IVS cause the fetus to become slightly acidotic, as reflected by lower plasma and capillary blood pH values. The accessibility of the fetal presenting part in advanced labor could facilitate the application of instruments to assess this acid–base status.

Electrocardiogram

The electrical activity generated by each contraction of the fetal heart, although clearly present by the ninth week of gestation, can be recorded from the maternal abdomen only several weeks later. The possibility of so doing depends upon the availability of good instruments. When obtained, the signals are superimposed on maternal ECGs. There is a marked difference in voltage generated by the two hearts, the fetal heart giving a maximum of 100 microvolts while the maternal is, in general, on the order of ≥ 1 millivolt, or about tenfold greater. Furthermore, there are intrinsic differences in rhythm, the fetal heart beating faster by approximately two to one. The electrical activity in the fetal heart starts and spreads in much the same manner as in the adult. The pacemaker is located at the sinoatrial node, which is formed by a specialized group of myocardial cells that generate action potentials at approximately 140 times in one minute. Its automaticity is controlled by the sympathetic system, which tends to accelerate it, and the parasympathetic (vagus), which tends to decrease the frequency of spikes. The action potential generated at the pacemaker is propagated over both auricles, which contract. The stimulus thus reaches the atrioventricular (AV) node, formed of a tissue similar to the sinoatrial node but set to a slower automatic pace. The stimulus then propagates, following the bundle of His and its branches, the fibers of Purkinje, which spread over both ventricles carrying to them the stimulus for the heart to contract almost simultaneously. The electrical activity generated by the contraction of the auricles triggers the P wave. The electrical activity of the ventricles (which overshadows the repolarization of the atria) produces the QRS complex; the ventricular repolarization is represented by the T wave. The conductive velocity of the impulse may be estimated by measuring the P-R interval and the width of the QRS complex. Both are usually stable regardless of heart rate but can be altered by pathologic conditions or pharmacologic agents. These electrical activities, very clearly observed and recorded by electrodes applied directly over the fetal heart, are attenuated when the recording electrodes are placed farther from the heart on the body surface of the fetus. They are further attenuated when the recording electrodes are applied over the maternal abdomen, the electrical signal having to pass through several layers of tissue. For these reasons, the fetal ECGs obtained with *abdominal electrodes* produce small signals, much smaller than the maternal complexes that are inevitably recorded simultaneously (Figure 3-1). To be able to use this external recording to feed a cardiotachometer and record the FHR, the maternal complexes must be eliminated, usually by cancellation (see Figure 1-17).

To overcome the problem created by the large maternal complex, it is necessary to apply the electrodes directly on the fetus. Under normal circumstances this may be done only during active labor when the cervix is in the process of dilatation and the membranes are ruptured, allowing application of the *electrodes on the presenting part* (internal or direct method). In this manner one may obtain an excellent fetal signal, much larger than the maternal; such signals need minimal processing or filtering before being used to trigger the tachometer (Figure 3-2). In fact, these signals are sometimes so good that they allow assessment of changes in conduction time and duration of QRS complexes.

Phonocardiogram

The sounds produced by the fetal heart valves during a contraction cycle—closing of AV valves (S_1) at the beginning of the ventricular systole and the closing of the aortic and pulmonary valves (S_2) at the end of it—occur in a low frequency, which creates significant problems for adequate recording and processing to trigger a ratemeter. Furthermore, these heart sounds do not occur in an environment free from extraneous noise, which interferes greatly with the quality of signal suitable for the tachometer. By necessity the microphones must be highly sensitive, thus capable of being triggered by sounds occurring either inside the mother (blood flow, placental souffles, fetal movements) or in her vicinity. This drawback may be partly overcome by shielding

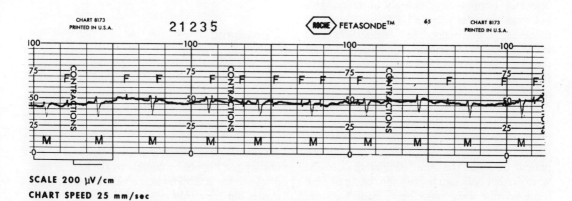

SCALE 200 μV/cm
CHART SPEED 25 mm/sec

Figure 3-1 Fetal ECG recorded with abdominal electrodes, with a single preamplifier. Note the large maternal complex (M) and the very small fetal (F) QRS waves. Significant fetal arrhythmia. Courtesy Roche Medical Electronics.

28

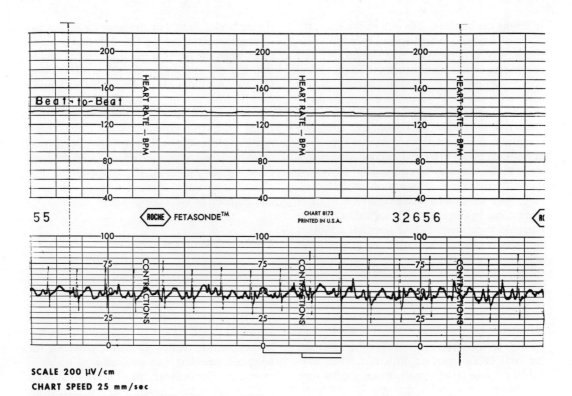

SCALE 200 µV/cm
CHART SPEED 25 mm/sec

Figure 3-2 Fetal ECG recorded with electrode applied directly on fetal skin (scalp). In the lower tracing, after minimal processing, the tracing shows a large QRS complex, more than adequate to trigger the tachometer. The corresponding beat-to-beat FHR is shown in the upper tracing. Courtesy Roche Medical Electronics.

the microphone, the remainder "noise" being filtered and processed. The effect of adequately filtered signals may make a tracing, either processed or unfiltered, completely unrecognizable one from the other (Figure 3-3). The filtering, or processing, is essentially done by using differences in frequency as bases for suppression. Unfortunately, many noises have frequencies similar to fetal heart sounds, hence the need for other manipulations to obtain reliable data. These difficulties are overcome by knowing that the noises are random, whereas fetal heart sounds occur at predictable intervals (particularly first and second sounds). The time intervals are computed and passed through the time-comparing circuits, which accept only signals with the timing of fetal heart activity while rejecting "parasite" sounds (Figure 3-4). These electronic manipulations markedly alter the shape of the recorded sounds but cannot change their timing—a crucial consideration in the study of the FHR. They are then

satisfactory signals to trigger a ratemeter, which, when sensitive enough, may record instantaneously the changes in rate.

Ultrasound

The opening and closing movements of the heart valves with each contraction may be used as signals to trigger a ratemeter if the movements can be adequately recorded. This is done by applying the Doppler principle of ultrasonic waves aimed at those valves. The technique is based on the principle that ultrasound waves (sound waves of a frequency too high to be audible by the human ear, on the order of 2 MHz) are capable of penetrating tissues but are partly reflected, depending on the density of the tissues. There is no change in the frequency of the return wave when the reflecting surface is not in motion. However, when the ultrasound waves encounter a moving surface, the

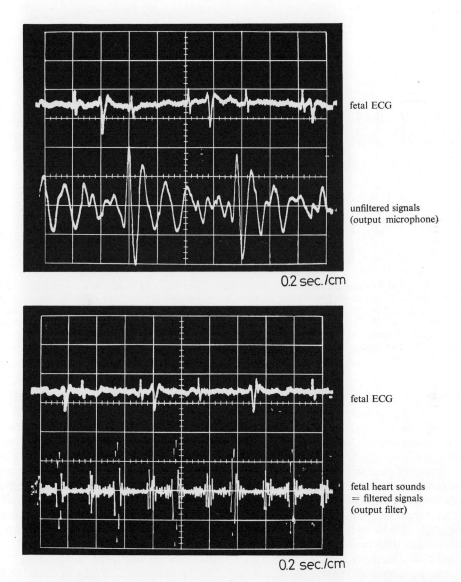

fetal ECG

unfiltered signals
(output microphone)

0.2 sec./cm

fetal ECG

fetal heart sounds
= filtered signals
(output filter)

0.2 sec./cm

Figure 3-3 *(Above)* Simultaneous recording of fetal ECG and (bottom) unfiltered fetal heart sounds picked up with an abdominal microphone. *(Below)* The same type of ECG and simultaneously obtained fetal heart sound after filtering and processing. Reprinted from Hammcher K: The diagnosis of fetal distress with an electronic fetal heart monitor, in Horský J, Stembera ZK (eds): *Intrauterine Dangers to the Fetus.* Amsterdam, Excerpta Medica, 1967, pp 228–233.

reflected part of the sound beam will have a different frequency (Figure 3-5). This is the Doppler principle and its application permits the recording of the FHR. A beam of ultrasound waves, generated by a transducer applied over the maternal abdomen, is directed at the heart of the fetus. The reflected part of the beam—with a change in frequency—is detected by the receptor crystal situated beside the emitting one. Because the heart valves may move toward and away from the ultrasound source, there will be a difference in the frequency shift of the reflected waves, and thus at least two groups of waves for each cardiac cycle (those reflected while the valves move toward, increased frequency; those reflected when the valves move away, lower frequency). These signals need

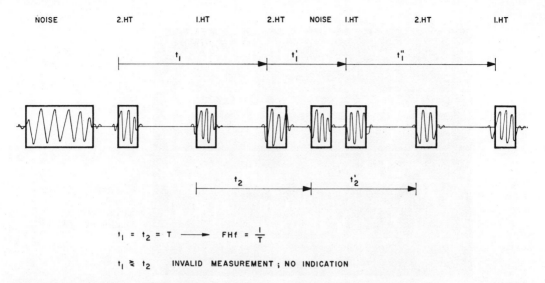

Figure 3-4 Schematic of electronic programming to accept or reject incoming signals. When the duration of these exceed that of the fetal heart tones (first waves), or when they appear in a sequence too close following a sound (fifth waves), they are rejected. Only sounds that appear with a time sequence equal to that between the first and second heart sounds, or with their normal duration, are recorded. Reprinted from Hammacher K: The diagnosis of fetal distress with an electronic fetal heart monitor, in Horský J, Stembera ZK (eds): *Intrauterine Dangers to the Fetus*. Amsterdam, Excerpta Medica, 1967, pp 228–233.

to be filtered in much the same manner as those perceived by the phonocardiograph. The same circuitry and principles may be applied to process and record them by time-comparing circuits that should accept only signals with the timing of the heart activity (Figure 3-6). When the ultrasonic beam is not directed at the heart valves, it will still be able to pick up the signals reflected by the fetal heart apex movement, the aortic blood flow, or the umbilical cord blood flow. Although all these actions produce shifts in reflected wave frequency, they will differ. Furthermore, the reflected wave may also be converted to audible signals of variable pitch depending on the moving speed of the reflecting object. Since the sound-emitting crystal and receiver are mounted close together, they can detect only moving surfaces perpendicular (or nearly so) to the sound beam.

Improved designs in recent years have made it possible to feed cleaner, or purer, signals to the ratemeter. The use of several transmitters around a central receiving crystal has made it possible to have less artifact from fetal movements because the area "covered" by the ultrasonic waves is significantly enlarged (Figure 3-7). In addition, this development is coupled with a "depth ranging" capability added to the transmitted ultrasonic

waves by using the known propagation time of the waves through the tissues. This principle allows for selection of waves reflected at specific depths and, in this manner, markedly diminishes the number of sounds received. The result is cleaner signals and better tracings. However, in spite of impressive improvements, these signals are not yet totally comparable to the single R wave of a direct ECG for which another unique characteristic of the Doppler principle had to be utilized to further improve the quality of the signals. The predictable difference in wavelengths produced by the motion of the heart valves is used to select the reflected sounds of a given wavelength only, depending on the *direction of movement* of the heart valves (Figure 3-8). The sharpness of the signal produced by the "ranged-directional" signal may be appreciated on the oscilloscope or in tracings (Figure 3-9). When these signals are fed to the cardiotachometer, it is possible to obtain tracings indistinguishable from those recorded from direct ECGs (Figure 3-10).

This method allows heart valve movements to be detected very early in gestation, permitting continuous monitoring, at almost any stage of gestation. The great advantage of phonocardiography and ultrasound is that both may be effectively used

THE DOPPLER PRINCIPLE

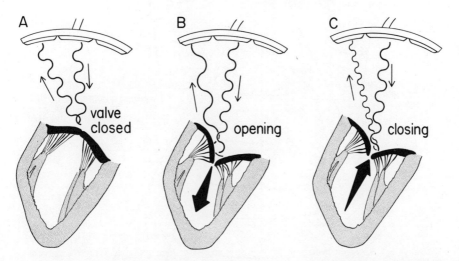

Figure 3-5 Schematic of the Doppler principle. *(A)* When the valves are *not moving,* the ultrasound waves are reflected without changes in frequency. *(B)* When waves emitted by the crystal encounter the heart valves *moving away,* they are reflected with lower frequency. *(C)* When they are interrupted by the heart valves moving *toward them,* they are reflected and shifted to a higher frequency. The receptor crystal is located next to the emitter.

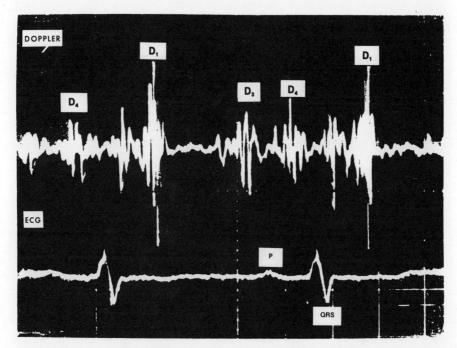

Oscilloscope Photograph of Doppler and ECG from the Fetal Heart

Figure 3-6 Simultaneous recording of *(above)* Doppler ultrasound waves and *(below)* fetal electrocardiogram. In spite of processing, the ultrasound tracing produces a series of signals that may interfere with good recording and thus give false baseline oscillations. Reprinted from Lauersen NH, et al: Evaluation of the accuracy of a new ultrasonic fetal heart rate monitor. *Am J Obstet Gynecol* 123:1125, 1976.

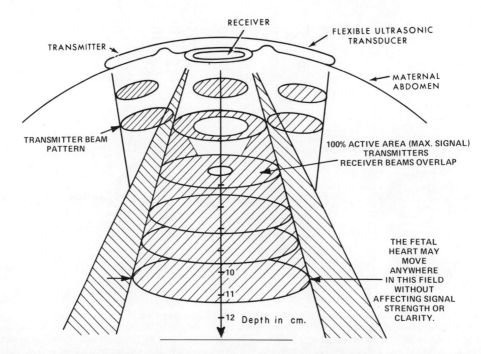

Figure 3-7 Schematic of distribution of transmitters and receiver in the wide-beam ultrasonic transducer. Note overlap of transmitted waves and area maximally covered at 10 to 11 cm depth. Waves emitted by three different crystals reflect on the centrally placed receiver. Courtesy Roche Medical Electronics.

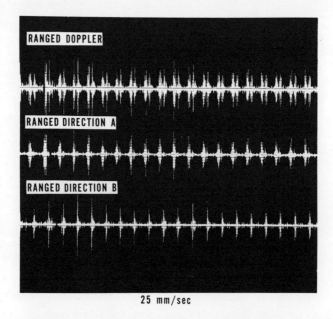

Figure 3-8 Separation of reflected sound waves by ranging in depth and selecting the directional waves. *(Above)* Ranged Doppler sound receiving all reflected waves. *(Center)* Waves reflected by the valves *moving away. (Below)* Waves reflected by the valves *moving toward* the emitting crystal. Note clarity of the signals in both lower tracings and compare with the top, which is a composite. Reprinted from Lauersen (1978).

33

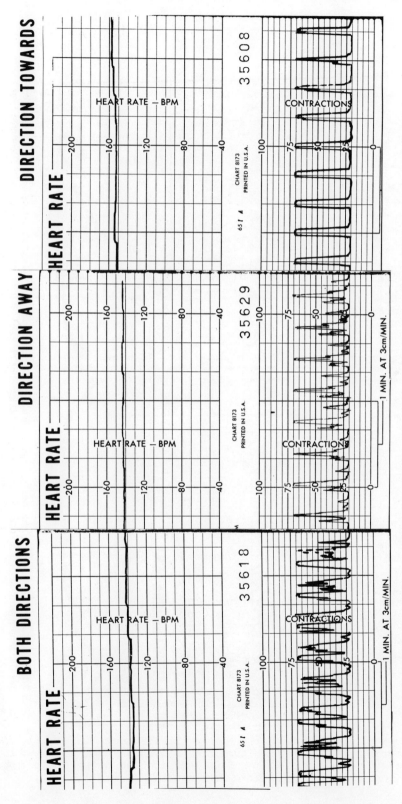

Figure 3-9 Simultaneous tracings of ranged Doppler signals *(bottom)* and the beat-to-beat FHR obtained from them. The lower tracings are the processed signals fed to the ratemeter. *(Left)* Record of Doppler signals from heart valves moving in both directions (less clear than the others). *(Center)* Signals reflected from the valves moving away. *(Right)* Signals from the valves moving toward the sound-emitting crystals. Clearly the directional Doppler system produces excellent and clean signals. Reprinted from Lauersen NH, et al: A new technique for improving the Doppler ultrasound signal for fetal heart rate monitoring. *Am J Obstet Gynecol* 128:300, 1977.

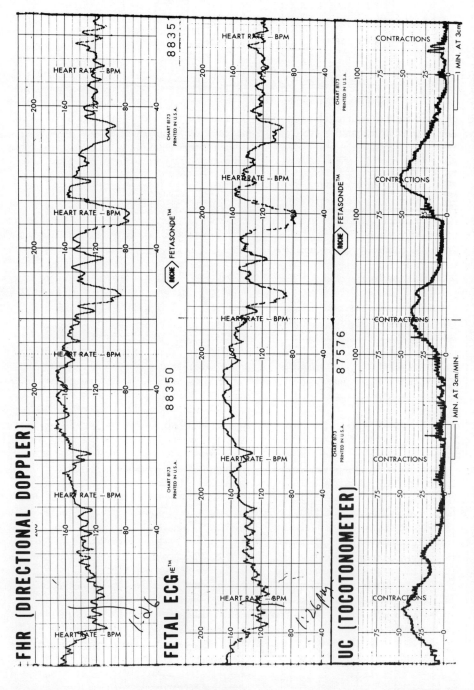

Figure 3-10 Simultaneous FHR tracings obtained from ranged-directional Doppler and direct ECG signals and uterine contractions (external). Note the almost identical FHR tracings of frequency and decelerations obtained by both methods independently. Reprinted from Lauersen (1978).

without disturbing the physical integrity of the ovular sac, that is to say they are noninvasive. This convenience permits one to repeat recording sessions many times during advanced gestation without significant discomfort for the mother or interference with the fetus.

Blood pH

During normal pregnancy and early labor fetal blood acid–base balance is maintained as in adults. The fetus has buffer mechanisms to compensate for transient alterations in the homeostatic equilibrium. However, under stressful conditions these compensatory safeguards may be overcome, and the fetus may develop acidosis. If this state is not corrected, the acidosis may progress more or less rapidly and possibly be lethal for the fetus. Acidosis may present itself late in gestation if a pathologic condition exists, or during first or second stages of labor. The only way to assess accurately fetal homeostasis is to analyze the ionic concentration of the fetal blood. The Saling (1967) method of intermittent testing of blood microsamples from the fetal scalp is now routine in most centers that treat high proportions of pathologic disorders of pregnancy and labor. However, this very useful technique provides information about only a transient moment of a very dynamic and changing condition of the fetus during the labor process.

It has recently been possible to record continuously the pH of the fetal tissues at the presenting part through an electrode capable of detecting the changes in ionic concentration of that tissue. The principle is relatively simple: the variations in concentration of hydrogen ions in tissue (expression of capillary values), with respect to a standard solution contained in the electrode, generate electric currents that are detected by appropriate preamplifiers and recorded on a moving chart (see Figure 4-6). Because of the necessity of penetrating fetal tissue, this procedure is invasive, requiring dilatation of the cervix and rupture of the membranes. It is thus applicable only during moderately advanced labor.

Blood pO$_2$

Although fetal blood oxygen pressure is significantly lower than in adults, it nevertheless needs to be maintained at a minimum level to supply the high requirements of the fetus. Under normal circumstances, the relatively low pressure is compensated for by a high dissociation capacity of the fetal hemoglobin and a very high fetal cardiac output that delivers sufficient oxygen to the fetal tissues. The fetal blood is resupplied with oxygen by its passage through the placenta, which receives it in the maternal blood flowing in the IVS. In pregnancy this flow is almost continuous, with only sporadic interruptions by Braxton Hicks contractions. In labor the condition changes radically because the continuous availability of oxygen to the fetal blood is frequently, and almost completely, interrupted by each uterine contraction, creating repetitive transient potential episodes of hypoxia during which the fetus must resort to its "reserves," which depend directly on its pO$_2$. If the interruptions are either too frequent, prolonged, or the reserves too low, the fetus will experience episodes of hypoxia during which it will have to sustain anaerobic metabolism with a challenge to its buffer system. Recovery will occur rapidly as the uterus relaxes and blood with high oxygenation is again available for exchange in the IVS.

Obviously, intermittent determinations of fetal capillary pO$_2$ are of only relative value, but a continuous recording may be helpful in evaluating the fetal condition. An electrode to be applied over the fetal skin has been developed; it is capable of continuously recording oxygen pressure changes in the blood circulating in the capillaries directly under the electrode. This instrument utilizes the great capacity of diffusion through tissues, which characterizes oxygen. To facilitate the manifestation of that quality, the electrode contains a heating thermostat that induces active capillary vasodilatation and thus constant blood flow. The fluctuations in pO$_2$ generate an electric current that is processed through a preamplifier and continuously recorded on a chart (Figure 3-11). Even though the electrode is noninvasive for the fetus because it is applied over the skin, the method should nevertheless be considered invasive because it requires that the membranes be ruptured for its application intrapartum.

With the continuous recording of fetal pO$_2$ one may follow the evolution of a pathologic labor and safely predict the fetal status as well as evaluate the benefits of therapeutic measures taken to correct untoward conditions.

36

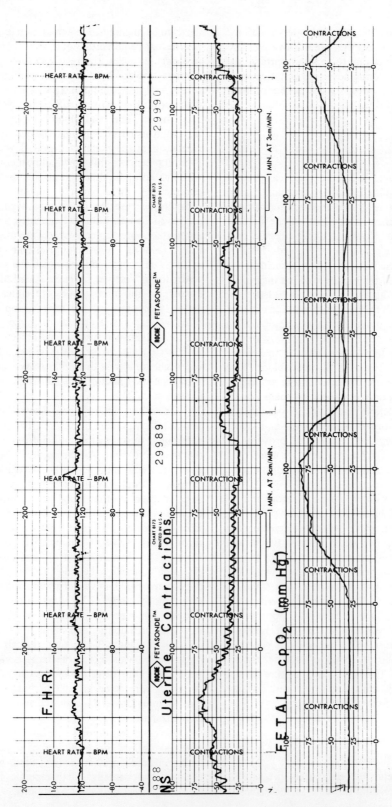

Figure 3-11 Continuous FHR, uterine contractions, and fetal cutaneous pO₂ recorded in advanced labor of primipara who was receiving oxygen by mask at 6 liters/min. Courtesy Roche Medical Electronics.

BIBLIOGRAPHY

Hammacher K: The diagnosis of fetal distress with an electronic fetal heart monitor, in *Intrauterine Dangers of the Fetus*. (Symposium, Prague, 1966) Amsterdam: Excerpta Medica, 1967, pp 228–233.

Hon EH, Hess OW: Instrumentation of fetal electrocardiography. *Science* 125:553, 1957.

Huch A, Huch R, Schneider N, et al: Continuous transcutaneous monitoring of fetal oxygen tension during labour. *Br J Obstet Gynaecol* 84(suppl 1): 1977.

Huch R, Lubbers DW, Huch A: Reliability of transcutaneous monitoring of arterial pO_2 in newborn infants. *Arch Dis Child* 49:213, 1974.

Larks SD: *Fetal Electrocardigraphy*. Springfield, Ill, Thomas, 1961.

Lauersen NH, Hochberg HM, George MED: Evaluation of the accuracy of a new ultrasonic fetal heart monitor. *Am J Obstet Gynecol* 123:1125, 1976.

Lauersen NH, Hochberg HM, George MED, et al: A new technique for improving the Doppler ultrasound signal for fetal heart rate monitoring. *Am J Obstet Gynecol* 128:300, 1977.

Lauersen NH, Hochberg HM, George MED, et al: Technical aspects of ranged directional Doppler: A new Doppler method of fetal heart rate monitoring. *J Reprod Med* 20:77, 1978.

Saling E: Neues Vorgehen zur Untersuchung des Kindes unter des Geburt. *Arch Gynaekol* 197:108, 1962.

Saling E, Schneider D: Biochemical supervision of the fetus during labour. *J Obstet Gynaecol Br Comwlth* 74:799, 1967.

Stamm O, Latscha U, Janacek P, et al: Development of a special electrode for continuous pH measurement in the infant scalp. *Am J Obstet Gynecol* 124:193, 1976.

Sturbois G, Uzan S, Rotten D, et al: Continuous subcutaneous pH measurement in human fetuses. Correlations with scalp and umbilical blood pH. *Am J Obstet Gynecol* 128:901, 1977.

Young BK, Hirschl IT, Klein SH, et al: Continuous fetal tissue pH monitoring in labor with high risk pregnancies. *Arch Gynaekol* 226:169, 1978.

CHAPTER 4
Instrumentation and Technique

Modern instruments to monitor maternal and fetal systems continuously during advanced gestation and labor are manufactured in an extraordinary variety of models, sizes, sensitivities, and potentials for simultaneous recordings. The most popular ones are the two-channel monitors designed to record uterine contractions (UC) and FHR. The accessory instruments and the techniques of application will be reviewed briefly, as well as the techniques to record a number of other physiologic phenomena of great importance to mother and fetus.

INSTRUMENTS

Recorders

Every manufacturer of electronic equipment has designed and marketed a fetal-maternal monitor to help evaluate the status of the patient in advanced gestation and labor. Figures 4-1, 4-2, and 4-3 show the three models of two-channel apparatuses available for routine use at the Chicago Lying-In Hospital. All have an upper channel on which the FHR is recorded on paper. The differences in the ranges of paper scales and speeds account for the apparent disparity in fluctuations of the baseline on each monitor for equivalent oscillations. (This point is of no negligible importance, as the study of the FHR baseline oscillations is significant in the diagnosis of some pathologic conditions during gestation and labor.) All manufacturers claim to record instantaneous heart rate (that is, no electronic manipulation of the original signal includes averaging of the heart frequency) by processing the signal through an amplifier that has a wave threshold detector.

In the *direct recording,* as the ECG obtained with an intrafetal electrode is also called, the detected signal is the R wave, which triggers the tachometer from which a rate display and chart recorder are fed. However, often there are artifacts and noise that need to be eliminated to obtain a clear tracing because they may have a voltage almost as high as that of the R wave. For that purpose, the preamplifiers are provided with an automatic gain to set the R signal just above the threshold and overlook the signals with lesser voltage. Then the tachometer calculates the time elapsed between R waves (or detected signals) and expresses it as beats per minute (or, in real elapsed time, milliseconds) for each heartbeat. In this manner the tracings obtained record the instantaneous heart rate or so-called true beat-to-beat frequency (Figure 4-4).

The *indirect recordings* (external methods) — abdominal ECG, phonocardiogram, and Doppler ultrasound — detect a much more complex set of waves, which are filtered and processed electronically before they are fed to the amplifiers. The amplifiers then select the waves, either by intensity or timed sequence, and trigger the rate-meter. It is often postulated that, because of the processing these signals must go through, the tracings obtained do not truly reflect instantaneous changes or beat-to-beat variations. In some instances rapid fluctuations are not recorded, while in others, artifacts that have not been eliminated are responsible for apparent oscillations that in reality do not exist. However, with a moderately good electrode application on the abdomen, an appropriately placed ultrasound crystal, or a well-insulated microphone, it is possible to obtain acceptable tracings with variations or oscillations similar to those recorded with an intrafetal electrode (Figure 4-5). The signals are then displayed in the upper channel of the recording paper at variable speeds; the usual is 1 cm/min, but it can vary to as fast as 3 cm/min or more.

These tracings show reasonable baseline oscillations when adequately obtained, but the

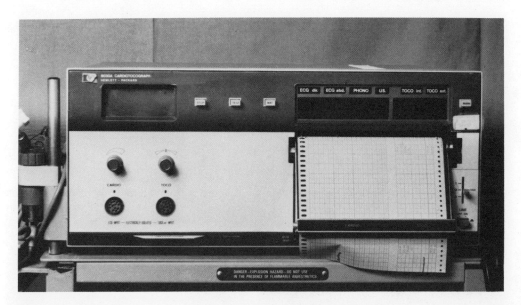

Figure 4-1 Two-channel monitor (Hewlett-Packard) can record signals from external and internal transducers and electrodes. The FHR channel has a range of 50 to 210 beats/min over 8 cm paper, and the UC has 0 to 100 mm Hg pressure on 4 cm paper. The recorder runs at 1 and 3 cm/min. A small oscilloscope may be seen on upper left side.

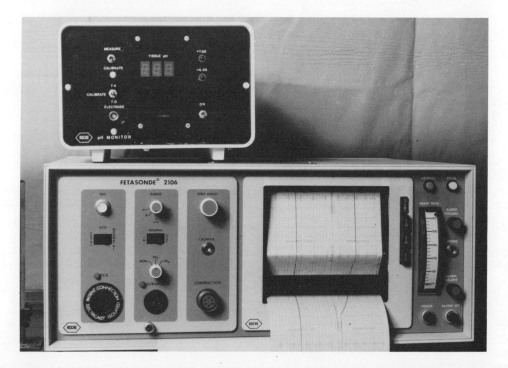

Figure 4-2 Two-channel monitor (Roche) can record from internal and external transducers and electrodes. The FHR ranges from 40 to 220 beats/min over 6 cm paper, and the UC has 0 to 100 mm Hg pressure on 4 cm paper. In addition, the small box on top is the pH preamplifier, with a digital display, the signals of which are recorded in the lower channel with a range of 7.00 to 7.40 on 4 cm paper, superimposed to the UC signal. It may run at from 1 to 3 cm/min paper speed.

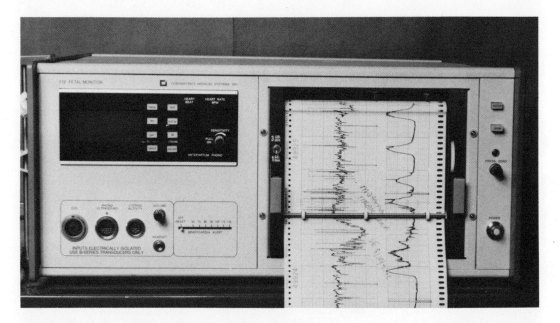

Figure 4-3 Two-channel monitor (Corometrics) can record from internal and external electrodes and transducers. The FHR channel has a range of 30 to 240 beats/min over 7 cm paper. The UC track ranges from 0 to 100 mm Hg pressure on 4 cm paper. The recorder runs at 1 and 3 cm/min. A small oscilloscope is provided on the left upper side.

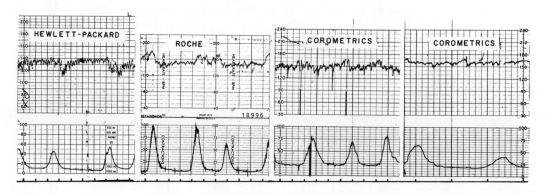

Figure 4-4 FHR and UC tracings obtained with intrafetal electrode and intrauterine catheter (direct methods). Recordings were obtained with the three monitors to illustrate the different appearance of equivalent tracings, particularly the FHR baseline oscillations around a normal frequency rate, when the scales are different. Note the faster paper speed on the last tracing on the right. The UC tracing shows the fluctuations of the resting pressure (or tonus) and the intensity of contractions, both in actual, accurate values.

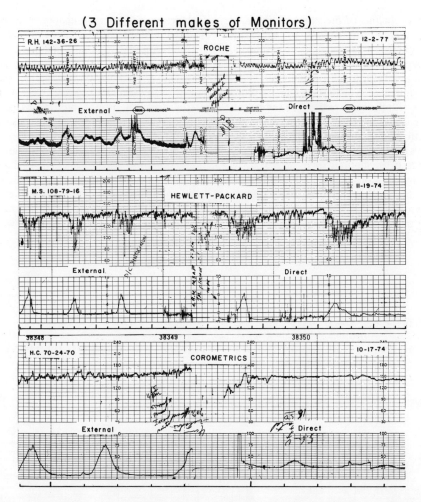

Figure 4-5 Tracings obtained with three different monitors. Uterine contractions and FHR recordings obtained with tocotransducers and Doppler ultrasound (indirect methods) seen on the left side. The quality of the FHR tracing obtained by Doppler ultrasound is not the same for all makes. In the middle of the tracings, scalp electrodes and catheters (direct methods) were connected. In the FHR tracings from the top and middle recorders there is very little visible difference between the FHR tracings obtained by external and internal methods. In the lower recorder, the external tracing has oscillations and variations not seen with the internal. (In the top and bottom recorders a brief period of faster running paper is seen at the time of connection to internal techniques.)

sounds detected by the phonocardiogram and the movements "seen" by the Doppler ultrasound are complex phenomena that create conditions which make possible the recording of some true oscillations with superimposed artifacts induced by setting the amplifiers to pick up only one of the many pulses generated by the fetal heart contraction. Since the regularity and/or intensity of these pulses may vary, the true beat-to-beat variations may be exaggerated, and thus falsely increased

oscillations will be recorded. The direct ECG has less chance of producing these types of artifacts but nevertheless it is not completely free of them. Rapid spikes recorded above the baseline generally indicate a shortened beat-to-beat time, while the spike below the baseline indicates a longer period, perhaps a missed signal or a compensatory pause following a premature ventricular contraction.

42

The lower channel of the standard monitors records the uterine contractions by either intrauterine catheters or external tocotransducers. The latter are applied over the abdominal (and uterine) wall and held in place by an elastic belt. When the equipment is maintained in the same position and with the same tension on the belt, it will record changes in the consistency of the abdominal wall during uterine contractions, the intensity of which will be relatively well indicated by the degree of oscillations in the tracings. It, therefore, cannot record actual intrauterine pressures as has been claimed by some investigators. When the recording transducer is connected to an intrauterine catheter, the tracing will represent actual pressures (generally calibrated in mm Hg). The fluctuations observed in the intensity of contractions are real variations that occur in normal labors. When care is taken to level the transducer with the upper level of the uterine hydrostatic system, an accurate tracing of variations in uterine tonus or resting pressure as part of the intrauterine pressure tracing is recorded (see Figure 4-4).

In addition to recording the uterine contractions, the lower channel of the Roche monitor is capable of inscribing the tracing of the subcutaneous fetal pH (tpH) when the pertinent electrode is implanted in the skin of the presenting part (Figure 4-6). Although this tracing writes only

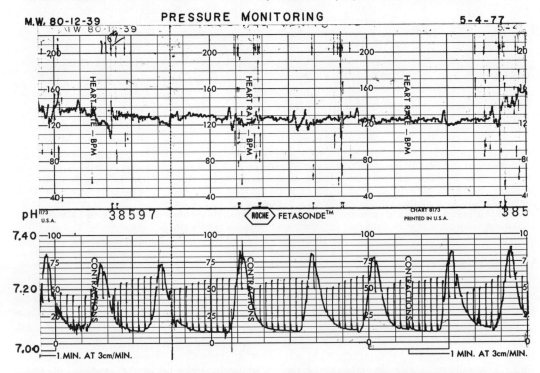

Figure 4-6 Tracings obtained with intrauterine catheter, direct ECG electrode, and subcutaneous pH electrode. The upper channel displays the FHR tracing, while in the lower channel the UC tracing is interrupted every 15 sec by the deflection of the stylus to mark the tissue pH at that moment. The overall tracing illustrates well the continuous changes occurring in the parameters recorded and their temporal relationships. Advanced labor in vertex presentation of term pregnancy.

every 15 seconds, from a practical standpoint it is as good as a continuous one because the tissue (or the plasma for that matter) pH does not change as rapidly as pO_2 or pCO_2. The new models of monitors are equipped with digital readings of all parameters recorded which, in a way, facilitate the interpretation of the recordings.

There is also available at the Chicago Lying-In Hospital a six-channel recorder, equipped with a taping system, with which more elaborate or detailed monitoring has been conducted (Figure 4-7). On it are recorded simultaneously, the FHR and UC; the maternal arterial, venous, and/or cerebrospinal fluid pressures; the maternal heart rate or ECG; and the maternal temperature if appropriate transducers and/or amplifiers are used. The paper can run as slow as 0.5 cm/min, or as fast as 2.5 cm/min.

Electrodes

ECG electrodes The electrodes used to detect the fetal heart electrical activity are applied over the abdominal skin or directly on the fetus. The *external ECG electrodes* are small round steel plates firmly applied over the maternal skin, after thorough cleaning and the application of an electrolyte-rich conductive paste (Figure 4-8, *left*). To obtain the highest possible voltage, they should be placed over the fetal shoulder and hip, that is to say, close to the midline above the pubis, and slightly above the umbilicus. It is critical that a good signal be seen on the screen of the oscilloscope before affixing the electrode to the skin. Minor fetal movements should not significantly alter the quality of the signals obtained; however, in some circumstances reapplication may be necessary to recover good complexes. In general, in spite of claims to the contrary, external electrodes produce a good FHR tracing in about one-half of attempted cases, and then only after spending some time finding the best place for the electrodes.

Internal ECG (or direct) electrodes are now simplified (Figure 4-8, *right*) and consist of a stainless steel needle, spiral shaped and implanted in the subcutaneous tissue. Electrodes made of simple metal are highly polarizable, meaning that, in order to transmit the electric current produced by the fetal heart, they must accumulate a more or less high ionic concentration gradient at their interface with the tissues in which they are implanted. An important drawback is that any movement of the electrode will alter the local ionic concentration and thus interfere with the pickup of current, the consequence of which will be the production of artifacts in the tracing. This hurdle is overcome by minimizing the amount of current flowing through the electrode with which the polarization phenomenon is directly proportional. A high input

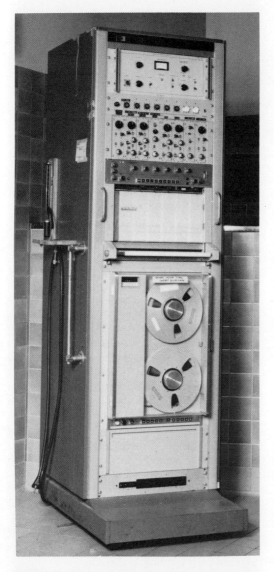

Figure 4-7 Six-channel Hewlett-Packard monitoring Polyviso with eight preamplifiers. On top is a custom-made Corometrics FHR preamplifier while the others are standard, interchangeable, and used to record pressures, heart rates, ECG, temperatures, and so on. At the bottom, under the recorder, is the tape-recording system for data storage.

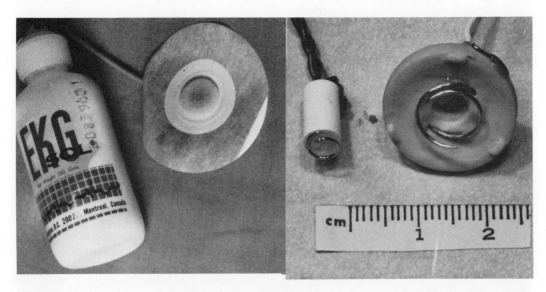

Figure 4-8 Various electrodes used to pick up the fetal ECG. *(Left)* Small round metal electrode covered by a jelly-rich sponge in the center of a reel of adhesive tape for abdominal application. Next to it, a container with extra jelly. *(Right)* A closer view of two types of internal screw subcutaneous electrodes: the small one is the standard made by Corometrics; the larger one, with two helixes and a wide base, has a central hole with a screw system into which the tissue pH electrode must be inserted and affixed.

resistance of the amplifier will prevent the passage of a large current, with minimal polarization of the electrode. This electronic trick is necessary because the nonpolarizable electrodes, like the silver–silver chloride electrode, are delicate and much more difficult to maintain than the ones made of simple metal. The reference electrode is situated on top of the small plastic cylinder that holds and insulates the spiral electrode. The wires from the electrodes are then attached to the leg plate that contains the grounding circuit. Thorough contact of the leg plate with maternal skin, by means of good electrolyte paste, is also mandatory to obtain a good tracing.

pH electrode The pH electrode is based on the principle that an electrical potential is generated when there are different hydrogen ion concentrations across a thin-walled glass membrane. The voltage generated may be measured and is proportional to the pH change. The glass is used as one pole of a battery, the other pole being a reference electrode, usually made of a silver wire coated with silver chloride. It is therefore important to understand that the determination of the charge will be accomplished by measuring the difference in charge against the known constant of the reference electrode immersed in an electrolyte

solution. The reference electrode is of silver–silver chloride, which is known to be electricaly stable. The electrode used for clinical application consists of a very small cone-shaped glass electrode, with the glass membrane at the tip, and a capillary channel filled with electrolyte solution (KCl) bridging between the tissue to be measured and the reference electrode (Figure 4-9). The wires coming from both electrodes are connected to an amplifier, and from this the signals are fed to the recording paper. For accurate monitoring, this electrode needs to be properly inserted and fixed in the intradermic tissue of the presenting part. Placement is done by means of a small stab wound and screw system attached to a double-helix electrode used to detect the fetal ECG and the heart rate pattern. The total unit thus will obtain the FHR and fetal subcutaneous tissue pH. Artifacts may be recorded when penetration is not satisfactory or when the electrode moves from its perpendicular position in the skin.

pO_2 electrode The electrode used to detect oxygen tension in the fetal capillary blood is based on the polarographic technique of measuring oxygen pressures. It is called the Clark principle and is based on the reactions in a cell constituted by a noble metal cathode (gold or platinum) and a

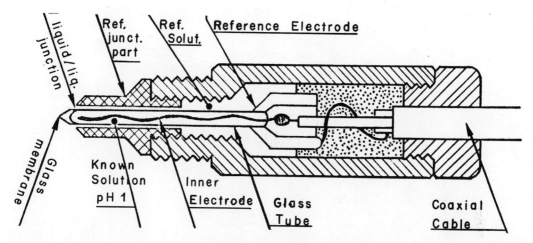

Figure 4-9 Diagram of the tissue pH electrode for subcutaneous insertion and continuous recording. The small plastic case houses the reference electrode, which is in contact with the reference solution. This, by means of a capillary layer around the glass tube, creates a liquid–liquid junction near the glass membrane, which is in contact with the inner electrode encased in the glass tube. The voltage difference between the reference electrode and the inner electrode measures the pH at the external surface of the glass membrane. The information is generated by the effects of hydrogen ions in tissue on the glass membrane and the liquid junction. Only this tip of the instrument needs to reach the deep dermis or subcutaneous tissue to measure the tissue pH. Reprinted from Hochberg HM, et al: Evaluation of continuous monitoring of tissue pH in cats. *Am J Obstet Gynecol* 131:770, 1978.

reference anode connected by an electrolyte, all covered by an oxygen-permeable membrane. When voltage is applied, the oxygen molecules are reduced at the cathode (exchange of electrons), and a measurable current is produced. By slowly changing the potential applied to the cathode to decreasing negative values, the produced current increases, and the current–voltage curve is called a polarogram. This curve has a plateau to which the potential may be adjusted, and then the current measured between the anode and cathode is proportional to the pO_2 in the medium outside of the membrane. The current of the polarographic cell is the result of the reactions that occur at the cathode and are dependent on the number of oxygen molecules available (these depend directly on the oxygen pressure).

The basic arrangement of the electrode consists in the complete separation of the anode, cathode, and electrolyte solution from the external medium by a membrane permeable to oxygen but impermeable to water and ions (Figure 4-10). To avoid polarization effects, the reference anode is made of silver–silver chloride, and the cathode of gold with a relatively large surface (4 mm diameter). To measure the pO_2 of the subcutaneous capillaries it is necessary to produce an adequate and sustained vasodilatation, which is

obtained by heating the skin. The heating system incorporated in the electrode consists of a resistor and two thermistors to control the temperature at 43 C to 44 C, sufficient for good vasodilatation, and still below the burning threshold. In this manner "arterialized' blood is circulating in the subcutaneous capillaries and its pO_2 is measured by the electrode. The membrane separating the electrode from the skin is 6 to 12 μ thick and made of Mylar or Teflon.

The compact electrode is connected to the preamplifier and to the recording system. Appropriate calibrations are mandatory to obtain reliable readings.

Transducers

The instruments used to detect and transmit the movements of the fetal heart valves are *ultrasound transducers,* which utilize the Doppler principle. The transducer consists of a crystal that produces sound waves of a frequency above the audible level and directed at the fetal heart valves. The reflected waves are bounced back with a changed frequency and are detected by a sensor crystal placed very close to the emitting crystal. New transducers have a series of emitting crystals

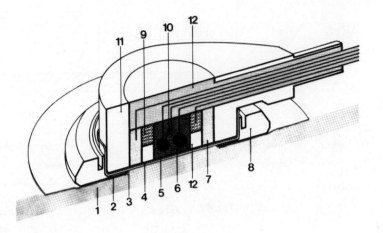

1) skin
2) adhesive ring
3) contact fluid
4) membrane
5) electrolyte
6) cathode

7) anode
8) membrane retainer ring
9) heating element
10) thermistors
11) encapsulation
12) encapsulation

Cross-section of cutaneous oxygen sensor

Figure 4-10 Schematic of the working elements of the cutaneous oxygen sensor applied directly over the skin (1). It is firmly affixed by an adhesive ring (2). Contact with the skin surface through a contact fluid (3) is facilitated by the flat membrane (4) which is permeable to oxygen and retained by a ring (8). The sensor itself has the cathode (6) and anode (7) separated by encapsulation material (12) and the heating elements (9). The temperature is controlled by thermistors (10) and the whole encapsulated in a sturdy small epoxy body (11) from which the connecting cables protrude. Courtesy Roche Medical Electronics.

placed around the receiving sensor, which allows for displacement of the target while still being able to record the movements without artifacts (Figure 4-11). Each receiving crystal is connected to an amplifier provided with the special circuits set to detect only one of the many pulsations produced by each fetal heartbeat. These ultrasound transducers must be attached with elastic belts to the area where the best signals are detected. In addition, because the small air layer between skin and the surface of the crystal is a very poor conductor of sound waves, a small amount of special jelly is used to fill that space and obtain good transmission. The amplifiers are set to determine that the signals received are within the logical time sequence observable in the physiologic phenomenon investigated, in this case the intervals between fetal heartbeats. It is said that the systems perform "electronic logical operations." They reject

signals from an interval different from the average being recorded, or from previously set arbitrary values.

Microphone The microphone used to detect the fetal heart sounds through the maternal abdomen is an extremely sensitive instrument that needs to be heavily insulated to avoid recording too many other sounds (Figure 4-12). Like the ultrasound transducer it must be placed over the best spot on the abdomen. The tracing produced by a single fetal cardiac cycle is complex with at least two distinct sounds recurring at almost precise intervals. They represent the closing of the mitral valve, and the closing of the pulmonary and aortic valves. The signals produced by the microphone are sharper than those originated by the ultrasonic Doppler system and after processing are clean enough to detect the time intervals between cardiac contractions. However, they still

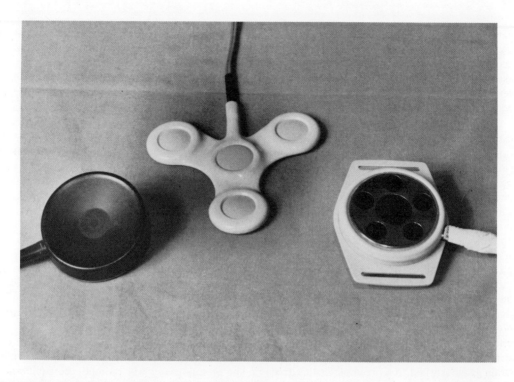

Figure 4-11 Ultrasound transducers viewed from the side applied over the abdomen. *(Left)* Hewlett-Packard. *(Center)* Roche. *(Right)* Corometrics. All have multicrystals.

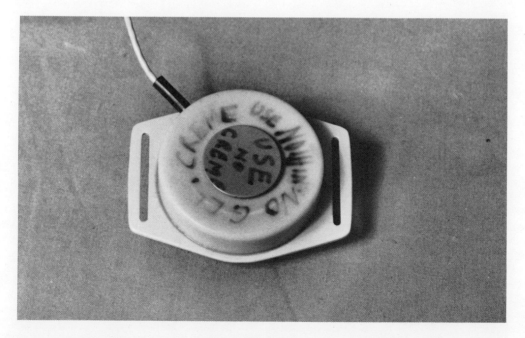

Figure 4-12 The microphone (Corometrics) viewed from the abdominal side that should be applied over the skin. It is a compact but heavy piece.

48

have to be subjected to the circuit of electronic logical operations because there are two sounds per cardiac cycle out of which only one should be used. The circuitry for phonocardiography is thus very similar to that used for ultrasound and abdominal electrocardiography.

External tocotransducers External tocotransducers actually are advanced models of the original, primitive external recorders. They consist basically of a spring-operated plunger that protrudes from a concave surface (toward the abdominal-uterine wall) and attached to a strain gauge. The strain gauge originates electric signals proportional to the displacement of the plunger and the pressure exerted over the transducer (Figure 4-13). This outward movement of the plunger is, in general, in direct proportion to the increase in resistance of the uterine wall, a consequence of a contraction. The action of the spring during relaxation returns the plunger to its resting position. The plunger is slightly indented in the abdomino-uterine wall; the contractions straighten the wall and displace the plunger. The strain gauge is wired to a preamplifier that feeds the signal to a recorder where it is picked up as a tracing. Although there is a relative proportion

between the intensity of the contractions and the hardening of the uterine wall as detected by the tocodynamometer and its tracing, only an approximate idea of the intensity of each contraction is given. On the other hand, it records the activity of a small area of the uterus and therefore cannot truly reflect the quality of contractions. Numerous external tocotransducers exist (Figure 4-14), and all are attached to the abdomen with elastic belts or mesh girdles.

Pressure transducers The pressure transducers for internal monitoring are constructed of a metal diaphragm that separates a leak-proof chamber from the strain gauge to which it is connected (Figure 4-15). The chamber above the diaphragm is filled with fluid, and, by a system of fluid-filled nonelastic catheters, connectedc to the amniotic cavity. By the law of communicating vessels (Pascal's law in an open system) the intraluminal pressures will be the same at equal levels when open to atmospheric pressure. But because this constitutes a closed system, it will also follow Pascal's law, and any change within the uterine cavity will promptly be equilibrated and transmitted to the transducer when it is connected to the catheter that closes the system. To

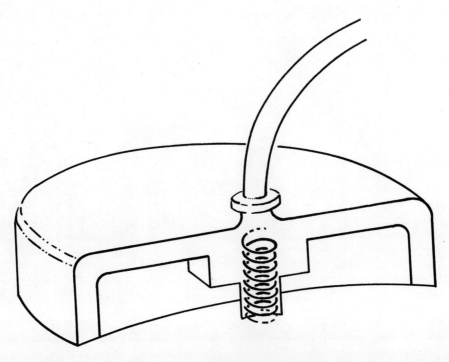

Figure 4-13 Tocotransducer section. The plunger is controlled by a spring and connected to a strain gauge that is wired to the preamplifier.

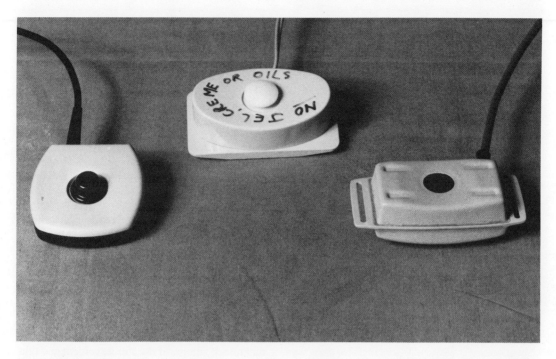

Figure 4-14 Different types of tocotransducers viewed from the side of the plunger. *(Left)* Hewlett-Packard. *(Center)* Roche. *(Right)* Corometrics.

obtain an accurate reading of the intrauterine pressure, the system must be neither elastic (the metal chamber and connecting catheter are not), nor have within it bubbles of air, which, being compressible, create undesirable elasticity and a source of artifacts.

An accurate recording depends on an uninterrupted connection between the uterine cavity and the chamber of the transducer, but often an intrauterine catheter may be obstructed by small pieces of vernix or simply by having the tip applied against a solid surface (uterine wall, fetal parts, placenta). It is then necessary to flush the obstructing substance by injecting extra saline through the catheter at sufficiently high pressure to displace it from its lumen (see Figure 4-23). With appropriate care taken to avoid obstructed catheters it is relatively easy to obtain accurate intrauterine pressure tracings over many hours or even days. The values recorded are representative of the pressure obtained during a contraction equally distributed within the uterus—a closed system which thus follows Pascal's law. However, the fluid system that fills the uterus also follows the law of gravity: when the patient is in the supine position, the posterior aspect of the uterine wall supports the hydrostatic pressure of the fluid directly above it (approximately 15 cm H_2O, 11 mm Hg), (Figure 4-16); when the pregnant patient is standing, the recorded pressure at the lower segment will support the pressure of the fluid column above, up to the dome of the fundus (approximately 30 cm H_2O, 22 mm Hg), (Figure 4-17).

This observation is critical when one wants an accurate record of the resting pressure of the uterus in addition to the increases produced by the contractions. The transducer must then be positioned at the same level as the tip of the catheter. The operator needs to have a good idea of this location (preferably around the middle of the uterus); the leveling of the two should represent the zero reading. This statement is valid for positioning the pressure transducer used to record pressures in any fluid system: it must be level with the atria for arterial or venous pressures, with the highest part of the skull for cerebrospinal fluid pressures, etc. These basic physical principles make it easy to understand that the pressure changes recorded with intrauterine open-end fluid-filled catheters represent the effect of contractions occurring in any (or all) of the uterine wall, and that the changes recorded simultaneously

50

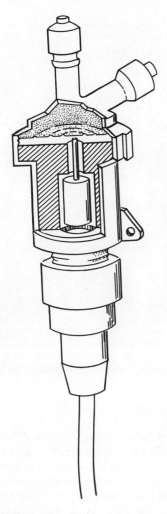

Figure 4-15 Diagram of a pressure transducer. Note that the diaphragm is situated between the strain gauge (below) and the fluid chamber (above). The latter must be connected to the intrauterine catheter and a syringe filled with saline for flushing. The wire leading to the preamplifier and the recording apparatus emerges from the bottom.

by several catheters will all be of equal value (see Figure 1-13). Therefore, any differences that are produced are caused by artifacts of one kind or another.

The most widely used method to record intrauterine pressure is the *transvaginal catheter,* introduced by means of a guide after rupture of the membranes. The tip of the catheter must be above the equator of the presenting part, and the other end connected to the fluid chamber of the pressure transducer. This description suggests that the intrauterine cavity is no longer a closed system after the membranes have been ruptured and that,

as a consequence, there must be a significant leak of pressure through the point where the membranes are interrupted. However, empiric observation indicates that there is no difference in the value of either the resting pressure or the intensity of contractions immediately before or after artificial or spontaneous rupture of the membranes (Figures 4-18 and 4-19). (Only the contractility pattern may change for reasons unrelated to possible leaks of fluid.) It is likely that the lower segment of the uterus adapts tightly around the presenting part during the contractions and therefore still maintains the physical characteristics of a closed system. It is possible to "feel" this tight adaptation by doing a pelvic examination during a contraction with an effaced cervix and attempting to "slip" the finger between the os and the presenting part. The exception to this general rule is seen when there is significant loss of fluid in cases of excess amniotic fluid or tone, as may often be seen in cases of polyhydramnios. When either one of these conditions is present, there is a marked increase in the intensity of contractions due to a diminished volume of the uterine content and thus of the radius of the circumference that constitutes the uterine wall (Laplace's law). Had there been a leak of pressure, a drop in pressure would be recorded. The resting pressure may not change or may drop only in cases of polyhydramnios with hypertonus (Figure 4-20). The latter observations may be confirmed by performing withdrawal of amniotic fluid by amniocentesis instead of by rupture of the membranes, in which case variations equal to those observed after amniotomy will be recorded (Figure 4-21).

Catheters

Some authors have recommended the use of *transvaginal extraovular catheters* provided with a small balloon at the tip to bypass the need for rupturing the membranes to obtain intrauterine pressures. But, in fact, this method is more prone to recording artifacts because the actual pressures are modified by "the other" closed system—the small balloon and its radius. Furthermore, the balloon may be directly compressed between fetal parts and the uterine walls, causing marked distortion in recording. It appears, therefore, that the only means to record accurately the intrauterine pressure is with an intrauterine open-end catheter appropriately attached to a pressure transducer.

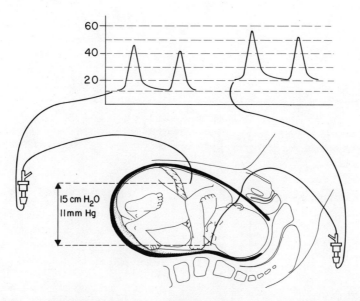

Figure 4-16 Schematic sagittal section of a full-term pregnant patient in *supine position* with two transabdominal catheters placed at different levels. The tip of each one is level with its respective pressure transducer chamber. The tracings obtained illustrate the difference in resting pressure (or tone) recorded depending on how far from the upper level of the fluid the tips are situated. The difference represents the excess hydrostatic pressure of the fluid above the deeper catheter (arrows). The intensity of contractions measured above the tone is the same in both tracings, as seen in the upper section (Pascal's law).

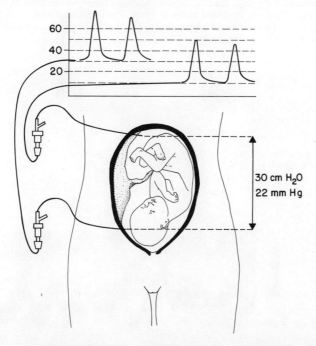

Figure 4-17 Schematic frontal section of a full-term pregnant patient in *standing position* with two abdominal catheters placed at upper and lower parts of the uterine cavity. The tip of each has been level with its respective pressure transducer chamber. The tracings illustrate the difference in pressure recorded at the resting state (or tone), which depends on the relationship of the tip and the upper level of the amniotic fluid. The difference represents the excess hydrostatic pressure of the fluid above the catheter in the lower segment with the value shown by the arrows. The intensity of contractions above the resting pressure is the same in both tracings (Pascal's law).

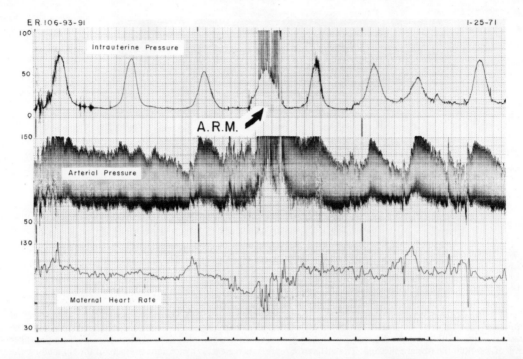

Figure 4-18 Simultaneous recordings obtained during elective induction of labor at term. The upper channel records the intrauterine pressure obtained by *transabdominal catheter* (intraamniotic); the middle channel records the arterial pressure obtained with a catheter placed in the *left femoral artery;* and the lower channel records the *maternal heart rate* obtained from the systolic wave of the blood pressure signal. The membranes were artificially ruptured (arrow) with passage of amniotic fluid. There is no noticeable change in either resting pressure or intensity of contractions. Blood pressure and pulse have normal fluctuations.

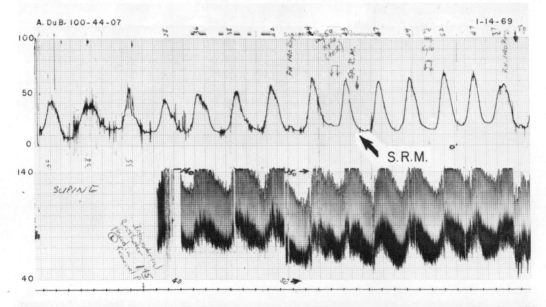

Figure 4-19 Simultaneous recording of intrauterine pressure obtained by *transabdominal catheter* (IVS) and arterial pressure with a catheter in the *left femoral artery*. The patient had spontaneous rupture of membranes (arrow) ascertained by pelvic examination. The steady increase in intensity started five contractions earlier and did not change. There is no significant variation in tone. Fluctuations in arterial pressure are normal responses to contractions.

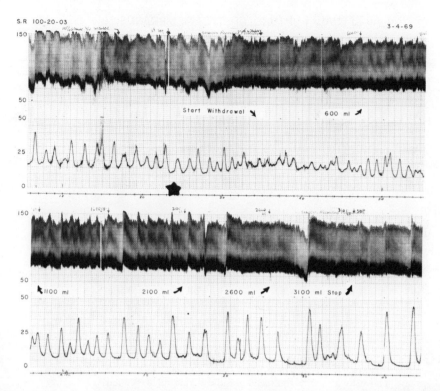

Figure 4-20 Intrauterine (transabdominal catheter) pressure recording from a full-term pregnant patient with polyhydramnios. *(Left)* The high tone and contractions of mild intensity. After amniotomy and passage of 1100 ml amniotic fluid, the tone dropped markedly, and the intensity of contractions increased noticeably (calculated figures shown below). Note the similarity with Figure 4-21, in which case the membranes were kept intact. Reprinted from Caldeyro-Barcia R, et al: Uterine contractility in polyhydramnios and the effects of withdrawal of the excess of amniotic fluid. *Am J Obstet Gynecol* 73:1238, 1957.

The insertion of a *transabdominal catheter* has not received the same acceptance as the transvaginal catheter, even though it is done with a truly aseptic technique, perhaps because it is possible to injure the placenta, and even the fetus, with the guiding needle at the time of the insertion. These catheters are of very fine caliber (1 mm external diameter), and are made of resistant nonelastic material (vinyl, polyethylene) but are flexible passing through an 18-gauge thin-walled needle. The actual recordings are not different from those obtained with the transvaginal catheter, since the physical conditions are the same or even better. Because of their smaller lumen they have a tendency to become obstructed more easily, but the same flushing technique used for the transvaginal catheter reestablishes the continuity of the fluid system between uterine cavity and recording transducer.

A similar system may be adapted to record the *intraarterial or intravenous pressures* by placing the catheter tip in the lumen of the vessel. Of course the fluid system filling the catheter and the transducer must contain a small amount of anticoagulant to avoid clot formation at the intraluminal tip. By extension, this method has been used to record the pressure within the spinal canal, *cerebrospinal fluid pressure,* and it may, likewise, be used to record pressures from any cavity with a fluid content. The open-end fluid-filled catheter has been found to be a good method to record the *intramyometrial pressure* when the tip is lying within the myometrial wall. A continuity is established between the fluid filling the lumen of the catheter and the interstitial fluid, making possible the accurate transmission of the pressure developed locally, at the site of the catheter tip.

54

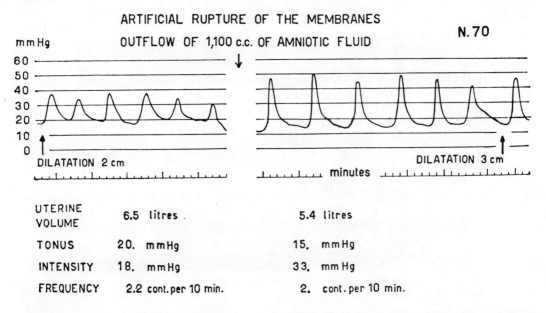

Figure 4-21 Continuous recordings of intrauterine (transabdominal catheter) and arterial (femoral artery) pressures obtained from a 33-week pregnant patient who had subacute polyhydramnios and was carrying an anencephalic fetus. *(Top)* The spontaneous uterine contractility with an increased tonus. By transabdominal tap, withdrawal of amniotic fluid was begun (first arrow). By the second arrow 600 ml had been withdrawn, and, at subsequent arrows (bottom tracing), the gradual withdrawal is indicated until 3100 ml were removed. Note the gradual drop in resting pressure and the marked increase in intensity of uterine contractions as the uterine volume diminished (Laplace's law). There is a mild drop of 10 mm Hg systolic and diastolic on arterial pressure tracing.

The *maternal heart rate* may be recorded by utilizing signals obtained from the R wave of the ECG to trigger the tachometer, or by having pulse waves recorded by a photoelectric cell applied over the earlobe to detect arteriolar pulsations. This signal may then be fed to the ratemeter, which can either send the instantaneous rate or average it.

The higher the number of parameters recorded simultaneously, the better the understanding of physiologic phenomena or pharmacologic responses observed. However, the higher the number of parameters recorded, the more difficult it is to obtain artifact-free tracings.

TECHNIQUES

External Methods

The aplication of the *external tocotransducer* is one of the most simple maneuvers in monitoring. It needs only to be placed over the uterus and affixed with an elastic belt or a girdle made of elastic mesh. The application must be over a spot on the uterus free from fetal parts and soft enough to allow a small indentation of the plunger. The baseline must then be adjusted on the paper; a knob is provided on the recorder or directly on the tocotransducer, depending on the make. The ideal point of application should be close to the midline and around the maximum uterine "bulging" (usually near the umbilicus) making sure that it is not over the fetal back, which is a nice smooth surface but too hard. A frequent error is applying the transducer near the uterine fundus where it has a natural tendency to slide up and away from the uterus and therefore produce totally unsatisfactory, if any, tracings. With the tocotransducer in the same place, the patient in the same position, and the writing stylus not readjusted, the tracing obtained will reflect very well the *relative* changes in the intensity of contractions, and accurately their frequency. To maintain the quality of the information recorded, the belt or the baseline or both must be readjusted every time the patient changes position, particularly when turning to her side. Of course, the appropriate notations must be made on the recording paper at the exact time when the changes occurred to enable the clinician to review the tracing, when needed, with all the potential variables clearly outlined.

The *ECG electrodes* should be applied tentatively, one over the anterior shoulder of the fetus and the other close to the hip. For a good recording it is mandatory to have an oscilloscope on which the clinician should assess the quality of the QRS wave and the presence or absence of artifacts or interferences. Moving the electrodes around should facilitate finding the combination of the highest voltage and fewest artifacts. The generous use of electrolyte jelly facilitates this objective. When the best spot has been found, the electrodes should be firmly taped. The inconvenience of this technique is that there is nearly a 50% failure rate in obtaining a good tracing, in spite of spending significant time finding the best place for the electrodes. Its advantages are that the tracing gives a very good beat-to-beat tracing, when obtained, and that the normal minor fetal movements will not distort the tracing or produce important artifacts.

The *microphone of the phonocardiograph* must be placed over the spot where the fetal heart sounds are best heard. It is of critical importance that the sounds heard not be "contaminated" by arterial hisses or placental souffles, which may occur with the repetitive frequency of the fetal heartbeats to be recorded. Once a good spot has been found, the microphone must be fixed with an elastic belt or the girdle used for the toco-transducer. To minimize the influence of extraneous noise, the room must be closed and soundproofed if possible because hospital noise, particularly on labor and delivery floors, is impossible to avoid. Readjustment may not be necessary following minor fetal movements, but it may be required when the patient turns, or when the position of the heart changes in relation to the microphone.

The *ultrasound transducer* must be applied over the spot where the sounds of the fetal heart valves are best heard. As for the microphone, it should be affixed with an elastic belt or girdle. Fetal movements should not significantly affect the quality of the recording because all modern transducers are equipped with multicrystal emitters, which ensure that the target (the valves) stays within their range if there is a displacment of the heart with respect to the sound-emitting crystal. Other models have several wide-beam emitting crystals placed around a single receiver, an arrangement that allows for significant fetal movement without loss of quality in the detected signals. Furthermore, refinements in technique have made it possible to select the type of wave to be recorded: either the ones reflected by the valves moving *away* from the emitting crystal, or those reflected by movements *toward* it. This characteristic has made the ultrasound technique the most widely used method for external monitoring in the United States. However, one possible drawback is the possibility of recording movements generated by blood flow in the maternal arteries, IVS, or umbilical cord. It is possible to filter out many of these extraneous sounds, but they may cause poor records and create difficulties for good interpretation. The great advantage of Doppler ultrasound is that it allows for movements of the patient without the need to readjust or reposition the transducer.

Internal Methods

The application of the so-called internal monitoring techniques requires the most *meticulous aseptic procedures,* from good sterilization of materials to handling of materials at the time of insertion.

Transabdominal catheter The insertion of the transabdominal catheter is a relatively simple procedure, when the operator knows the placental location as previously obtained by ultrasound. Preparation of the abdominal skin with an antiseptic solution containing iodine is generally done before draping. The tray with all necessary material is shown in Figure 4-22. The use of local anesthetic for infiltration of the abdominal wall through the parietal peritoneum will make the procedure painless. After infiltration, the No. 17 Tuohy thin-walled needle is inserted until the operator has the sensation of having penetrated the amniotic cavity; then the lead is removed. Often amniotic fluid will flow immediately, while in other instances there is no indication of having penetrated the amniotic sac. The needle should then be turned around or gently moved laterally to find a pool of fluid to indicate that the puncture has reached the cavity. Rarely it will be necessary to withdraw the needle and retap at a point close to the first one. The area of choice for puncture is at the midline, from the umbilicus to the pubis, between the fetal head and anterior

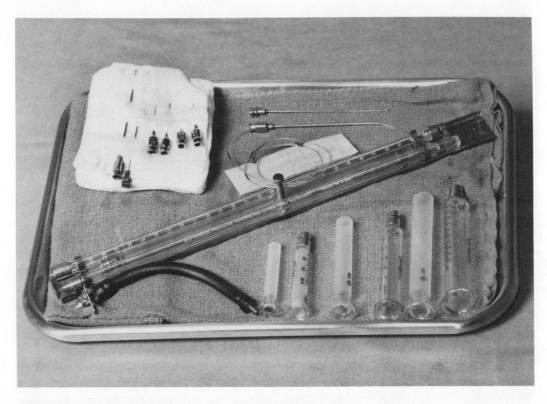

Figure 4-22 Essential elements for transabdominal tap: syringes, needles, catheter, sponges, venous pressure manometer tubes, and stopcocks.

shoulder in cephalic presentations. Only under exceptional circumstances should one attempt to tap away from the midline because of the possibility of injuring branches of the epigastric arteries, or exposing the uterine pedicles to the needle because of rotation of the uterus.

When there is certainty that the tip of the needle is free in a pool of amniotic fluid the catheter is threaded, about 25 to 30 cm, and the needle removed. The catheter should be taped to the abdomen and connected to the pressure transducer. Of course, the system must be filled with a solution of sterile saline. Every attempt should be made to have the pressure transducer at the same level of the uterine fundus to be able to obtain a good approximate value of the resting pressure. If one is interested in a very accurate measurement, before inserting the catheter, a venous pressure tube may be connected to the needle and a direct reading obtained. The baseline of the recording paper may then be set at that value, but it should be adjusted every time the patient changes posi-

tion and alters the level of the uterine fundus. It is always *mandatory to auscultate* the fetus after completing this procedure, as is after any amniocentesis.

Obviously, the technique of inserting a transabdominal catheter is not different from that used in performing an amniocentesis in the outpatient office, a procedure done routinely and repeatedly by obstetricians. However, there is very strong resistance to using the transabdominal route to insert a pressure recording catheter, for not very convincing reasons. When there is need to obtain an accurate reading of the intensity of contractions, it is probably the best approach. In advanced gestation, and when dealing with obese subjects, it is often necessary to resort to it to have an acceptable "contraction stress test."

Insertion of a catheter is not necessarily contraindicated if the placenta is anterior. Hendricks (1959) demonstrated that the insertion of a thin *catheter in the IVS* is safe and provides accurate intrauterine pressure readings. The only additional technical requirements are that one needs to observe free blood flow through the needle (instead of amniotic fluid) and that the sterile saline solution must have a small amount of heparin to prevent clotting at the catheter tip and blocking of the fluid connection (Figure 4-23).

A similar setup and technique is used to insert *catheters into arteries, veins,* and the *spinal canal.* The site of puncture is, of course, dictated by the vessel from which the pressures are to be recorded: wrist for radial, elbow for brachial, groin for femoral or iliac. When vessels are punctured all steps must be taken to avoid the formation of hematomas. The most effective is the simplest: continuous moderate pressure after the needle has been withdrawn and more prolonged pressure at the time the catheter is removed. If these steps are carefully followed, there should not be complications as a consequence of inserting the recording catheter at any of these sites.

The insertion of catheters for recording the *intramyometrial pressure* requires the same technique as for intraamniotic pressure, with the added difficulty that the Tuohy needle has to be directed in a slanted, oblique upward direction as soon as the operator feels it is in the myometrium. The catheter is then inserted and the needle carefully pulled. It is easy to understand how unstable the setup is; the catheters have a great tendency to slip out of the myometrium. The only way to prevent this problem is to tie the catheter to the myometrium to secure proper anchorage.

This has been done postpartum at the time of tubal ligation; the catheters are inserted by means of short No. 18 needles and tied in palce with 000 catgut (Figure 4-24). With this procedure it is possible to know precisely how deep the catheter has been implanted, and to choose the areas of implantation. This technique has been instrumental in elucidating the postpartum contractility patterns, and the relationships between intrauterine pressures and the pressures at different depths in the myometrium. Of course, this technique is strictly a research tool rather than having any application in routine clinical work.

Transvaginal catheter The transvaginal catheter obviously requires that the membranes be ruptured, and because of the impossibility of complete vaginal preparation, the technique is not as aseptic as the transabdominal route. The materials needed are shown in Figure 4-25. The important differences, compared to the transabdominal setup, are that the catheter is considerably thicker with a larger lumen, and that it is inserted through a semirigid plastic guide. The perineum must be thoroughly prepared with an antiseptic solution and draped. All instruments should be readied before starting, including the catheter already filled with saline.

The operator proceeds in the same manner as when rupturing the membranes—during a contraction when the membranes are bulging, and after amniotomy one finger is inserted into the rent. The fluid is allowed to escape slowly and

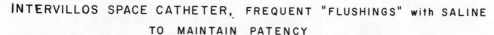

INTERVILLOS SPACE CATHETER, FREQUENT "FLUSHINGS" with SALINE TO MAINTAIN PATENCY

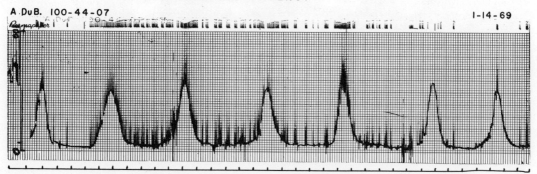

Figure 4-23 Excellent intrauterine pressure recording obtained with a *catheter in the IVS.* In the first five contractions the shade above the tracing was produced by the stylus moving fast, responding to flushing at high pressure, and the line on top, where the stylus remains until the pressure is discontinued. There was minimal flushing in the last two contractions. Marks below indicate minutes.

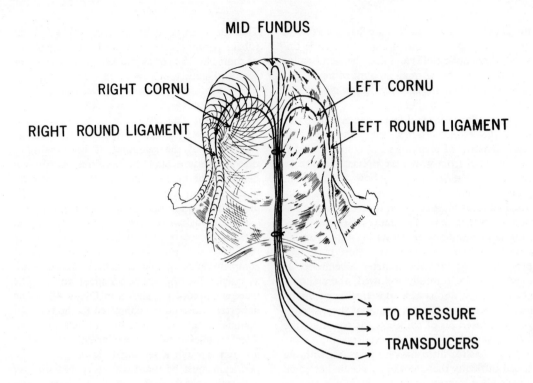

Figure 4-24 Schematic representation of implantation of intramyometrial catheters at laparotomy. Each catheter was tied to secure the anchorage firmly. The catheters inserted in various regions of the uterus are passed through the abdominal wall, identified, and connected to the pressure transducers. Reprinted from Hendricks CH, Moawad AH: Round ligament motility in vivo studies in man. *J Obstet Gynaecol Br Comwlth* 72:618, 1965.

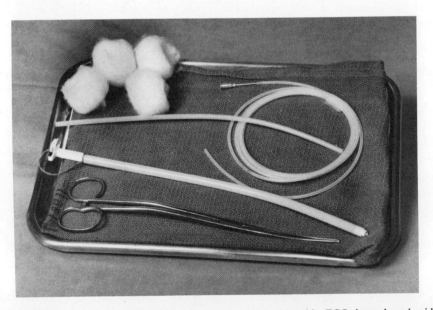

Figure 4-25 Essential elements for transvaginal monitoring: catheter with guide, ECG electrode and guide, sponge, forceps, cotton balls.

when it has reached the desired amount, the semi-rigid catheter guide is slipped in the groove formed by the index and middle fingers and *gently pushed* between the presenting part and the cervix (Figure 4-26). It should never pass beyond the control of the fingers usually placed in the sacral concavity of the birth canal. This position is facilitated by the small curvature of the guide. With its tip between the presenting part and cervix, the operator threads the catheter *between contractions* when he should not feel any significant resistance, up to a mark usually made at about 50 cm from the tip. After insertion, a gentle suction should be applied on the catheter, with the syringe attached to its free end, and free flow of amniotic fluid should be obtained. When the fluid is not obtained, the catheter should be slightly withdrawn, flushed, and again suction applied. When no flow is obtained it is convenient to remove the catheter, reposition the guide, and reinsertion is performed according to the same

steps. Only after good free flow has been obtained should the catheter be connected to the transducer, the stopcock switched, and the recording started. The baseline must be adjusted at this point to accurately record the resting pressure (or tone).

Scalp electrode The scalp electrode is applied in the subcutaneous tissue of the fetus. It has either one or two spiral screw-like needles mounted on a plastic body and connected to thin cables. The whole is enclosed in a plastic, hollow, slightly curved guide to be slipped along the groove formed by the two examining fingers and firmly pushed against the presenting part. This is usually the scalp, but it may be the gluteal area or the heel of a fetal foot in a case of breech presentation. It is very important to avoid the area immediately over the fontanelles or the sutures under which run large venous sinuses. With an assistant firmly holding the uterine fundus the operator turns the piece holding the electrode

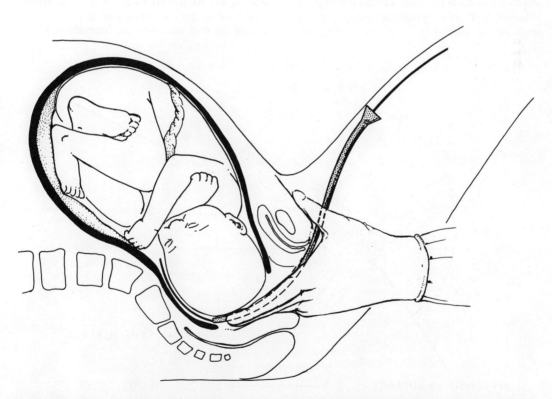

Figure 4-26 Technique of inserting a transvaginal intrauterine catheter. The *semirigid guide has been advanced only a few millimeters beyond the tips of the guiding fingers,* which have been placed between the presenting part and the cervix. With the guide properly set, during relaxation of the uterus, the catheter can be threaded to pass the equator of the presenting part into the amniotic cavity.

clockwise until it springs back. At this moment the locking system is released and both the holding piece and the guide are removed, leaving the electrode firmly attached to the presenting part. The cables are then connected to the leg plate and the FHR is recorded in the appropriate channel. Artifacts may be recorded if the electrode has taken part of the cervix at the insertion or the electronic system functions improperly (poor electrode or faulty preamplifier).

pH electrode The application of the pH electrode, a much more elaborate procedure, must be done under direct visual control. The patient must be placed in the lithotomy position with the perineum thoroughly prepared and draped. The electrode is mounted and calibrated with meticulous aseptic technique maintained. When all instruments are ready and in order, a pelvic examination is done to map precisely the location of the fontanelles and the sutures, which should be avoided when hooking the electrode. Because an amnioscope has to be used, a minimum of 4 to 4.5 cm cervical dilatation is required through which the amnioscope has to be gently introduced and pushed against the presenting part.

An assistant firmly holds the uterine fundus to prevent disengagement or upward movement of the fetus. The double-helix fetal ECG electrode is then introduced and screwed away from the fontanelles or sutures. The hold is tested by gently pulling from the handle of the applicator forceps. Then the knife-carrying handle is inserted within the hole of the plastic body that holds the actual electrodes. With a quick, clean push a small stab wound is made on the scalp, the depth of which is controlled by the length of the protruding knife. The handle is removed and the electrode-carrying handle is slowly and gently introduced through the amnioscope and into the hole of the plastic part of the ECG electrode on which the pH electrode is screwed. The relationship between the different parts is such that the glass tip of the pH electrode should be about 2 mm beneath the skin surface when the instrument has been well applied (Figure 4-27). The applicator handle and amnioscope are then removed, the FHR electrode wires connected to the leg plate, and the pH electrode cable to the electronic measuring system connected to the main recording apparatus. The signals of this electrode are intermittently re-

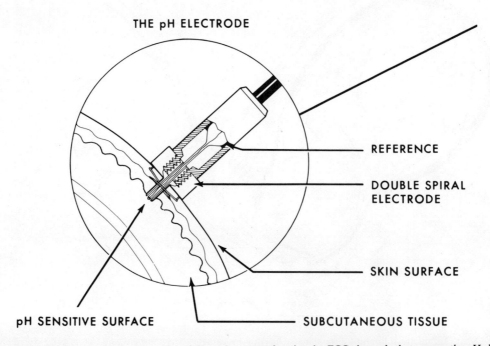

THE pH ELECTRODE

REFERENCE

DOUBLE SPIRAL ELECTRODE

SKIN SURFACE

pH SENSITIVE SURFACE

SUBCUTANEOUS TISSUE

Figure 4-27 Illustration of the relationships of the various parts forming the *ECG electrode that secures the pH electrode,* and the layers of the scalp after a good application. Only the very tip of the glass cone has penetrated the deep part of the dermis. It is also seen that the pH electrode has been screwed on the pastic body of the ECG electrode, which is hooked by the two helixes in the superficial part of the skin.

corded (every 15 sec) in the same channel as the uterine contractions. In this manner one may have three different phenomena recorded on only two channels. Furthermore, the pH meter is provided with a continuous digital readout for direct visual information.

There are a number of reasons for unwanted signals, the first of which could be an unstable electrode. Inadequate penetration into the dermis causes a false low reading. A "bobbling" electrode, insecurely fixed, causes wide, wild oscillations of the values. The substitution of a triangular shaped knife (Figure 4-28) for the standard blade knife routinely used to obtain scalp blood samples for intermittent blood gas measurements may overcome most problems of improper penetration and unstable holding.

Oxygen electrode The oxygen electrode, like the pH electrode, has to be applied under direct visual control with the help of an amnioscope or special speculum. The calibration is undertaken with careful sterile technique before application. To assure a good recording, the fetal scalp must be shaved, with a special blade, over an area larger than that covered by the electrode of 3 cm² but only about 1 cm² is covered by the active area. The electrode is affixed by means of a special glue that hardens when in contact with wet surfaces. Others use dental cement with equal success. These substances are applied on small holes evenly distributed over the fetal side of the ring surrounding the anode; the scalp is moistened just before application of the electrode. A specially designed forceps presses the electrode against the fetal head for several seconds until the glue or cement hardens sufficiently to hold it firmly (Figure 4-29). In general it remains in position for up to a few hours but it may be displaced by movements of the fetal head against the cervix or in the birth canal. When this happens, the recording becomes clearly out of all reasonable range, an indication to check and confirm the displacement of the instrument. Another important cause of false recording occurs when the electrode is pressed against the scalp, a circumstance often present in advanced stages of dilatation or in second stage of labor.

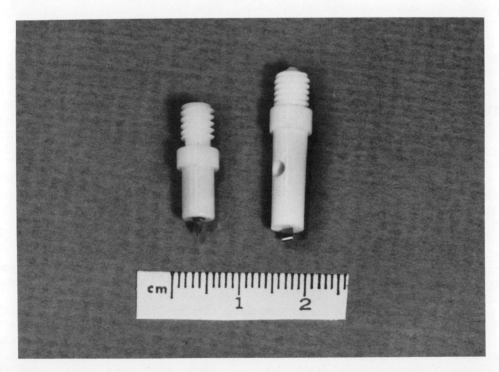

Figure 4-28 Two kinds of knives used to make the stab wound on the skin of the presenting part. *(Left)* Pyramidal shaped blade 2 mm length and 1.5 mm each side of the triangular base. *(Right)* The standard flat blade of 2 mm width and protruding 2 mm.

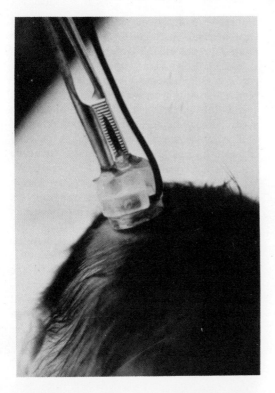

Figure 4-29 The oxygen electrode held with the applicator forceps pressed against the shaved scalp waiting for glue (cement) to harden. Reprinted from Huch A, et al: Continuous transcutaneous monitoring of fetal oxygen tension during labour. *Br J Obstet Gynaecol* 84(suppl 1): 1977.

STERILIZATION

The use of flexible catheters made from synthetic material, and electrodes mounted in plastic, precludes the standard sterilization technique of autoclaving. Thus, all the nondisposable material made of synthetics shown in the figures in this chapter are subjected to *gas sterilization*. All glass and metal instruments, gauze, and cotton may be *autoclaved* without any problem, provided the other elements of the tray are added at the time of preparation for insertion, particularly when the very thin catheters are used for transabdominal, intrauterine, and intravascular recordings.

The large transvaginal catheter and guide, as well as the ECG electrodes and plastic syringes, come as disposable equipment, sterilized and ready to use. The newest scalp electrodes with the helix made of stainless steel are resterilizable a few times — in the gas sterilizer because of their plastic body and connecting cable.

The pH electrode cannot be subjected to autoclaving or gas sterilization because it may be damaged by the heat. It is necessary to *cold sterilize* it; the most convenient agent is activated dialdehyde, which is believed to produce bacterial sterilization after 10 min of soaking but requires several hours of immersion to eliminate spores and reach true bacteriologic sterilization. In the limited number of subcutaneous pH recordings there has not been any report of infection attributable to the instrument. However, it remains to be seen what will occur with a larger experience. Because this electrode (and that for the ECG) is applied in a nonsterile area it it difficult to evaluate the actual cause of an infection. This particular problem is discussed in more detail in Chapter 19, Complications. The various ampules containing the buffer and reference solutions utilized to calibrate the pH electrode may be autoclaved.

The pO_2 electrode, after complete assembly, may be sterilized in ethylene oxide vapor at 55 C. This should alter neither the properties of the membrane nor the balance of the electrode, and it gives satisfactory sterilization.

BIBLIOGRAPHY

Alvarez H, Caldeyro-Barcia R: Estudios sobre la fisiologia de la actividad contractil del utero humano. Tercera communicacion: Estudios de los valores absolutos de la presion intrauterina como medida de la activadad contractil del utero. El tono uterino. *Arch Ginecol Obstet (Uruguay)* 7:139, 1948.

Alvarez H, Caldeyro-Barcia R: Fisiopatologia de la contraccion uterina y sus aplicaciones en clinica obstetrica. *II Cong Lat-Am Obstet Ginecol (Brasil)* 1:1, 1954.

Bishop EH: Ultrasonic fetal monitoring. *Clin Obstet Gynecol* 11:1154, 1968.

Caldeyro-Barcia R, Alvarez H: Abnormal uterine action in labour. *J Obstet Gynaecol Br Emp* 59:646, 1952.

Caldeyro-Barcia R, Pose SV, Alvarez H: Uterine contractility in polyhydramnios and the effects of withdrawal of the excess of amniotic fluid. *Am J Obstet Gynecol* 73:1238, 1957.

Cibils LA: Efecto de la rotura de mambranas en el parto inducido con ocitocina. *II Cong Uruguayo Ginecotocol* 2:346, 1957.

Cibils LA, Caldeyro-Barcia R: Efectos de la ocitocina sobre el tono uterino. *Proc I Meet Lat-Am Assoc Physiol Sci* (Punta del Este) 53, 1957.

Cibils LA, Hendricks CH: Uterine contractility in the first day of puerperium. *Am J Obstet Gynecol* 103:238, 1969.

Cibils LA, Pose SV, Zuspan FP: Effect of *L*-norepinephrine infusion on uterine contractility and cardiovascular system. *Am J Obstet Gynecol* 84:307, 1962.

Hammcher K: The diagnosis of fetal distress with an electronic fetal monitor, in *Intrauterine Dangers to the Fetus*. Amsterdam, Excerpta Medica, 1967, pp 228–233.

Hendricks CH, Eskes TKAB, Saameli K: Uterine contractility at delivery and the puerperium. *Am J Obstet Gynecol* 83:890, 1962.

Hendricks CH, Moawad AH: Round ligament motility in vivo studies in man. *J Obstet Gynaecol Br Comwlth* 72:618, 1965.

Hendricks CH, Quilligan EJ, Tyler CW, et al: Pressure relationships between the intervillous space and the amniotic fluid in human term pregnancy. *Am J Obstet Gynecol* 77:1028, 1959.

Hochberg HM, Lauersen NH, George MED, et al: Evaluation of continuous monitoring of tissue pH in cats. *Am J Obstet Gynecol* 131:770, 1978.

Hon EH: Electronic evaluation of the fetal heart rate. *Am J Obstet Gynecol* 83:333, 1962.

Hon EH, Hess OW: Instrumentation of fetal electrocardiography. *Science* 125:553, 1957.

Hopkins E, Hendricks CH, Cibils LA: Cerebrospinal fluid pressure in labor. *Am J Obstet Gynecol* 93:907, 1965.

Huch A, Huch R, Schneider N, et al: Continuous transcutaneous monitoring of fetal oxygen tension during labour. *Br J Obstet Gynaecol* 84(suppl 1): 1977.

Lauersen NH, Hochberg HM, George MED, et al: A new technique for improving the Doppler ultrasound signal for fetal heart rate monitoring. *Am J Obstet Gynecol* 128:300, 1977.

Lauersen NH, Hochberg HM, George MED, et al: Technical aspects of directional Doppler: A new method of fetal heart rate monitoring. *J Reprod Med* 20:77, 1978.

Pose SV, Alvarez H, Caldeyro-Barcia R: Contractilidad uterina de los polihidramnios. *Ann Ginecotocol (Uruguay)* 2:116, 1955.

Schuler R, Kreuzer F: Properties and performance of membrane-covered rapid polaragraphic oxygen catheter electrodes for continuous oxygen recording in-vivo. *Prog Respir Res* 3:64, 1969.

Stamm O, Latscha U, Janecek P, et al: Development of a special electrode for continuous subcutaneous pH measurement in the infant scalp. *Am J Obstet Gynecol* 124:193, 1976.

Sturbois G, Uzan S, Rotten D, et al: Continuous subcutaneous pH measurement in human fetuses. Correlations with scalp and umbilical blood pH. *Am J Obstet Gynecol* 128:901, 1977.

Young BK, Hirschl IT, Klein SH, et al: Continuous fetal tissue pH monitoring in labor with high risk pregnancies. *Arch Gynecol* 226:169, 1978.

CHAPTER 5
Normal Uterine Contractility

EARLY PREGNANCY

Contrary to the classically held concept that the uterus is at rest during pregnancy, Alvarez and Caldeyro-Barcia demonstrated early in their work that the uterus is never completely relaxed and that it is constantly having small contractions periodically interrupted by stronger ones. Much later in gestation (at about the sixth month) these contractions may be palpated. Described by John Braxton Hicks in 1872, they are now named after him. In Chapter 2 (Figure 2-2) it was shown that the nonpregnant uterus is never at rest during the reproductive age of the patient. In fact it is *never quiescent*, not even around *implantation time* (Figure 5-1) or in the *early weeks of gestation* (Figure 5-2). Later in pregnancy the periods of apparent quiescence may be longer, but with intrauterine catheters it is possible to record clear activity in early and middle second trimester of gestation (Figures 5-3 and 5-4). These contractions are not palpable and their function and significance are not known.

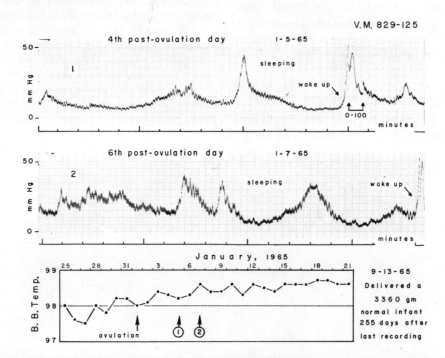

Figure 5-1 Uterine contracility recorded in early luteal phase as indicated by the arrow on basal body temperature shown below. The pattern illustrated on top is typical of the phase, as well as the almost instantaneous strong contraction triggered by waking up. The lower tracing obtained two days later, at the estimated sixth day postovulation, shows the same characteristic luteal phase pattern and the wake-up response. Interestingly, this patient was in early stage of gestation, around the *estimated implantation time*. Reprinted from Cibils LA: Contractility of the nonpregnant human uterus. *Obstet Gynecol* 30:441, 1967.

64

5 MONTHS POST-PARTUM, and early AFTER IMPLANTATION

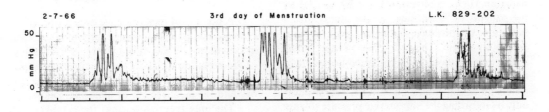

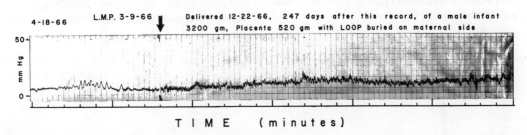

T I M E   (m i n u t e s)

Figure 5-2 Uterine contractility in a patient wearing a Lippes loop five months postpartum. *(Above)* Intramenstrual tracing with characteristic strong contractions. *(Below)* Nine weeks later without intervening menstruation, on the left a short burst of mild contractions of around 10 mm Hg intensity. The range was changed to 0 to 25 mm Hg (arrow), and three mild contractions were recorded in 20 minutes (arrow). The patient had conceived before this recording and probably had already implanted. Reprinted from Cibils (1970).

Contractility of Early Mid-trimester of Pregnancy

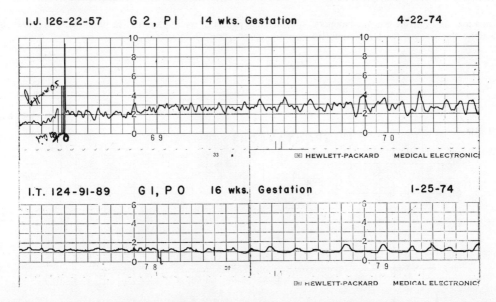

Figure 5-3 Intrauterine (amniotic) pressures obtained in two patients at 14 and 16 weeks gestation before injection of prostaglandin and hypertonic saline respectively. Spontaneous contractions of moderate intensity recur with an irregular pattern. The uterus seems to be always contracting in some area in both patients. Pressure range, 0 to 100 mm Hg; paper speed, 1 cm/min (between heavy lines).

In *early third trimester* the sporadic strong contractions are clearly palpable by an observer (Braxton Hicks contractions) and recognized by the patients as "hardening" of the uterus with a sensation of pressure; however, pain is conspicuously absent. They may come in short bursts a few times a day, or they may be isolated and recurring regularly. The latter type usually alternate with small, nonpalpable ones, recognizable only by recording the intrauterine pressure (Figure 5-5).

The factors that control this contractility and the possible conversion to pathologic contractions will be discussed in Chapter 8.

ANALYSIS OF UTERINE CONTRACTILITY TRACINGS

A number of methods have been proposed to evaluate the tracings obtained during labor. This information would enable a better understanding of the evolution of labor, and the ability to apply that knowledge to the study of uterine pharmacology and the management of abnormal labors.

The only accurate tracings for reliable analysis are records obtained by internal methods, particularly open-end and fluid-filled catheter systems, which should not record unwanted signals. *The internal method is the only method*

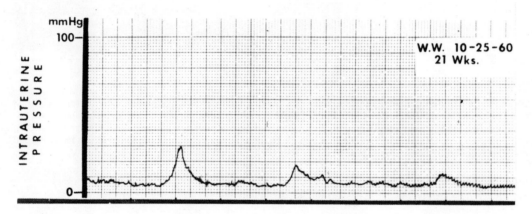

Figure 5-4 Intrauterine pressure (amniotic) obtained in a patient 21 weeks pregnant. In 10 min there are three contractions, the first one reaching 25 mm Hg intensity. (Paper speed, 3 lines/min).

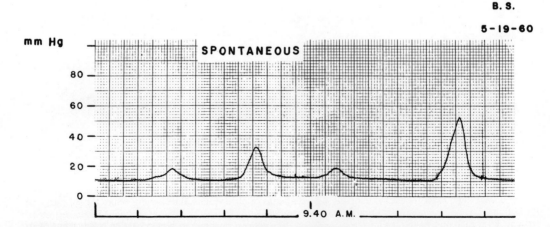

Figure 5-5 Intraamniotic pressure tracing of a patient 28 weeks pregnant before medically indicated induction of labor. Note the fluctuating intensity of contractions, one reaching 50 mm Hg.

that *gives precise values*. The intrauterine but closed methods, like the balloon-tipped catheter, are all subject to inevitable flaws inherent in the technique (see Chapter 4). The external methods, by definition, do not provide information about intrauterine pressure values, and therefore any attempt at calculating their significance from that standpoint is a waste of time and effort.

The first method proposed was an adaptation of a well-known technique to study in vitro muscle strips. Reynolds, Harris, and Kaiser (1954), in their book on uterine physiology, applied the measurement of the *area under the curve* by using the weighing technique: careful reproduction of the tracing on a special paper, with the planimeter, and then cutting and weighing the paper. It gave them grams per centimeter as unit of measure. Several subsequent authors proposed variants of this same concept as ways to analyze a record. Csapo and Sauvage (1968), using the extraovular balloon-tipped catheter, as a revival of the Reynolds' method, measured the area under the curve by calculating it in square millimeters and called it active pressure area (APA). Of course the concept may be applied to true intrauterine pressure tracings.

Caldeyro-Barcia and collaborators (1957) published their work based on consideration of *intensity and frequency of contractions* as parameters for analysis and called them *Montevideo Units*. Essentially, it consists of measuring the intensity of the contraction (in mm Hg) from the resting pressure to the peak, and multiplying it for its frequency in 10 min. The latter is calculated by measuring the time from the preceding contraction peak and extrapolating to a theoretical number of contractions occurring with the exact same frequency in 10 min (Figure 5-6).

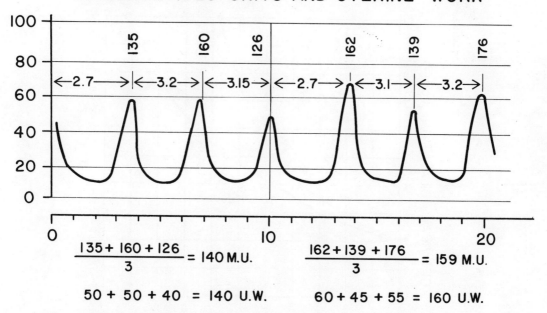

Figure 5-6 Two methods to analyze uterine activity in a 20-min tracing. There are three contractions in each period. The *frequency per 10 min* for each is measured between peaks of contractions: the *intensity* in mm Hg for each is in the last line. The *product of intensity and frequency* gives the *uterine activity* for that contraction (Montevideo Units) written above each one. In the lower part of the figure the three contractions per 10 min have been added and averaged to find the *uterine activity for that period*. The *simple sum* of the three contractions gives the *uterine work* for that period, in the last line. Uterine work in 10 min is equal to uterine activity in Montevideo Units.

Some investigators object to this method because it takes into account neither the tone nor the duration of the contractions. It will be seen that these objections have very little bearing when tracings within a wide range of normal contractility patterns are evaluated. This method is particularly useful for the study of fluctuations in contractility occurring within reasonably short periods of time, and to study the effect of drugs or maneuvers that may either increase or decrease uterine activity.

Shortly thereafter and working in the same laboratory Cibils (1957) proposed that the frequency with which the contractions occurred be disregarded, and suggested a simple calculation of the arithmetic sum of the intensity of contractions (in mm Hg), which he called *uterine work*. Of course this is not work in the strict physical sense, but the word conveys the idea that whatever the uterus is doing represents a mechanical action, spending energy and enhancing the progress of labor. The uterine work may be calculated for the total period monitored, *total uterine work,* or applied to phases of the period recorded. *Prelabor*

uterine work would thus be the total pressure (in mm Hg) added from the beginning of the recording until dilatation advances above 3 cm; *uterine work of first stage* would be that added from 3 cm to the moment dilatation is complete. When uterine work, as defined here, is tabulated against cervical dilatation (Figure 5-7) it becomes useful in assessing the efficiency of the contractions to dilate the cervix. When the same information is tabulated on semilog paper (Figure 5-8) it becomes *a straight line, the slope of which measures the efficiency of the uterine work to accomplish cervical dilatation.* Because the slope does not change under stable conditions, it is an excellent guide to study the effect of potential variables influencing the efficiency of the contractions such as amniotomy, drugs, anesthetics, sedatives, maternal position changes, parity, variety of position of the presenting part, and so on. Furthermore, because the technique does not take into consideration the frequency of the contractions, it is possible to use it to compare the efficiency of contractions among patients. Some

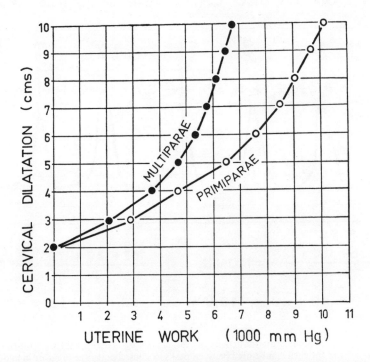

Figure 5-7 Cervical dilatation tabulated against the uterine work calculated between 2 and 10 cm dilatation. Mean curves of 46 multiparas and 9 primiparas. Primiparas required significantly more uterine work to complete dilatation. Reprinted from Alvarez H, et al: Cervical dilatation and uterine "work" in labour induced by oxytocin infusion, in Caldeyro-Barcia R, Heller H (eds): *Oxytocin.* NY, Pergamon, 1961, pp 203–211.

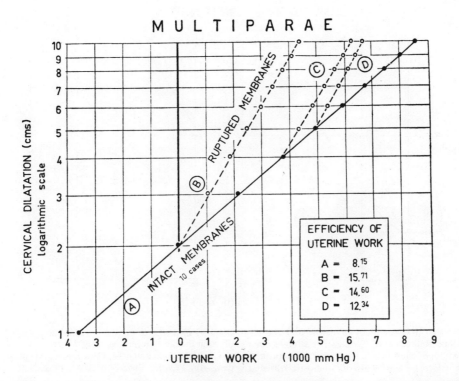

Figure 5-8 Cervical dilatation tabulated on semilog paper against uterine work. The full line A groups the cases evolving with intact membranes. The cases with membranes ruptured at 2 cm (B), 4 cm (C) and 5 cm (D) are shown with interrupted lines. Note the straight lines obtained in each case, the slope of which measures the efficiency of the contractions to dilate the cervix (the actual calculated figures framed on the lower right side). Note the parallelism after amniotomy irrespective of the stage at which it took place. Reprinted from Alvarez H, et al: Cervical dilatation and uterine "work" in labour induced by oxytocin infusion, in Caldeyro-Barcia R, Heller H (eds): *Oxytocin.* NY, Pergamon, 1961, pp 203–211.

have a high frequency of contractions while others contract every several minutes. For this last reason it seems a more accurate method of comparison than tabulation of dilatation against time which is, in cases of differing contractility patterns and particularly frequency, open to misleading impressions.

A somewhat different way of using the added intensity of contractions was utilized by Cibils and Spackman (1962), when they plotted the *cumulative intensity* (in mm Hg) against time and found that in normal, uninterfered labors the slope of the curve does not change (Figure 5-9) as labor progresses.

The acceptance of the Montevideo Units as a method to assess uterine activity did not preclude the exploration of applying new techniques to old ideas. It was in this context that Sala et al, (1959) used an electronic pressure–time integrator to calculate *on-line the total area beneath the curve*

of the pressure tracing. They fed the input from the preamplifier that received the signals from the pressure transducer connected to the intrauterine catheter to the integrator and had a continuous digital display of the values. The result was expressed in mm Hg times seconds (mm Hg × sec) as the figure accumulated. To compare with Montevideo Units for the same contractions, they took the total figure per ten contractions and subtracted the area under the tonus; the remainder figure was divided by the elapsed time, and the mean pressure of the contractions (MPC) was obtained. While this method had a linear relationship with the Montevideo Units under all circumstances, the total area maintained a linear relationship with Montevideo Units only when the contractility patterns were regular and there was good relaxation between contractions (the fluctuations of the baseline or coupled contractions altered the parallelism).

70

CUMULATIVE INTENSITY

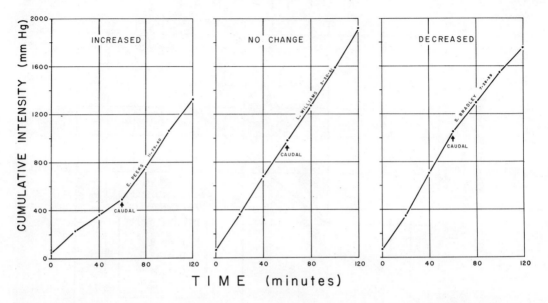

Figure 5-9 Arithmetic sum of all uterine contractions *(cumulative intensity,* or uterine work) tabulated against time for 120 min in three cases. *(Center)* The *straight line* usually seen in stable conditions. *(Left)* Increased, and *(right)* decreased slope following caudal anesthesia. Reprinted from Cibils LA, Spackman TJ: Caudal analgesia in first stage of labor: Effect on uterine activity and cardiovascular system. *Am J Obstet Gynecol* 84:1042, 1962.

The concept that duration of contraction might have an important influence made El-Sahwi and co-workers (1967) propose the inclusion of this parameter in the calculation of uterine activity. They expressed the result in *Alexandria Units*. However, their results may not be considered valid because their recordings were obtained with an external tocotransducer, and thus (in spite of all claims) useless to assess intrauterine pressure. Nevertheless, it is an interesting concept, which is applied (although not specifically so expressed) in the methods of calculating the area under the curve.

More recently Hon and Paul (1973) introduced an on-line method to calculate (in mm Hg/unit of time) the *"area under the uterine pressure curve,"* which they expressed in 1 min and called *uterine activity unit* (UAU). Clearly, this method is exactly the same as the one used by Sala et al (1959), including its on-line application. On the other hand, when the results are plotted against time (Figure 5-10) the curve bears close resemblance to the one obtained by the "cumulative intensity" method published by Cibils and Spackman (compare with Figure 5-9). The similarity of

this method with the one used by Sala et al is corroborated by a comparative study with Montevideo Units done most recently in multiparous patients (Huey and Miller, 1979), which arrived at the same conclusion: both methods are equivalent.

PRELABOR

All the changes occurring in the cervix and lower segment in the last several weeks of gestation are the consequence of the physiologic process of preparation for labor, or *prelabor*. Danforth (1954) carefully studied the changes in the anatomic components of the cervix in advanced gestation and early labor. He found that striking shifts take place in the relative concentrations of some amino acids and in the constitution of collagen fibers. It is not clear whether the changes are due to the mechanical effect of the contractions, the hormonal changes occurring in late pregnancy, or both. Important physical changes may be induced in the cervix by carefully stimulated uterine contractions during relatively short periods of time, but they do not prove that

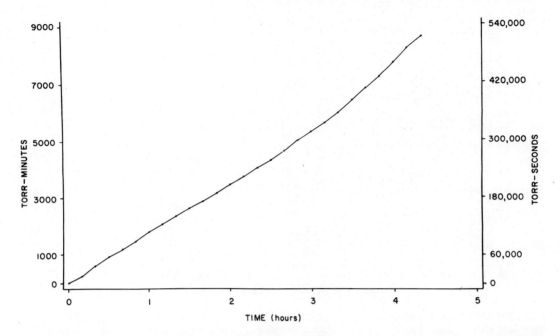

Figure 5-10 Uterine activity units (mm Hg/min intrauterine pressure) plotted against time (hours) to show a straight ascending line indicating effectiveness of uterine work. Reprinted from Hon EH, Paul R: Quantitation of uterine activity. *Obstet Gynecol* 42:368, 1973.

other factors may not significantly contribute to the changes occurring in spontaneous prelabor.

The process of prelabor may be clinically followed by *five important converging cervical physical changes:* 1) *centering* of the cervix, the gradual pull from back in the sacral concavity to the center of the birth canal; 2) *softening* of the cervix, taking place simultaneously with the described migration, as well as 3) *effacement,* with clear shortening of the distance between external and internal os; 4) at the same time *dilatation* of the internal os, which progresses slowly in reverse proportion to the resistance of the ring that forms that internal os. These four changes are preconditions to 5) *formation of the lower segment,* which is physically manifested by deepening of the vaginal fornices and thinning of the uterine wall with easier palpation, through them, of the presenting part. These aspects of the cervical condition, assessed at the time of pelvic examinations, tend to change in parallel (or in converging) fashion, as if there were an interdependency among them or they all change because of the same factor. That those changes occur slowly in the *last weeks of pregnancy* has been shown by

Hendricks and collaborators (1970) by separate evaluation of each of them (Figure 5-11). Cervical effacement (Figure 5-12), and dilatation (Figure 5-13) in prelabor occur in different degrees according to the parity of the patient. In addition, slightly higher incidence of multiparas have equivalent dilatation when compared to primiparas (Figure 5-14). These observations may be corroborated by anyone who takes the time to examine his patients at each visit in the last weeks of gestation—an excellent way to predict the approximate date of active first-stage labor. Rightfully Hendricks stated that "the persistent idea that all cervical dilatation is performed during a period of a few hours is a myth."

Thus, prelabor starts at an undetermined date several weeks before term but it ends when the first stage begins, at the onset of clinical labor. Because the onset of clinical labor varies from patient to patient, and because the majority go into it with at least 2.5 cm dilatation (see Figure 5-11) it was arbitrarily decided to consider the *end of prelabor* and the onset of first stage to be when *dilatation progresses beyond 3 cm.* This facilitates the comparison of cases when undertaking clinical studies

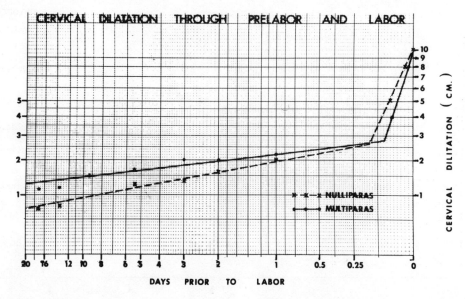

Figure 5-11 Mean cervical dilatation throughout the last 3 weeks of pregnancy (including labor) tabulated on logarithmic paper against time. The patients grouped according to parity; the cervix starts to dilate several weeks before labor and continues to do so in a slow but pregressive manner. Reprinted from Hendricks CH, et al: Normal cervical dilatation pattern in late pregnancy and labor. *Am J Obstet Gynecol* 106:1065, 1970.

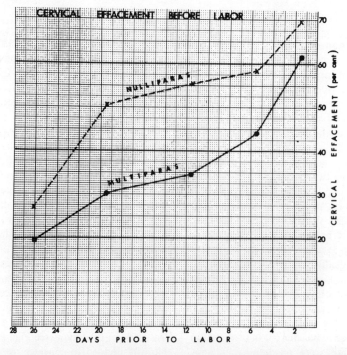

Figure 5-12 Curves of mean cervical effacement the last 4 weeks before onset of spontaneous labor. Patients grouped by parity show that effacement is already evident several weeks before term. Note the degree of effacement accomplished 2 days before labor. Reprinted from Hendricks CH, et al: Normal cervical dilatation pattern in late pregnancy and labor. *Am J Obstet Gynecol* 106:1065, 1970.

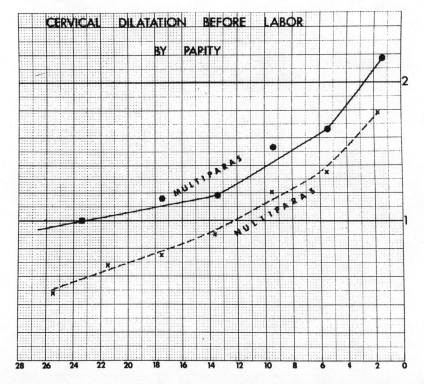

Figure 5-13 Curves of mean cervical dilatation the last 4 weeks before onset of spontaneous labor in multiparas and primiparas show the early start and steady progress during subclinical prelabor. Reprinted from Hendricks CH, et al: Normal cervical dilatation pattern in late pregnancy and labor. *Am J Obstet Gynecol* 106:1065, 1970.

and makes them more comparable by removing the patient's subjective symptom of "painful contractions" as the moment when labor starts or the moment when prelabor has been completed.

These slow anatomic changes observed in the cervix with their gradual evolution are essential to the concept of *cervical ripening* or readiness for labor. Without prelabor a cervix will be long, posterior, closed, relatively firm, and the vaginal fornices will be shallow with a nonformed lower segment; in other words, it will be *unripe,* not ready, or unfavorable for labor. On the other hand, a cervix that is shortened, centered, soft, and partially dilated with a loose internal os and with deep fornices for a good lower segment is quite ready, ripe, or favorable. Often one may face an intermediate condition, particularly if the internal os feels of rubbery resistance and still somewhat thick. For this condition the label of *partially ripe* is reserved (Figure 5-15).

Because there are significant differences between primiparous and multiparous cervices, it is important to establish that the description (or definition) of a ripe cervix will not be the same for both. It is common knowledge among clinicians that a very high percentage of primiparas enter first stage with effaced cervices (see Figure 5-12). On the other hand, multiparas are usually in rather moderate dilatation but only partially effaced (see Figures 5-12 and 5-14). These two conditions affect the consistency of the internal os and are not comparable. Therefore, when assessing a cervix for readiness it is of utmost importance to take into consideration the parity of the patient. Once a classification has been given, then the cases are comparable because parity has already been taken into account. With this in mind, and a good knowledge of uterine physiology, it is possible to make a reasonable prediction of how a given labor should evolve, considering

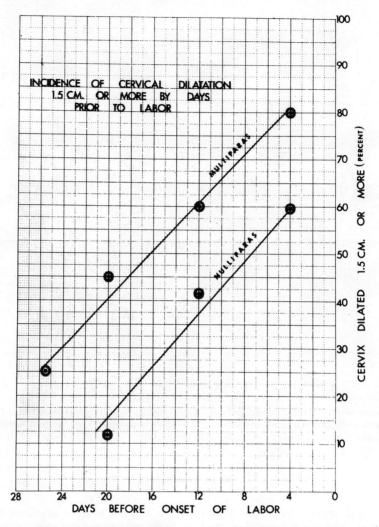

Figure 5-14 Incidence of patients, grouped by parity, with cervix dilated at least 1.5 cm, in the last 4 weeks of pregnancy. Courtesy C.H. Hendricks.

the quality of contractions and the physical relationship between the presenting part and the birth canal.

A clarification is essential at this point, to indicate that the concept of prelabor is not the same as the "latent phase" described by Friedman, which, according to his labor curves, starts only a few hours before progressive dilatation. The latent phase, at best, may be part of the last stages of prelabor. However, other differences exist between the two concepts: *prelabor* results from a slow protracted process producing *cervical dilatation* and effacement several days prior to active labor; the *latent phase* is depicted in Friedman's curves as starting with a *closed cervix* in primiparas and multiparas.

Bishop (1964) proposed a scoring system with which a reasonable prediction of evolution of first stage may be established. In it he proposed to consider dilatation, effacement, consistency, and position (all included in the present evaluation) in addition to station of the presenting part. Not included are resistance of the internal os and quality of lower segment. There should be good correspondence between the Bishop scoring system and the evaluation proposed here.

The *contractility pattern of a spontaneous prelabor* resembles that of midgestation, the dif-

STAGES OF CERVICAL READINESS

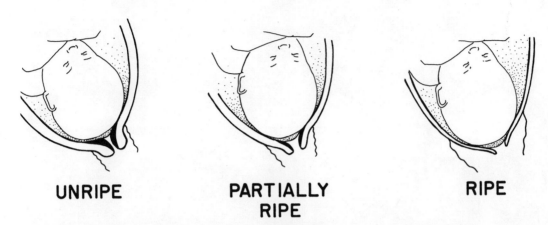

UNRIPE   **PARTIALLY RIPE**   **RIPE**

Figure 5-15 Cervical readiness schematically represented. *(Left)* The *unripe* cervix is still formed, the black area representing resistance of the internal os. The vaginal fornices are very shallow. *(Center)* The shorter, *partially ripe,* cervix is beginning to open; it has less resistance at the internal os, and deeper fornices. *(Right)* An almost effaced and open cervix with deep fornices is *ripe,* allowing a small hourglass bag of water to form.

ference being that its rate is much faster. The contractions are irregular in intensity and frequency, predominantly mild ones (Figure 5-16). This irregular pattern is still very much present at the beginning of first stage (Figure 5-17).

The same pattern may be expected when labor is *induced* with intravenous infusion of oxytocin at physiologic doses in patients with *unripe cervices.* The physical changes accomplished with the contractions are subtle and occur very slowly. These changes are evaluated by pelvic examination and usually consist of a little shortening of the cervix, slight position change toward the center of the birth canal, and increased softening and/or lessening of the resistance at the internal os. An inherent high resistance of the internal os is the major factor that must be overcome by the uterine contractions. This factor is responsible for the apparent slow progress of labor after induction with unfavorable cervices. Several hours of good contractions are needed to bring about any appreciable change; thus frequent pelvic examinations are useless at this stage.

The *uterine work* required to ripen a cervix depends, of course, on what has already been accomplished spontaneously before the monitoring started. Experience indicates that there is a wide range for clinically labelled *unripe cervices;* a range

of 7000 to 18,000 mm Hg (Figure 5-18) with an average of over 10,000 mm Hg (Table 5-1) uterine work has been found to be necessary to complete prelabor. Noriega-Guerra and collaborators recorded slightly higher figures for a somewhat smaller series of patients, but the concept has been clearly confirmed by their work. A *partially ripe cervix* will require less uterine work, about 4200 mm Hg, and a *ripe cervix* may start dilating over 3 cm immediately or require a number of contractions before that process is started, the average being slightly over 1600 mm Hg.

Table 5-1
Prelabor (371 Cases)

Condition of Cervix	No. of Cases	Uterine Work (mm Hg)
Unripe	75	10,850 ± 2900
Partially ripe	93	4230 ± 1100
Ripe	203	1670 ± 1150

It is convenient to reemphasize that parity has no influence on the uterine work needed to ripen the cervix. That should have already been taken into consideration when the case was classified.

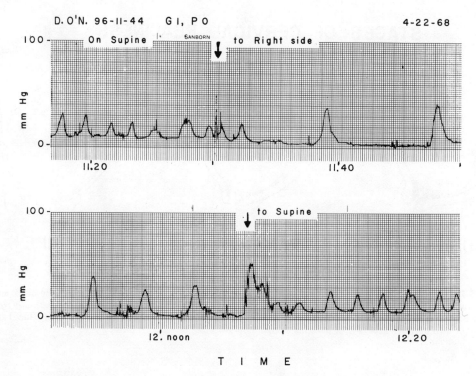

Figure 5-16 Continuous intrauterine pressure tracing of full-term pregnant patient in spontaneous prelabor. Small uterine contractions and marked change follow the adoption of the lateral position. The change reverses when the patient returns to supine. Reprinted from Cibils LA: Enhancement and induction of labor, in Aladjem S (ed): *Risks in the Practice of Modern Obstetrics, II*. St. Louis, Mosby, 1975, pp 182–210.

SPONTANEOUS LABOR at TERM

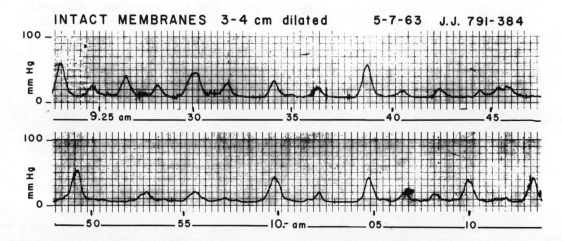

Figure 5-17 Uterine contractility pattern in spontaneous early labor at term. Continuous 50-min tracing illustrates the irregular pattern of frequency and intensity. Reprinted from Cibils and Hendricks (1969).

Unripe   Partially Ripe   Ripe

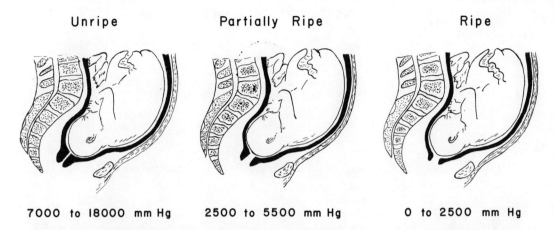

7000 to 18000 mm Hg   2500 to 5500 mm Hg   0 to 2500 mm Hg

Figure 5-18 Uterine work required to accomplish prelabor (to reach and progress over 3 cm dilatation) according to the degree of cervical readiness reached before monitoring was begun. Ranges for each group are minimum and maximum observed in normal cases. Reprinted from Cibils LA: Enhancement and induction of labor, in Aladjem S (ed): *Risks in the Practice of Modern Obstetrics, II*. St. Louis, Mosby, 1975, pp 182–210.

FIRST STAGE

The contractility pattern of early first-stage labor is indistinguishable from that of late prelabor, as may be observed in Figures 5-16 and 5-17 compared with the upper two parts of Figure 5-19. The intrinsic irregularity and cyclic pattern of the contractions evolves subtly from late prelabor into labor and demonstrates that the divisions introduced in the study of contractility are artificial. However, these patterns help to study better the various clinical stages of labor. With slow progress of dilatation the long, slow contractility cycles become shorter and the contractions acquire a certain regularity or uniformity; the intensity and frequency fluctuate within a more narrow range (see the lower two parts of Figure 5-19). There seems to be a constantly accelerating process that brings about better coordinated and more regular contractions, which reach their maximum efficiency at the end of first stage. Nevertheless, a detailed analysis of the tracings always reveals some irregularity of contractions even under the most stable and undisturbed conditions. This assertion becomes obvious when calculations are made and uterine activity is tabulated for individual contractions; a repetitive wavy cycle is characteristic of all stages of labor. In addition to this intrinsic variability, numerous factors influence the contractility pattern, some of them well studied and with predictable effect, others less well understood. All will be considered in the forthcoming pages.

The Normal Contraction

Contraction waves (recorded with an intrauterine catheter) are the result of the force of the contracting myometrium on the intrauterine, noncompressible contents. A good artifact-free tracing records a wave that allows the physician to study tone, intensity, duration, frequency, and coordination of each contraction. To gain this information, one may take an average good contraction of advanced first stage and analyze it in detail (Figure 5-20).

Shape The shape of a curve representing a contraction varies, of course, with the speed of the recording paper and the range of sensitivity of the preamplifier (standard recorders run at 1 to 3 cm/min, and display 100 mm Hg over 4 cm paper). However, regardless of the apparent look, there is a constant relationship among the various components of the wave. The *ascending* part of the wave, which responds to the active *contraction*, starts rather abruptly and rises rapidly in a steep line to reach the acme in about 25 to 30 sec. The *acme* or peak is always short (only a few seconds), and looks very pointed at the regular paper speeds. It is then followed by the descending leg of the wave as *relaxation* takes place. This leg has two clearly different phases: the first (rapid relaxation) descends rather rapidly (although less steep than the ascending one), to about the lower one-third of the attained height and is reached in about 30 to 35 sec. This is followed by slow relaxation, a much smoother curve tending gradually

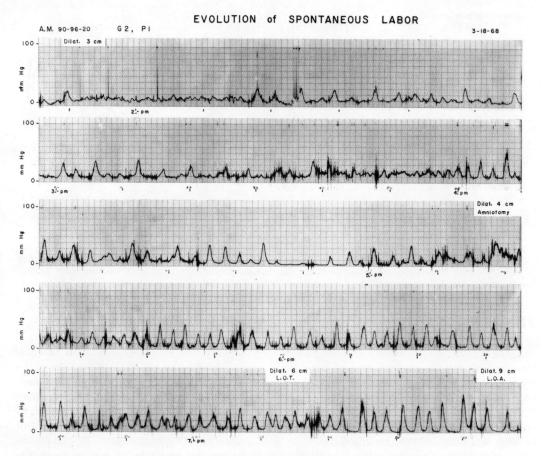

Figure 5-19 Six hours of continuous intrauterine pressure tracing of spontaneous labor that progressed with contractions of *very low intensity* averaging less than 30 mm Hg. For several hours, until amniotomy, the contractions had the pattern of prelabor. Even in advanced first stage, after 6 cm dilatation, the contractions had periods of irregularity and very low intensity. Reprinted from Cibils LA: Enchancement and induction of labor, in Aladjem S (ed): *Risks in the Practice of Modern Obstetrics, II.* St. Louis, Mosby, 1975, pp 182–210.

toward the horizontal, and lasting about 70 sec. When the tracing reaches the level of *resting pressure* or *tone* it represents a period of noncontractile activity or rest (remember that in muscle physiology the tone is controlled by a mechanism different from the one controlling the contraction). This period may last until the next contraction repeats the cycle.

Duration The duration of the cycle covered by the active part of the contraction wave lasts about 60 sec, and the slow relaxation phase lasts about 70 sec, gving a total of slightly more than 2 min before it is ready for a restart. Of course the duration of each of these phases, and thus the total duration, depends on the intensity of the contractions. Mild ones reach the acme much

faster than very strong ones. Palpation of the contractions is never a reliable means to assess quality or duration of the contractions because so much depends on the thickenss of the subcutaneous tissue and the resistance of abdominal muscles. In general, contractions are palpable during a time much shorter than the duration of the total active phase. How good they are can be ascertained only by attempting to "indent" the uterus at the peak of the contraction, generally impossible to do when the intensity is 40 mm Hg or greater.

Intensity The intensity of contractions, ranging between 35 and 55 mm Hg (average about 45 mm Hg) is measured from the resting pressure to the acme (Tables 5-2 and 5-3). However, some labors progress reasonably well with contractions

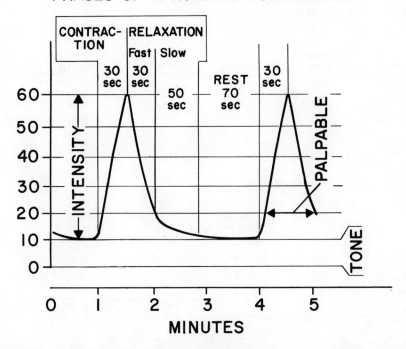

PHASES OF A NORMAL CONTRACTION

Figure 5-20   Phases of a normal contraction. An average uterine contraction of 50 mm Hg intensity (measured from the resting pressure to the peak), and 10 mm Hg tone (measured from the 0 line to the resting value) is analyzed in its various components. The ascending part, *active contraction,* reaches the peak rapidly, and *relaxes* in two stages. A period of rest follows when the frequency is moderate (every 3 min on the diagram), after which the next contraction starts the cycle of rapidly rising pressure. The palpable part of the contraction is usually shorter than its actual duration.

averaging less than 30 mm Hg (see Figure 5-19), while others average very high intensities of over 60 mm Hg (see Figure 5-27). Contractions of less than 20 mm Hg in a uterus of term size will not advance cervical dilatation, and, for the same size uteri, contractions of over 100 mm Hg intensity are rarely seen. Distended or small uteri will differ but Laplace's law applies equally to all of them.

The pain produced by contractions is not generally in direct proportion to their intensity. It relates more to the state of cervical dilatation and to the pain threshold of each individual. The claims that myometrial ischemia induced by the contraction is the cause of pain have never been substantiated. Study of the propagation of a contractile wave shows that the shape of the wave is of great importance, and its changes may be diagnostic of some abnormalities.

Frequency   Ordinarily during spontaneous labor the frequency of contractions varies from two to four in 10 min (that is, they recur every 2.5 to 5 min). Slower patterns tend to be seen in cases with very slow progress while frequencies higher than every 2 to 2.5 min are present in cases of polysystoly or hypercontractility. As during prelabor, the frequencies fluctuate cyclically in each case, with a tendency to increase as dilatation progresses. The very high frequencies, polysystoly, interfere with complete relaxation and thereby cause an increase of the resting pressure due to incomplete relaxation. The contraction starts before the slow phase of relaxation reaches the level of the resting pressure. The higher the frequency the shorter the slow relaxation phase will appear, and the higher the tone will be. Furthermore, with a very high frequency the intensity of the contractions diminishes (see Figures 5-29 and 5-30) and probably with it their efficiency to dilate the cervix. One may speculate that this could be due to the incomplete recovery of the myometrium after each contraction. Contractions that occur too frequently have other deleterious effects, particularly on the fetus (see Chapter 14).

Table 5-2
Average Values in First-Stage Primiparas

Variety of Position of Fetus	No. of Cases	Average Intensity (mm Hg)	Average No. of Contractions	Uterine Work (mm Hg)	Time (hours)
Occiput anterior	181	42	122	5120	5.45
Occiput transverse	51	47	131	6350	6.55
Occiput posterior	103	45	207	9300	9.20
			χ^2(2d.f.)	14.2 = < 0.001	11.3 = < 0.005

Table 5-3
Average Values in First-Stage Multiparas

Variety of Position of Fetus	No. of Cases	Average Intensity (mm Hg)	Average No. of Contractions	Uterine Work (mm Hg)	Time (hours)
Occiput anterior	283	44	68	2990	3.05
Occiput transverse	85	45	103	4630	4.10
Occiput posterior	182	48	105	5040	4.30
			χ^2(2d.f.)	9.2 = < 0.01	8.2 = < 0.025

Tonus Expressed in intrauterine pressure recording, the tonus is the lowest value obtained between contractions. With a very low frequency, as in prelabor, it probably represents the effect of some localized contractions. However, during periods of active contractility, the lowest part of the tracing may be a point just preceding the rise of the contraction curve. The tonus ranges between 8 and 10 mm Hg for a normal pattern which may be calculated by averaging the lowest points preceding the contractions in a given period of time. A high frequency increases the tonus by interrupting the completion of the slow phase of relaxation. If this circumstance is present, one faces the condition of *hypertonus due to polysystoly*. However, there may be other times when the high tonus could be due to other causes. When the uterus is overdistended by multiple pregnancy or polyhydramnios the myometrium generally adapts to the excess volume and maintains the tonus within the average range. Nevertheless, on occasions the myometrium does not adapt to the increased content, and the tonus rises creating the condition of *hypertonus due to overdistension* (see Figures 4-20 and 4-21). A further possibility is realized when the contractions are of such irregularity that the baseline never reaches normal values: to this condition is given the name of *hypertonus due to incoordination or hypercontractility* (see Figures 6-4 and 6-10). As here defined, the normal tonus has very little influence on the process of cervical dilatation and probably is negligible during gestation or prelabor or both.

The Normal Contractile Wave

With the TKD, Reynolds (1947) was able to obtain multiple simultaneous external tracings and postulate a mechanism of action of the uterine contraction summarized in the concept of *fundal dominance*. Using the intraamniotic and multiple intramyometrial catheter methods simultaneously, Alvarez and Caldeyro-Barcia (1947–1952) were able to "map" precisely the characteristics of the normal and abnormal contractions of labor and outline their concept of *triple descending gradient* of the normal contractions. Some refinements in the interpretation and perhaps more accurate determination of certain values were later contributed by Hendricks (1962). Essentially, what is known about this aspect of uterine pathophysiology is due to the work of these investigators.

By implanting catheters in several areas of the myometrium during labor, it is possible to observe the general area where the contractions originate and begin to spread, their speed of propagation and its direction, their duration, relative strength, and the process of relaxation (Figure 5-21).

Origin Normal contractions tend to start in the fundal area of the corpus. Since catheters have been implanted close to the cornual region, it has been postulated (Alvarez and Caldeyro-Barcia, 1954) that therein are the uterine "pacemakers." However, it has never been demonstrated that specialized tissue, which could be called or characterized as pacemaker, exists in any area of the uterus. Nevertheless, contractions do start in the fundal region, the area with the highest concentration of myocells per unit of weight and the thickest uterine wall. Together these two circumstances establish that, by statistical chances, the contractions should start in that area if all the cells have the same capability of firing. In fact, a characteristic of myometrial cells of several species studied in vitro is the capacity to behave as pacemaker.

Propagation From its area of origin the stimulus propagates in all directions along the myometrial cells, which contract as the stimulus reaches them. When this reaches successively the area where the catheters are implanted the local pressure increases and the contraction curves are recorded sequentially (Figure 5-22). The relative intensity of the local pressure may also be analyzed in the record. Finally, the slow process of relaxation may be observed and evaluated. From the study of the isolated wave it has been stated (see Figure 5-20) that the contraction reaches its peak in approximately 25 sec. From the analysis of intramyometrial pressures it was found that the stimulus propagates at 1 to 2 cm/sec to cover the uterus completely in about 20 to 30 sec. As the contraction wave propagates, the intrauterine pressure increases in a smooth, steady fashion and reaches its acme simultaneously in all the intramyometrial catheters (i.e., all the uterus).

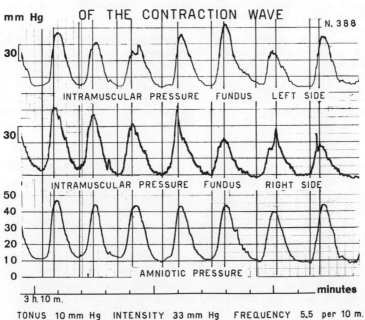

Figure 5-21 Simultaneous intraamniotic and intramyometrial pressure (microballoons) before cesarean section of term pregnancy. The contractions start slightly earlier on the right side (middle tracing). Note the regularity of the contractions and the good coordination recurring with every contraction. There is good intensity and borderline high frequency. Reprinted from Alvarez and Caldeyro-Barcia (1954).

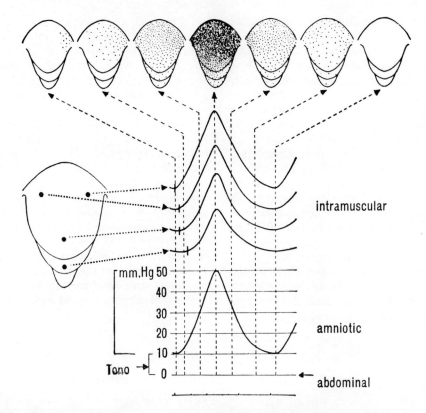

mm.Hg 50
40
30
20
10
Tono → 0

intramuscular

amniotic

abdominal

Figure 5-22 Schematic representation of a *normal, well-coordinated uterine contraction* recorded with intraamniotic catheter (bottom tracing) and four intramyometrial microballoons. In the top part of the figure in the small uteri the *dotted areas* represent the *myometrium contracting,* and concentration of dots represents *strength.* On the extreme left the contraction starts and reaches the area where the microballoon is implanted as increasing pressure is recorded in the top tracing (at the same time the intraamniotic pressure starts to rise above the tonus). The contraction *propagates and reaches* successively the other three microballoons *in sequence* with evidence of rising local pressure in the other tracings. The maximum pressure is achieved simultaneously in all recording catheters (darkened uterus) and relaxation follows also in a uniform manner until it is completed. Intramyometrial pressure is strongest in both fundal catheters and diminishes in middle corpus, to be lowest in the lower segment. At the same time the fundal contractions last longer. Reprinted from Caldeyro-Barcia R, et al: *Triangle, Sandoz Journal of Medical Science* 2:41, 1955.

Duration   Relaxation occurs in all areas at the same time, indicating then that contractions last longer where the stimulus started.

Strength   In addition, careful evaluation of individual pressures reveals that pressures are higher in the fundus, less in the middle corpus, and lowest in the lower segment. As the contractions start in the fundal area, they propagate downward to spread over all the uterus.

In this manner, in the normal contraction, three of its elements predominate in the fundus and progressively diminish as they travel toward the cervix: origin and propagation, strength, and duration—the three components of the *triple descending gradient.* The anatomy and biochem-istry of the myometrium—thicker, richer in cells per unit of weight, and cells richer in acto-myosin—all predispose to the *fundal dominance.* The actual pressures within the myometrium diminish exponentially from the decidua toward the peritoneum (Figure 5-23). The very deep layers of myometrium have the same pressures as are in the uterine cavity—shown by Hendricks (1962) and confirmed by Cibils and Hendricks (1969) (see Figure 5-52). This finding conflicts with the paradoxical reports of Alvarez and Caldeyro-Barcia (1954) that the intramyometrial pressure is several times higher than that within the uterine cavity.

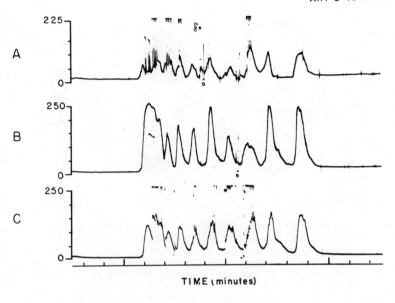

A.F. 8-10-61

INTRAMYOMETRIAL PRESSURE (mm Hg)

A : in SUPERFICIAL layer

B : in DEEP layer

C : in MIDDLE layer

after Ergotrate 122 µg i.v. (60 hours post partum)

Figure 5-23 Simultaneous recordings of intramyometrial pressure with open-end fluid-filled catheters placed over the same area at three different known depths. *(A)* Superficial. *(B)* Deep. *(C)* Middle. The sensitivity is the same in all three channels. The intravenous administration of ergotrate triggers a burst of strong contractions lasting 9 min. Note that the deepest catheter (B) records much stronger contractions than the more superficially placed ones; values in (C) are about one-half of (B), and in (A) about one-third. Courtesy C.H. Hendricks.

Effect of contractions The ultimate function of the contractions is to dilate the cervix completely and expel the fetus. To reach the last stage, the resistance of the cervix needs to be overcome —a slow process which, as it goes along, requires the formation of the lower segment and the gradual dilatation of the cervix. Normal contractions are indispensable to that process as well as to the subsequent dilatation. The physical conditions predispose to that final outcome. The stronger and longer lasting fundal component of the contraction (Figure 5-24) pulls from the weaker lower regions that stretch, giving up a little at a time. With each contraction the lower segment thins out, thus becoming still weaker, and by extension, it pulls the cervix. The cervix is pulled at the peak

of each contraction by the powerful muscular structure of the fundal area. Having no muscle to contract and counteract the pull from above, it thins out completely and then dilates.

The stretching effect of the contractions on the cervix has been recorded with cervimeters by some authors (Siener, 1964), who measured the intensity of the pull (Figure 5-25). In general this intensity is proportional to the intensity of the contractions. An additional element of fundamental importance is the bag of waters (or the presenting part) pushing from the uterine cavity against the cervical os, with a strong force directly transmitted from the fundus by the fetal body. With each period of relaxation (Figure 5-26), some retraction remains due to the elasticity of the

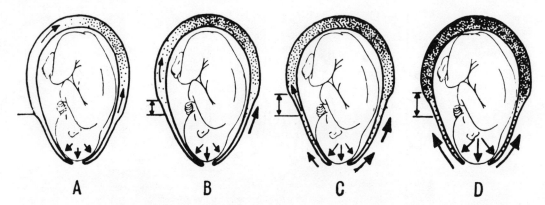

Figure 5-24 Schematic representation of the *normal wave of contraction* and its effect on the lower segment and cervix. Dotted areas represent contracting myometrium and concentration of dots represents force exerted. The cervix is effaced and in early dilatation. *(A)* Contraction starts in the fundus and *pulls* (arrows) from the noncontracting, elastic areas below. *(B)* As the contraction propagates, the thinner *lower segment begins to stretch* (small arrow outside). *(C)* and *(D)* The process continues with maximum pulling away from the lesser muscular lower segment, and the cervix, mainly constituted of connective tissue. Note the stretching of the lower segment. Also note the *direct pressure* exerted by the *fetal head* against the opening cervix. Reprinted from Caldeyro-Barcia R, et al: *Triangle, Sandoz Journal of Medical Science* 2:41, 1955.

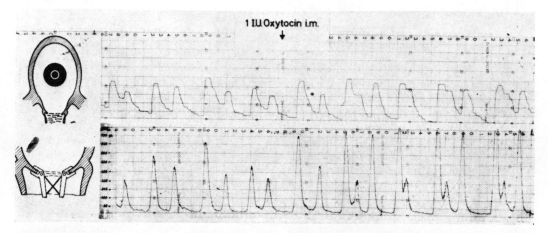

Figure 5-25 Recording of uterine contractions. *(Above)* By external tocogram. *(Below)* Cervical stretching (or strain) by a dynamometer applied against the internal os in a patient in early labor (calibration in grams). Each uterine contraction exerts a strong pull on the internal os in proportion to the intensity of contractions. The stronger contractions after 1 unit oxytocin IM have a marked effect on the pattern of pull, as recorded by the dynamometer. After Siener H: Cervical dynamometry. *Am J Obstet Gynecol* 89:579, 1964.

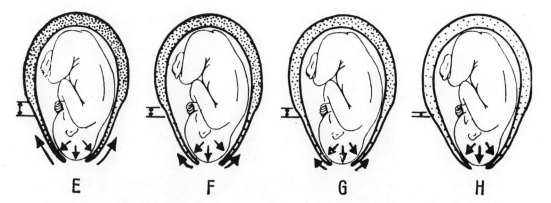

Figure 5-26 Schematic representation of the *relaxation* phase of a *normal contraction*. The relaxation occurs simultaneously. The lower regions regain part of their original position because of their elasticity. However in *(H)* at the completion of relaxation some stretch remains in the lower segment, and the cervix is more open. Reprinted from Caldeyro-Barcia R, et al: *Triangle, Sandoz Journal of Medical Science* 2:41, 1955.

myometrial cells and the connective tissue of the lower segment and cervix. The regular repetition of this process succeeds in accomplishing the dilatation, provided that all the elements described for the normal contraction are present. In other words, *good coordination of all factors* is necessary for the contraction to be efficient. Contractions should start in the fundal area, propagate symmetrically downward to reach maximum intensity simultaneously over the whole uterus, be stronger in the fundus, and relax slowly and evenly. The propagation of the wave is symmetrical and complete when the myometrium receives the impulse and is capable of responding after recovery from the previous contraction and is beyond the refractory period that follows muscular contractions. The total organ responds harmoniously to the impulse originating in one population of fundal cells whose resting membrane potential has reached the threshold of firing.

However, there are other factors, in addition to basic coordination, that significantly affect the contractility pattern in prelabor or labor and thereby, perhaps, the progress of labor.

Position The position of the parturient woman predictably influences the pattern of contractions at any stage of labor. Noriega-Guerra and co-workers (1959) first recognized that when a patient lies in the *supine position* her contractions have a higher frequency and lesser intensity than when she is in a *lateral position* (Figure 5-27). This they called the law of position. This reponse is predictable in over 90% of cases if either intensity or frequency of contractions is considered separately. However, the simultaneous change of both in the direction dictated by the law varies from 60% to 90% depending on the stage or the type of labor. In spontaneous prelabor (see Figure 5-16) only 4% do not respond as predicted whereas in induced prelabor (Figure 5-28) 13% fail to show the changed pattern. In spontaneous first stage (Figure 5-27) all cases studied followed the law, while in the group of induced labors 11% did not respond with some change in the pattern along the established prediction. The mechanism governing this conspicuous phenomenon is unknown; the state of the membranes, the presentation of the fetus, the variety of position, the side of the fetal back, or the type of labor do not have any influence on this peculiar response, which is reversible when the patient returns to her prior position (see Figures 5-27 and 5-28).

The knowledge of this particular response of the uterus is useful in clinical practice when episodes of spontaneous hypercontractility jeopardize fetal oxygenation (Figure 5-29). The reverse may be observed on certain occasions, such as sudden polysystoly and fetal distress when the patient turns to her back. This may simulate an episode of iatrogenic hypercontractility (Figure 5-30) even though it does not exist. Prompt return to the lateral position should correct the "hyperstimulation."

Mendez-Bauer and co-workers (1975) observed the significant changes in contractility pattern when a patient lying in the supine position adopts

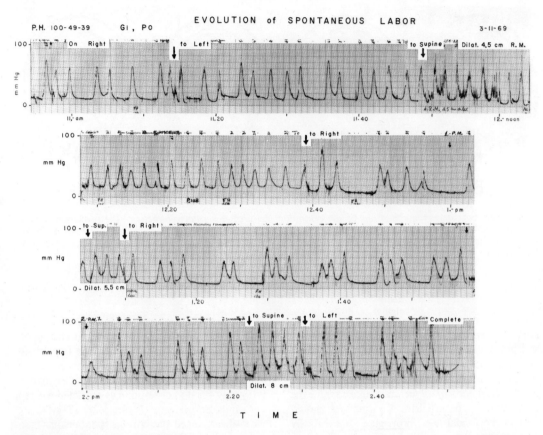

Figure 5-27 Contracility and evolution of first-stage spontaneous labor completed in 4 hours. Two elements are outstanding in this tracing: (1) the very strong contractions averaging almost 60 mm Hg, and (2) the remarkable effect of the patient's position on the contracility pattern. Position changes are indicated by arrows. Note the immediate *decrease in intensity and increase in frequency* when the patient turns from lateral to supine. *The reverse is true when turning to lateral.* Observe at the beginning of the tracing *(top, left)* no change is seen when the patient turns from one lateral side to the other. Reprinted from Cibils LA: Enhancement and induction of labor, in Aladjem S (ed): *Risks in the Practice of Modern Obstetrics, II.* St. Louis, Mosby, 1975, pp 182–210.

the standing position. They demonstrated that the intensity increased predictably in three-quarters of the patients, while the frequency was unchanged in more than one-half of them. This phenomenon occurs whether the patient moves from standing to supine (Figure 5-31) or vice versa. As in the case of lateral position, the changes are predictable, reversible, and are not influenced by parity or state of the membranes.

Comparison of these works indicates that the degree of increase in intensity seems roughly equivalent when the patient changes from supine to either the lateral or standing position. If there is any difference between these two it is in favor of the lateral position, in which the intensity in-

creases slightly more (Figure 5-32). However, other important effects on the progress of labor following adoption of the standing position by the parturient patient may not be present when she is in the lateral position (see below).

Efficiency of the Contractions

The classic method of assessing the efficiency of contractions in dilating the cervix has been tabulating the progress of dilatation against time. Friedman (1955) divided this curve into several phases to follow and evaluate labors, clinically. In

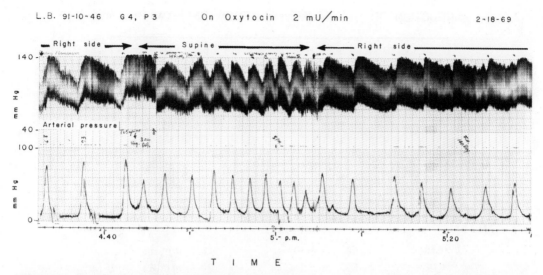

Figure 5-28 Intrauterine and arterial pressure tracings obtained in induced prelabor. The contractility pattern changes immediately and markedly when the patient turns (position shown at top). The changes reversed when the position changed back to the original. Note the very important fluctuations in blood pressure coinciding with the contractions, and how these are sharper in supine position. Note also that the fluctuations of the systolic pressure are consistently more important than those of the diastolic. Reprinted from Cibils LA: Enhancement and induction of labor, in Aladjem S (ed): *Risks in the Practice of Modern Obstetrics, II.* St. Louis, Mosby, 1975, pp 182–210.

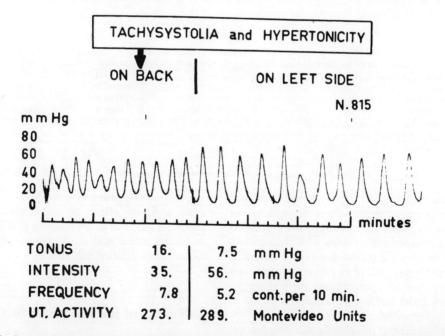

Figure 5-29 Intrauterine pressure tracing of *full-term spontaneous labor,* at 6 cm dilatation. When the patient was supine the contractions were very frequent and of mild intensity. At the same time the tonus increased, and there was fetal distress. Turning the patient to her side brought about an immediate change in pattern with diminished frequency and increased intensity; the tonus diminished also. (The calculated values for each period are shown in the lower part of the figure.) Reprinted from Caldeyro-Barcia R, et al: Effect of position changes on the intensity and frequency of uterine contractions during labor. *Am J Obstet Gynecol* 80:284, 1960.

88

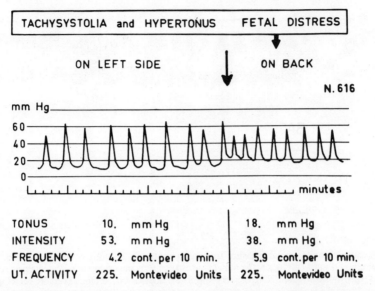

INDUCTION OF LABOR WITH OXYTOCIN INFUSION 2 mU/min.

TACHYSYSTOLIA and HYPERTONUS   FETAL DISTRESS

ON LEFT SIDE   ON BACK

N. 616

TONUS	10. mm Hg	18.	mm Hg
INTENSITY	53. mm Hg	38.	mm Hg
FREQUENCY	4.2 cont. per 10 min.	5.9	cont. per 10 min.
UT. ACTIVITY	225. Montevideo Units	225.	Montevideo Units

Figure 5-30 Intrauterine pressure tracing of a *term labor* at 5 cm dilatation *induced with 2 mU/min* oxytocin infusion. A normal contractility pattern changes suddenly, becoming polysystolic and hypertonic as the patient turns from lateral to supine (first arrow). The abnormality was corrected when the patient returned to a lateral position. (The calculated values for each period are shown in the lower part of the figure.) Reprinted from Caldeyro-Barcia R, et al: Effect of position changes on the intensity and frequency of uterine contractions during labor. *Am J Obstet Gynecol* 80:284, 1960.

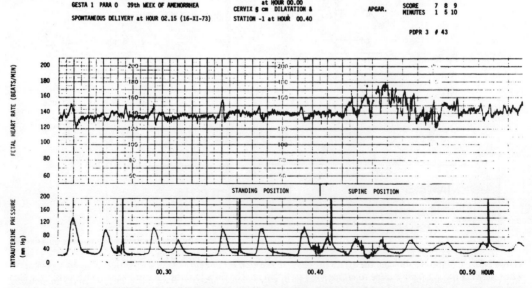

Figure 5-31 Intrauterine pressure and FHR tracings from a term primipara in spontaneous labor, middle of first stage. Until hour 00.40 the patient was in *standing position,* when the contractions were strong and with moderate frequency. Recumbency in *supine position* coincided with increased frequency and diminished intensity of contractions. Reprinted from Mendez-Bauer C, et al: Effects of standing position on spontaneous uterine contractility and other aspects of labor. *J Perinat Med* 3:89, 1975.

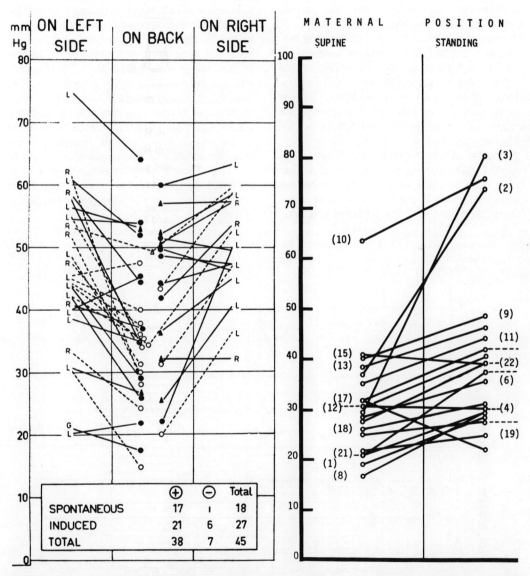

Figure 5-32 Composite showing the *effect of maternal position on intensity* of contractions. *(Left)* Changes observed when patients turned *from supine to either right or left side*. The lines join the pressure values observed in the same patients (scale in mm Hg) and are rather steep. *(Right)* Changes observed when the patients changed from *supine to standing position;* the lines join the pressures observed in each case (scale in mm Hg). Note overall lesser steepness. (The calculated values are shown at the lower part of the figure.) Reprinted from Caldeyro-Barcia R, et al: Effect of position changes on the intensity and frequency of uterine contractions during labor. *Am J Obstet Gynecol* 80:284, 1960; Mendez-Bauer, et al: Effects of standing position on spontaneous uterine contractility and other aspects of labor. *J Perinat Med* 3:89, 1975.

90

spite of its deficiencies, it did fulfill the important function of drawing attention to the need to correlate the several elements involved in labor and to some of the variables influencing its progress. With the current availability of labor monitors, one should be able to make an assessment based on the analysis of contraction tracings and cervical dilatation rather than basing it solely on the dilatation curve against time. The various methods of analysis reviewed at the beginning of this chapter will be used to study the several factors that may affect the efficiency of contractions as a dilating force or alter the contracility pattern in a favorable or unfavorable way. Particular emphasis will be put on *cervical dilatation plotted against uterine work and time*. The slope of the uterine work curve thus tabulated defines the efficiency of the contractions as a dilating force.

Parity Through the years clinicians have reported that labors in primiparas tend to last longer than in multiparas as demonstrated by curves of cervical dilatation against time. That classic observation has been confirmed in a study of the patients delivering at the Chicago Lying-In Hospital (Figures 5-33 and 55-34). For all positions studied the *duration of first stage* from 3 cm to completion is significantly *longer in primiparas than in multiparas*.

Only Hendricks and collaborators (1970) reported that there is no appreciable difference in duration of dilatation due to parity. This difference in duration of first stage might be because of a number of factors some of which have been studied in detail; the pattern of contractions appears not to be influenced by the parity in term pregnancies (Figures 5-35, 5-36, 5-37). The contractions early in the period of dilation or close to completion have the same characteristics within the range of normal. It is not possible to distinguish a primipara from a multipara by analyzing the tracing of the contractions. Another possible factor could be the difference in *frequency of contractions*. There is no difference, as indicated by the similar pattern as well as by the higher number of contractions required by the groups with longer labors (Tables 5-2 and 5-3).

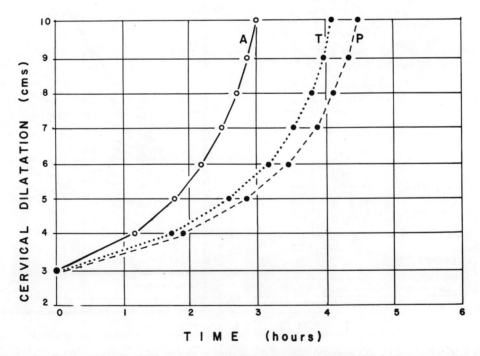

Figure 5-33 Average cervical dilatation curves of first stage in 550 multiparas grouped according to variety of position. Fetal anterior positions *(A)* were so diagnosed throughout first stage. Transverse (T) and posterior (P) positions were so diagnosed at some time during the study period and tabulated as such even though they may have later rotated to the anterior position. Reprinted from Cibils LA: Enhancement and induction of labor, in Aladjem S (ed): *Risks in the Practice of Modern Obstetrics, II.* St. Louis, Mosby, 1975, pp 182–210.

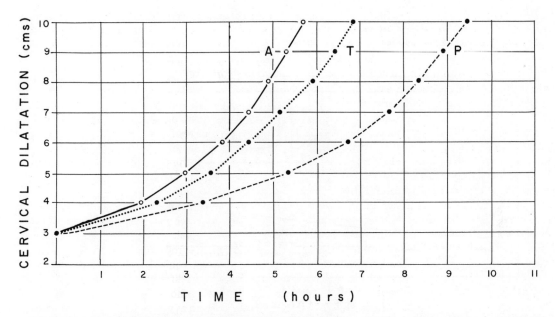

Figure 5-34 Average cervical dilatation curves of first stage in 335 primiparas grouped according to variety of position (same symbols as in Figure 5-33). Reprinted from Cibils LA: Enhancement and induction of labor, in Aladjem S (ed): *Risks in the Practice of Modern Obstetrics, II.* St. Louis, Mosby, 1975, pp 182–210.

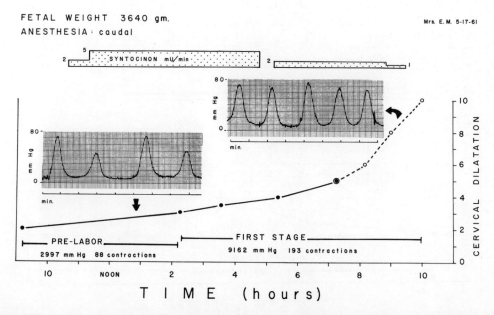

Figure 5-35 Uterine work and evolution of cervical dilatation in *induced labor, primipara, left occipito-anterior position.* The representative patterns of uterine contractility for *prelabor* and *first stage* are shown with arrows indicating the moment to which they correspond. Amniotomy was performed at 5 cm dilatation (where interrupted line starts). The calculated values of uterine work and number of contractions for each of the two periods appear at the lower part of the figure. Reprinted from Cibils LA, Hendricks CH: Normal labor in vertex presentation. *Am J Obstet Gynecol* 91:385, 1965.

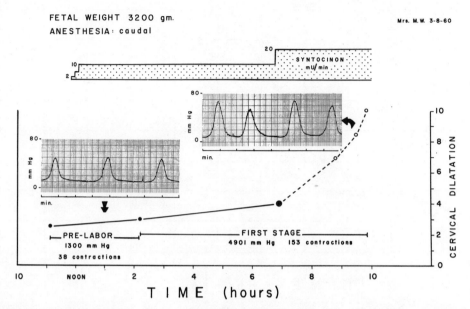

FETAL WEIGHT 3200 gm.
ANESTHESIA: caudal

Mrs. M.W. 3-8-60

Figure 5-36 Uterine work and evolution of cervical dilatation in *induced labor, multipara, left occipitotransverse position*. The representative patterns of uterine contractility for *prelabor* and *first stage* are shown, with arrows indicating the moment to which they correspond. Amniotomy was performed at 4 cm dilatation (where interrupted line starts). The calculated values of uterine work and number of contractions for each of the two periods appear at the lower part of the figure. Reprinted from Cibils LA, Hendricks CH: Normal labor in vertex presentation. *Am J Obstet Gynecol* 91:385, 1965.

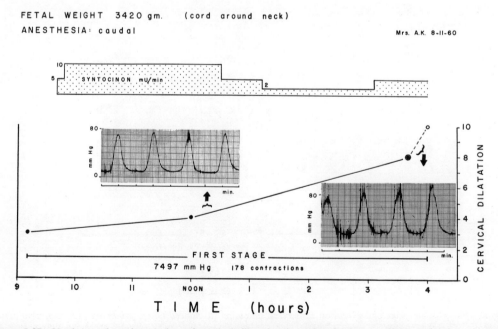

FETAL WEIGHT 3420 gm. (cord around neck)
ANESTHESIA: caudal

Mrs. A.K. 8-11-60

Figure 5-37 Uterine work and evolution of cervical dilatation in *induced labor, multipara* with fetus in *right occipitoposterior position*. Representative patterns of uterine contractility of early and late *first stage,* with arrows indicating the moment to which they correspond. Amniotomy was performed at 8 cm dilatation (where interrupted line starts). The calculated uterine work and number of contractions appear at the lower part of the figure. Reprinted from Cibils LA, Hendricks, CH: Normal labor in vertex presentation. *Am J Obstet Gynecol* 91:385, 1965.

The tables confirm the various factors discussed here: no significant difference in the average intensity of contractions, and therefore the number of contractions is higher among those who required significantly longer time. The *uterine work* from 3 cm to complete dilatation averaged 3920 mm Hg for multiparas, and 6890 mm Hg for primiparas ($p = < 0.001$), indicating that the efficiency of the contractions is higher in multiparas (Figure 5-38).

Variety of fetal position The incidence of fetal posterior positions among the general obstetric population ranges from 10% to 50%. In this material only 55% of primiparas had a fetal head in the *anterior position* while in multiparas only slightly over 51% were in the anterior position when first examined. The variety of position of the presenting part has important implications for the progress of labor. Opinions to the contrary notwithstanding, when the fetus is in the anterior position, the efficiency of uterine contractions is better; this position requires less uterine work than the transverse or posterior positions (see Tables 5-2 and 5-3). This observation is valid regardless of the type of labor (spontaneous or induced), (Tables 5-4 and 5-5). The same conclusion may be reached when comparing the *duration* of first stage in either multipara (see Figure 5-33) or primiparas (see Figure 5-34). A good demonstration of the influence of the variety of position on the efficiency of the contractions is seen when cervical dilatation of single cases that rotated during first stage is tabulated against uterine work (Figure 5-39). The relatively poor efficiency when the occiput is posterior improves somewhat with the rotation to transverse, and it becomes maximal with the rotation to anterior as the slope of the curve (which measures the efficiency) becomes steeper with every step of rotation. How the variety of position affects the efficiency of the contractions is unknown. However, the physical relationships of the birth canal and the presenting part vary with the variety of position. It is equally true that those relationships are clearly altered by the degree of flexion and synclitism of the presenting part. It may well be that, with the rotation, there

UTERINE WORK REQUIRED TO
ACCOMPLISH FIRST STAGE

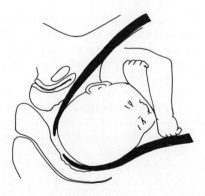 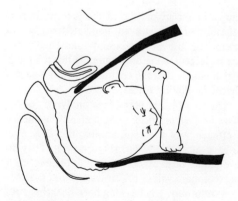

Primiparas 6,300 mm Hg (3,500 to 12,000)

Multiparas 3,500 mm Hg (1,200 to 7,000)

Figure 5-38 Schematic representation of cervical changes observed during first stage of labor (from 3 cm to completion) and the *uterine work required to accomplish it*. Cases grouped by parity with average figures and ranges given in parentheses.

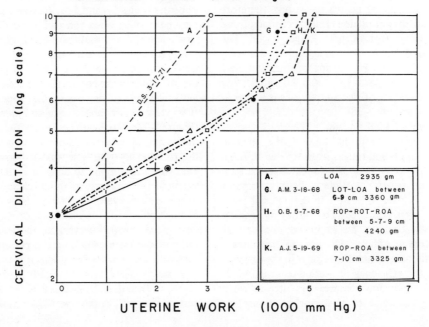

EFFECT of ROTATION upon EFFICIENCY of
UTERINE WORK (first stage)

Figure 5-39 Cervical dilatation curves of four term labors plotted on semilog paper against uterine work. All start at 3 cm dilatation with subsequent examinations indicated by each point. The clinical characteristics of the cases are shown on the right side enclosure. Case G had amniotomy at 4 cm while all others had it at 3 cm. The slope of the curve changes when there is a change in the variety of position of the fetal head (Cases G, H, K). All curves become almost parallel when the heads are in the anterior position. Reprinted from Cibils LA: Enhancement and induction of labor, in Aladjem S (ed): *Risks in the Practice of Modern Obstetrics, II.* St. Louis, Mosby, 1975, pp 182–210.

occurs a better adaptation of the presenting part to the birth canal with an associated better application against the cervix and a lessened resistance to descent in the birth canal. If this is so, it is understandable that the contractions will be more efficient as dilating forces.

The two factors heretofore analyzed, *parity and variety of position,* independently influence the efficiency of the contractions, but they may also have an additive effect (Figure 5-40). They do not exclude each other but can influence each other (compare values of Tables 5-4 and 5-5).

Amniotomy   It has long been held that rupture of the membranes is a maneuver that facilitates the progress of labor by improving the contractility pattern. But that concept was strongly challeneged by some, notably Friedman and Sachtleben (1963), who thought the state of membranes had no influence on the efficiency of the contractions. However, the majority of studies carried out in recent times, using different methods to assess efficiency of contractions either by calculating the uterine work (see Figure 5-8) or including the cervical dilatation against time method applied to large populations (Schwarcz et al, 1976), have clearly shown that contractions after amniotomy are far better dilating forces. This effect is predictable regardless of parity of the mother or position of the fetal head (Figure 5-41). The sequential and additive effect of *amniotomy and rotation* of the head to a more favorable position may be appreciated in Figure 5-42.

The effect of amniotomy on the contractility pattern may be very clear when there is some lack of coordination or irregularity of contractions (see Figure 5-19). In those cases the quality of the contractions improves and with it their efficiency. However, in most circumstances when a good active labor pattern has been established, the rupture of the membranes has no appreciable effect on the contractility patterns (see Figures 4-18 and 4-19).

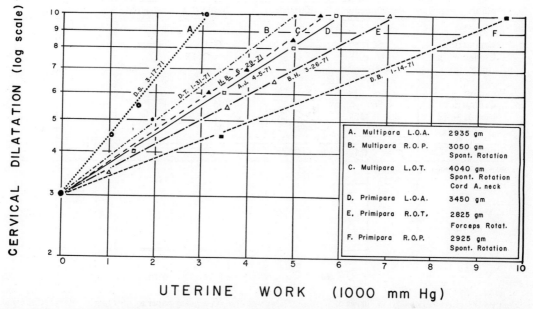

Figure 5-40 Cervical dilatation curves from six term labors plotted on semilog paper against uterine work. All cases start at 3 cm with individual progress indicated by points in each curve that fall on the straight lines. The slope of the curves measures the efficiency of uterine work, and the differences show the influence of parity and variety of position on the efficiency to dilate the cervix. All cases had membranes ruptured at 3 cm or before. The individual clinical data are shown on the inset. Reprinted from Cibils LA: Enhancement and induction of labor, in Aladjem S (ed): *Risks in the Practice of Modern Obstetrics, II.* St. Louis, Mosby, 1975, pp 182–210.

Table 5-4
Effect of Fetal Position on First-Stage Labor of Primiparas

Position	Labor			Statistical Significance	
	Spontaneous[a]	Enhanced	Induced	χ^2(2d.f.)	p
Anterior					
Contractions	88	131	143		
Uterine work	(54)	(62)	(65)		
(mm Hg)	3550	5100	6600	8.1	< 0.025
Posterior					
Contractions	138	184	242		
Uterine	(12)	(43)	(48)		
(mm Hg)	5800	8100	11,400	9.5	< 0.01
Student's T Test	p = < 0.05	< 0.05	< 0.001		

[a]Number of patients in parentheses.

Table 5-5
Effect of Fetal Position on First-Stage Labor of Multiparas

Position	Labor			Statistical Significance	
	Spontaneous[a]	Enhanced	Induced	χ^2(2d.f.)	p
Anterior					
Contractions	56	61	73		
Uterine work	(61)	(37)	(185)		
(mm Hg)	2300	2650	3290	6.1	< 0.05
Posterior					
Contractions	96	97	106		
Uterine work	(21)	(26)	(135)		
(mm Hg)	4340	4690	5180	7.0	< 0.05
Student's T Test	$p =$ < 0.001	< 0.001	< 0.001		

[a]Number of patients in parentheses.

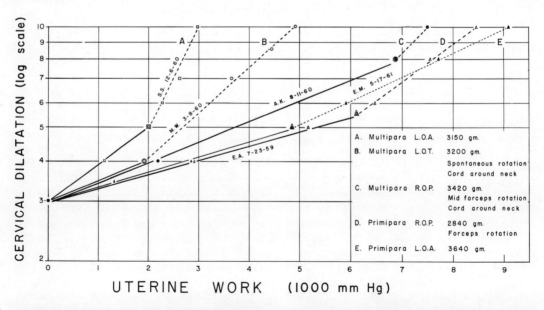

Figure 5-41 Cervical dilatation curves of five representative cases plotted on semilog paper against uterine work. The continuous lines indicate labors proceeding with intact membranes; interrupted lines are after amniotomy. The clinical data for each case are summarized on the inset. *All curves increase their slope after amniotomy.* Reprinted from Cibils LA, Hendricks CH: Normal labor in vertex presentation. *Am J Obstet Gynecol* 91:385, 1965.

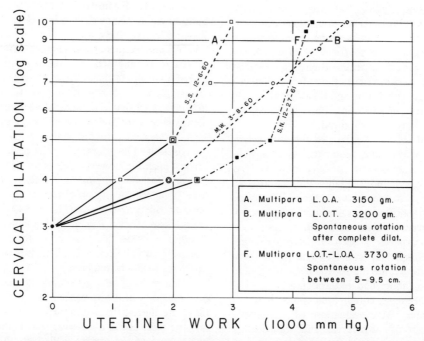

Figure 5-42 Cervical dilatation curves of three cases plotted on semilog paper against uterine work. The continuous lines indicate labors with intact membranes; ruptured membranes are interrupted lines. Note in all cases the *increase in slop after amniotomy,* and in case F a *further increase after the head rotated to anterior position.* Note the parallelism of the lines with case A when the variety of position was the same. (Clinical data on inset.) Reprinted from Cibils LA, Hendricks CH: Normal labor in vertex presentation. *Am J Obstet Gynecol* 91:385, 1965.

The most notable effect of amniotomy is the physical change created by the missing part of the contractile ovoid wall—over its weakest point: the lower segment–internal os area. As shown in Chapter 2 the radius of the uterine wall is smallest over this area, therefore exercising the least tension and resistance to stretching (which is a direct function of the radius of the curved wall) during a coordinated contraction. The formula T = pr/2 indicates that, predictably, the lower segment–cervical area must give in to the pulling forces of the powerfully built muscular corpus-fundus area. The lower segment and cervix can offer mainly passive resistance because they are formed predominantly by connective tissue, thus further facilitating the thinning out process. As there is no wall over the area of dilated cervix, no resistance may be offered; in addition, the pulling force of the contraction overcomes little by little the passive resistance of the cervix.

When the membranes are still intact they "absorb" the pressure exerted over the area; that is, they oppose some "counterpressure" manifested by the tension of the bag of forewaters palpable during a contraction (particularly evident when the bag has an "hourglass" shape). The counterpressure tends particularly to oppose the action of the presenting part, which tends to protrude through the lower segment and cervical area. This local pressure produced by the presenting part acts unopposed after amniotomy and thus contributes significantly to overcoming the resistance of the weakest area of the uterus.

The protrusion of the small bag of waters seems to be important in the early stages of dilatation. In other words, the *hourglass shape* seems to be important because, when the *membranes are flat,* the contractions are inefficient in dilating the cervix. This fact becomes evident in these latter cases when the membranes are ruptured and an extraordinary increase in the efficiency of the contractions follows. One has the impression that the flat membranes (or flat bag of waters) hold the presenting part and prevent its application and pushing action against the cervix.

Cervical dilatation requires less uterine work

as it progresses, as shown by the exponential curve of uterine work, because the ever-increasing opening in the wall of the contracting ovoid gives less and less resistance to contractions of equivalent intensity. Physical principles then easily explain the increase in the efficiency of uterine contractions to dilate the cervix, and therefore the more rapid progress of dilatation observed after the membranes have been ruptured.

Type of labor Analysis of the characteristics of the uterine contraction tracing of a well-coordinated spontaneous labor compared with that of a properly induced labor shows hardly an appreciable difference between them. The shape of the contraction is the same, and the slow but constant increase in intensity and frequency as dilatation advances is seen in both (compare Figures 5-19 and 5-27 with 10-1 and 10-4). From this observation it has mistakenly been said that in spontaneous labors and induced labors cervical dilatation progresses equally well and both are indistinguishable. The evaluation of reasonably large numbers of cases reveals that significantly more uterine work is required for enhanced labors, and still more for induced labors when they are compared to spontaneous labors (see Tables 5-4 and 5-5). This observation is true for primiparas and multiparas regardless of the variety of position of the presenting part.

If the observation is clear, the reason for the difference is less obvious. A possible explanation must take into consideration that there are unknown factors controlling cervical readiness, and some of their effects are not physically appreciable with our current means of observation. It seems that cervical resistance is lessened in spontaneous compared to induced labors, even though a cervix may feel very ripe before an induction is started.

Maternal position Most observations and studies carried out on uterine contractions have been conducted on patients laboring in recumbent positions—as much the consequence of the necessity to maintain the patients in bed to facilitate studies as of the tradition that patients need to undergo the process of labor lying comfortably in bed. The observations about uterine contracility patterns and efficiency, as well as duration and characteristics of various types of labors, are all valid for the patient in the recumbent position. However, patients may also request or be invited to stand, sit, or walk while undergoing first stage, which may influence the progress of labor.

A review of contractility patterns related to position changes showed that *between supine and lateral positions* there are predictable changes in intensity and frequency with minimal effect on the calculated uterine activity. The only study conducted to evaluate the effect of these changes on the progress of cervical dilatation (Cibils et al, 1959) revealed that regardless of whether the patient is supine or lateral, the efficiency of uterine work is the same provided that all other variables are constant. The adoption by the patient of the *vertical position,* however, seems to have not only a clear effect on the pattern but also is a significant influence on the efficiency of the contractions to dilate the cervix (Figure 5-43). Uterine contraction efficiency is greatly enhanced in the standing position. This is not so for the sitting position in which there is a high incidence of labor problems (Mendez-Bauer et al, 1976).

The physical laws governing the distribution of pressures within the uterine cavity help to explain the more effective labors when the uterus and the fetus are in a quasivertical position. The lowest part of the uterine walls (cervix) receives the hydrostatic pressure of the fluid column above it, that is, the amniotic fluid from the internal os to the fundus. This pressure is approximately 20 mm Hg, which should be added to the pressure exerted by the tonus (see Figure 4-17). When the patient is standing and the membranes are ruptured, much more pressure is constantly exerted against the internal os by the presenting part and therefore the cervix should dilate faster.

Uterine Size

Multiple pregnancy The distended uterus of twin (or more) gestation creates physical conditions somewhat different from those observed in the single pregnancy. The calculated *augmented intrauterine volume* expands the cavity and stretches the walls, thereby *increasing the diameter* of the ovoid. The consequence of a *larger radius* is that, for forces of equal values exerted by the contractions, the intrauterine pressure is of lesser intensity (Laplace's law) in the uterus carrying twins than in the one carrying a single fetus (for chronologically comparable pregnancies), (Figure 5-44). The intrauterine pressure values of the overdistended uterus are then not comparable to those of normal size. The values of the intensity of contractions being lower, the calculations based on them will understandably be lower because all methods use intensity as the most critical element for calculation.

When there is a twin gestation, it is important to assess properly the size of the uterine contents to make an adequate interpretation of the tracings. If the total volume is close to double of the term single pregnancy (Figure 5-44) poor looking contractions may be very effective in inducing

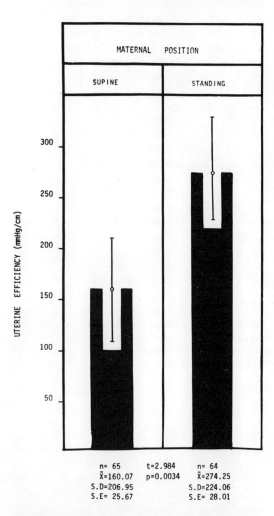

Figure 5-43 Comparison of efficiency of uterine work to dilate the cervix in patients laboring in *supine* and *standing positions*. The work necessary to dilate each centimeter of cervical dilatation has been calculated. It required significantly more work (less efficiency) when the patients were in supine position. Reprinted from Mendez-Bauer C, et al: Maternal standing position in first stage of labor, in Scarpelli EM, Cosmi E (eds): *Reviews in Perinatal Medicine.* Baltimore, University Park Press, 1976, pp 281–293.

progress; when the total of both fetuses is only equivalent to a large single fetus, the contractility pattern should be similar to that of a singleton (Figure 5-45). With extreme distension, the contractility will appear exceptionally poor looking as in triplet gestations (Figure 5-46) where contractions of very low intensity will induce normal progress of labor.

Preterm pregnancy   Laplace's principle applies equally to the uterus with small content and therefore with a smaller radius of the wall curvature. Often the recorded intensity of the contractions surpasses 100 mm Hg (Figure 5-47), something rarely seen in term-size uteri. The smaller the pregnant uterus in labor, the higher the recorded pressure. As for overdistended uteri, the calculations made with these pressure values are not comparable with those of term size.

SECOND, THIRD, AND FOURTH STAGES

Second Stage

The frequency and intensity of contractions in the second stage differ very little from those of first stage. At second stage they usually reach their highest intensity, best coordination, and highest frequency. In addition, these contractions are superimposed on the increase in pressure brought about by the bearing-down efforts (Figure 5-48). There are about two or three bearing-down efforts (value range of 30 to 40 mm Hg) for each uterine contraction. Rested patients and those with no anesthesia push better and record the highest pressures. By and large, they record beyond the standard paper recording ranges giving the tracing a flat-top appearance. Contractions last about 10 sec, drop quickly to the peak of the contraction pressure, and repeat the cycle. Their effect on further descent and rotation is important for the progress of second stage. Depending on the position and attitude of the fetal head, the fetopelvic relationship, and parity, the number of second stage contractions may vary from a few to several dozen if the expulsion of the fetus is difficult.

Third Stage

As soon as the infant is delivered, the unanesthetized patient feels much relief. But if the

100

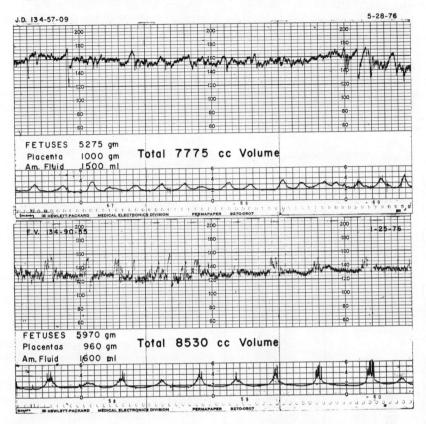

Figure 5-44 Uterine contractility and FHR tracings of *advanced twin gestations* recorded by direct methods. *(Above)* Patient with intrauterine content of 7775 ml (overdistended uterus). *(Below)* Tracing from a uterus with 8530 ml content. Note the very low intensity of contractions of around 20 mm Hg that occasionally reach 30 mm Hg. (Pressure tracing range is 20 mm Hg between each ordinate.)

appropriate recording methods are used, it may be observed that the *uterus continues to contract at the same frequency* as during second stage. Furthermore, the intensity of these contractions, as assessed by intrauterine pressure, is significantly higher than those of second stage (Figure 5-49). This is of course the result of the marked diminution in size of the uterine cavity and its contents: the corpus, filled only by the placenta, has an average volume of approximately 700 ml. The function of these contractions is as follows:

1. They separate the placenta from the uterine wall and push it down to the lower segment. This part is usually completed in about three to four contractions within 15 min after the birth of the infant. When the placenta is not separated within this period the third stage may be considered prolonged. In about 5% of unmedicated patients, the placenta may be retained (Figure 5-50) (see Chapter 6, Abnormal Uterine Contractility). The separation of the placenta occurs because physically the uterus retracts markedly while the placenta, implanted over its wall, cannot adapt to the diminution in surface of implantation; thus it separates over the decidual layer. Danforth et al (1942) showed that in higher nonhuman primates the placenta begins its separation during second stage in some cases, and there is no reason to believe that the same thing does not occur in normal third stage in humans.

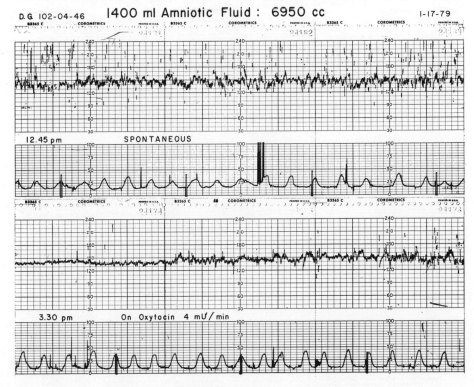

Figure 5-45 Direct recordings of uterine contractility and FHR tracings of *preterm twin gestation* with total intrauterine content of 6950 ml (moderate overdistention). *(Above)* Contractions up to 20 mm Hg. *(Below)* Two hours later, after oxytocin infusion, increased frequency, and intensity up to 35 mm Hg.

2. When the placenta separates, the spiral arterioles of the myometrium supplying the IVS are severed. The mechanical clamping of the myometrium by the powerful third-stage contractions prevents what would otherwise be severe blood loss. This process takes place simultaneously with the "retraction" of the arterioles, a step not too well understood but assumed to include actual physical retraction of the remainder of the vessels by their marked coiling. In between the contractions the tone and/or the retraction mechanism avoid the blood loss.

Fourth Stage

The period covering *the first 24 hours after delivery of the placenta* is defined as fourth stage. The important function ascribed to the postpar-

tum contractions in the hemostatic mechanism of the uterus suggests that the study of these contractions is no idle academic exercise. The very large placental bed with its numerous spiral arteriole openings (estimated to be between 20 and 40) could be the site of potentially severe hemorrhages if the physiologic mechanisms were deranged; among these, altered quality of contractions may be fundamental.

The contractility pattern has been studied in the puerperium by many authors using intrauterine balloons of various sizes and Voorhees' bags connected to recording apparatuses. For a detailed and fine study of the elements participating in the contractility of the puerperium, the use of balloons seems to introduce the same artifacts and unreliability as during intrapartum monitoring. This has been conclusively shown by Cibils and Hendricks (1969) who used open-end fluid-filled catheters to record the pressures within the

102

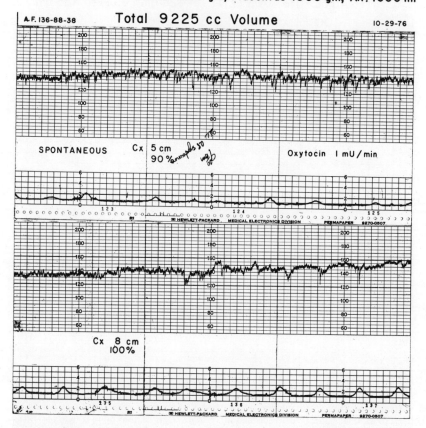

Figure 5-46 Uterine contractility and FHR tracing of *term triplet gestation* with a total intrauterine content of 9225 ml (overdistended uterus). *(Above)* Spontaneous activity in early first stage, recorded with intrauterine catheter, produces progress in spite of very low intensity. *(Below)* Stronger contractions induced with oxytocin, 1 mU/min, but still of low intensity (20 to 30 mm Hg). Low intensity values are due to the *large diameter of the uterine ovoid.* (Pressure scale 20 mm Hg between each ordinate line.)

virtual uterine cavity and several areas of the myometrium simultaneously.

Postpartum intrauterine pressure is extremely high, normally between 80 and 200 mm Hg (Figure 5-51) with the tracing having a smooth-looking profile in the first few hours postdelivery. If judged by the same standards of interpreting pressures during gestation, the majority of them might be thought to be coordinated and encompassing the whole uterus. The fact that one is dealing with a virtual cavity creates different physical conditions, the extent of which can be elucidated only with several intramyometrial catheters recording simultaneously. These demon-

strate that relatively early in the postpartum period the uterus may have strong localized contractions with minimal expression in the former cavity (Figures 5-52 and 5-53) suggesting that a constant "fibrillatory-like" activity may be occurring under those circumstances. Those regional contractions may be so localized and spread so slowly that regions relatively close to each other may have asynchronous patterns. However, it seems that there is good propagation over any particular area of the wall and that all layers contract at about the same time, with the deep areas having significantly higher pressures during the majority of recorded contractions (Figure 5-53).

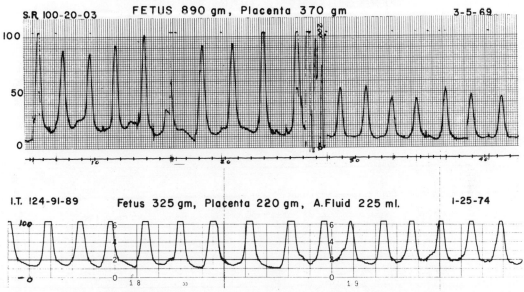

Figure 5-47 Uterine contractility in advanced first stage of two *preterm single pregnancies*. *(Below)* At 16 weeks gestation with uterine content of 770 ml. *(Above)* At 33 weeks gestation, anencephalic, with uterine content of 1260 ml. Pressure ranges shown at left. Strong contractions, well over 100 mm Hg. High intensity values are due to a relatively *small diameter of the uterine ovoid*. (In the upper tracing the pressure range was changed to 0 to 2000 mm Hg, in the middle, to be able to record the peak of the contractions.)

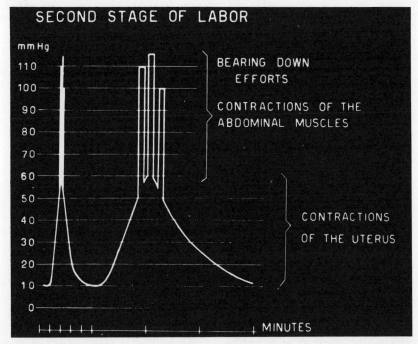

Figure 5-48 Schematic representation of two contractions of second stage. *(Left)* At normal paper speed showing lines produced by the pushing efforts on top of the contraction. *(Right)* At higher paper speed, showing duration and individual intensity of three bearing-down efforts on top of the contraction. Courtesy R. Caldeyro-Barcia.

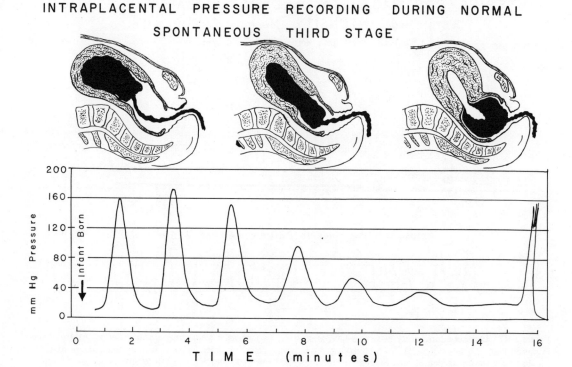

Figure 5-49 Uterine contractility (intraplacental pressure) of normal spontaneous third stage. *(Above)* Drawings illustrate the process of placental separation and its progressive passage to the lower segment. *(Below)* Less pressure is transmitted because of lack of contractility in the lower segment. Three or four contractions are sufficient to complete third stage. Reprinted from Alvarez and Caldeyro-Barcia (1954).

These puerperal contractions resemble the characteristics of prelabor or labor contractions in this aspect only. The very localized contractions can be triggered by pharmacologic stimulation, the response being maximal expression of disorganized activity if one considers the whole organ (Figure 5-54). The slow propagation of the wave is also clearly seen when it may take more than 10 min to have a complete contraction of the organ. In fourth stage, the uterine cavity seems to have become "compartmentalized" by contractions of the deep myometrium, which may then lock areas of the uterus and prevent the transmission of pressure.

The complete cycle of activity from advanced pregnancy to late puerperium suggests that in fact it is a process of incoordinated activity (prelabor), becoming slowly better organized (first stage), reaching maximum coordination and strength during second and third stage, and following with a slow process of "deceleration" in which the contractions become less and less coordinated (fourth stage) as the hours pass. This cycle is summarized in Figure 5-55. The reason for the extremely incoordinated activity during puerperium may have a physiologic role in hemostasis and the subsequent uterine involution when retention of lochia may predispose to complications.

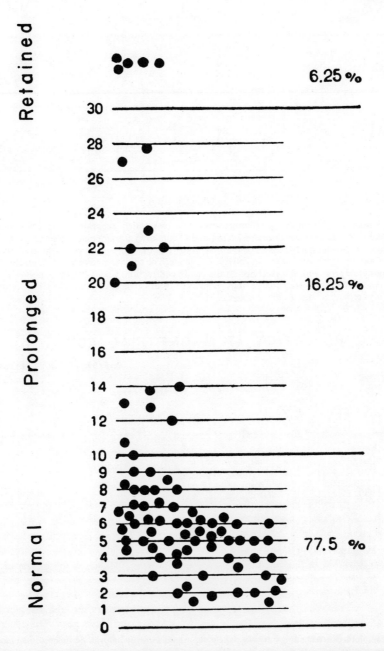

Figure 5-50 Duration of spontaneous *third stage* in 80 patients who were given no drugs. The numbers on the left are minutes elapsed between delivery of the fetus and expulsion of the placenta. Those completing within 10 min were considered *normal;* between 10 and 30 min, prolonged; longer than 30 mintues, *retained placentas.* Reprinted from Alvarez and Caldeyro-Barcia (1954).

106

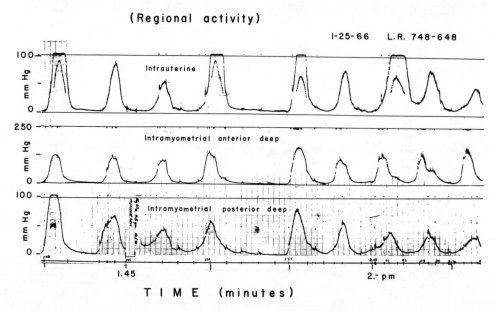

Figure 5-51 Simultaneous recordings of *intrauterine* and two widely separated *intramyometrial pressures* in a *postdelivery uterus,* 4½ hours after cesarean section and 45 min after intramyometrial injection of 20 mU oxytocin. (Pressure ranges are shown on left.) Peaks of the first, fourth, fifth, and seventh contractions of the top tracing and the first of the bottom were recorded at 0 to 250 mm Hg range. The contractions seem coordinated, occurring slightly earlier in the posterior area, with the exception of the eighth contraction. The intrauterine pressure is always equal to or higher than intramyometrial pressure readings. Reprinted from Cibils LA, Hendricks CH: Uterine contractility in the first day of puerperium. *Am J Obstet Gynecol* 103:238, 1969.

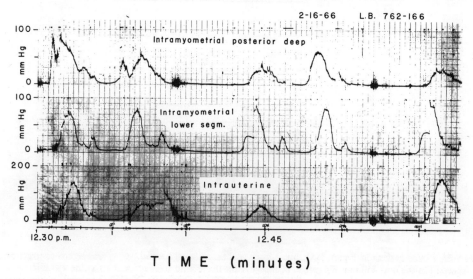

Figure 5-52 Simultaneous recordings of two widely separated *intramyometrial areas* and *intrauterine pressures* 17 hours after term vaginal delivery showing incoordination of myometrial activity. There is not good coincidence of peak contractions or regular proportion of contractions. Note the higher range and the small third and fourth contractions in the intrauterine tracing. Reprinted from Cibils LA, Hendricks CH: Uterine contractility in the first day of puerperium. *Am J Obstet Gynecol* 103:238, 1969.

INCOORDINATED MYOMETRIAL CONTRACTIONS EFFECT UNPREDICTABLY the INTRAUTERINE PRESSURE

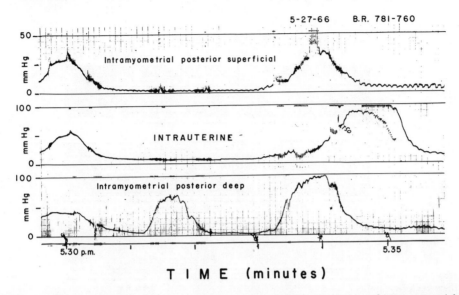

Figure 5-53 Simultaneous recordings of pressures of *intrauterine* and two *closely located intramyometrial* areas 6 hours after term delivery by cesarean section. The range in the top tracing is 0 to 50 mm Hg but in the others it is 0 to 100; the peak of the second intrauterine contraction was recorded at 0 to 250 mm Hg range. The paper was running faster than usual. The small contraction in deep myometrium is not expressed in the other recorded areas. Reprinted from Cibils LA, Hendricks CH: Uterine contractility in the first day of puerperium. *Am J Obstet Gynecol* 103:238, 1969.

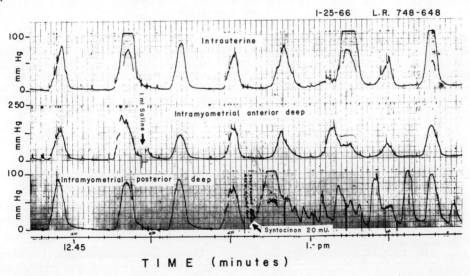

Figure 5-54 Same case as in Figure 5-51, but 1 hour earlier. *(Above)* Second, sixth, and eighth contraction peaks were recorded in the 0 to 250 mm Hg range. *(Center)* After the second contraction 1 ml saline was injected into the myometrium through the recording catheter without visible effect on pressures. Note the apparent coordination of the first four contractions with pressures starting on posterior catheter. *(Below)* At arrow 20 mU oxytocin in 0.5 ml saline was injected, followed by a very strong local contraction, the peak of which was recorded at 0 to 250 mm Hg. The series of rapid contractions does not seem to be reflected in the uterine cavity until the last strong one, when all three channels record a synchronized contraction. Reprinted from Cibils LA, Hendricks CH: Uterine contractility in the first day of puerperium. *Am J Obstet Gynecol* 103:238, 1969.

Evolution of Uterine Contractility throughout Pre-labor, Labor, and Post-Partum

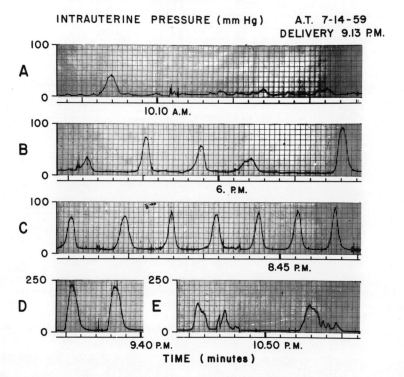

Figure 5-55 *First postpartum recording with open-end intrauterine catheter.* Representative tracings of various stages of uterine contractility in advanced pregnancy. *(A)* Typical *prelabor* pattern, followed in *(B)* by *early first stage* pattern. *(C)* Regular, maximally active pattern of *advanced first stage*. *(D) Early fourth stage,* followed in *(E)* by the breaking down pattern seen *several hours* after delivery. Here is shown the complete evolution of uterine contractility, from poorly effective prelabor pattern, increasing coordination and efficiency, followed by slow return to incoordination. Reprinted from Hendricks CH, et al: Uterine contractility at delivery and the puerperium. *Am J Obstet Gynecol* 83:890, 1962.

BIBLIOGRAPHY

Alvarez H, Caldeyro-Barcia R: Fisiopatología de la contracción uterina y sus aplicaciones en clínica obstétrica. *II Cong Lat-Am Obstet Ginecol (Brasil)* 1:1, 1954.

Alvarez H, Cibils LA, Gonzalez-Panizza VH: Cervical dilatation and uterine "work" in labour induced by oxytocin infusion, in Caldeyro-Barcia R, Heller H (eds): *Oxytocin.* NY, Pergamon, 1961, pp 203–211.

Arroyo J, Mendez-Bauer C: The maintenance of a stable baseline in intrauterine pressure with varying maternal position. A practical approach. *J Perinat Med* 3:129, 1975.

Bishop EH: Pelvic scoring for elective induction. *Obstet Gynecol* 24:266, 1964.

Caldeyro-Barcia R, Alvarez H, Poseiro JJ: Normal and abnormal uterine contractility in labor. *Triangle* 2:41, 1955.

Caldeyro-Barcia R, Alvarez H, Reynolds SRM: A better understanding of uterine contractility through simultaneous recording with an internal and seven channel external method. *Surg Gynecol Obstet* 91:641, 1950.

Caldeyro-Barcia R, Noriega-Guerra L, Cibils LA, et al: Effect of position changes on the intensity and frequency of uterine contractions during labor. *Am J Obstet Gynecol* 84:284, 1960.

Caldeyro-Barcia R, Sica-Blanco Y, Poseiro JJ, et al: A quantitative study of the action of synthetic oxytocin on the pregnant human uterus. *J Pharmacol Exp Ther* 121:18, 1957.

Cibils LA: Efecto de la rotura de las membranas en el parto inducido con ocitocina. *II Cong Uruguayo Ginecotocol* 2:346, 1957.

Cibils LA: Contractility of the non-pregnant human uterus. *Obstet Gynecol* 30:441, 1967.

Cibils LA: Effect of intrauterine contraceptive devices upon human uterine contractility. *J Reprod Med* 5:242, 1970.

Cibils LA: Enhancement and induction of labor, in Aladjem S (ed): *Risks in the Practice of Modern Obstetrics. II*. St Louis, Mosby, 1975, pp 182–210.

Cibils LA, Caldeyro-Barcia R, Carballo MA, et al: Uterine work during labor. *Proc 21st Int Cong Physiol (Buenos Aires)*, 1959, p 65.

Cibils LA, Hendricks CH: Normal labor in vertex presentation. *Am J Obstet Gynecol* 91:385, 1965.

Cibils LA, Hendricks CH: Uterine contractility in the first day of puerperium. *Am J Obstet Gynecol* 103:238, 1969.

Cibils LA, Hendricks CH: Effect of ergot derivatives and sparteine sulfate upon the human uterus. *J Reprod Med* 2:147, 1969.

Cibils LA, Noriega-Guerra L, Sala NL: Trabajo uterino y dilatacion cervical. Efectos de los cambios de posicion de la parturienta. *Proc V Jorn Rioplat Obstet Ginecol (Montevideo)*, Dec 1959.

Cibils LA, Spackman TJ: Caudal analgesia in first stage labor: Effect of uterine activity on the cardiovascular system. *Am J Obstet Gynecol* 84:1042, 1962.

Csapo A, Sauvage J: The evolution of uterine activity during human pregnancy. *Acta Obstet Gynecol Scand* 47:181, 1968.

Danforth DN: The distribution and functional activity of the cervical musculature. *Am J Obstet Gynecol* 68:1261, 1954.

Danforth DN, Buckingham JC: Connective tissue mechanisms and their relation to pregnancy. *Obstet Gynecol Surv* 19:715, 1964.

Danforth DN, Graham RL, Ivy AC: Functional anatomy of labor as revealed by frozen sagittal sections in Macaca rhesus monkeys. *Surg Gynecol Obstet* 74:188, 1942.

El-Sahwi S, Gaafar AA, Toppozada HK: A new unit for evaluation of uterine activity. *Am J Obstet Gynecol* 98:900, 1967.

Friedman EA: Primigravid labor: A graphico-statistical analysis. *Obstet Gynecol* 6:567, 1955.

Friedman EA: Labor in multiparas: A graphicostatistical analysis. *Obstet Gynecol* 8:691, 1956.

Friedman EA: *Labor: Clinical Evaluation and Management*. New York, Appleton-Century-Crofts, 1967.

Friedman EA, Sachtleben MR: Amniotomy and the course of labor. *Obstet Gynecol* 22:775, 1963.

Friedman EA, Von Wicsky LI: Electronic cervimeter: A research instrument for the study of cervical dilatation in labor. *Am J Obstet Gynecol* 87:789, 1963.

Haughton S: *Principles of Animal Mechanics*. London, Longmans, Green, 1873, pp 151–164.

Hendricks CH, Brenner WE, Kraus G: Normal cervical dilatation pattern in late pregnancy and labor. *Am J Obstet Gynecol* 106:1065, 1970.

Hendricks CH, Eskes TKAB, Saameli K: Uterine contractility at delivery and the puerperium. *Am J Obstet Gynecol* 83:890, 1962.

Hicks JB: On the contractions of the uterus throughout pregnancy. *Trans Obstet Soc Lond* 13:216, 1872.

Hon EH, Paul RH: Quantitation of uterine activity. *Obstet Gynecol* 42:368, 1973.

Huey JR, Miller FC: The evaluation of uterine activity. A comparative analysis. *Am J Obstet Gynecol* 135:252, 1979.

Langlois PL: The size of the normal uterus. *J Reprod Med* 4:220, 1970.

Lindgren L, Siener H: Cervical tension during labor. *Am J Obstet Gynecol* 95:414, 1966.

Mendez-Bauer C, Arroyo J, Garcia-Ramos C, et al: Effects of standing position on spontaneous uterine contractility and other aspects of labor. *J Perinat Med* 3:89, 1975.

Mendez-Bauer C, Arroyo J, Menendez A, et al: Effects of different maternal positions during labor, in Rooth G, Lars-Bratevy E (eds): *Perinatal Medicine*. Stockholm, Almqvist and Wiksell, 1976, pp 233–237.

Mendez-Bauer C, Arroyo J, Zamarriego J: Maternal standing position in first stage of labor, in Scarpelli EM, Cosmi E (eds): *Reviews in Perinatal Medicine*. Baltimore, University Park Press, 1976, pp 281–293.

Noriega-Guerra L, Cibils LA, Alvarez H, et al. Efectos de los cambios de posicion de la parturienta sobre la intensidad y frecuencia de las contracciones uterinas. *An Fac Med Montevideo (Uruguay)* 44:383, 1959.

Noriega-Guerra L, Pastelin JF, Arevalo N, et al: Las modificaciones cervicales producidas por la contraccion uterina. *Ginecol Obstet Mex* 22:1071, 1967.

Parikh MN, Mehta AC: Internal cervical os during the second half of pregnancy. *J Obstet Gynaecol Br Comwlth* 68:818, 1961.

Reynolds SRM, Harris JS, Kaiser IH: *Clinical Measurement of Uterine Forces in Pregnancy and Labor.* Springfield, Ill, Thomas, 1954.

Reynolds SRM, Heard OO, Burns P: Recording uterine contraction patterns in pregnant women: Application of the strain-gauge in a multichannel tokodynamometer. *Science* 106:427, 1947.

Sala N, Fielitz C, Mendez-Bauer CJ, et al: Quantitative relationship between uterine activity and the area beneath the amniotic pressure tracing. *Proc 21st Int Cong Physiol Sci (Buenos Aires)* 1959, p 241.

Schaffner F, Schanzer SN: Cervical dilatation in the early third trimester. *Obstet Gynecol* 27:130, 1966.

Schwalm H, Dubrauszky V: The structure of the musculature of the human uterus, muscles and connective tissue. *Am J Obstet Gynecol* 94:391, 1966.

Schwarcz R, Diaz AG, Belizan JM, et al: Influence of amniotomy and maternal position on labor. *Proc 8th World Cong Gynecol Obstet (Mexico).* Amsterdam, Excerpta Medica, 1976, pp 377–389.

Siener H: Cervical dynamometry. *Am J Obstet Gynecol* 89:579, 1964.

Van Praagh I, Hendricks CH: Effect of amniotomy during labor in multiparas. *Obstet Gynecol* 24:258, 1964.

CHAPTER 6
Abnormal Uterine Contractility

Although the range of normal contractions varies widely in the different stages of gestation, patterns clearly outside of those ranges have been recorded. When these patterns are analyzed in relation to the clinical condition under which they are observed, it is obvious that they are abnormal contractility patterns. Contractility can be abnormally low, excessive, or extremely irregular.

HYPOCONTRACTILITY

When recorded (or palpated) contractions during labor are of low intensity or poor frequency, the syndrome has been clinically defined as *hypotonic inertia*. Although it is a poor term, which refers to tonus rather than to effective labor contractility, it should be maintained for lack of a better one and because its meaning is well understood by clinicians. When the uterus is of term size (approximately 5000 ml intrauterine content) and *the intensity of contractions is less than 30 mm Hg* or *recurring less often than every 5 min* in presumed established labor, the pattern is clearly of *hypocontracility*. Even if these contractions effectively dilate the cervix every time they occur, the uterine work per hour will be in the range of 300 to 400 mm Hg, much below the calculated one of 1000 to 1500 mm Hg in normal labors. Uterine activity may be inadequate from the moment a labor is presumed to have started; this is called *primary uterine inertia. Secondary uterine inertia* occurs more often and may follow periods of satisfactory contractility.

It is not very well understood why the activity of some uteri does not develop spontaneously. Several hypotheses have been propounded to attempt to explain this phenomenon, from postulates that implicate insufficient glucose supply to the myometrium, to exhaustion of the muscle, or

the protective response of a uterus to a mechanical obstruction that may lead to its rupture. There is no scientific observation that supports any of the numerous proposed explanations for primary or secondary inertia. These uteri are capable of regaining their ability to contract effectively, with normal strength and frequency, when they are stimulated by the proper dose of indicated medications (see Chapters 9 and 10). Clinically, the two types of inertia are similar: patients feel very little discomfort, the contractions are weak and sporadic, and, for practical purposes, *the labor has been arrested*. When the curve of cervical dilatation is plotted against time, one sees that a plateau is established and that it can be corrected only by the active intervention of the obstetrician by either mechanical interference or pharmacologic stimulation.

External recordings are not adequate to make a definitive diagnosis of uterine hypocontractility unless the clinician palpates each contraction recorded and estimates its quality and duration. Internal monitoring without extraneous noise is ideal for making the diagnosis because it yields precise measurement of the intensity of contractions.

INCOORDINATED ACTIVITY

As shown in Chapter 5, the normal contraction is characterized by the *triple descending gradient*, or *fundal dominance*. When one or more of the elements constituting the gradient is absent in a contraction it is said that it is *incoordinated*. Thus there may be several types of incoordination—a possibility that, in fact, is confirmed by experience. Furthermore, the incoordinated contractions may be either localized or generalized (that is, involving the whole uterus).

Generalized Contractions

These contractions do not appear much different from normal contractions when both are recorded by an intrauterine catheter. They may be distinguished only by simultaneous intramyometrial pressures. The abnormal contraction does not start in the fundal region but in a lower area of the corpus. It propagates in all directions with normal speed. Therefore, the pulling effect against the cervix is dampened by a similar pulling effect against the not yet contracting (and elastic) fundal myometrium, which consequently gives up until enough stimulation reaches it to make it contract firmly, and even then it pulls only from the weaker lower regions (Figure 6-1). The complete contraction cycle usually lasts as long as a normal one; therefore, the effective pulling from the lower segment is shorter and thus of diminished efficiency. The *time gradient* (duration) is abnormal because the contraction lasts longer around the middle of the corpus where the contraction started. It follows that the *propagation gradient* is also abnormal because, in part, the stimulus spreads upward to reach the fundus. The only *gradient normally* maintained is *strength,* which is responsible for the slow but observable progress seen in these cases. This description explains why these contractions do not look abnormal in an intrauterine tracing.

Localized Contractions

The failure of a contraction stimulus to propagate over the whole uterus determines the occurrence of regional or localized contractions, which are unable to effect the pulling action over the lower segment; their tension is dampened by the elasticity of the noncontracting areas of the myometrium. This irregular or incomplete contraction, which may be locally very strong, results in only a moderate increase in intrauterine pressure. Furthermore, if the noncontracting region starts a contraction while the other area is relaxing, the intrauterine pressure will not reach the "resting" level seen under normal circumstances. The occurrence of contractions limited to partial areas of the myometrium constitutes the *syndrome of incoordinated uterine contractility,* which has a characteristic appearance on intrauterine pressure tracings (Figure 6-2). A representation of the observations made in cases of moderate incoordination depicts alternating contractions of uneven extent and distribution, which produce an irregular pattern of intrauterine pressure changes (Figure 6-3). It has been postulated that this pattern of contractions could be caused by the fact that the propagated contraction wave reaches an area in the *refractory period* that is unable to respond and thus blocking it. Because of their alternating manner of occur-

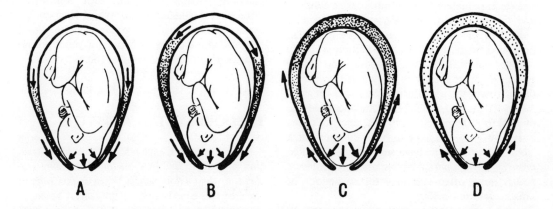

Figure 6-1 Diagram representing a contraction starting in the middle of the corpus. Dotted area indicates contraction, and concentration of dots, the *strength* of the contraction. *(A)* Arrows point in the direction of the pull with the noncontracting and elastic fundus giving in. *(B)* Contraction propagates upward, and less area of elastic muscle dampens the pulling effect. *(C)* Arrows change direction because the whole organ is contracting as in a normal, well-coordinated contraction; the stronger fundus predominates. *(D)* Relaxation is uniform and simultaneous. Size of arrows depicts degree of pulling and, when over the fetal head, degree of pushing against the cervix. Reprinted from Caldeyro-Barcia R, et al: *Triangle, Sandoz Journal of Medical Science* 2:41, 1955.

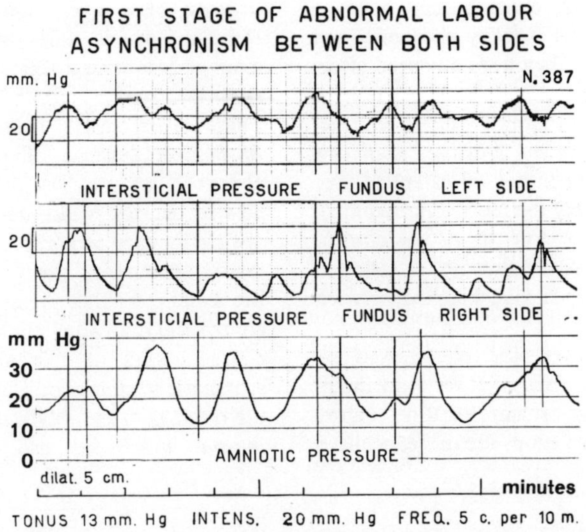

FIRST STAGE OF ABNORMAL LABOUR
ASYNCHRONISM BETWEEN BOTH SIDES

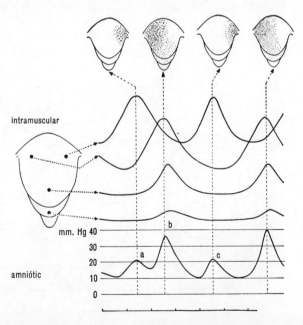

Figure 6-2 Simultaneous recordings during first stage of abnormal term labor. *(Above and center)* Tracings with intramyometrial microballoons, left and right sides of fundus. *(Below)* With intrauterine open-end catheter. Note the irregular profile of intramniotic pressure changes with its high resting pressure (points preceding the contraction) and the unequal duration of the contractions. The careful study of intramyometrial catheters reveals independent contractions that only occasionally coincide in relaxing simultaneously. The calculated values of activity are given at the bottom. This tracing is *characteristic of incoorindated activity.* Reprinted from Alvarez and Caldeyro-Barcia (1954).

Figure 6-3 Diagrammatic summary of the concept of *moderate incoordinated contraction* recorded with intramyometrial catheters. *(Above)* Uteri with dotted areas representing contracting activity. *(Left)* Points where the intramyometrial catheters were implanted and connected to the respective tracings. *(Below)* Intraamniotic pressure tracing. At *(a)* and *(c)* localized contraction of the left cornual region produces a high local pressure but with only minor effect on the amniotic pressure. At *(b)* contraction of right cornual region, of equal intensity, propagates to a larger area including lower corpus and lower segment thus having a much higher pressure reading in the amniotic tracing. Propagation is blocked at the left cornu because it is probably in refractory period. The pattern is characteristic of moderate incoordinated activity. Reprinted from Caldeyro-Barcia R et al: *Triangle, Sandoz Journal of Medical Science* 2:41, 1955.

114

rence these localized contractions have a pendular-like pattern of activity that may not change spontaneously. They have a limited effect over the lower uterine segment (compare Figures 6-3 and 5-22) because the intensity of the contraction, measured by recorded pressure, is of low amplitude even for the contraction extended over the largest area. Probably the most common incoordinated pattern observed in clinical obstetrics is that of a weak contraction following, or followed by, a stronger one with a high baseline between them.

A still more abnormal pattern, observed less often, is frequent contractions of very low intensity with a high resting pressure or tone (Figure 6-4). The areas of contractions are more localized because there is very limited propagation of the stimulus, which starts in a completely erratic manner over several regions of the uterus. For this type of severe incoordination, Alvarez and Caldeyro-Barcia (1954) reserved the label *uterine fibrillation* because of its similarity with the abnormal contractility of the myocardium thus labeled. In this syndrome an area of the uterus is always in state of contraction, and therefore the lowest intrauterine pressure is significantly above the average resting pressure observed in normal contractility; an apparent hypertonus is one of the characteristics of this abnormal pattern. The schematic summary of Figure 6-4 looks similar to the tracings often obtained in cases of *hypertonic inertia,* which are also characterized by high

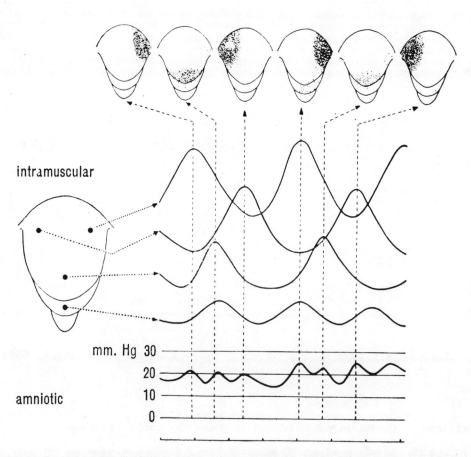

Figure 6-4 Diagram and symbols as in Figure 6-3. *Severe incoordination* characteristic of *hypertonic inertia.* Localized contractions have only minimal **expression** on the amniotic pressure. Because all four areas contract independently, the resting pressure is never less than 15 mm Hg and the amniotic pressure tracing shows only minimal contractions of very high frequency. Reprinted from Caldeyro-Barcia R, et al: *Triangle, Sandoz Journal of Medical Science* 2:41, 1955.

resting pressure, small, frequent, and irregular contractions that usually cause marked discomfort to the patient during a very ineffective labor. This inefficiency is a logical consequence of the localized contractions, which, although strong, pull from noncontracting and thus elastic myometrium without affecting the lower segment (Figure 6-5). This elasticity is also responsible for the very marked dampening effect on the intensity of the intrauterine pressure and the irregular profile of the contractility pattern (Figure 6-6).

The diagnosis of incoordinated patterns can be made from an adequate artifact-free intrauterine tracing as long as all its elements are studied

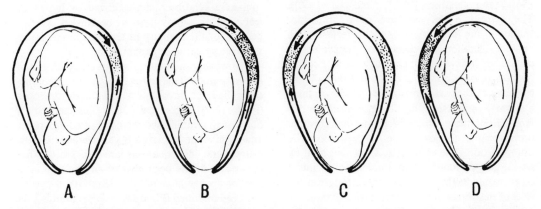

Figure 6-5 Diagram and symbols as in Figure 6-1. *Severe incoordination*. Localized contractions pull from the neighboring myometrium (arrows) with negligible effect on the lower segment and cervix. Reprinted from Caldeyro-Barcia R, et al: *Triangle, Sandoz Journal of Medical Science* 2:41, 1955.

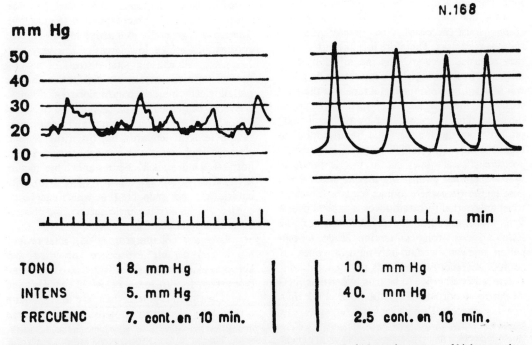

Figure 6-6 Intrauterine pressure tracings during labor, term pregnancy. *(Left)* Irregular pattern of high tonus, low intensity, and high frequency very much like one of hypertonic inertia. *(Right)* Change to one of normal-looking activity after receiving spinal anesthesia. Reprinted from Alvarez and Caldeyro-Barcia (1954).

carefully. There is a complete range of incoordinated patterns, from the most simple, characterized by bigeminal unequal contractions, to classic fully established hypertonic inertia. An accurate diagnosis is essential before taking the therapeutic steps aimed at correcting the abnormality.

A different type of incoordinated activity has been described by a number of Swedish authors (Borell and Ferstrom [1959], Lindgren [1960]). They postulate the existence of a "muscular spasm" in the *lower segment* that interferes with cervical dilatation and descent of the presenting part. They believe that this pattern is, as a consequence, responsible for prolonged labors. Interestingly, in their judgment, the effects of these abnormal contractions on the fetal head are different from those produced by normal contractions trying to overcome a cephalopelvic disproportion. The contractions, as measured by strain gauges mounted in tandem over metal tapes, would be three to four times stronger at the level of maximum head circumference than in the uterine cavity. However, since the lower segment is significantly thinner and poorer in muscle cells per unit of weight than the corpus, it is difficult to understand the interpretation they advance for their observations. Furthermore, the radius of the lower segment is smaller than in the areas situated above it, and therefore the *tension exerted* by the *corpus* must necessarily be *greater* than in the lower segment. Therefore it is likely that what they recorded were artifacts magnified by their method of measuring the pressures: their gauge was situated between the metal tape and the hard surface of the skull and received the pressure of the head directly transmitted by the fetal body pushed from the fundus. This finding does not represent the real, evenly distributed, intrauterine pressure (Pascal's law) but in fact is the *local pressure exerted against the uterine wall* by the head on the areas where contact is made. (Similarly when an external tocotransducer is applied over a fetal limb, extraordinary displacement of the stylus suggests strong contractions when, by palpation, one can ascertain only moderate ones.) If appropriate recording methods are used, this syndrome may well prove to be true hypertonic inertia due to incoordinated contractions rather than one of paradoxically high regional pressure.

HYPERCONTRACILITY

Contractions characterized by *excessive intensity or exaggerated frequency* constitute the syndrome of *uterine hypercontractility*—which may be either iatrogenic or observed to appear spontaneously without an apparent trigger. Its spontaneous occurrence may represent the symptom of a syndrome characterized by hypercontractility, or it may have to be labeled *essential* because of the inability of the clinician to find a satisfactory cause to explain it.

Probably the most frequent cause of *uterine hypercontractility is iatrogenic,* the excessive, uncontrolled, or involuntary misuse of oxytocics (Figure 6-7). These cases are characterized by polysystoly, diminished intensity of contractions, and significant hypertonus, all leading to fetal distress and inadequate progress of labor. They may occur at the beginning of an oxytocin infusion or appear later after an established pattern has been obtained (Figure 6-8). Discontinuing the exogenous stimulus is generally followed by recovery of a normal pattern of contractions.

One of the most severe syndromes observed in obstetrics, *abruptio placentae* (separation of a normally implanted placenta), is typically manifested by excessive uterine activity with the most classic pattern of hypercontractility (Figure 6-9). The tonus is generally well above 15 mm Hg; the contractions are of low intensity and very high frequency, all causing fetal distress of varying degree. Both the excessively high tonus and the pathologically frequent contractions contribute to a severely decreased IVS blood flow and thus fetal hypoxia and asphyxia. Prompt intervention may save a fetus in jeopardy but often the fetus is already dead when the patient arrives at the hospital. Under such circumstances the picture is classical—*board-like* uterus (Figure 6-10), with contractions not palpable (but which can be recorded with an intrauterine catheter), and absence of audible fetal heart tones.

Cobo and collaborators (1965), after reviewing a considerable experience, observed that abruptio placentae may be divided into two broad types: type I, with tonus below 30 mm Hg, and type II, with tonus greater than 30 mm Hg (Figure 6-11). They described moreover, the different

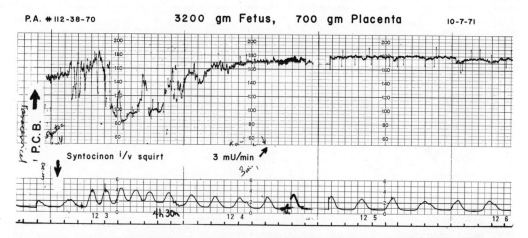

P.A. # 112-38-70   3200 gm Fetus,   7oo gm Placenta   10-7-71

Syntocinon i/v squirt   3 mU/min

Figure 6-7 *Transient iatrongenic hypercontractility* at the beginning of an oxytocin infusion in term multipara at 6 cm dilatation; 37-min tracing illustrates sudden hypertonus and polysystoly (hypercontractility). The excessive amount of the drug triggered the dangerous response with corresponding transient fetal distress (top tracing). Uterine activity became normal after oxytocin infusion was decreased. Reprinted from Cibils LA, Santonja-Lucas JJ: Clinical significance of fetal heart rate patterns during labor. III. Effect of parcervical block. *Am J Obstet Gynecol* 130:73, 1978.

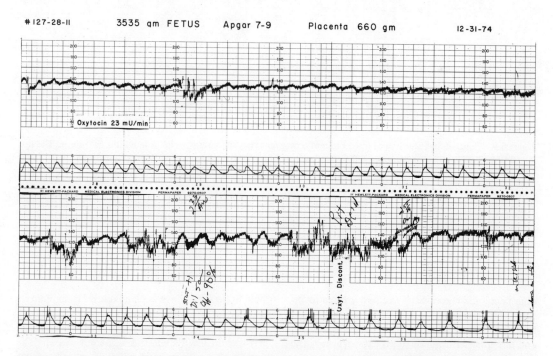

127-28-11   3535 gm FETUS   Apgar 7-9   Placenta 660 gm   12-31-74

Oxytocin 23 mU/min

Figure 6-8 *Prolonged iatrogenic hypercontractility.* Enhanced labor in term multipara receiving oxytocin 23 mU/min. Continuous 100-min recording illustrates, upper tracing, the polysystoly (6 contractions/10 min) and hypertonus (average 20 mm Hg) produced by unphysiologic infusion of oxytocin. The same pattern continues on the left side of lower tracing. The excessive activity diminished only after the oxytocin infusion was discontinued. Note rapid drop of frequency and tonus and improvement of FHR tracing, which had had signs of distress during the period of hypercontractility.

118

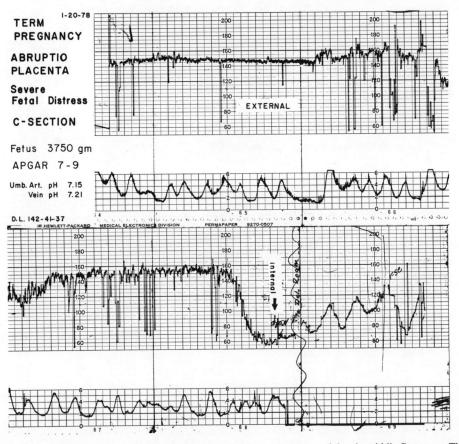

Figure 6-9 Continuous recording of last 53 min of term pregnancy, spontaneous labor in middle first stage. The upper tracing (external recordings) illustrates marked uterine polysystoly with a high fluctuating baseline and fixed FHR baseline. Same pattern on left half of lower tracing until severe fetal bradycardia mandated amniotomy and internal monitoring. The patient was rushed to the delivery room; the direct FHR recorded severe bradycardia with superimposed late decelerations and fixed baseline (severe fetal distress). Immediate cesarean section produced a moderately acidotic infant with good Apgar scores. A retroplacental clot of moderate size was found when the placenta was removed confirming the diagnosis of *abruptio placentae*.

pharmacologic response of the two groups to intravenous oxytocin. A few cases with minimal hypertonus may be found (Figure 6-12) but, by and large, hypertonus of significant degree is the characteristic of this syndrome. The cause of the hypercontractility seems to be that the retroplacental clot acting as a foreign body irritates the myometrium. This explanation is supported by the observation that hypercontractility and hypertonus are usually in direct proportion to the size of the retroplacental clot (Figure 6-13). However, there is no known cause for the actual separation of the placenta even though innumer-

able hypotheses have been advanced to explain it.

Occurring less often, but with a frequency that constitutes a serious problem, is *essential hypercontractility* without apparent cause. The condition covers a wide range of severity, from benign and easily correctable with a change in patient's position (see Figure 5-29), to the really severe requiring immediate intervention to save the fetus (Figure 6-14). From studying the tracings, it is impossible to distinguish these cases from genuine abruptio placentae, which are ruled out only after third stage when the absence of retroplacental clots can be demonstrated.

INTRAUTERINE FETAL DEATH VAGINAL DELIVERY
Fetus 2690 gm   Placenta 650 gm
8000 gm RETROPLACENTAL CLOT

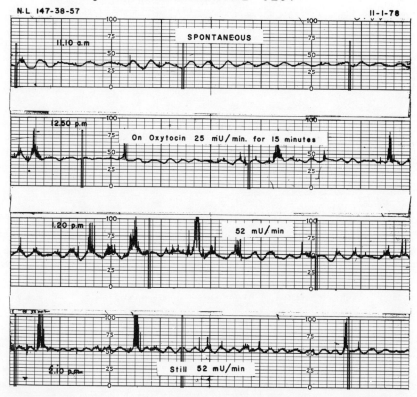

Figure 6-10 *Severe abruptio placentae* at 36 weeks gestation. Multipara admitted in spontaneous labor, fetus was dead. Four different sections, each 32 minutes uterine activity, show increasingly severe hypertonus (from 22 mm Hg to 50 mm Hg) and extreme polysystoly. Clinical observation was "board-like sustained tetanic contraction." Complete lack of response to very high doses of oxytocin. The total blood behind the placenta weighed 8000 gm.

OBSTRUCTED LABOR

The mechanical interference with the engagement and/or descent of the presenting part is the cause of arrest of labor, called *obstructed labor* because a *physical obstacle prevents its further progress*. A pathologic relationship between the birth passage and fetus is the direct cause of obstruction of labor, such as a birth canal of small diameter, tumors preventing the engagement or descent of the presenting part, malposition of the presenting part (deflections, asynclitism) offering diameters too large for a normal birth canal, or abnormal fetal lies (oblique, transverse) with absolute mechanical obstruction.

The most frequently observed is the syndrome of cephalopelvic disproportion (CPD) in which relatively minor alterations in shape and/or diameter of the birth canal create too tight a passage for a presenting part, also may have altered mechanical adaptation, compounding the situation. Regardless of the degree of disproportion or maladaptation, the problem for the "powers" (uterine corpus) is the same: a struggle against a mechanical obstacle that does not permit the passage of the presenting part. Under those circumstances and with a uterus in good condition, the lower segment will be steadily thinned out and the cervix dilated as a consequence of the coordinated contractions recurring with regularity. The slow but continued upward stretching of the lower segment is simultaneously accompanied

120

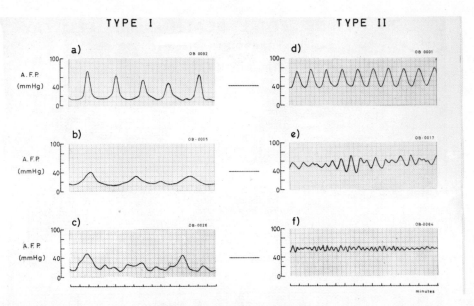

Figure 6-11 The two broad groups of abruptio placentae, classified by uterine activity. Type I: *(a)* normal-appearing, *(b)* low, and *(c)* incoordinated activity. Type II: the severe hypertonus group with increasing polysystoly and diminished intensity from *(d)* to *(f)*. Reprinted from Cobo E, et al: Uterine behavior in abruptio placentae. *Am J Obstet Gynecol* 93:1151, 1965.

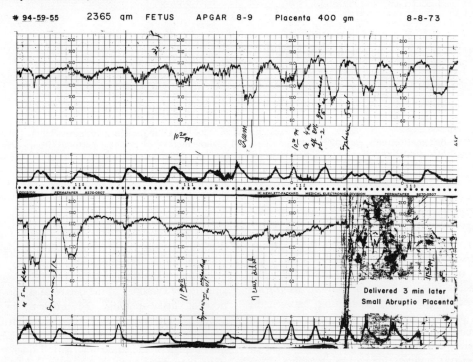

Figure 6-12 Continuous 80-min recording of enhanced labor in patient with vaginal bleeding at 34 weeks gestation. On the upper tracing, with 5 mU/min oxytocin, moderate intensity and frequency of contractions trigger worsening late decelerations and rising baseline (fetal hypoxia, placental insufficiency?). When oxytocin was discontinued, start of lower tracing, the frequency diminished drastically, but oxytocin had to be restarted 14 minutes later; labor progressed rapidly with delivery of an infant with very good Apgar score. Small abruptio placentae was confirmed at delivery of the placenta. Reprinted from Cibils LA: Clinical significance of fetal heart rate patterns during labor. II. Late decelerations. *Am J Obstet Gynecol* 123:473, 1975.

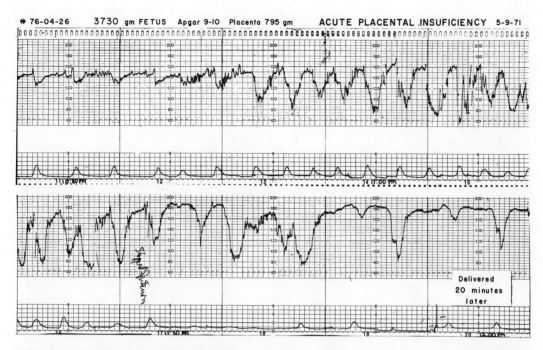

Figure 6-13 Continuous 100 minutes of uterine contractions and FHR monitoring of a term induced labor. Moderate uterine activity and rather unimpressive FHR pattern suddenly changes into one of deteriorating fetal distress. There is some increase in uterine activity but well within a normal pattern of intensity, frequency, and tonus. Oxytocin was discontinued, (lower left), and the contractions diminished in frequency and intensity (note three unrecorded contractions because of catheter obstruction). Cesarean section performed 20 min later revealed an *occult abruptio placentae* not suggested by the contractility pattern. Reprinted from Cibils LA: Clinical significance of fetal heart rate patterns during labor. II. Late decelerations. *Am J Obstet Gynecol* 123:473, 1975.

by a *retraction* of the corpus, which increases in thickness little by little with each contraction. As the presenting part cannot move downward, the inevitable consequence is the disproportionate thinning of the lower segment (formed predominantly by connective tissue at this stage), and the exaggerated thickness of the powerful muscular walls of the corpus. This unequal struggle promotes an ever-accelerating development of the described pathologic condition of the uterine walls (Figure 6-15). Usually the uterine contractions continue with the same frequency and increased intensity, further accelerating the process of reaching the inevitable outcome: rupture of the lower segment unless there is intervention to prevent it. The syndrome thus developed is characterized, clinically, by the appearance over the anterior uterine wall of a clear division *between the corpus and the lower segment* in the form of a transverse depression, *Bandl's ring.* At the same time, the round ligaments are visible and palpable

because the retraction of the fundal area pulls their insertion upward — a sign of the same syndrome originally described by Frommel. These elements together — appearance of the Bandl's ring, palpation of the round ligaments, vigorous uterine contractions, and arrest of the descent of the presenting parts — constitute the *syndrome of distended lower segment,* a most dangerous condition because it ends in disaster unless timely intervention prevents it. It may present itself with dilatation at any stage, from minimal to complete (Figures 6-16 and 6-17), in spite of the popular mythical belief that somehow the uterus will recognize early in labor the presence of the obstruction and will go into secondary inertia.

Among the many causes of spontaneously diminished uterine activity (and they are probably numerous) obstructed labor is definitely not one of them. Were it so, it would be impossible to observe spontaneous rupture of the uterus, a most serious condition still periodically observed in the

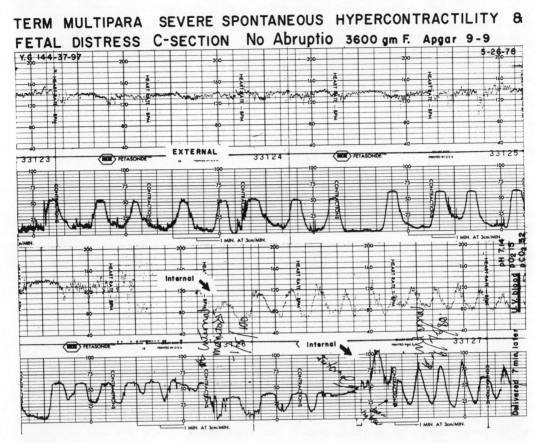

Figure 6-14 Continuous 65 min uterine contractions and FHR monitoring of a term spontaneous labor. The upper tracings, obtained by external methods, illustrate a good FHR and completely normal contractility pattern, three to four per 10 min, and good relaxation. This followed, in the lower tracings, by sudden *hypercontractility* with contractions recurring every 90 sec and marked *hypertonus*. Direct monitoring of FHR revealed overlapping late decelerations; the intrauterine recording of contractions *(right)* confirmed the *polysystoly* and *hypertonus*. Cesarean section, 7 min later, produced an acidotic infant with good Apgar scores. Surprisingly, there was *no evidence of abruptio placentae*. The preoperative diagnosis had to be changed to idiopathic hypercontractility.

practice of clinical obstetrics. Very often, one may see the contractions in an obstructed labor becoming stronger as the time goes by, reaching unusually high values in spite of clearly irregular patterns. Of course, obstructed labors with the fetus in the longitudinal lie are seen mainly with term size fetuses (and thus term size uterine volume). In other words, the high intrauterine pressure recorded is not due to the small diameter of the uterine ovoid but to the strength of the contracting muscle.

Another popularized myth is the so-called *uterine contracture*. The uterus, by its nature, cannot sustain an isotonic contraction for a prolonged period of time and therefore its contracture is a physiologic impossibility. It is possible to

see a uterus with exceedingly high tonus (see Figure 6-10), which, on palpation, feels as if it is in a state of continuous uninterrupted contraction, but in fact has superimposed a rhythmic activity clearly recorded with intrauterine catheters.

PROBLEMS OF THIRD STAGE

The abnormal contrctility of the uterus after delivery of the infant may create series problems related to the third stage of labor and the period immediately following it. The causes may be related to either excessive and/or irregular contractility or to insufficient uterine contractions.

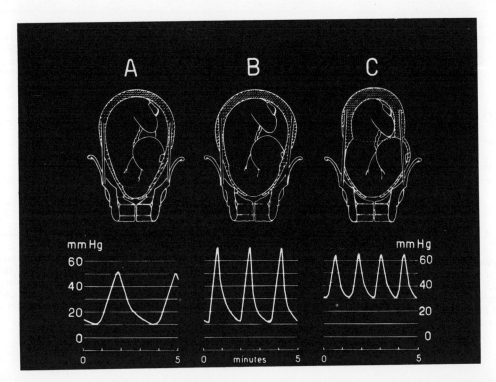

Figure 6-15 Schematic representation of uterine contractions and myometrial changes occurring in *obstructed labor* (shoulder presentation). *(A)* Normal relationships of corpus and lower segment (dotted line above the cervix), with early labor pattern of contractions, accomplishing cervical effacement. *(B)* The mechanical obstacle causes arrest in descent, but the strong uterine contractions continue and with them the lower segment is further thinned out and the corpus gains in thickness; the limit between the two rises (dotted line). *(C)* Fully developed prerupture syndrome: extremely thin lower segment, limit with corpus very high and marked by an external groove (Bandl's ring) further exaggerated by the fetus through the very thin lower segment. The insertion of the round ligaments has been pulled upward, and they become tense (Frommel's sign). The contractility is exaggerated, with polysystoly on occasions. Reprinted from Caldeyro-Barcia (1958).

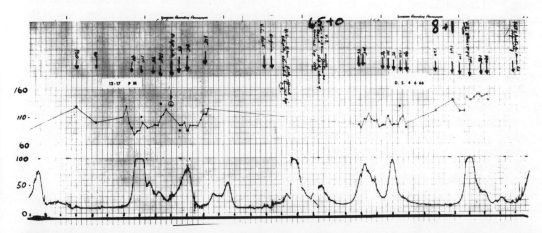

Figure 6-16 Advanced first stage in term spontaneous labor. Thirty-two minutes of intrauterine pressure recording showing extremely strong contractions, some above the range of 100 mm Hg, and a strikingly irregular pattern. The FHR recorded by ECG and calculated has been marked on the middle channel, and the FHR obtained by auscultation noted at the arrows in the upper channel. At the end of the tracing, dilatation is 8 cm, + 1 station.

124

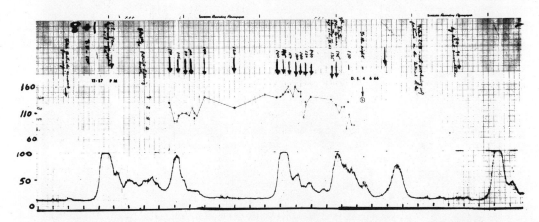

Figure 6-17 Continuation of tracing shown in Figure 6-16 after a 10-min interruption. The extremely strong contractions are extremely irregular and last over 2 min, causing sustained baseline elevations for prolonged periods of time. The FHR continued to be irregular with episodes of bradycardia. The bizarre pattern accomplished full dilatation but the *fetus failed to descend.* Cesarean section for *obstructed labor* through a *very thin lower segment* produced a 4100 gm mildly depressed infant with significant caput succedaneum. These extremely high intrauterine pressures are almost never seen in term size uteri.

Retained Placenta

The failure of the placenta to be expelled within 30 min of delivery of the infant determines the diagnosis of *retention of the placenta* (see Figure 5-49). This syndrome is caused by either *incomplete separation* of the placenta or by its *incarceration* after separation. The normal physiology of the process of third stage (see Figure 5-48) is coordinated to avoid this type of complication: the normal coordinated contractions of second stage continue uninterrupted after the fetus is born but with a marked retraction all around of the corpus, which promotes the "sliding" separation of the placenta from its area of implanation. *If contraction of the myometrium* over the placental bed is *inadequate,* local retraction will be insufficient, and the placenta will fail to separate in the absence of the normal mechanical disruption that leads to the "sliding" of the adjacent uterine-placental surfaces. Of course, this type of abnormality ranges in severity, the extreme being labeled *uterine atony.* In these cases, intraplacental pressures are recorded as mild contractions (remember the small size of the cavity at this stage) of low frequency—a pattern that may continue for a long time unless the clinician intervenes. Most frequently, the cause of this syndrome is unknown (spontaneous) but occasionally it may be caused by exogenously administered uterine relaxants (see Chapter 9).

The other mechanism of retained placenta is irregular hypercontractility in which the placenta, either partly or completely separated, is *trapped* within the uterus by bands or rings of contractions that compartmentalize its cavity. It is as if the contractility pattern that will develop later in postpartum, (see Chapter 5, Fourth Stage) sets in prematurely, and thus causes the pathologic syndrome. Frequently, the ring is located low in the corpus, trapping only part of the placenta, the remainder being palpated in the lower segment. It is not possible to say whether there is a combination of two patterns of abnormal contractility: partial hypocontractility over the placental insertion and irregular bands in lower regions. It is certainly theoretically possible and it may well occur in a number of cases.

Postpartum Atony

The insufficient, inadequate, and poor contractions of the uterus observed after the delivery of the fetus may or may not be accompanied by severe bleeding. When there is no separation of the placenta, there is no disruption of the spiral arterioles, and therefore no bleeding occurs; this is often labelled *placental retention*. Frequently, however, contractility becomes inadequate or absent and occurs after the placenta has been partially separated, in which case severe bleeding takes place. This is the classic manifestation of the syndrome known as *uterine atony*. The failure of the myometrium to clamp the spiral arterioles (and perhaps also their failure to retract) causes them to remain wide open and therefore to bleed profusely. The most frequent cause of the latter abnormal pattern is the injudicious use of uterine relaxant drugs (anesthetics) at the time of mechanical (manual) separation of the placenta and thus opening of the spiral arteriolar bed.

The insertion of the placenta in the lower segment may partly mimic the syndrome of uterine atony because it can cause significant bleeding from the spiral arteriolar bed, which occupies the lower segment. This, being mainly collagenous, does not contract, and therefore hemostasis depends entirely on the retraction of the spiral arterioles, which constitutes only part of the normal mechanism involved in postpartum hemostasis. Usually the corpus is in a state of firm contraction, which may be ascertained by palpation. The history of the pregnency and the inspection of the placenta should help in making the diagnosis of the cause of this severe bleeding complication.

BIBLIOGRAPHY

Alvarez H, Caldeyro-Barcia R: Fisiopatologia de la contraccion uterina y sus aplicaciones en clinica obstetrica. *II Cong Lat-Am Obstet Ginecol (Brasil)* 1:1, 1954.

Borell U, Fernstrom I: X-ray diagnosis of muscular spasm in the lower part of the uterus from the degree of moulding of the fetal head. *Acta Obstet Gynecol Scand* 38:181, 1959.

Caldeyro-Barcia R: Uterine contractility in obstetrics. *II Int Cong Gynecol Obstet (Montreal)* 1:65, 1958.

Caldeyro-Barcia R, Alvarez H, Poseiro JJ: Normal and abnormal uterine contractility in labor. *Triangle* 2:41, 1955.

Cibils LA: Clinical significance of fetal heart rate patterns during labor. II. Late decelerations. *Am J Obstet Gynecol* 123:473, 1975.

Cibils LA, Santonja-Lucas JJ: Clinical significance of fetal heart rate patterns during labor. III. Effect of paracervical block. *Am J Obstet Gynecol* 130:73, 1978.

Cobo E, Quintero CA, Strada G, et al: Uterine behavior in abruptio placentae. *Am J Obstet Gynecol* 93:1151, 1965.

Lindgren L: The causes of fetal head moulding in labour. *Acta Obstet Gynecol Scand* 39:46, 1960.

CHAPTER 7
Systemic Effects of Contractions

The contraction of a large muscular organ like the uterus has to have significant systemic repercussions particularly because a very large proportion of the cardiac output, supplying the IVS circulation, passes through it. Almost every bodily system or apparatus is affected by the contractions of the uterus, but only those directly involved in sustaining fetal life (cardiovascular system) and those related to the painful reactions produced by the contractions or interventions to control the pain (central nervous system) are reviewed here.

CARDIOVASCULAR SYSTEM

Intervillous Space

A specialized part of the cardiovascular tree, the IVS depends completely on the activity of the uterine muscle, because its blood supply is furnished through the uterine walls penetrated by the branches of the uterine artery. Thus a strong contraction of the myometrium clamps the arteries and stops the blood flow to the IVS. This aspect of the placental circulation has been extensively studied in pregnant monkeys (Ramsey et al, 1963, 1966; Freese et al, 1966) and in various stages of human pregnancy (Borell et al, 1964, 1965; Bieniarz et al, 1966, 1968) who injected a radio-opaque contrast medium in the lower aorta and obtained either rapid serial angiographic or cineradiographic films. The following paragraphs summarize the basic physiologic process clarified by those investigators.

A strong uterine contraction in *midgestation* is capable of blocking the blood flow to the IVS and the outflow of the uteroplacental veins (Figure 7-1), a flow that is free and wide open when the uterus is in a state of relaxation. In a very few seconds the dye injected in the aorta clears the main arterial trunks and appears in the veins draining the placental bed. In *term gestation* the vascular tree and the IVS space are outlined in perfect detail when the contrast medium is injected with the uterus in a state of relaxation (Figure 7-2); the number of arterial entries and cotyledons may be mapped and counted, and the time to clear the dye may be studied. The effect of contraction is a drastic curtailment by fewer vascular tree elements visualized and far fewer cotyledons injected (Figure 7-3).

In general, the stronger the contraction, the more evident these effects. However, there have been occasions when even moderate contractions have succeeded in blocking much of the IVS blood supply. When a contraction compounds its local intramyometrial effect with a compression of the aorta and/or iliac arteries the blood cutoff to the IVS may be nearly complete (Figure 7-4). This single effect of strong contractions has two important and different results: 1) By temporarily cutting the supply of oxygenated blood to the IVS, it puts the fetus in the position to utilize its own oxygen reserves until new fresh blood flows again for exchange; 2) the blood flow through the low-resistance arteriovenous fistula IVS constitutes about 17% of the cardiac output which, when cut off, has to be redistributed immediately or rerouted, causing major problems of hemodynamic adaptation. These are expressed in the cardiovascular reponse to the contractions reviewed below.

Blood Pressure and Pulse Rate

The most striking systemic effect of a strong uterine contraction is the marked increase in systolic and diastolic pressures with the concomitant slowing down in pulse rate (Figure 7-5). The range of responses is wide, depending on the sub-

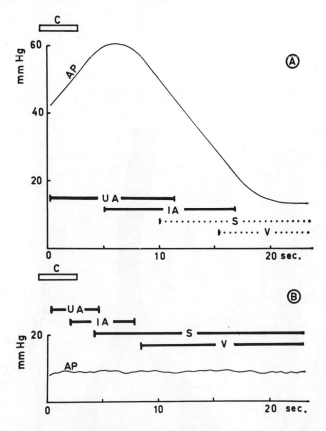

Figure 7-1 Schematic representation of blood flow taken from serial arterioplacentograms during *(A)* a *uterine contraction* and *(B) relaxation in midpregnancy.* The thin lines AP are the tracing of intrauterine pressure. The bars C, left, are the time of contrast injection. UA is the time the uterine artery is visulaized, and IA the intramural arteries. S indicates seeing contrast in the IVS: and V in the uterine veins. In *(A)* S and V are indicated by dotted lines because they are faintly visible in only a few cases studied. Reprinted from Borell U, et al: Effect of uterine contractions on the human uteroplacental blood circulation. *Am J Obstet Gynecol* 89:881, 1964.

ject, her position, the type and amount of medication received, and so on. It has been estimated that between 10% and 15% of pregnant women in advanced gestation have the supine hypotensive syndrome—that is, a significant drop in both systolic and diastolic pressures when they adopt the supine position while recumbent. (The absence of this response in the majority of cases indicates variations that have no clear explanation.) However, a given subject, when maintaining a position, will have the repetitive arterial pressure changes which will be in proportion to the intensity of the contractions (Figure 7-6). On the other hand, by and large a change of position of the subject brings about clear alterations in that regular pattern recorded, and a distinct new pattern is established (Figure 7-7; see also Figure

5-16). The pulse rate tends to mirror the changes observed in the blood pressure (Figures 7-6 and 7-7) but in rare cases marked pressure changes are accompanied by only modest fluctuations in pulse rate (Figure 7-5) and therefore significant alterations in the workload of the myocardium.

The recording of blood pressure in the upper and lower limbs is important in understanding some otherwise unexplained alterations in fetal condition—crucial because the uterus exerts pressure over the lumbar spine (when the patient lies supine) and thereby over the vena cava, interfering with blood return, and over the lower aorta, interfering with blood supply to the iliac and uterine arteries. This mechanical circumstance creates physical conditions that may alter the blood pressure relationships otherwise

BETWEEN CONTRACTIONS

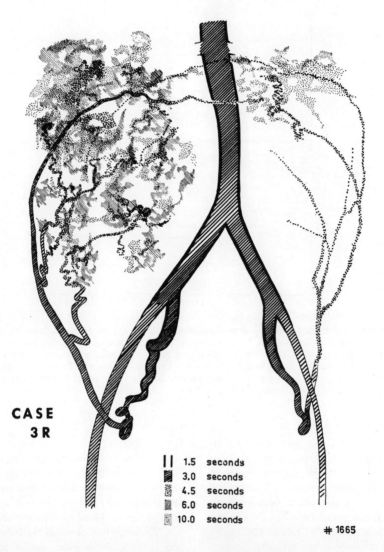

CASE
3R

‖	1.5	seconds
▰	3.0	seconds
▦	4.5	seconds
▨	6.0	seconds
▩	10.0	seconds

1665

Figure 7-2 Drawing made from sequential arterioplacentograms to demonstrate the progress and clearance of contrast medium injected in the aorta of a *pregnant patient at term with relaxed uterus*. The signs in middle lower part of the figure indicate the time between injecting the dye and taking the film; the areas marked with those characteristics indicate the filling in the corresponding film. Note that at 1.5 sec only the aorta, common iliac, internal iliac, and part of the external iliac arteries were filled. After 10 sec (very fine dots) the contrast was still distinguished only in the IVS. The placenta is well outlined on the upper right part of the fundus. Reprinted from Bieniarz J, et al: Aortocaval compression by the uterus in late human pregnancy. *Am J Obstet Gynecol* 100:203, 1968.

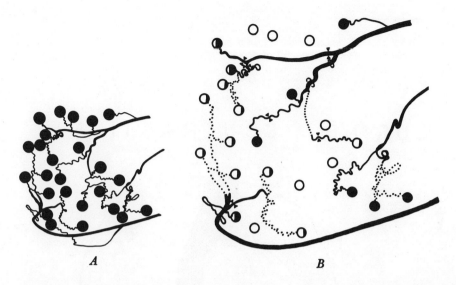

A   *B*

Figure 7-3 Reconstruction from serial radiographs taken from *term pregnant uteri. (A)* In state of *relaxation.* The filled arteries are drawn, and the black dots represent well-filled intracotyledonary spaces (IVS). *(B)* During *contraction.* The dotted lines are arteries only faintly outlined; black dots are cotyledons with slightly reduced contrast — two-thirds black, moderately reduced; one-third black, markedly reduced in contrast. Clear circles are cotyledons not visualized during contractions. The diminished blood supply to the IVS during the contraction is clear. Reprinted from Borell U, et al: Influence of uterine contractions on the uteroplacental blood flow at term. *Am J Obstet Gynecol* 93:44, 1965.

observed between the femoral arteries and the brachial arteries (usual site for taking blood pressure). In normotensive patients the two pressures will be nearly equal, with slightly higher values in the femoral vessels (Figure 7-8). The fluctuations caused by contractions are much the same in both tracings. However, in hypertensive patients the readings in the femoral artery tend to be consistently and clearly higher (Figure 7-9). The opposite has been observed to occur during episodes of hypotension when borderline hypotension in the brachial artery may be accompanied by extremely low systolic and diastolic readings in the femoral arteries. Because the blood supply to the IVS depends on the pressure below the uterine compression, this finding is particularly important in cases of hypotension produced by sympathetic blockade of the lower abdomen and limbs (see Chapter 18).

Depending on the position of the patient during a contraction, the uterus may exert a localized pressure over the iliac vessels and markedly curtail the blood flowing beyond that spot: in a pressure tracing obtained below the area of compression the record may suggest that the patient is in collapse, while in all other areas the pressure is not only satisfactory but high (Figure 7-10). This curious phenomenon was originally observed by Poseiro and is now called the Poseiro effect of contractions. Needless to say, when the side of the compressed vessel supplies the blood to the uterine artery carrying most of the blood to the IVS, major problems for the fetus may be created. In general, the average systolic and diastolic pressure increases are relatively modest but are high enough to influence cardiac output (Figure 7-11), and thus be of significance in the hemodynamics of the patient in labor (Hendricks, 1958).

DURING   CONTRACTION

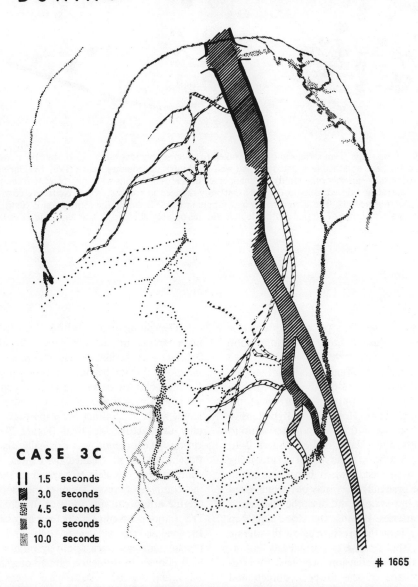

CASE 3C

‖	1.5	seconds
▮	3.0	seconds
▦	4.5	seconds
▨	6.0	seconds
▩	10.0	seconds

1665

Figure 7-4 (Same case and symbols as Figure 7-2.) Injection of contrast medium *during a contraction*. Note the total exclusion of the right iliac artery and its branches (compression against the vertebrae). Furthermore, the injection failed to visualize the placenta or even the right uterine artery, but it did visualize the left gluteal and obturator arteries at 3 sec. Reprinted from Bieniarz J, et al: Aortocaval compression by the uterus in late human pregnancy. *Am J Obstet Gynecol* 100:203, 1968.

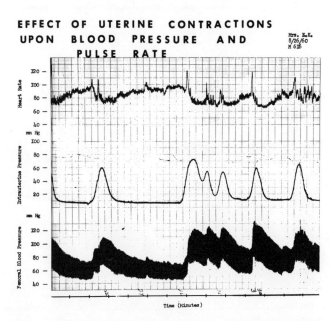

Figure 7-5 Tracings obtained during spontaneous labor at term. *(Above)* Maternal heart rate obtained with a photoelectric cell applied on the earlobe. *(Center)* Intrauterine pressure. *(Below)* Femoral artery pressure. Sharp rise in systolic and diastolic pressures coincides with uterine contractions and the slow fall following relaxation. The pulse rate drops somewhat with the hypertensive response but not in equivalent proportion to the rise in blood pressure. An incoordinated contraction *(middle)* is reflected on the blood pressure all the same.

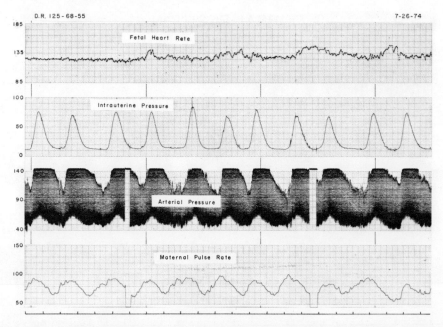

Figure 7-6 Effect of uterine contractions on blood pressure and heart rate. Recordings during induced labor at term with patient in supine position. *(Top)* FHR. *(Second channel)* Intrauterine pressure. *(Third channel)* Femoral artery pressure—maximum systolic pressures not recorded because the peak goes off the scale. *(Bottom)* Maternal heart rate obtained from the systolic wave of the blood pressure recording. The blood pressure responds to the contractions with a marked systolic rise and a lesser diastolic rise, while the pulse rate tends to mirror those changes in a slightly delayed fashion. The FHR is apparently not influenced by either the contractions or the blood pressure changes. (Scales in ordinates are in mm Hg and beats/min; abscissa, in minutes.)

132

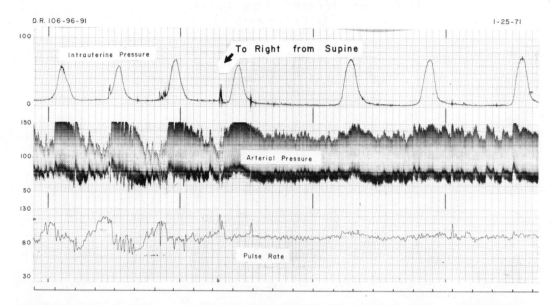

Figure 7-7 Effect of uterine contractions on blood pressure and heart rate and the influence of the patient's position on this response. Tracings were taken with an enhanced labor of a term pregnancy. (Scales are as in Figure 7-6.) The supine patient was turned (arrow). The blood pressure and heart rate had lesser fluctuations with the contractions while the patient was in lateral position. Between contractions, in both positions, oscillations of the blood pressure recur approximately two to three per min ("vasomotor oscillations").

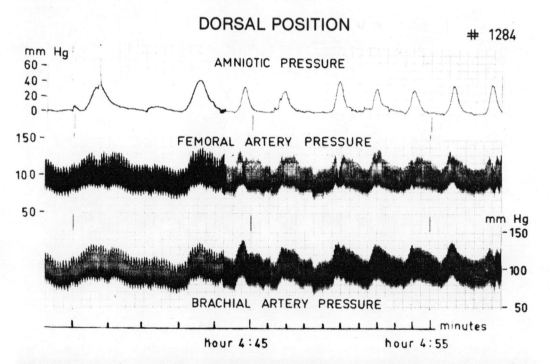

Figure 7-8 Simultaneous intrauterine, femoral artery, and brachial artery pressures, in a 34 week gestation preeclamptic patient in *supine position,* with blood pressure within normal ranges. Note the effect of contractions on blood pressure, and the nearly equal readings in both vessels. In the left third of the figure, the paper speed is doubled, to see better the blood pressure fluctuations produced by the respiratory movements. Reprinted from Bieniarz J, et al: Compression of the aorta by the uterus in late human pregnancy. *Am J Obstet Gynecol* 95:795, 1966.

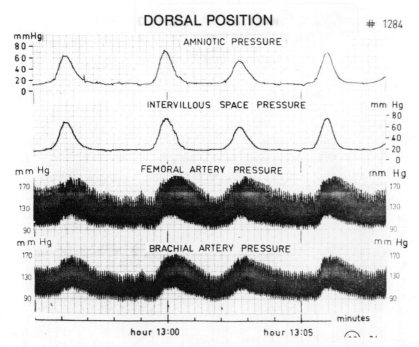

Figure 7-9 Same case and position as Figure 7-8 but with blood pressure in hypertensive range. In the *femoral artery* the systolic is 5 mm Hg and the diastolic 5 mm Hg *higher than in the brachial artery*. The top two channels show that the IVS and amniotic fluid pressures are equal. Reprinted from Bieniarz J, et al: Compression of the aorta by the uterus in late human pregnancy. *Am J Obstet Gynecol* 95:795, 1966.

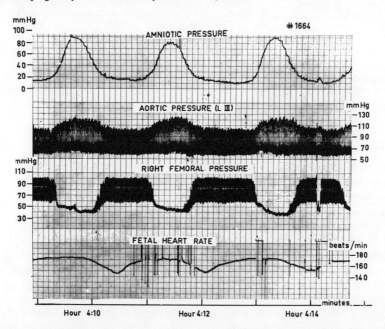

Figure 7-10 Simultaneous intrauterine, aortic, and femoral pressures and FHR recorded in the patient studies in Figures 7-2 and 7-4. The compression of the right common iliac artery seen in the serial radiographs (Figure 7-4) explains the severe hypotension recorded in the femoral catheter below the compression (Poseiro effect), and the increased pressures recorded in the lumbar aorta. The FHR shows a deceleration following each contraction, indicating that the diminished IVS blood supply significantly affects fetal oxygenation. Reprinted from Bieniarz J, et al: Aorto-caval compression by the uterus in late human pregnancy. *Am J Obstet Gynecol* 100:203, 1968.

134

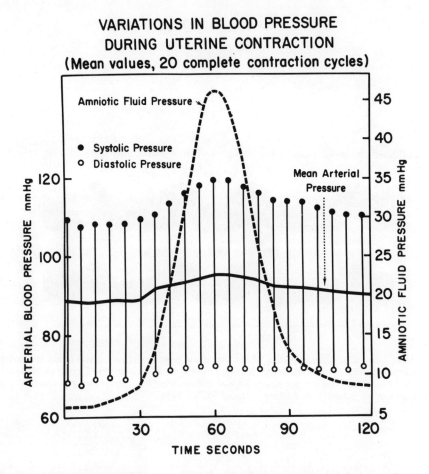

**VARIATIONS IN BLOOD PRESSURE
DURING UTERINE CONTRACTION
(Mean values, 20 complete contraction cycles)**

Figure 7-11 Mean values of systolic, diastolic, and mean arterial pressures recorded during uterine contractions. Although there are variations among the blood pressure responses to uterine contractions, the normal response is as illustrated here, with a higher rise in the systolic than in the diastolic pressure. Reprinted from Hendricks CH: The hemodynamics of a uterine contraction. *Am J Obstet Gynecol* 76:969, 1958.

The predictable increase in blood pressure during a contraction is almost certainly due to a combination of several mechanisms; the predominant one must be the sudden severe diminution of the IVS blood flow (shutting off the "arteriovenous fistula") with a dramatic increase in peripheral resistance. An almost instantaneous hypertensive response to muscular activity has been demonstrated to occur in patients whose autonomic nerves have been blocked (Guyton et al, 1962) suggesting that the response is an intrinsic hemodynamic adaptation to the increased peripheral resistance. In the pregnant patient, furthermore, the baroreceptors must play an important part in regulating the bradycardia that accompanies this transient hypertension. Other aspects of cardiac function are altered simultaneously.

Venous Pressure

The pressures in the venous system undergo extreme fluctuations with changes in patient position. When the uterus is relaxed and the patient is supine, the pressure readings are much higher in the femoral and iliac veins then in the lower vena cava. They are approximately the same in the retrohepatic part of the vena cava and the brachial veins; the pressure is slightly negative in the superior vena cava. When the patient is in lateral position, the venous pressure values below the promontory are lower, while all others remain about the same.

The contraction of the uterus causes marked changes. When the patient is supine, the pressure in the iliac veins increases by an average of 25 mm Hg; it is greater in the retrouterine part of the vena cava, while in the retrohepatic region there is a slight drop. At the same time, the pressure in the superior vena cava becomes positive, on the order of 6 mm Hg. When the patient lies in the lateral position there is a mild increase in all values of venous pressure, including the superior vena cava, which becomes slightly positive. The causes of these very different values, depending on the position of the patient, are related to the pressure exerted by the pregnant uterus on the lower lumbar spine. When the patient is supine, this pressure over the spine is increased during the contraction, causing a still further compression of the vena cava. With an augmented venous pressure below the obstacle created by the pressing uterus, there is a diminished pressure above it and a significant compensatory increase of the collateral circulation, particularly in the paravertebral venous plexus. These veins contribute to the blood supply of the superior vena cava—a likely explanation for its significantly positive pressure during contractions.

Cardiac Output

All the hemodynamic alterations heretofore described necessarily affect the work of the myocardium, which must adapt to the changes in resistance as well as to the inflow of blood from the venous system. This adaptation is manifested by a gradual increase in cardiac output paralleling the ascending intrauterine pressure but which peaks before the acme of contraction. The slow return to precontraction values parallels uterine relaxation (Figure 7-12).

The factors directly affecting the cardiac output are: 1) *increased stroke volume* manifested by a widening of the pulse-pressure tracing achieved by a larger increase in systolic than diastolic pressure; 2) *diminution in pulse rate* not sufficient to compensate for the increased stroke volume and thus the augmented output; 3) relative hypertension as the consequence of the *sudden increase in peripheral resistance* as the uterine contraction obliterates the low resistance arteriovenous fistula, which is the IVS. It has been postulated that the contraction extrudes some blood from the IVS and thus contributes to an increased venous return (Hendricks, 1956). However, radiographic studies have failed to document this phenomenon during a strong contraction (Ramsey et al, 1966).

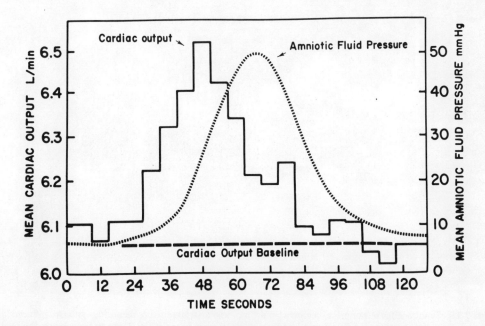

Figure 7-12 Effect of uterine contraction on cardiac output (calculated by the pulse-pressure method). Cardiac output reaches maximum shortly before the contraction reaches its highest intensity. Reprinted from Hendricks CH: The hemodynamics of a uterine contraction. *Am J Obstet Gynecol* 76:969, 1958.

136

The sudden increase in peripheral resistance, eliminating almost 20% of the arteriolar bed for the same blood volume, imposes a drastic need for immediate adaptation. Increased cardiac output with increased blood velocity (faster circulation time) and venous pressure seem to be adequate stopgap measures until a redistribution of blood can be effected.

CENTRAL NERVOUS SYSTEM

Cerebrospinal Fluid Pressure

The cranium and vertebral column completely wrap the central nervous system and its protecting and nutrient elements (dura, vessels, blood, and cerebrospinal fluid). Because there is a direct communication with the vascular bed, it should be expected that the hemodynamic changes observed with uterine contractions would trigger changes in that closed system, which is sensitive to pressure and/or volume changes. In spite of this logical reasoning it is still believed that only minimal or no changes are produced in the cerebrospinal fluid pressure (CSFP) by the contractions, and that these changes occur only when the contractions are painful.

The careful, simultaneous recording of several parameters during labor proves that the CSFP (average about 13 mm Hg), is predictably increased with each contraction (Figure 7-13), and

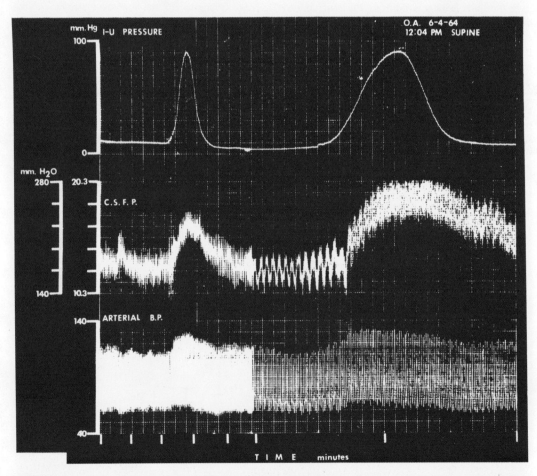

Figure 7-13 Simultaneous intrauterine, cerebrospinal fluid, and arterial pressure recordings at term, induced labor. Slow, regular paper speed for the first 5 min and four times the speed for the last 2 min to show better the relationships among the pressures studied. Note parallel increase in blood pressure and CSFP seen in the middle as the uterus contracts. Fluctuations in CSFP coincide with respiratory movements. Reprinted from Hopkins EL, et al: Cerebrospinal fluid pressure in labor. *Am J Obstet Gynecol* 93:907, 1965.

that there is a close parallelism between blood pressure and CSF pressure increases. The increase in CSFP is proportionally very significant, approximately 20% over the resting pressure. Even the small fluctuations or "vasomotor oscillations" often observed in blood pressure recordings are represented in CSFP tracings (Figure 7-14). So sensitive is the CSF hydraulic system to volume and pressure changes that the intrathoracic pressure variations produced by normal respirations are instantaneously transmitted, in proportion to the depth of their fluctuations (Figure 7-15).

All these various responses of CSFP to contractions are predictable, regardless of the patient's position or stage of labor. Furthermore, unlike what many have said, the responses are independent of any pain produced by contractions. There may be other added effects, such as movement or straining, which are as variable as the causes may be. However, the basic fact remains: the hemodynamic effects of uterine contractions are reflected in the CSFP because the CSF is enclosed in a rigid bony container. The increase in arterial and venous pressures and particularly, rerouting of venous blood through the paravertebral venous plexuses, when the patient is in the supine position, directly affect the volume to be accommodated within the unexpansible bony case housing the CNS and its protective fluid cushion. The implications of these observations are important in the technique and execution of conduction anesthesia, very frequently used in obstetrics.

Bearing-Down Efforts

The bearing-down reflex, triggered by completion of dilatation and simultaneous contraction, is essentially a prolonged Valsalva maneuver with all its hemodynamic implications. All the other systems already described are further affected by these efforts, except the IVS circulation.

The *arterial pressure* rises immediately with the increase in intrathoracic and intrauterine

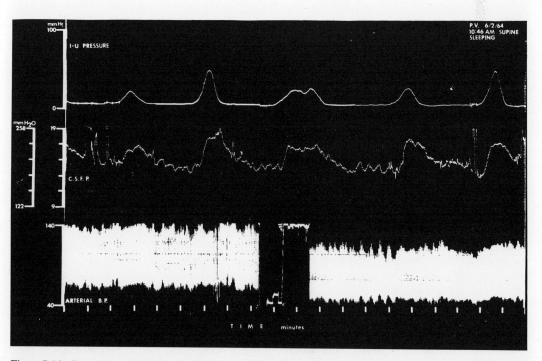

Figure 7-14 Recordings obtained as for Figure 7-13. Blood pressure scale was adjusted in the middle of the record to pick up the top of the tracing. Note the regular response of CSFP to contractions (more so than the blood pressure), and the parallelism of its small fluctuations with the vasomotor oscillations of the blood pressure. Reprinted from Hopkins EL, et al: Cerebrospinal fluid pressure in labor. *Am J Obstet Gynecol* 93:907, 1965.

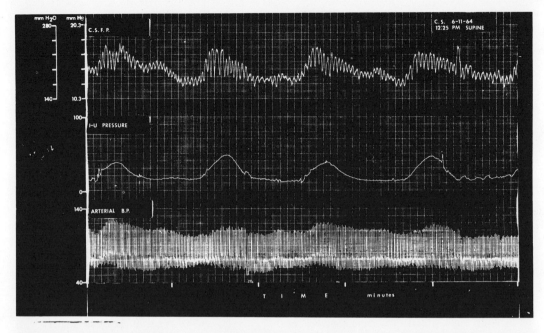

Figure 7-15 Cerebrospinal fluid, intrauterine, and arterial pressures in term spontaneous labor. High-speed recording illustrates the effect of respiratory movements on CSFP and effect of contractions on both blood pressure and CSFP. Reprinted from Hopkins EL, et al: Cerebrospinal fluid pressure in labor. *Am J Obstet Gynecol* 93:907, 1965.

pressures, to be followed by a slow decline toward the precontraction diastolic with a gradual drop accompanied by a diminishing pulse pressure. A corresponding *bradycardia* occurs during this transient hypertension. When the patient interrupts the Valsalva maneuver to take another deep breath there is a rapid fall in blood pressure followed by a recovery completed in about four or five beats. The process is repeated as many times as the patient bears down (Figure 7-16). The *venous pressures* also rise markedly as the intrathoracic pressure increases, and with the latter the venous return flow is interrupted, or at least severely disrupted. The transient interruption of the Valsalva maneuver opens up the venous return, and a dramatic fall in pressure takes place, followed by repetition of the cycle with the next pushing effort.

The CSFP also rises to very high levels, in keeping with what is observed in the cardiovascular system. In fact, the parallelism is similar to the one seen during a simple contraction (Figure 7-17).

The drastic, albeit transient, alterations in hemodynamics produced by the pushing efforts of second stage are all clearly the consequence of the physical relationships of changing pressures and movement of blood. When the glottis closes and the intrathoracic pressure increases markedly, there is interruption of venous return (rise in venous pressure), but at the same time the blood contained in the lungs (estimated to be about 600 ml) is rapidly extruded toward the left atrium, promoting a transient increase in cardiac output and hypertension. Because the amount of blood in the lungs is not replaced (the venous return has been severely diminished) the blood pressure and pulse pressure start to fall, with a corresponding drop in cardiac output. When the deep inspiratory effort terminates the Valsalva maneuver, the venous return is widely reopened, but the cardiac output and stroke volume do not recover immediately because the depleted pulmonary bed has to be refilled before the blood reaches the left atrium. This requires a few seconds, and only after that vascular bed has been replenished do stroke volume and cardiac output return to control levels. These hemodynamic alterations are directly and instantaneously reflected in the CSFP because they constitute a hydraulic unity.

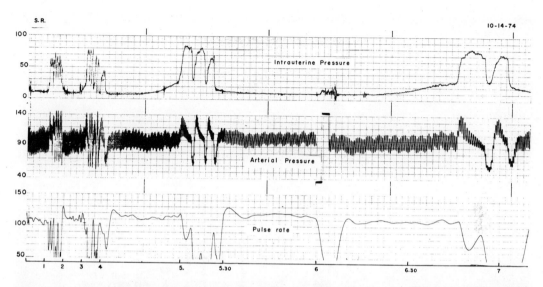

Figure 7-16 Second stage in term, spontaneous labor with patient under epidural anesthesia. Effect of bearing-down efforts on intrauterine pressure, arterial pressure, and pulse rate. Note the rapid rise at the beginning of the bearing-down effort with slow decline, and the sharp fall with the inspiratory movement. On the extreme right is shown the recovery of the blood pressure at the end of the contraction-pushing cycle (the loss of the pulse tracing when the blood pressure tracing drops below 80 is an artifact of the recording technique. (In the abscissa, the time scale in minutes shows three different speeds: the first 4 min at regular 1.5 cm/min speed; the next 1½ min at 7 cm/min; and the last 1½ min, from 5.30 on, at 15 cm/min.)

Postpartum

The expulsion of the fetus relieves the abdomen of a large space-occupying mass and the large prevertebral vessels form a compression that interferes with free blood flow. The result of this physical change is a redistribution of blood, and with it changes in arterial and venous pressures. The expected change would be an increase in blood pressure (because of the obliteration of the IVS and its functional arteriovenous fistula) but in fact this does not occur. A small proportion of the circulating volume is lost during the process of separation and expulsion of the placenta (third stage), and much more is distributed into the splanchnic capillary and venous beds now free from the compression of the pregnant uterus. The result is a *moderate drop in systolic and diastolic blood pressures,* increased pulse pressure, and moderate tachycardia (Figure 7-18).

The CSFP, as in all other circumstances, parallels the alterations in blood pressure: a mild drop follows the delivery of the infant, but a relatively rapid recovery takes place when the venous pressures reequilibrate shortly thereafter (see Figure 7-17).

The postpartum contractions after expulsion of the placenta continue to affect these hydraulic systems because the large uterus, although no longer receiving a very large part of the cardiac output with its IVS, is still a large, well-vascularized muscular organ, interrupting its circulation with each contraction.

Pain

The so-called vasomotor oscillations observed in the blood pressure tracings (see Figures 7-7 and 7-14) do not correspond to either respiratory movements or changes produced by the contractions. The label given them implies that they represent periodic "pulses" of the vasomotor center that maintain the oscillating characters of the blood pressure. The existence of these pulses is strongly suggested by observations in animals, by recording electrical potentials from the areas where these centers are presumed to be located. It has further been postulated that these periodic impulses are intrinsic to the function of the centers.

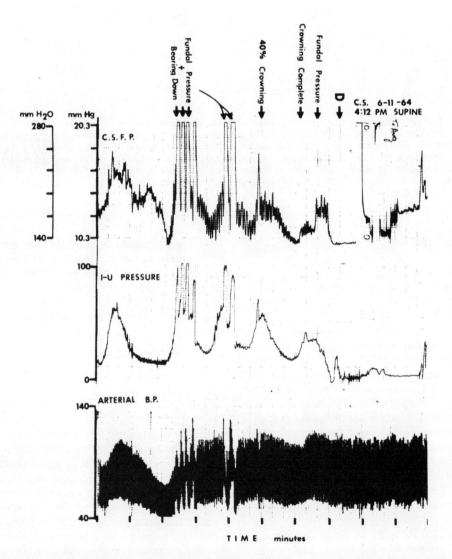

Figure 7-17 Second stage and delivery, term pregnancy, with patient under continuous epidural anesthesia. Recorded as for Figure 7-15 to observe the effect of pushing on CSFP. Note the perfect parallelism in the three channels, the transient drop in CSFP at delivery, and the almost immediate recovery that follows. The blood pressure stabilizes with a large pulse pressure. Reprinted from Hopkins EL, et al: Cerebrospinal fluid pressure in labor. *Am J Obstet Gynecol* 93:907, 1965.

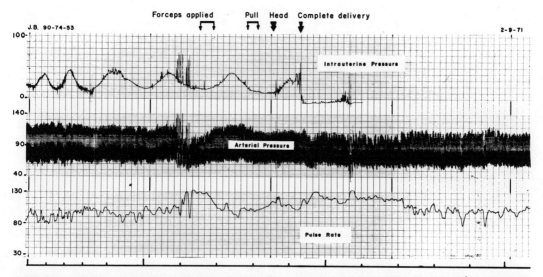

Figure 7-18 Effect of delivery on blood pressure and pulse rate—15½-min recording of second stage and outlet forceps delivery, term spontaneous labor with patient under epidural anesthesia. The first 4 min were run at 1.5 cm/min paper speed; the rest of the tracing at 3 cm/min. Birth process (arrows). Following delivery there is a drop in systolic (10 mm Hg) and diastolic (5 mm Hg) average pressures, and an increase of 5 beats/min in the average pulse rate.

However, indirect observations may be interpreted to indicate that extrinsic stimuli significantly influence the response of the target system of those impulses. Among those stimuli, pain must be considered of paramount importance because it indirectly triggers the release of a number of vasoactive hormones and by these it influences the blood pressure and pulse rate. The diminution or disappearance of the oscillations may clearly be observed following administration of conduction anesthesia (see Chapter 18). However, it may be argued that the sympathetic block interferes with the pathways whereby the vasomotor center controls peripheral vessel response.

An effective paracervical block does not block the sympathetic reflexes but it may succeed in decreasing the oscillations observed in the blood pressure (Figure 7-19). Furthermore, with this decrease, the block often promotes a decrease in systolic and diastolic pressures, which slowly recover when the effect of the anesthesia subsides. These clinical observations would suggest that the liberation of endogenous catecholamines may be a common consequence of painful stimuli (including labor pains) and that, their obliteration, the systemic effect of these amines is eliminated. It is possible to postulate that the vasomotor oscillations may be peripheral vascular responses to *pulsatile liberation of vasoactive amines.*

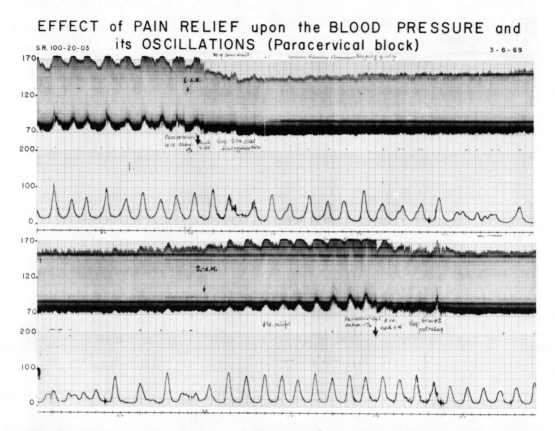

Figure 7-19 Tracing of an enhanced labor at 33 weeks gestation with an anencephalic fetus. Continuous 2-hour recordings of arterial and intrauterine pressures are shown. *(Above, left)* Blood pressure fluctuations not quite corresponding to intrauterine pressure changes. Effective paracervical block with 200 mg mepivacaine produced a marked effect on the blood pressure as soon as pain relief was apparent: disappearance of the fluctuations and a significant drop in systolic and diastolic pressures. *(Lower, middle)* Return of the fluctuations following a gradual recovery of the blood pressure. When the contractions were again painful (small arrow) the pattern was the same as that of the preanesthetic period. Repetition of the paracervical block with 160 mg mepivacaine produced the same effect as the first one, both on pain and blood pressure patterns.

BIBLIOGRAPHY

Bieniarz J, Cibils LA, Caldeyro-Barcia R: La presion venosa en distintas regiones vasculares en estado gravido puerperal. *IV Cong Uruguayo Ginecotocol* 1:482, 1964.

Bieniarz J, Crottogini JJ, Curuchet E, et al: Aortocaval compression by the uterus in late human pregnancy. *Am J Obstet Gynecol* 100:203, 1968.

Bieniarz J, Maqueda E, Caldeyro-Barcia R: Compression of aorta by the uterus in late human pregnancy. I. *Am J Obstet Gynecol* 95:795, 1966.

Borell U, Fernstrom I, Ohlson L, Wiqvist N: Effect of uterine contractions on the human uteroplacental blood circulation. *Am J Obstet Gynecol* 89:881, 1964.

Borell U, Fernstrom I, Ohlson L, et al: Influence of uterine contractions on the uteroplacental blood flow at term. *Am J Obstet Gynecol* 93:44, 1965.

Eskes T, Stolte L, Seelen J, et al: Radio-angiographic studies of the maternal circulation in the human placenta. *Arch Gynaekol* 200:735, 1965.

Freese UE, Ranniger K, Kaplan H: The fetal maternal circulation of the placenta. II. An x-ray cinematographic study of pregnant rhesus monkeys. *Am J Obstet Gynecol* 94:361, 1966.

Guyton AC, Douglas BH, Langston JB, et al: Instantaneous increase in mean circulatory pressure and cardiac output at onset of muscular activity. *Circ Res* 11:431, 1962.

Hendricks CH: The hemodynamics of a uterine contraction. *Am J Obstet Gynecol* 76:969, 1958.

Hendricks CH, Quilligan EJ: Cardiac output during labor. *Am J Obstet Gynecol* 71:953, 1956.

Hopkins EL, Hendricks CH, Cibils LA: Cerebrospinal fluid pressure in labor. *Am J Obstet Gynecol* 93:907, 1965.

Ramsey EM, Corner GW, Donner MW: Serial and cineradioangiographic visualization of maternal circulation in the primate (hemochorial) placenta. *Am J Obstet Gynecol* 86:213, 1963.

Ramsey EM, Martin CB, McGaughey HS, et al: Venous drainage of the placenta in rhesus monkeys: Radiographic studies. *Am J Obstet Gynecol* 95:948, 1966.

CHAPTER 8
Initiation of Labor

The extraordinary hormonal and physical changes that occur in the pregnant subject and her uterus are the ultimate expression of the wonders of adaptation. Pregnancy brings a complete turnabout of the hormonal status of the individual with the appearance of the placenta, a new, large, and potent endocrine organ that secretes a number of new hormones and metabolizes others produced by the patient or her conceptus. In addition, the physical changes of a growing uterus—a potent, contractile, hollow viscus receiving a large proportion of the cardiac output to supply the enlarged vascular bed (IVS)—constitute constant threats to interruption of the growing conceptus. Why pregnancy terminates at a given stage, and what triggers labor are fundamental biologic problems that, so far, have not been solved (an equally monumental problem, possibly closely related, is why the conceptus—a partial homograft—is not rejected by the maternal organism).

SPONTANEOUS LABOR

Several hypotheses have been proposed to explain the onset of spontaneous labor and, indirectly, why the products of conception are not expelled from the uterus before term. Some of the more pertinent hypotheses dealing with the onset of spontaneous labor will be reviewed here. Since experimental studies have been conducted on a variety of animals, some hypotheses are limited to specific species and will be discussed in that context. Others purport to have a wider biologic application.

Progesterone Block

Based on his studies on uterine physiology of rabbits Csapo (1961) postulated that the uterus is quiescent during the whole period of gestation because of the effect of progesterone on the myometrium, which would hyperpolarize the cells and thereby make them incapable of propagating the stimulus, which may be triggered in any area of the myometrium. In humans, because the progesterone is secreted mainly by the placenta, it would exert its effect particularly over the area of placental implantation and thereby create an imbalance among the various regions of the myometrium. The *functional asymmetry* would make the human uterus incapable of coordinated contractions, which are a prerequisite for effective cervical effacement and dilatation. The hormonal differences between humans and rabbits imposed the necessity of reviewing this hypothesis because progesterone levels do not seem to drop significantly in humans in the days or hours preceding spontaneous labor.

The see-saw theory This updated hypothesis incorporates the investigations carried out to evaluate the role of prostaglandins in the initiation of labor in humans. It basically states, "The factors which promote the termination of pregnancy must be opposed by those which prohibit it." This concept implies a balance among the various factors, the loss of which is inevitably followed by labor and expulsion of the conceptus. Some of these balances are maintained as follows:

1. Progesterone is the blocking agent of the myometrium against the stimulatory effect of prostaglandin $F_2\alpha$.
2. The distension or stretching of the myometrium as pregnancy advances is another strong stimulant of contractions, but is is counterbalanced by increasing progesterone levels, which thus prevent the onset of coordinated contractions.

3. The actions of estradiol, other fetal hormones, and oxytocin on the myometrium are not yet clear, but if they have such an action it may be mediated through prostaglandins or progesterone.

The protective effect of progesterone is graphically shown in Figure 8-1. As long as the threshold for stimulation and propagation is high, the action of oxytocins will be transient and ineffective, and the *uterus* will continue to be *refractory*. Only when the *progesterone* effect on the myometrium has been *withdrawn* do the contractions become effective and labor progresses; prostaglandins break the balance and predominate (Csapo, 1975). It is not clear what determines the progesterone withdrawal that ultimately promotes spontaneous labor and delivery.

In spite of the claims by its supporters, this hypothesis has a number of elements that are inconsistent with known pathophysiologic and hormonal observations in humans. It needs a revision or an updating to adjust properly to current concepts of perinatal endocrinology and pathophysiology.

Oxytocin Sensitivity

Independently, Caldeyro-Barcia (1959) and Theobald (1969) postulated that the known refractoriness of the myometrium to oxytocin is maintained through most of gestation, and that it decreases only in the last week preceding labor (Caldeyro-Barcia) or just in the hours before it starts (Theobald) (Figure 8-2). All through pregnancy there is a normal blood oxytocin level well below that capable of stimulating the refractory myometrium. Thus pregnancy is protected from extemporaneous contractions, which are triggered, when labor starts, by a marked increase in the sensitivity of the myometrium to oxytocin and the steady blood level of this neuropituitary hormone.

Recent contributions to this hypothesis have been made by a number of authors who investigated the blood levels of oxytocin in mother and fetus, and found that the fetal contribution to oxytocinemia might be considerable. However, those investigators did not consider either the significant dilutional faction when fetal secretions pass to the maternal circulation, or the inactivation of the oxytocin by the placental tissue, which is extremely rich in oxytocinase.

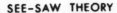

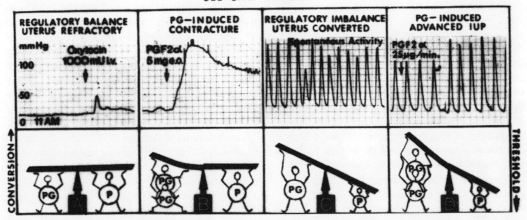

Figure 8-1 The see-saw theory of maintenace of pregnancy. *(A)* Prostaglandin (PG) and progesterone (P) are in balance, and therefore a large dose of oxytocin cannot stimulate the uterus. *(B)* Exogenous PGF$_2\alpha$ tends to break the equilibrium but succeeds only in bending the arm because P is still high. *(C)* With lower P, PG predominates and a large uterine activity (above) is recorded. *(D)* An already imbalanced state can be further pushed by exogenous PGF$_2\alpha$ to increase the uterine activity. Not shown in the figure is the possibility of regressing the uterine activity by large amounts of exogenous P. Reprinted from Csapo AI: The "seesaw" theory of the regulatory mechanism of pregnancy. *Am J Obstet Gynecol* 121:578, 1975.

INITIATION OF LABOR IN HUMANS
Oxytocin Sensitivity Hypothesis
(Caldeyro-Barcia & Theobald)

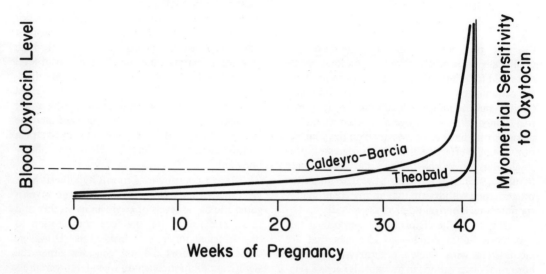

Figure 8-2 Schematic representation of uterine reactivity to oxytocin throughout pregnancy. In the abscissa, weeks of gestation; in the ordinates, a steady blood oxytocin level that does not change, and two curves indicating the sensitivity of the myometrium to oxytocin. For Caldeyro-Barcia, it begins to rise steadily in the last several weeks of gestation, and for Theobald, the rise is sudden and sharp, increasing only in the hours preceding labor.

Labor in Animals

It appears that a simple hypothesis to explain the onset of labor in humans may not be satisfactory because it cannot consider the very numerous, intimately related, alterations observed to occur before labor. Other hypotheses (results of thorough and lengthy investigations), proposed to explain the onset of labor in animals, are much more complex and therefore coordinate a higher number of phenomena. Because of their biologic importance they will be briefly summarized in the following pages before discussing the last one postulated for the human.

Labor in sheep The first to postulate a hypothesis in which the fetus seems to control the onset of labor was Liggins (1967, 1968, 1973). It is based on his extensive studies on the sheep, an animal with a high placental secretion of progesterone. In simple terms, the *fetal pituitary-adrenal axis* controls the first significant endocrine changes leading to spontaneous labor;

however, the signal that originates the functional changes observed in the pituitary has not yet been determined. Even though the fetal blood level of ACTH has not been shown to change immediately before labor, the adrenal secretion of cortisol rises sharply in the days preceding labor and thereby triggers a cascade of reactions terminating in regular uterine contractions and labor (Figure 8-3). It has not been clarified whether the increased adrenal sensitivity to ACTH is due to activation of more receptors or to maturation of other systems that influence their capacity to secrete steroids.

Be that as it may, the high levels of cortisol act on the placenta, where they stimulate the activity of 17α and 11β hydroxylase on progesterone and pregnenolone to synthesize androstenedione. Under the effect of aromatase this androgen is very rapidly converted to estrogens estrone and estradiol-17β. These then would act on the estrogen receptors of the placenta to enhance the production of prostaglandin $F_2\alpha$; at the same time

INITIATION OF LABOR IN SHEEP
(Liggins)

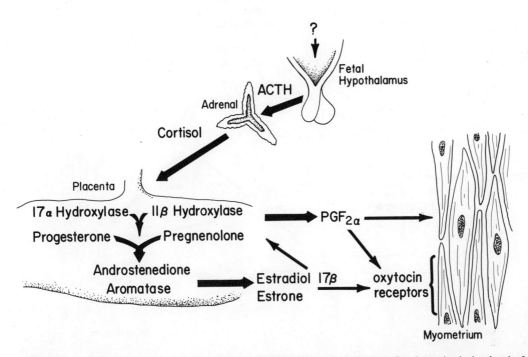

Figure 8-3 Initiation of labor in sheep accoridng to Liggins. Under the influence of undetermined stimulus the fetal hypothalamus stimulates the pituitary to release more ACTH, which acts on the adrenals. These secrete large quantities of cortisol, which stimulates the placental enzymes to convert progesterone and pregnenolone into androstenedione. The aromatization of this steroid converts it into estrone and estradiol-17β. These estrogens enhance the placental production of PGF₂α and activate oxytocin receptors in myometrium, which contract under the stimulus of these oxytocics.

the estrogens seem to increase or activate the oxytocin receptors of the myometrium. A reciprocally potentiating oxytocic effect seems to exist between oxytocin and prostaglandin $F_2\alpha$. The poor uterine sensitivity to oxytocin observed in early gestation evolves to a sensitivity exquisite enough to trigger contractions by circulating oxytocin, when the prostaglandin seems accelerated under the influence of infused oxytocin. The final effect of these two potent oxytocics on the myometrium is the continuous accelerating stimulatory action observed in labor.

Labor in monkeys After Liggins' excellent demonstration that the fetus may be the controlling factor in the onset of labor, other investigators entertained applying the same idea to other species. Recently Challis and Manning (1978) summarized their work with monkeys and

pointed out the similarities and differences of the factors operating in sheep and subhuman primates. There seem to be some important differences, particularly in *adrenal and placental* metabolic participation in the chain of events terminating in labor (Figure 8-4). The fetal hypothalamus, by undetermined stimulus, enhances the production of ACTH by the pituitary. This trophic hormone acts on the fetal adrenals, which seem to undergo a burst of maturation in the days preceding labor. They respond by increasing the production of C-19 steroids (androstenedione and dehydroepiandrosterone) that are then rapidly aromatized into estrogens (estradiol-17β and especially estrone) by the placental aromatases. There may not be a drop in progesterone concentration but there is an increase of estrogens that affects three different systems: the production of

INITIATION OF LABOR IN MONKEYS
(Challis)

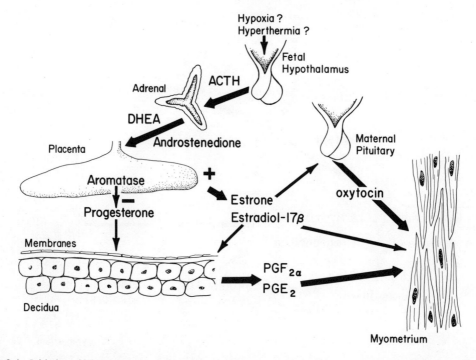

Figure 8-4 Initiation of labor in monkeys according to Challis. Unknown factors stimulate the hypothalamus to trigger the release of ACTH by the pituitary. The stimulated adrenals increase their output of dehydroepiandrosterone and androstenedione. These androgens are aromatized by the placenta preferentially into estrone and, to a lesser degree, estradiol-17β (at the same time there seems to be a decrease in placental progesterone). The rise in estrogen concentration sensitizes the myometrium to oxytocin, its release by the maternal pituitary, and the synthesis of PGF$_2\alpha$ by the fetal membranes and decidua. Eventually the myometrium is stimulated.

prostaglandin F$_2\alpha$ by the fetal membranes and decidua, the myometrium sensitivity to oxytocin, and the production and release of oxytocin by the maternal pituitary. The result of the convergent action of these oxytocic substances on the myometrium is the onset of labor contractions.

The experimental studies and hormonal measurements in monkeys, mother and fetus, have been carefully done by many investigators, and the hypothesis described takes into account the most relevant findings. However, the trigger that stimulates the hypothalamus still remains to be found.

The investigations conducted to test the applicability of these hypotheses to the human female have been much more difficult, for obvious reasons. From those observations it is irrefutable that many of those postulates fail to be

relevant in the chain of events known to occur when *spontaneous labor starts in the human;* conversely, other human mechanisms are not represented in animal observations.

Labor in Humans

After a long series of carefully planned and executed experiments, MacDonald and collaborators (1978) have put together a hypothesis that attempts to explain the puzzle of human labor. In their opinion, the emphasis is shifted from the fetal hypothalamus–pituitary, or the adrenal-placenta, to "the *amniotic fluid–membranes-decidua* complex as a metabolically active unit that may transmit or respond to signals that lead to the onset of labor." The action of the very high levels of estrogens, particularly estriol, in late pregnancy stimulates the synthesis of phospholipids and the incorporation of arachidonic acid into phospholipids, as well as the biosynthesis of prostaglandins, and the formation of lysosomes in the endometrium (decidua?, membranes?). This very high estrogen level is the product of rapid fetal adrenal growth stimulated by increased prolactin levels, and ultimately the secretion of dehydroisandrosterone sulfate rapidly converted to estradiol and estriol by the placenta. Basically, the fetal membranes are richly charged with arachidonic acid, the natural precursor of prostaglandins, but this is esterified and stored in the form of arachidonoyl esters as phosphatidylethanolamine. Its utilization for prostaglandin synthesis is possible only if it is available in free form. On the other hand, the chorion cell lysosomes are richly charged with lipid substances that may well be accumulated phospholipids. One of the effects of progesterone may well be to prevent the action of phospholipase A_2 on the phospholipids by stabilizing the lysosomes and thus preventing the formation and release of free arachidonic acid (Figure 8-5). The destabilization of the lysosomes is probably triggered by a *progesterone binding protein* that specifically binds progesterone, thus creating an alteration in the progesterone concentration and permitting the action of phospholipase A_2 to hydrolyze phosphatidylethanolamine. The cascade of reaction follows: 1) Lysoglycerophospholipid, product of the hydrolysis, is a potent cytolitic agent that may initiate a vicious cycle by disrupting more lysosomes to provide more substrate and more phospholipase A_2; 2) the free arachidonic acid released by the hydrolysis diffuses to the amniotic fluid and the decidua, which is rich in prostaglandin synthetases serving as the substrate for the synthesis of prostaglandin $F_2\alpha$. This potent oxytocic, in part, diffuses into the amniotic fluid, and also stimulates the contractility of the myometrium.

INITIATION OF LABOR IN HUMAN
(MacDonald)

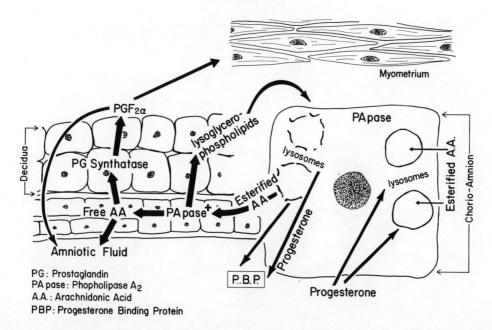

PG: Prostaglandin
PA pase: Phopholipase A_2
A.A.: Arachnidonic Acid
PBP: Progesterone Binding Protein

Figure 8-5 Initiation of labor in humans according to MacDonald. The high progesterone levels recorded in pregnancy stabilize the lysosomes, which contain esterified arachidonic acid and/or phospholipase A_2, in the chorioamniotic cells. The binding of progesterone by a specific binding protein breaks the stability and promotes the release of phospholipase A_2, the hydrolysis of phospholipids, and the release of free arachidonic acid and lysoglycerophospholipids. These initiate a vicious cycle by increasing lysosomal destabilization. The decidual prostaglandin synthetases utilize arachidonic acid as substrate for synthesis of $PDF_2\alpha$, which diffuses into amniotic fluid and toward the myometrium, which is thus stimulated.

The only missing link in this hypothesis based strictly on findings observed in human investation is this: what controls the production of the progesterone-binding protein that is found in significant quantities in the membranes only after the 37th week of gestation?

THE MYOMETRIAL CONTRACTION

As seen in Chapter 2, the uterine contraction results from activation of the contractile proteins actin and myosin by several ions and the energy supplying compound adenosintriphosphate (ATP). The resting membrane potential, under which the muscle is quiescent, is maintained by an equilibrium between a high sodium ion and low potassium ion concentration outside of the cell membrane, and a low sodium ion and high intracellular potassium ion concentration. In addition calcium ion is of fundamental importance in the contractile process because when calcium ions are free within the cell they bind to the contractile proteins and activate their property to slide on each other and thus produce a contraction. Calcium is abundant within the muscle cells, but it is sequestered or bound in mitochondria, sarcoplasmic reticulum, and the cell membrane. The myometrial cells are rich in these intracellular organelles and as a consequence depend on them to supply the free calcium ions required to start and sustain a contraction. Binding of calcium ions by the sarcoplasmic reticulum is inhibited by oxytocic substances: oxytocin, prostaglandin $F_2\alpha$, prostaglandin E_2. Their action seems to be mediated by 1) stimulation of phosphodiesterase to convert cyclic adenosinmonphosphate (cAMP), which stimulates calcium ion binding in sarcoplasmic reticulum, into adenylic acid; and 2) inhibition of adenylcyclase, which catalyzes the synthesis of cAMP. The decrease in cAMP could activate the release of free calcium ion from the sarcoplasmic reticulum, break the balance of the membrane potential, and trigger the contraction by its action on the *contractile proteins* (Figure 8-6).

THE EXCITATION-CONTRACTION MECHANISM IN MYOMETRIUM
(Effect of Oxytocics)

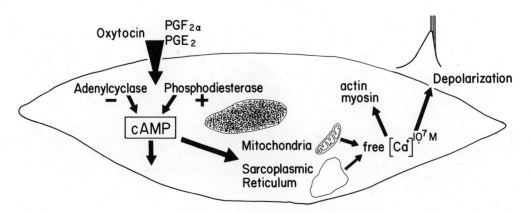

Figure 8-6 The excitation–contraction mechanism in myometrium. Simple diagram of intramyometrial events when the cells are stimulated by oxytocic substances (oxytocin, $PGF_2\alpha$, PGE_2). There is a decrease in adenylcyclase, and a stimulation of phosphodiesterase. The latter converts cAMP to adenylic acid; the lower cAMP activates the release of calcium ion from mitochondria and sarcoplasmic reticulum. The free calcium ions act on actin and myosin and trigger the contraction, and at the same time contribute to depolarization of the membrane and the firing of action potentials.

It becomes then very clear that the synthesis of prostaglandin $F_2\alpha$, its reciprocal synergistic effect with oxytocin, and the activation of the oxytocin receptors by estrogens all tend to stimulate contractions of the myometrium. Nevertheless, isolated contractions at various uterine regions are neither sufficient nor effective to produce labor. To have an effect upon the lower segment and cervix (see Chapter 5), the contractions must encompass the whole uterus and be coordinated. This effect is obtained by good and synchronized propagation of the action potentials starting in the fundal area, an ideal condition that does not seem to occur until labor starts. There is an anatomic barrier to the propagation of action potentials during gestation: there are gaps between the myometrial cells that are not in contact with each and therefore cannot function as a multicellular bundle coupled through low resistance pathways. They must do this to propagate the action potentials synchronically and produce a harmonious, effective contraction. However, during labor and the stages immediately preceding it, the myometrial cells are provided with "gap-junctions" (Figures 8-7 , 8-8), which then bridge the contiguous myometrial cells with low resistance contacts and serve to propagate the contraction wave (Garfield et al, 1979). It is not known what controls the activation of these gap-junctions, but their presence has been shown in laboring human myometrium, and they have been conspicuously absent in specimens obtained from nonlaboring uteri.

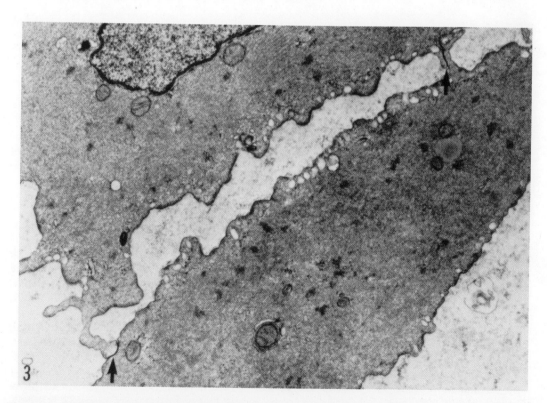

Figure 8-7 Electron micrograph of human myometrium in labor. Two gap-junctions (arrows) bridge the separation between muscle cells ($\times$ 28,000). Reprinted from Garfield RE, et al: Ultrastructural basis for maintenance and termination of pregnancy. *Am J Obstet Gynecol* 133:308, 1979.

152

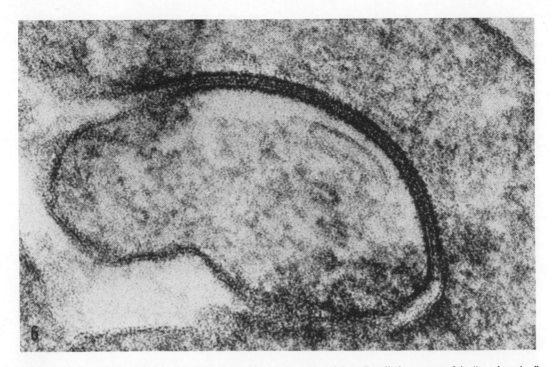

Figure 8-8   Electron micrograph of human myometrium in premature labor. Detailed structure of the "gap-junction" between two myometrial cells; the membranes seem fused by seven-line structure (× 252,000). Reprinted from Garfield RE, et al: Ultrastructural basis for maintenance and termination of pregnancy. *Am J Obstet Gynecol* 133:308, 1979.

BIBLIOGRAPHY

Caldeyro-Barcia R, Poseiro JJ: Oxytocin and contractility of the human uterus. *Ann NY Acad Sci* 75:813, 1959.

Caldeyro-Barcia R, Sereno JA: The response of the human uterus to oxytocin throughout pregnancy, in Caldeyro-Barcia R, Heller H (eds): *Oxytocin*. NY, Pergamon, 1961, pp 177–202.

Challis JRG, Manning FA: Control of parturition in subhuman primates. *Semin Perinatol* 2:247, 1978.

Csapo AI: The onset of labor. *Lancet* 1:277, 1961.

Csapo AI: The prospects of PGs in postconceptional therapy. *Prostaglandins* 3:245, 1973.

Csapo AI: The "seesaw" theory of the regulatory mechanism of pregnancy. *Am J Obstet Gynecol* 121:578, 1975.

Csapo AI, Takeda H: Effect of progesterone on the electric activity and intrauterine pressure of pregnant and parturient rabbits. *Am J Obstet Gynecol* 91:221, 1965.

Farr CJ, Robards MF, Theobald GW: Changes in myometrial sensitivity to oxytocin in man during the last six weeks of pregnancy. *J Physiol* 196:58, 1968.

Flint APF, Anderson ABM, Patten PT, et al: Control of utero-ovarian venous prostaglandin F during labour in sheep: acute effects of vaginal and cervical stimulation. *J Endocrinol* 63:67, 1974.

Garfield RE, Rabideau S, Challis JRG, et al: Ultrastructural basis for maintenance and termination of pregnancy. *Am J Obstet Gynecol* 133:308, 1979.

Kuriyama H, Csapo AI: Placenta and myometrial block. *Am J Obstet Gynecol* 82:592, 1961.

Liggins GC: Premature parturition after infusion of coritcotropin or cortisol into fetal lambs. *J Endocrinol* 42:323, 1968.

Liggins GC, Fairclogh RJ, Grieves SA, et al: The mechanism of initiation of parturition in the ewe. *Recent Prog Horm Res* 29:111, 1973.

Liggins GC, Kennedy PC, Holm LW: Failure of initiation of parturition after electrocoagulation of the pituitary of the fetal lamb. *Am J Obstet Gynecol* 98:1080, 1967.

MacDonald PC, Porter JC, Schwarz BE, et al: Initiation of parturition in the human female. *Semin Perinatol* 2:273, 1978.

Theobald GW, Robards MF, Suter PEN: Changes in myometrial sensitivity to oxytocin in man during the last six weeks of pregnancy. *J Obstet Gynaecol Br Comwlth* 76:385, 1969.

Thorburn GD: Hormonal control of parturition in the sheep and goat. *Semin Perinatol* 2:235, 1978.

CHAPTER 9
Pharmacology of the Uterus

The proper management of labor, at any stage of gestation, requires a thorough knowledge of the pharmacologic response of the uterus to drugs and their side effects manifested on other maternal systems or on fetal well-being. The great number of substances employed in modern obstetrics imposes a systematization that may be based on 1) stage of gestation, 2) aim of the clinician, or 3) the most predictable response of the uterus. For practical considerations the drugs discussed here are grouped according to the last and are generally divided as oxytocics, uterine relaxants, and a miscellaneous group of all others used in clinical obstetrics, the aim of which is not to alter uterine function but to exert systemic effects on the central nervous system, the cardiovascular system, the peripheral nervous system, and so on. Potential *untoward* effects on the fetus will be mentioned only briefly here, because the detailed evaluation will be done in the corresponding chapters on the FHR analysis. The same approach will be taken with the anesthetic drugs, which have a direct effect on the myometrium, while all the others will be discussed in Chapter 18, dealing with anesthesia in obstetrics.

OXYTOCICS

The so-called oxytocic substances have the outstanding characteristic of stimulating uterine contractions. Their mechanism of action may vary from one group of drugs to the other, and therefore their clinical indication may be guided by that characteristic. Some have a prolonged effect, while the action of others is transient. Likewise, the side effects of certain drugs are dramatic while others create a negligible response, if any, in other organ systems.

Oxytocin

One of the two known neurohormones released by the posterior pituitary, oxytocin is an octapeptide with a potent effect on the pregnant human myometrium as its primary observed effect. It also affects other systems and organs, as the breasts and peripheral vessels—actions that will be reviewed in relation to the clinical application of this hormone.

It has been in clinical use for many years as the natural extract (Pituitrin), which contains oxytocin and vasopressin (antidiuretic hormone) in varying proportions. Subsequent techniques in purification facilitated its isolation in purer forms until it was synthetized (DuVigneaud, 1953, 1954). Its eventual industrial production (Syntocinon, Pitocin) led to studies that defined its role in labor, dosages, catabolism, and side effects.

In vitro studies of pregnant uteri have demonstrated that oxytocin has a triple effect on the myometrial cells: it is inotropic, bathmotropic, and chronotropic; that is, it increases the excitability of the muscle, the strength of the contraction, and the velocity of propagation of the contraction wave. The action on the myometrium seems to be exerted by indirect stimulation of the release of calcium ions, which is influenced by direct action on adenylcyclase and phosphodiesterase, and a fall in cAMP. As the free intracellular calcium ion facilitates the sliding of actin and myosin, it also contributes to the ionic imbalance and the activation of the sodium ion movement, thus affecting the membrane potential.

The development of radioimmunoassay techniques applied to oxytocin has not been too successful in clarifying the blood levels of the hormone in gestation or during labor. Widely different blood concentrations have been reported by the few investigators who claim to have developed a reproducible technique. It is probably wise to wait for further refinements in technique or confirmation of some of the values before accepting any of them. Theobald (1948) estimated that the circulating oxytocin concentration was on the order of 1 to 5 mU/liter of blood, a very modest concentration. Recent investigations suggest that the fetus has a higher concentration of circulating oxytocin than the mother. The significance of this observation remains to be elucidated after it has been confirmed.

The *nonpregnant uterus* is almost refractory to even large doses of oxytocin administered intravenously. Within this very low degree of sen-

sitivity there are some fluctuations during the ovarian cycle, the highest response being achieved during the menstrual period. An extraordinary change develops as pregnancy progresses: a steady increase in sensitivity to oxytocin is apparent, reaching its maximum during spontaneous labor at term. Pharmacologic observations have been instrumental in determining the degree of this sensitivity, which has direct implications in the clinical use of the hormone for enhancement or induction of labor.

The *pregnant human uterus,* from midgestation on, responds increasingly to the intravenous infusion of oxytocin (Figure 9-1). The modest

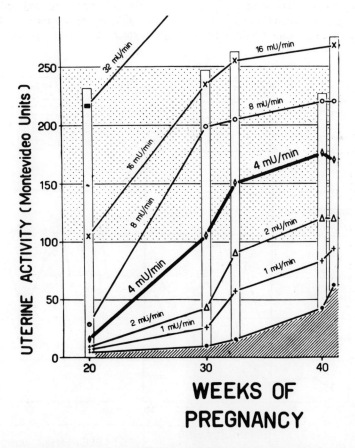

Figure 9-1 Mean values of *uterine activity* expressed in Montevideo Units (MU) plotted against duration of the second half of pregnancy, in weeks. The shaded area, lower part, represents normal spontaneous activity; the dotted area, between 100 and 250 MU, indicates the range of normal labor at term. Oxytocin infusion rates are shown in mU/min and the uterine reactivity indicated, for each gestational age in the columns. Note the rise after 30 weeks and only minimal increase after 32 weeks for 1 to 16 mU/min infusion rates, indicating the changes in myometrial sensitivity to oxytocin. This figure summarizes the concept of poor reactivity to oxytocin in early pregnancy and the sharp rise after 30 weeks. Reprinted from Caldeyro-Barcia R, Sereno JA: The response of the human uterus to oxytocin throughout pregnancy, in Caldeyro-Barcia R, Heller H (eds): *Oxytocin.* NY, Pergamon, 1961, pp 177-200.

156

reactivity demonstrated at 20 weeks gestation evolves steadily until about 35 weeks. There is no general agreement concerning the changes in uterine sensitivity to oxytocin beyond this period: Caldeyro-Barcia and his school (1961) believe that there no longer is an increase in sensitivity, while Theobald and others postulate that the sensitivity continues to increase steadily to make a sharp change immediately preceding labor.

Oxytocin should be administered only by the *intravenous route and in very diluted concentrations.* When the infusions are started at the physiologic rates and administered to term uteri, uterine activity rises slowly but does not reach maximum effect for at least 20 to 60 min, depending on the rate of infusion. The lower infusion rates take longer (Figure 9-2) than the higher rates (Figure 9-3) to reach a steady state. for this reason

it is not advisable to increase infusion rates more often than every 20 min; hyperstimulation may be the consequence of too hasty increases in rate. After the steady state has been reached—approximately 30 minutes—uterine activity remains fairly constant with only the normal slow oscillating fluctuations characteristic of its spontaneous action (Figure 9-4). However, with the progress of labor there is a small but continuous increase in spontaneous uterine activity (Figure 9-5) superimposed on which is the effect of the exogenous oxytocin. For this reason, constant monitoring is mandatory for a patient being given oxytocin, and the tracing must be frequently reviewed for appropriate adjustment of the dose.

The pregnant uterus responds with increased contractility when the rates of infused oxytocin are augmented in a stepwise manner; starting with

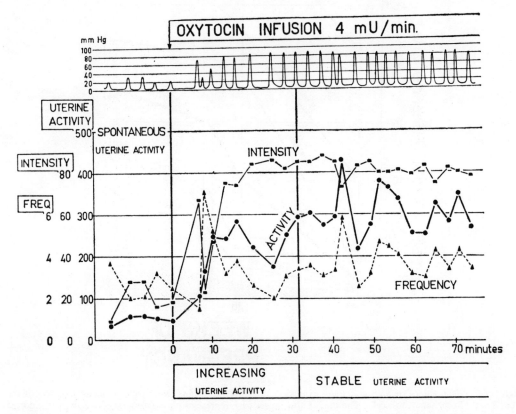

Figure 9-2 Uterine response to oxytocin infusion started at 4 mU/min on a term pregnant patient. *(Above)* Intrauterine pressure tracing. Frequency (per 10 minutes), intensity (in mm Hg), and uterine activity (in Montevideo Units) have been calculated and plotted for each contraction. Shortly after the oxytocin infusion was started, the uterine contractility increased regularly to reach stable values at 32 min. Note the fluctuations of all parameters even with stable activity. Only a minimal increase in tonus may be observed. Reprinted from Sica-Blanco, Y, Sala NL: Uterine contractility at the beginning and end of an oxytocin infusion, in Caldeyro-Barcia R, Heller H (eds): *Oxytocin.* NY, Pergamon, 1961, pp 127–136.

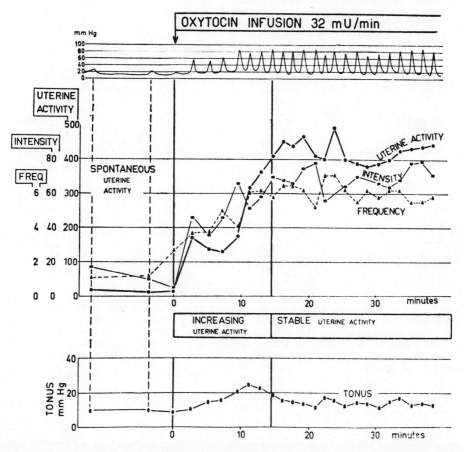

Figure 9-3 Uterine response to oxytocin infusion started at 32 mU/min in a term pregnant patient carrying a dead fetus. *(Above)* Intrauterine pressure tracing. Shortly after the oxytocin infusion was started the uterine activity increased rapidly. The rising contractility reached a stable level about 15 min after starting the oxytocin (much sooner than in Figure 9-2) and the fluctuations were still present thereafter. Note the rise of the tonus to pathologic levels followed by slow adaptation and return to normal. Reprinted from Sica-Blanco Y, Sala NL: Uterine contractility at the beginning and end of an oxytocin infusion, in Caldeyro-Barcia R, Heller H (eds): *Oxytocin.* NY, Pergamon, 1961, pp 127–136.

small doses (1 mU/min) they may be doubled (2,4,8 mU/min) approximately every 30 min. All the elements analyzed may show an increase (Figure 9-6), and therefore the calculated uterine activity will rise regularly.

The *frequency* of contractions increases steadily in about 75% of cases, as the oxytocin infusion rate is augmented within physiologic ranges. This is more clearly observed in prelabor with contractions occurring at moderate to low frequency. In approximately 25% of cases the spontaneous frequency is very high, when oxytocin may induce no change or even a slight decrease as the effects on intensity are established.

The *intensity* of contractions is likewise in-

fluenced according to preinfusion spontaneous values. In about 90% of cases the intensity increases as the oxytocin infusion rate is augmented in a stepwise fashion, until uterine activity reaches its maximum efficiency. If the infusion rate is further augmented, the intensity diminishes (Figure 9-6) as the tonus increases, and the frequency is so high that the relaxation phase of the contraction is interrupted by the next contraction (polysystoly). Only in 10% of cases is spontaneous intensity high enough so that no further increase is induced by the oxytocic.

The *tonus,* which at term ranges between 6 and 10 mm Hg, is always affected by infusions of oxytocin, even small doses. However, important

158

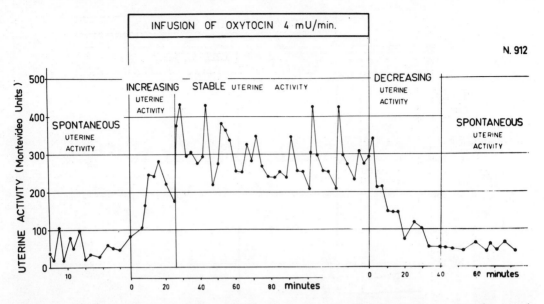

Figure 9-4 Uterine response, stable activity, and decreasing contractility of a term pregnant uterus under oxytocin infusion at 4 mU/min. Uterine activity plotted against time illustrates the rising contractility, which stabilizes at about 26 min; the normal fluctuating activity when uterus is in steady state; and the regular decline after discontinuing the infusion. Activity reached preinfusion values 40 min later. Reprinted from Sica-Blanco Y, Sala NL: Uterine contractility at the beginning and end of an oxytocin infusion, in Caldeyro-Barcia R, Heller H (eds): *Oxytocin.* NY, Pergamon, 1961, pp 127–136.

increases are seen only when the oxytocic is given with an already maximal normal contractility (Figure 9-6), or when starting an infusion at a very high rate (see Figure 9-3). When these infusion rates are not supraphysiologic, the tonus will slowly come down, "adapting" to the new conditions, and stabilize in about 15 min when the frequency of contractions normalizes. On the other hand, the infusion of supramaximal rates will trigger "tetanic" contractions, with very high tonus, which remain sustained as long as the infusion passes and for prolonged period of time after it has been discontinued (see Figure 9-18).

There is an interesting, and probably useful, reciprocal relationship between the intensity and frequency of contractions and the achievement of a steady state or stable uterine activity. The dose–response curve for uterine activity of the normal term pregnant uterus has been defined (Figure 9-7), and it is amazingly parallel to the curve of oxytocin blood levels measured during infusions of very high doses of oxytocin (Figures 9-8 and 9-18) under study conditions. When the infusion rate is above the physiologic concentra-

tions, the uterus will manifest overstimulation expressed as increased tonus, a significant rise in frequency, or a diminished intensity as a result of the hypertonus. The hypercontractility may severely compromise a living fetus. Experience has demonstrated that the sensitivity of the term uterus is such that infusion of more than 20 mU/min oxytocin to obtain a labor-like contractility is seldom required; usually between 1 and 5 mU/min is sufficient. A *preterm uterus requires higher infusion rates,* in reverse proportion to the age of gestation, to obtain comparable uterine activity.

When the oxytocin infusion is discontinued, uterine activity decreases exponentially until it reaches the preinfusion, or control, activity (Figures 9-4 and 9-9). The average time to reach the control activity level has been found to be in the range of 40 to 50 min for physiologic infusions in term pregnancies. Increasing and decreasing activity curves are clearly different and independent from each other but dependent on the infusion rate and the age of gestation: the greater the starting infusion rate, the shorter the time to reach

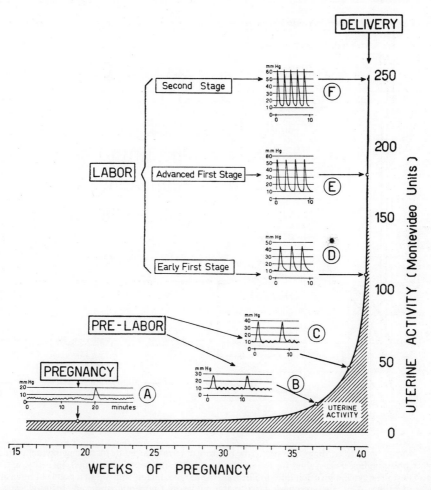

Figure 9-5 Schematic representation of spontaneous uterine activity during pregnancy and labor in Montevideo Units (shaded area) plotted against stage of gestation in weeks. Note slow rise after 35 weeks and the sharp increase during labor. Representative tracings for each stage are shown with arrows indicating the corresponding time. In labor (D,E,F) there is a steady increase in intensity and frequency as dilatation progresses. Reprinted from Caldeyro-Barcia, Poseiro JJ: Oxytocin and contractility of the pregnant human uterus. *Ann NY Acad Sci* 75:813, 1959.

stable uterine activity; the earlier the gestation, the faster the decline of activity toward preinfusion values.

The *half-life* of exogenous *circulating oxytocin* is very short, on the order of *3 min* (Figure 9-8), while the half-life of the uterine response is about *15 min* (Figures 9-9, 9-21). But the calculation of the half-life of oxytocin in the body of a patient gives a theoretical time of 9 min. Be that as it may, the important consideration is duration of uterine effects after the infusion is discontinued because the aim of the clinician is to control the contractility of the uterus.

The direct action of oxytocin on the myometrial cell facilitates the correction of irregular or ineffective contractions because it improves the three elements involved in the contractile process: excitability, strength, and propagation. Clinical use proves that the effects in vivo have confirmed in vitro studies (see Chapter 10).

160

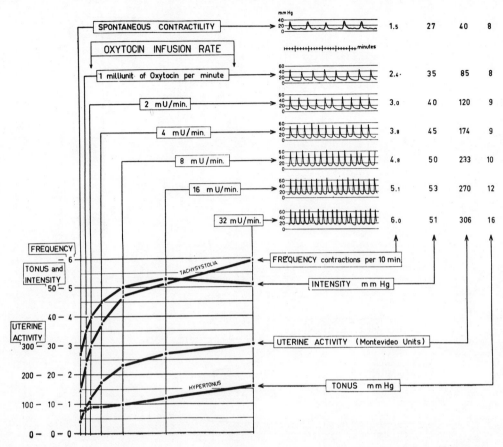

Figure 9-6 *(Above, right)* Recordings of intrauterine pressure at term induced by increasing oxytocin infusion rates. *(Below, left)* Corresponding mean values for tonus, uterine activity (in Montevideo Units), intensity, and frequency are plotted against the oxytocin infusion rates to illustrate the parallel increments (up to a point) of intensity and frequency of contractions. This dose–response curve is the one most frequently observed. Infusion rates above 16 mU/min induced polysystoly, hypertonus, and diminishing intensity. Reprinted from Poseiro JJ, Noriega-Guerra L: Dose-response relationships in uterine effects of oxytocin infusions, in Caldeyro-Barcia R, Heller H (eds): *Oxytocin.* NY, Pergamon, 1961, pp 158–174.

The intravenous infusion of oxytocin in physiologic amounts was introduced by Theobald (1948) but close to a decade elapsed before the dose–response relationships were studied for term pregnancies (normal and pathologic) or preterm gestations. Currently the intravenous route is used widely, and it should be used that way, with few exceptions. The *intramuscular* and *subcutaneous* routes should never be used with the intention of stimulating a uterus with a live fetus because they require the administration of large doses, which have unpredictable absorption rates, therefore creating the risk of inducing significant hypercontractility. These routes of administration may be used to stimulate the uterus after second stage has been completed, to facilitate separation of the placenta or control of postpartum bleeding. It should be understood that the oxytocin given by these ways will have a short-term effect because its half-life in the circulating blood is extremely short (only about 3 min).

Exceptionally the *intranasal route* may be used because the total dose given is small, and the absorption rate has been calculated to be equivalent to a single intravenous dose of 5 mU for each spray of 40 units/ml. The response is rapid, predicatable, and appears physiologic (Figure 9-10) when the sensitivity of the uterus

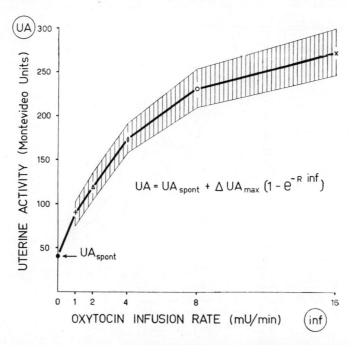

Figure 9-7 Dose–response curve of oxytocin infusion rates and uterine activity plotted in Montevideo Units. It represents the average and standard deviation of normal patients between 36 and 40 weeks gestation. Reprinted from Caldeyro-Barcia R, Poseiro JJ: Oxytocin and contractility of the pregnant human uterus. *Ann NY Acad Sci* 75:813, 1959.

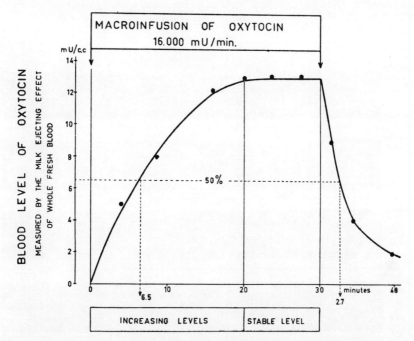

Figure 9-8 Increasing concentration of exogenous oxytocin plotted against time. Administered to a patient carrying a dead fetus. The supraphysiologic infusion was started and assays made at each point plotted. Blood level stabilized at 20 min but had reached 50% at 6.5 min. The infusion was discontinued, and the blood level of oxytocin fell very rapidly, reaching half-life in 2.7 min. Reprinted from Gonzalez-Panizza VH, et al: The fate of injected oxytocin in the pregnant woman near term, in Caldeyro-Barcia R, Heller H (eds): *Oxytocin*. NY, Pergamon, 1961, pp 347–357.

162

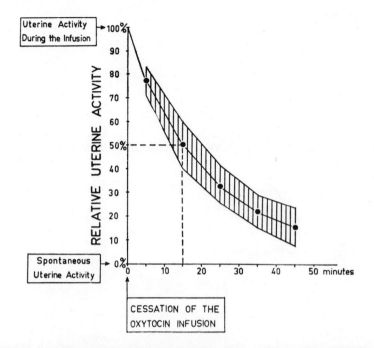

Figure 9-9 Average curve and standard deviation of decreasing *uterine activity* after discontinuing a physiologic ox-ytocin infusion in term pregnant patients not in labor. For comparison, the values of all cases were tabulated in per-cent of activity. The time required to drop the activity to 50% was 15 min, while that required to reach control was over 50 min. Reprinted from Sica-Blanco Y, Sala NL: Uterine contractility at the beginning and end of an oxytocin in-fusion, in Caldeyro-Barcia R, Heller H (eds): *Oxytocin*. NY, Pergamon, 1961, pp 127–136.

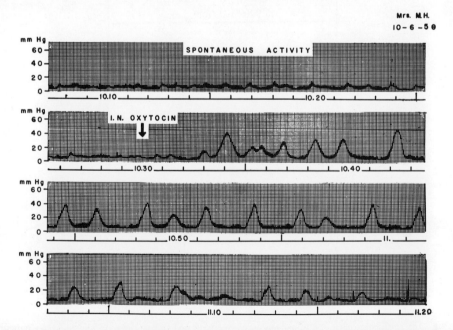

Figure 9-10 Continuous 72-min intrauterine pressure tracing of term patient not in labor. Intranasal spray of ox-ytocin (arrow) was given, and within 4 min the uterine contractility was stimulated. *(Bottom)* The decreasing activity after 30 min of excellent response. Reprinted from Hendricks CH, Pose SV: Intranasal oxytocin in obstetrics. *JAMA* 175:384, 1961. Copyright 1961, American Medical Association.

can respond to such small doses. In fact, in many circumstances very few applications are sufficient to trigger labor.

The uterine response to oxytocin is conditioned not only by the stage of gestation and the amount given but also by the preexisting uterine activity. When this activity is excessively high, the uterus is already contracting at supramaximal capacity and will not significantly increase in activity when physiologic infusions are given. This quality served Cobo et al (1965) as the basis for their classification of abruptio placentae in two types (Figure 9-11) and should be an important element to consider in the management of this syndrome.

Precautions in the use of oxytocin   The injudicious use of this hormone may jeopardize the life of the fetus, the mother, or both. Hyperstimulation of the uterus produces hypercontractility of

variable degree and diminution of IVS blood flow. Uterine hyperstimulation may occur at the onset of an infusion (Figures 9-12 and 9-13) if there is an error in technique or if the proportion of hormone is too great.

It may also occur when, during steady infusion, the underlying spontaneous uterine activity increases as dilatation progresses; the sum of both effects (spontaneous and induced) then becomes an exaggerated contractility manifested by polysystoly and hypertonus (Figures 9-14 and 9-15). The consequence of this excessive contractility will be diminished oxygen supply to the fetus, fetal distress expressed by altered FHR patterns, and eventual fetal death if the hypercontractility is prolonged (so-called tetanic contraction).

It is often reported that oxytocin is the principal cause of uterine rupture, but this occurs only when oxytocin is grossly misused or when the

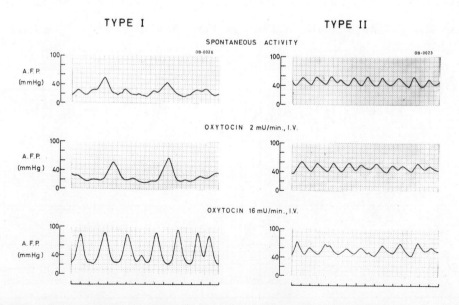

Figure 9-11   Uterine response to oxytocin in two cases of abruptio placentae. Type I responded to increasing infusion rates of oxytocin, having an excellent pattern with 16 mU/min. Type II illustrates a complete lack of response because the spontaneous activity *(top)* was already the maximal activity which that uterus could develop. Reprinted from Cobo E, et al: Uterine behavior in abruptio placentae. *Am J Obstet Gynecol* 93:1151, 1965.

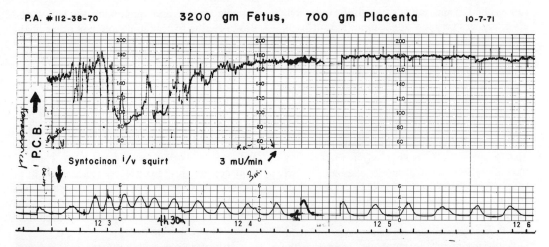

Figure 9-12 Continuous 37-min intrauterine pressure and FHR recordings of enhanced labor in term primipara, middle of first stage. When the oxytocin infusion was to be started (arrow) a large amount was inadvertently injected. Rapid uterine response with polysystoly and hypertonus triggered a severe fetal bradycardia. The hypertonus lasted 8 min after which the contractility resumed a more physiologic pattern and the FHR recovered with a rebound tachycardia and fixed baseline. Reprinted from Cibils LA, Santonja-Lucas JJ: Clinical significance of fetal heart rate patterns during labor. III. Effect of paracervical block anesthesia. *Am J Obstet Gynecol* 130:73, 1978.

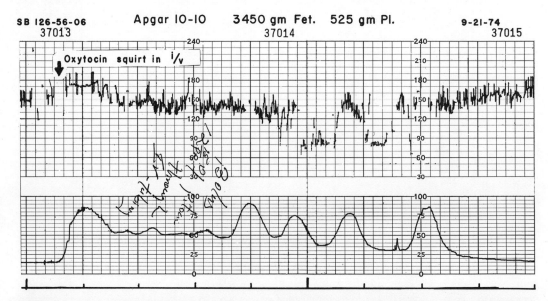

Figure 9-13 Nine minutes of intrauterine pressure and FHR tracings in term multipara with premature rupture of membranes. At the start of the induction of labor a bolus of oxytocin was unwittingly injected, and a severe episode of hypercontractility (hypertonus and polysystoly) was triggered. Note the moderate fetal bradycardia accompanying the hypertonus, which lasted over 7 min. The patient delivered 10 hours later.

"LATE" DECELERATIONS, REBOUND TACHYCARDIA and RECOVERY

118-22-64   3465 gm FETUS   Apgar 6-7   Placenta 740 gm   2-21-73

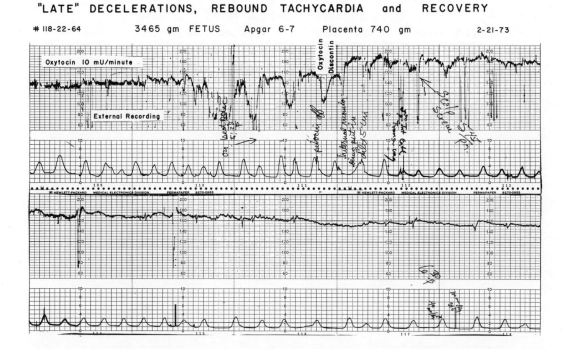

Figure 9-14 Continuous 100-min uterine contraction and FHR tracings at term, induced labor. *(Above)* With oxytocin running at 10 mU/min and with 5 cm dilatation, the frequency of contractions reached 6 to 7/10 min; later decelerations of FHR were recorded until oxytocin was discontinued. Rebound tachycardia and fixed baseline were thereafter recorded. *(Below)* Slow return to normal was observed with frequency of contractions around 5/10 min. Reprinted from Cibils LA: Clinical significance of fetal heart rate patterns during labor. II. Late decelerations. *Am J Obstet Gynecol* 123:473, 1975.

uterus is defective. Hypercontractility and rupture of course may occur only with a fetus in utero, but the implication that large amounts of oxytocin can be safely administered in the postpartum period is inaccurate and even dangerous. The *rapid intravenous* administration of oxytocin causes a significant episode of hypotension (Figure 9-16), the degree of which is in direct proportion to the amount of oxytocin given (Figure 9-17).

The mechanism of action seems to be due to peripheral vasodilatation, as shown by the study of the tidal and dicrotic waves in arterial pressure tracings. The potential toxic effects on myocardium have been denied by some, but the number of maternal deaths reported immediately following the intravenous administration of large doses of oxytocin requires a rational explanation. Lipton et al (1962) have shown that when intravenous

oxytocin in supraphysiologic doses is given simultaneously with certain anesthetics, it produces alarming alterations in the maternal ECG, suggesting a cardiotoxic effect. The hypotensive effect of large doses of intravenous oxytocin is reproducible even in patients with hypovolemic hypotension (Hendricks and Brenner, 1970), a particularly critical situation, often seen in postpartum or in postabortion hemorrhages.

The potentially dangerous effects and the disturbing hemodynamic action of large amounts of intravenous oxytocin are better seen by observing the alterations produced by macroinfusions (Figure 9-18). The hypotension triggered is not counterbalanced by the immediate uterine "tetanic" contraction, and it continues for several minutes. At the same time the central venous pressure rises and stays high even after recovery and rebound of blood pressure. The cardiovas-

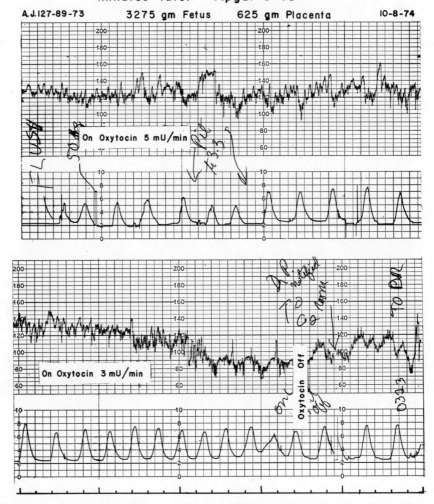

Figure 9-15 Continuous 50-min recording of intrauterine pressure and FHR tracings of induced labor in term multipara. *(Above)* Advanced first stage, 5 mU/min oxytocin, produced maximal uterine activity and was reduced to 3.3 mU/min, which was still too much. *(Below)* Hypercontractility (10 contractions in 15 min at one point) and hypertonus produced significant fetal bradycardia. Oxytocin was discontinued as dilatation completed, and shortly thereafter a normal infant with good Apgar scores was delivered.

cular system of the pregnant patient is much more sensitive to these large amounts of oxytocin than that of the male or the nonpregnant female. It is likely that the high steroid hormonal levels of pregnancy condition (or prime) the smooth muscle receptors to oxytocin in the various target organs (uterus, arteriolar smooth muscle)—as occurs with the sympathomimetic substances during the ovarian cycle (Cibils, 1971).

A very important and potentially severe side effect produced by large and sustained adminis-

tration of oxytocin is the syndrome of water intoxication. Essentially, it is the consequence of the injudicious use of oxytocin in electrolyte-free solutions given over prolonged periods of time. Oxytocin in sustained high-infusion rates has an antidiuretic effect, which, with large quantities of infused fluids, will trigger a severe electrolyte imbalance, water retention, and interstitial and brain edema. The condition is completely preventable by the careful administration of fluids when there is need to give large amounts of oxytocin.

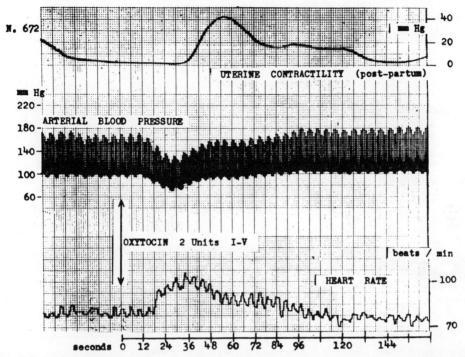

Figure 9-16 Arterial hypotension and tachycardia produced by the intravenous push of 2 IU oxytocin post-partum. *(Above)* Intrauterine pressure. *(Center)* Intraarterial catheter records blood pressure. *(Below)* Tachometer fed by systole signal records pulse rate. Within 15 sec of intravenous injection (circulation time) a significant hypotension is observed; it recovered 90 sec later. Reprinted from Caldeyro-Barcia and Poseiro (1958).

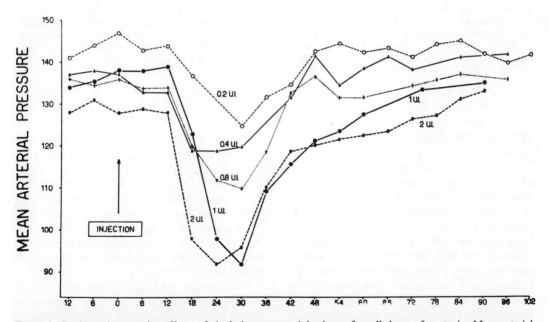

Figure 9-17 Acute hypotensive effects of single intravenous injections of small doses of oxytocin. Mean arterial pressure recordings from femoral artery in the immediate postpartum. The hypotensive effect is proportional to the dose injected: even very small doses triggered significant transient hypotension. Reprinted from Hendricks (1957).

168

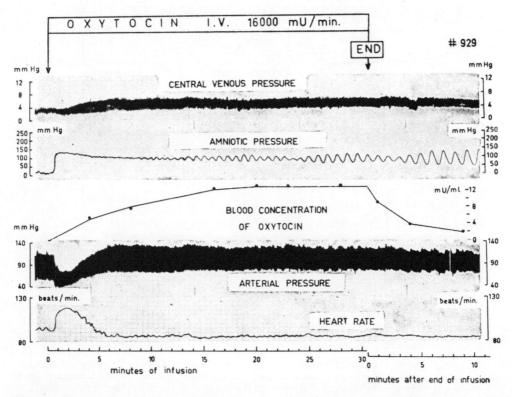

Figure 9-18 Continuous tracings, recorded from a 34-week pregnant patient carrying a dead fetus. *(Above)* Central venous and intrauterine pressures. *(Below)* Intraarterial pressure and pulse rate. *(Center)* Blood oxytocin levels during the infusion (similar curve as in Figure 9-8). The supraphysiologic infusion of 16,000 mU/min triggered at the start a dramatic hypotension and tachycardia, with small drop in CVP. The latter bounced up at 2 min, but the blood pressure recovered only after 5 min and was followed by hypertension and bradycardia. The intrauterine pressure responded almost instantly with a prolonged "tetanic contraction," but in spite of this increased peripheral resistance, the hypotension persisted several minutes. Infusion was discontinued after 30 min, triggering a small drop in blood pressure but still staying above control values. Reprinted from Bieniarz J: Cardiovascular effects of high doses of oxytocin, in Caldeyro-Barcia R, Heller H (eds): *Oxytocin*. NY, Pergamon, 1961, pp 80–83.

Oxytocin Derivatives

The original investigations on oxytocin were carried out with pituitary extracts of variable degrees of purity. The material consisted mainly of oxytocin and antidiuretic hormone (ADH) as significant contaminant. One extract (Pituitrin) contains about 20% of the ADH vasopressin, which affected the systemic response to it. Further purified substances were marketed as Pitocin and Pitressin, each one almost pure oxytocin and ADH. As a matter of practical importance, the response of these various preparations was studied and compared with the pure synthetic oxytocin then available. The highly purified marketed extract, a purified laboratory extract, and the synthetic preparation have equivalent oxytocic effects on the pregnant human uterus (Figure 9-19). Their action is so similar that they look almost indistinguishable. The period of increasing uterine activity and the time required to reach a stable effect are almost the same (Figure 9-20), as are the curve of decreasing activity and half-life of uterine activity after discontinuing the infusion (Figure 9-21).

Vasopressin (ADH) A natural posterior pituitary hormone with a chemical structure similar to oxytocin, vasopressin is a constituent of the neurohypophyseal extract Pituitrin. However, its effects on the uterus and the cardiovascular

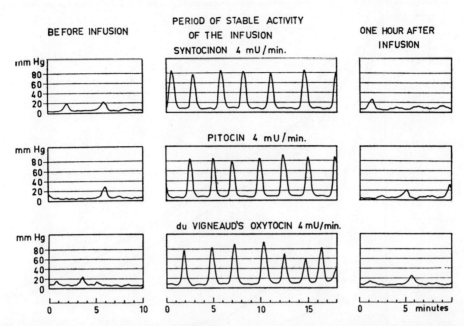

Figure 9-19 Uterine activity before, during stable response, and 1 hour after discontinuing the infusion of three different oxytocin preparations in a term pregnant patient with intact membranes. Note the remarkable similarity of responses to the same infusion rates. Reprinted from Cibils LA, et al: Comparison of the effects on the pregnant human uterus of highly purified natural oxytocin, Pitocin, synthetic oxytocin (Syntocinon) valyl-3-oxytocin and arginine vasopressin, in Caldeyro-Barcia R, Heller H (eds): *Oxytocin.* NY, Pergamon, 1961, pp 266–275.

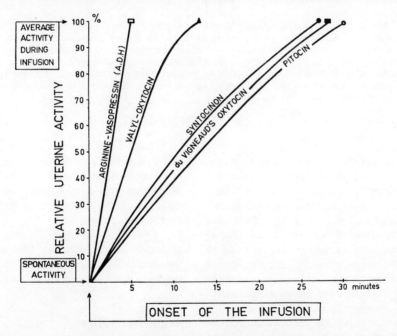

Figure 9-20 Period of increasing uterine activity until stabilization, plotted against time, for five oxytocic substances. Average of relative increases, the stabilized activity taken as 100% and the spontaneous activity preceding the infusion taken as zero. For the oxytocins, the settling time is similar (26 to 30 min), while the ADH and valyl-oxytocin the time is much shorter. Reprinted from Cibils LA, et al: Comparison of the effects on the pregnant human uterus of highly purified natural oxytocin, Pitocin, synthetic oxytocin (Syntocinon) valyl-3-oxytocin and arginine vasopressin, in Caldeyro-Barcia R, Heller H (eds): *Oxytocin.* NY, Pergamon, 1961, pp 266–275.

170

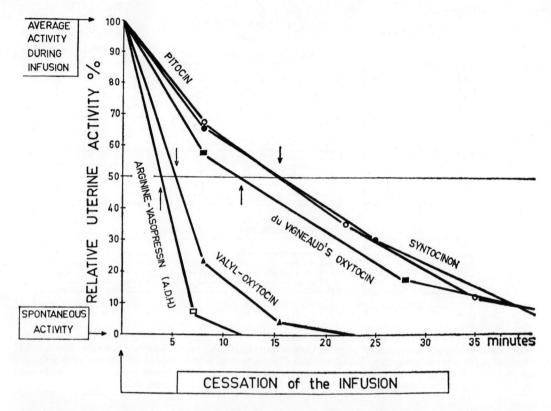

Figure 9-21   Rate of decline of uterine activity after discontinuing the infusion of various oxytocins in term pregnant uteri. The stable activity during infusion was taken as 100%, and the level of spontaneous activity after stabilization as zero. The arrows along the line of 50% indicate the half-life of uterine activity for each preparation. The oxytocins have a very similar curve (13 to 16 mm T 50%), while ADH and valyl-oxytocin have a much shorter time. Reprinted from Cibils LA, et al: Comparison of the effects on the pregnant human uterus of highly purified natural oxytocin, Pitocin, synthetic oxytocin (Syntocinon) valyl-3-oxytocin and arginine vasopressin, in Caldeyro-Barcia R, Heller H (eds): *Oxytocin.* NY, Pergamon, 1961, pp 266–275.

system are significantly different from oxytocin. As an oxytocic, it is approximately 30 times less effective than oxytocin (Figure 9-22) even though it requires a very short time to reach maximum effect (settling time), and it has a rapid decreasing activity with a half-life of only 5 min (Figure 9-21). Furthermore, it triggers contractions of incoordinated characteristics. Finally, the uterine sensitivity to vasopressin does not change with the progress of pregnancy; also, the menstrual uterus is exquisitely sensitive to ADH. All these distinctions point to important pharmacologic differences between vasopressin and oxytocin in spite of their similarity in chemical structure.

An equally different action is observed with blood pressure. Vasopressin is a hypertensive substance (Figure 9-23) in large and small doses

and is capable of partially counteracting the effect of oxytocin when a mixture of both is injected. This characteristic justifies the reluctance of the clinicians of the recent past to give Pituitrin to preeclamptic patients.

The recent synthesis of over 40 oxytocin analogues has extended this field immeasurably, but their clinical application has been very disappointing, none being as good as oxytocin.

Ergot Derivatives

Ergot was the first oxytocic substance used with the specific purpose of stimulating uterine contractions, a property originally observed to be effective in cows. In fact, the empiric use of

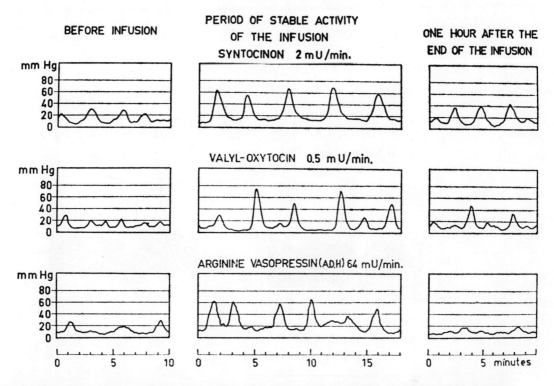

Figure 9-22 Uterine activity recorded before, during stable induced activity, and after discontinuing infusion of oxytocin, ADH, and valyl-oxytocin in the same term pregnant patient with intact membranes. Note the irregular, incoordinated pattern produced by ADH and the much higher infusion rate (than oxytocin) required to trigger a grossly equivalent response. Reprinted from Cibils LA, et al: Comparison of the effects on the pregnant human uterus of highly purified natural oxytocin, Pitocin, synthetic oxytocin (Syntocinon) valyl-3-oxytocin and arginine vasopressin, in Caldeyro-Barcia R, Heller H (eds): *Oxytocin.* NY, Pergamon, 1961, pp 266–275.

substances containing ergot was in regular use until the identification and crystallization of the pure principle (Dudley and Moir; Adair et al, 1935). Its action was well studied in the postpartum human uterus, and its use and benefits outlined.

However, the intrapartum use of ergot and its derivatives remained largely confusing, or controversial, because of the known potent oxytocic activity of some and the claimed sympatholitic (and thus "antispasmodic" or relaxant) properties of others, the latter presumably facilitating the progress of labor by "relaxing the lower segment and cervix." With the advent of intrauterine recording techniques and their application to study the effect of drugs, the latter properties were disproved for dihydroergotamine which in fact is a potent oxytocic causing severe hypertonus. This property is proportional to the dose given, irrespective of the route of administration.

Methergine   A synthetic ergot derivative,

Methergine, like all ergots, produces irregular contractions and hypertonus even in small doses. An important characteristic of all these drugs is their *long-lasting effect on the uterus* even when given intramuscularly in doses of 5 μg (1 ampule of standard preparation has 200 μg) (Figure 9-24). When Methergine is given in this manner its effect may not be immediate, but it will become apparent when the spontaneous activity increases or is stimulated by intravenous infusion of oxytocin at physiologic doses (Figure 9-25).

Ergotrate   The ergot derviative most commonly used has the same characteristics as Methergine. When infused intravenously, extremely small doses may be used to attempt induction of labor but are usually not effective because of the poor quality of the contractions thus obtained (Figure 9-26). For this reason, ergotrate should not be used to induce labor (at one time it was given orally to induce and stimulate labor).

172

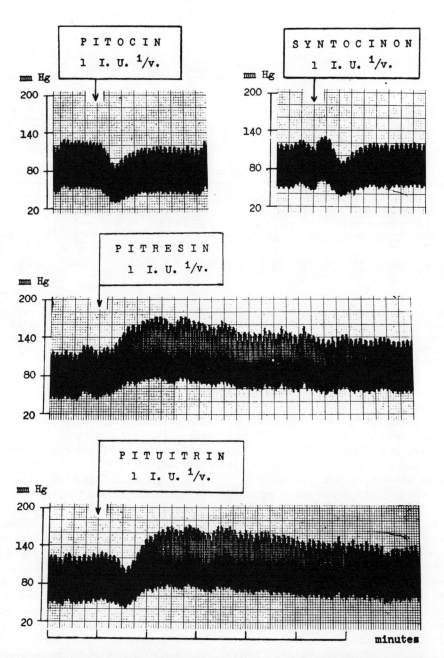

Figure 9-23 Comparison of cardiovascular effects of oxytocin *(top),* ADH *(middle),* and their mixture in natural extract *(bottom).* In each 1 IU was administered. The rapid intravenous injection of oxytocin produced hypotension and slow recovery; ADH triggered marked hypertension, lasting several minutes; and their mixture, a combination of both effects but the hypotension was less. Reprinted from Caldeyro-Barcia and Poseiro (1958).

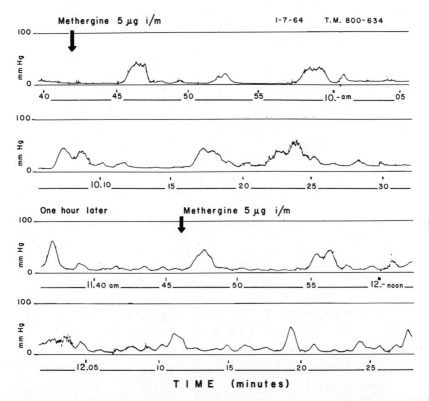

Figure 9-24 Intrauterine pressure tracings of term pregnant patient in prelabor. The top two tracings show continuous 53 min of contractility following the intramuscular injection of 5 μg of methylergonovine maleate. Note the long undulating contractions in the second tracing. In the bottom two tracings, after another dose of 5 μg, the contractility persisted as incoordinated and irregular. There was no apparent change in tonus. This activity continued for over 2 hours. Reprinted from Cibils and Hendricks (1969).

The *sensitivity of the pregnant* uterus to ergot derivatives increases as term approaches, but the long-lasting effect is the same at all stages. In addition, and because of the latter quality, it "sensitizes" the uterus of midgestation to oxytocin, making it responsive to doses that, when used without previous administration of ergots, would not trigger significant uterine activity (Figure 9-27). This characteristic may be applied to the clinical conditions in which the uterus manifests very poor reactivity to oxytocin (as in midgestation) and there is the compelling need to evacuate it of a nonviable (or already dead) fetus.

The intrinsic incoordinating effects of ergot derivatives on the uterus are better observed when they are given to a patient who has demonstrated good response to oxytocin (Figure 9-28). The characteristic of increasing the tone, and having a very long effect should be applied to good use in clinical application, reserving their use for the *postpartum period* when the uterus is empty and there is need for good hemostasis brought about by the contractions.

The use of ergot derivatives to stimulate the expulsion of the placenta is not effective because it has been shown that there is a higher rate of retained placentas with the use of ergots as compared to spontaneous third-stage delivery (Figure 9-29). It is likely that the incoordinated contractions generated in the pregnant uterus also occur after expulsion of the fetus, thus facilitating the trapping of the placenta.

Ergot derivatives should not be administered before the third stage of labor. Their proper place in obstetrics is after the expulsion of the placenta, when their long-lasting and hypertonic properties are most useful in preventing unnecessary blood loss.

174

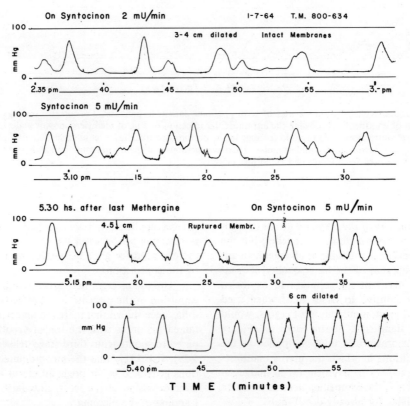

On Syntocinon   2 mU/min   1-7-64   T.M. 800-634

100

mm Hg

              3-4 cm dilated   Intact Membranes

0

2.35 pm____40_____45_____50_____55_____3.-pm

Syntocinon 5 mU/min

100

mm Hg

0

_____3.10 pm_____15_____20_____25_____30_____

5.30 hs. after last Methergine   On Syntocinon 5 mU/min

100

mm Hg

         4.5↓ cm   Ruptured Membr.

0

_____5.15 pm_____20_____25_____30_____35_____

100   6 cm dilated

mm Hg

0

_____5.40 pm_____45_____50_____55_____

T I M E   (minutes)

Figure 9-25   Same case as in Figure 9-24, 2 hours later at the beginning of an oxytocin infusion 2 mU/min *(top)*. In the second tracing the early response to oxytocin at 5 mU/min is characterized by marked irregularity, incoordination, and high tonus. The lower two tracings 2 hours later are continuous 48 min of middle first stage after amniotomy. The incoordinated contractions still persist more than 5 hours after the last small (5 μg) dose of ergot was given. Note the polysystoly during the last 15 min shown. Reprinted from Cibils LA, Hendricks CH: *J Reprod Med* 2:147, 1969.

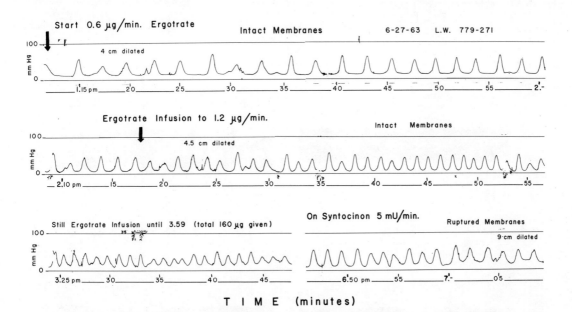

Figure 9-26 Uterine response to intravenous infusion or ergonovine maleate in a normal term pregnant patient. *(Above)* Response to the first 50 min of infusion at very slow rate. *(Center)* Increase in rate and uterine response. Note some irregularities in the pattern, absent in the top tracing, and the steady increase in frequency. *(Below, left)* Disrupted contractility pattern (compare with *above, right)* induced by the continuous infusion eventually discontinued after reaching 160 μg. *(Below, right)* Stable activity with incoordination and hypertonus still present in advanced first stage after 5 mU/min oxytocin is administered. Reprinted from Cibils LA, Hendricks CH: *J Reprod Med* 2:147, 1969.

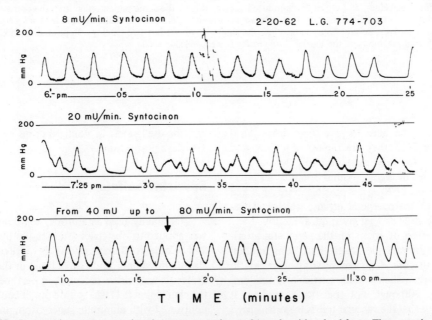

Figure 9-27 Intrauterine pressure tracings in pregnant patient at 24 weeks with a dead fetus. The oxytocin response 5 hours after administration of 48 μg of ergonovine. *(Above)* Response to only 8 mU/min of oxytocin evokes contractions of over 100 mm Hg at a frequency of 6/10 min. *(Center, and below)* Infusion increase to 20, 40, and 80 mU/min produced an extraordinary hypercontractility of one contraction per minute of very high intensity with hypertonus. Reprinted from Cibils LA, Hendricks CH: *J Reprod Med* 2:147, 1969.

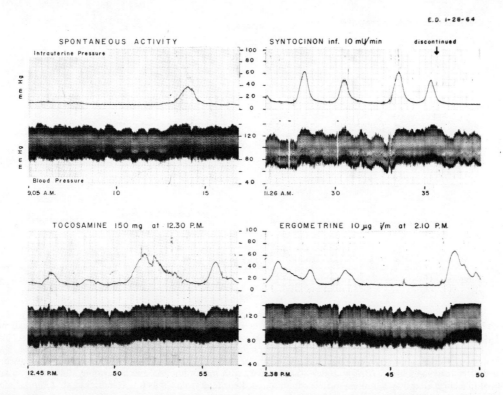

Figure 9-28 Uterine contractility and blood pressure tracings recorded in term pregnancy. Patterns of spontaneous, and oxytocin-, sparteine-, and ergometrine-induced contractility in the same patient. The smooth contractility produced by oxytocin is very different from that induced by intramuscular sparteine sulfate (lower left) or by ergometrine in very small amounts, several hours later. Note the similarity of the last two tracings. Reprinted from Cibils LA, Zuspan FP: Pharmacology of the uterus. *Clin Obstet Gynecol* 11:34, 1968.

There is no need to give these drugs intravenously because they are rapidly absorbed, and the term uterus is extraordinarily sensitive to minute doses of ergots. Within 3 min of an intramuscular dose of 20 μg it is possible to see a marked response of the puerperal uterus, which will respond to as little as 1 μg given intravenously.

The effect of ergots on the peripheral arterioles must always be taken into consideration because of the high sensitivity observed in hypertensive patients and particularly in preeclampsia. Although not specifically studied, it may well be that the vascular tree is hypersensitized to ergots as it has been shown to be for angiotensin II. Thus the use of ergot derivatives should not be recommended in the immediate postpartum period of patients with preeclampsia or chronic hypertension. However, experience has demonstrated that it

may be used safely in standard doses by mouth a few days postpartum.

Sparteine Sulfate

Originally used in Europe, sparteine sulfate was applied to obstetrics after studies by Alvarez and Caldeyro-Barcia (1954) in Uruguay and Plentl, Friedman, and Gray (1961) in the United States. It was widely accepted, in part, because of the claims that it 1) was so safe that it could be administered with minimum supervision, and 2) had practically no side effects. Subsequent clinical reports and laboratory studies prompted a reevaluation of its safety because of the unpredictability of its effects. The *intramuscular* administration of 150 mg may be sufficient to induce or enhance

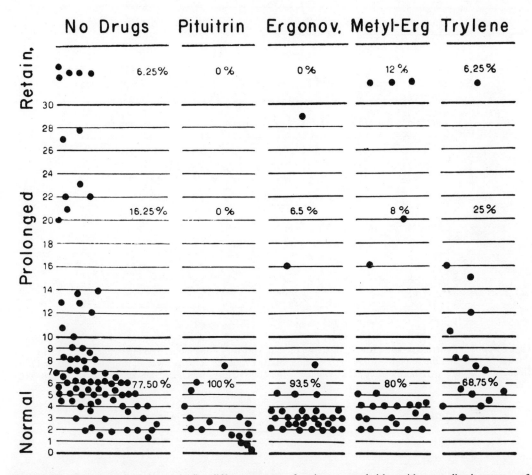

Figure 9-29 Duration of third stage in five different groups of patients treated either with no medication or one of four different preparations. Note the proportion of *retained* placentas and *prolonged third stage* when using some ergot preparations, and the best results obtained when using Pituitrin. Reprinted from Alvarez and Caldeyro-Barcia (1954).

labor (Figure 9-30). However, the uterine response cannot be predicted because contractions are smooth and coordinated in only one-third of the cases. In the other two-thirds, sparteine sulfate triggers irregular, incoordinated contractions particularly in advanced first stage when uterine activity is maximal. This abnormal pattern has been seen even several hours after giving the drug, with spontaneous or oxytocin-enhanced contractions. The *intravenous* administration in rates equivalent to the recommended intramuscular doses produces consistent hypercontractility with hypertonus and incoordinated contractions (Figure 9-31)—patterns very different from those recorded in spontaneous activity and accepted as normal.

Another unpublicized characteristic of the

uterine response to sparteine sulfate is the poor response observed in gestations not quite at term, when several injections of the drug are required to induce labor, indicating that, as for oxytocin and ergots, the sensitivity to sparteine sulfate increases as pregnancy progresses, becoming maximal during labor. Also, like ergots, sparteine sulfate has *very long lasting effects,* predisposing to abnormal contractility in advanced labor when the spontaneous activity increases.

The sequential administration of sparteine sulfate and ergotrate in the same patient triggers contractions that are similar in characteristics and effect: poor coordination, irregularity, and hypercontractility in advanced first stage (Figure 9-32). Furthermore, the efficiency of the contractions

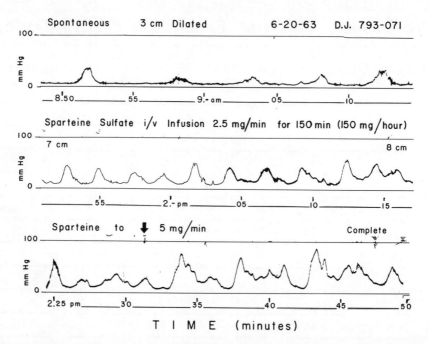

Figure 9-30 Intrauterine pressure tracing of term pregnant patient, during labor. The top two tracings record continuous 50 min, and the response to 150 mg sparteine sulfate IM (given at arrow) was an irregular pattern and high frequency. Amniotomy shortly after 10:25 enhanced the contractility, which became abnormal. Reprinted from Cibils LA, Hendricks CH: *J Reprod Med* 2:147, 1969.

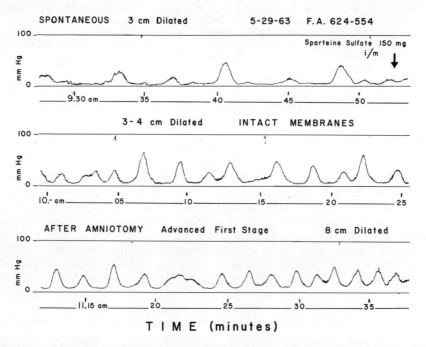

Figure 9-31 Intrauterine pressure tracings of term pregnant patient. *(Above)* Spontaneous prelabor. *(Center)* Contractility induced by 2.5 mg/min sparteine sulfate infusion for 150 min illustrates normal frequency but poor, slow relaxation of contractions in advanced first stage. *(Below)* increased, very irregular activity induced by 5 mg/min when dilatation is being completed. Reprinted from Cibils LA, Hendricks CH: *J Reprod Med* 2:147, 1969.

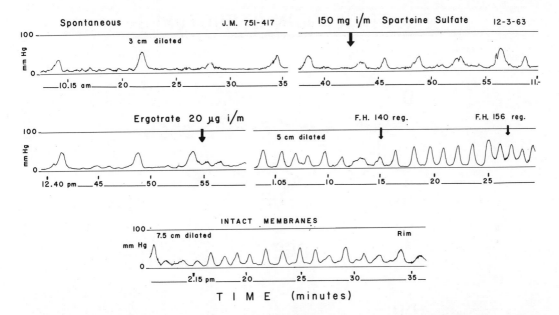

Figure 9-32 Intrauterine pressure tracing of normal term pregnancy. Evolution of uterine contractility in labor induced with sparteine sulfate and ergonovine. *(Above, left)* Characteristic spontaneous prelabor pattern. *(Above, right)* Early response to intramuscular sparteine: the average intensity remains the same but the frequency increases sharply from 1.5 to 3 contractions in 10 min. *(Center, left)* Persistent effect of sparteine with slightly diminished frequency after 2 hours, and the administration of intramuscular ergotrate. *(Center, right)* Rapid response, the outstanding feature being the marked polysystoly (up to 7 contractions in 10 min) and hypertonus due to hypercontractility. *(Below)* The effect was still very clear 1½ hours later, when incoordination seems more evident than hypercontractility, while hypertonus appears clearly as dilatation progresses. Reprinted from Cibils LA, Hendricks CH: *J Reprod Med* 2:147, 1969.

produced by these drugs cannot be compared to the more coordinated ones observed in spontaneous labor.

In essence, and in spite of the original claims, sparteine sulfate has uterine effects very much like those of ergot derivatives (Figure 9-28) although somewhat less violent, and therefore it *should not be used in human labor*.

Prostaglandins

The prostaglandins (PGs) are 20-carbon carboxylic, unsaturated fatty acids, derived from the prostanoic acid. They seem to be ubiquitous, produced in numerous tissues, and probably metabolized in situ. More than 500 compounds of this group and their analogues have been isolated or synthesized, but only a few have been studied regarding their effects on certain organ systems and still fewer with regard to their effects on the uterus.

They are classified according to the chemical structure of the ring, and the degree of unsaturation of the chains determines the subclassification (Figure 9-33) into mono-, bi-, or triunsaturated varieties. These are double-bond carbons located at specific points in the chain.

Synthesis PGs are probably synthesized from arachidonic acid, and apart from the seminal vesicles they do not seem to be stored anywhere else. It appears that only free polyunsaturated fatty acids serve as the substrate for their synthesis. PGs are mainly the product of the action of phospholipase A_2 on phospholipids rich in arachidonate in the 2 position. The subsequent synthesis is the product of a not-too-well defined group of enzymes collectively called *PG synthetase;* they are responsible for cyclization of the ring, hydroperoxydation, and hydrogen abstraction at various points of the chains. The two best studied preparations are PGE_2 and $PGF_2\alpha$, and there seems to be in certain tissues an enzyme that converts PGE_2 to $PGF_2\alpha$. This action may have

PROSTAGLANDIN STRUCTURES

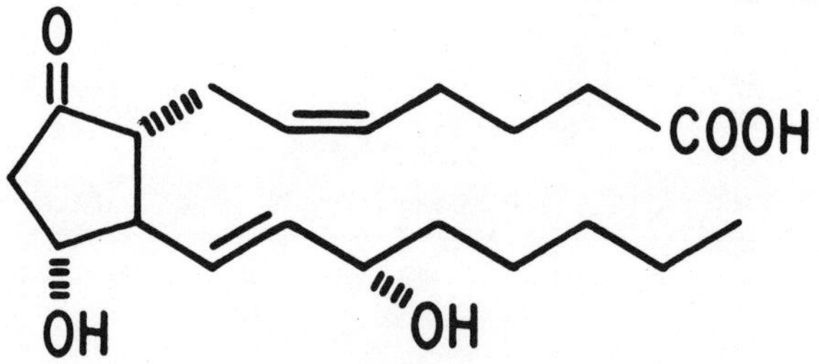

PGE₂

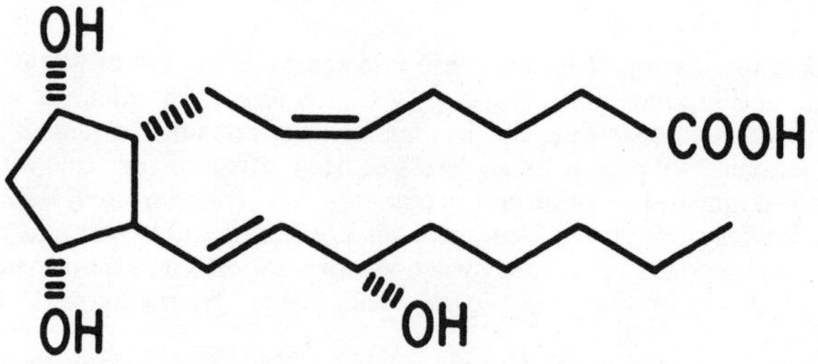

PGF₂α

Figure 9-33 Structure of the two better studied prostaglandins, showing the close similarity between the two.

important physiologic implications because they have antagonic effects on some organs. Recently a third PG with a possibly important physiologic function has been identified: prostaglandin PGI₂, or prostacyclin, with very interesting effects on smooth muscles.

Metabolism The prostaglandins are rapidly converted into inactive metabolites either within the cell or in more distant target tissues. The denaturation entails steps of oxydation and/or reduction, the major metabolite measurable in circulating blood or tissues being 15-keto, 13, 14 dehydro PGF₂α. The half-life in circulating plasma is less than 2 min when injected intravenously. A good quantity of metabolite is excreted in the urine.

Effects The endogenous synthesis of PG has specific action within the cells where receptor sites have been identified in the cell membranes. Furthermore, steroid hormones (estrogens and progesterone) seem to regulate the number of PG receptor sites in the myometrium, thus indirectly influencing the reactivity to its oxytocic action.

The action of PGS on the various systems is only partly known and understood. The cardio-vascular and renal systems, blood, gastrointestinal tract, lungs, and some basic regulatory mechanisms are all significantly affected by these compounds. However, the best known (and studied) effects are those observed on the reproductive tract, particularly the uterus and tubes. The actions on smooth muscles, excretory functions, neurotransmitters, and trophic hormones are very relevant and justify the reservations about the indiscriminate use of PGs for therapeutic purposes in obstetrics.

The direct effect on smooth muscles seems to be at the cellular level, affecting the metabolism and concentration of cAMP. The effect, however, depends on the specific type of PG, its dose, route of administration, and receptivity of the target organs often regulated by steroid hormones. From the clinical standpoint, the exogenous administration of PGs may produce the intended or desired actions as well as untoward effects of such magnitude that their use may be precluded under certain circumstances.

The use of PGs in obstetrics is, so far, based on the application of one of its outstanding actions: the *oxytocic effect* observed at any stage of gestation and the consequent property of expelling the products of conception (preterm or term). The following considerations are based on the experience gathered with PGF$_2\alpha$ and PGE$_2$ preparations.

PGs predictably *trigger uterine contractions* at any stage of gestation and, if these are maintained for a sufficiently long time, cause cervical changes and eventual expulsion of the fetus.

These effects have been observed regardless of the route of administration, which may be intravenous, oral, or intravaginal. PGs act on specific receptors located on call membranes and affect the intracellular organelles through action on cAMP. This effect is mediated by action on adenylcyclase and phosphodiesterase, decreasing the content of cAMP and facilitating the liberation of free calcium ions, which are ultimately responsible for the contraction process. Furthermore, it seems that PGs activate oxytocin receptors in the myometrium and thereby facilitate a vicious cycle of increasing contractility.

The use of intraamniotic prostaglandin F$_2\alpha$ in the second trimester of pregnancy is approved only in the United States. However, the other routes of administration and use of PGE$_2$ have been studied in limited observations in several countries, and their pharmacologic effect is well known. The uterus in early second trimester responds rather rapidly to the intraamniotic injection of PGF$_2\alpha$ (Figure 9-34). This action seems to stimulate a continuously increasing activity that

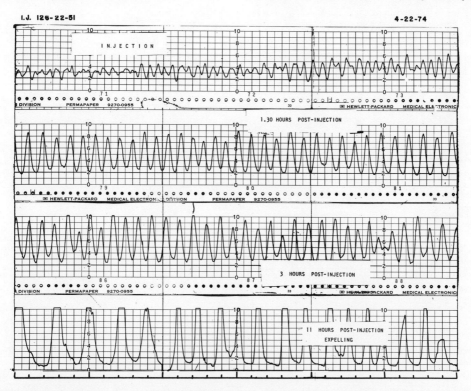

Figure 9-34 Effect of PGF$_2\alpha$ on uterine contractility in a 14-week primiparous pregnant uterus. *(Top)* The intraamniotic injection of 40 mg triggered small rapid contractions and rising tonus. Second and third tracings, the contractility is much higher and regular. *(Bottom)* Very strong contractions of over 100 mm Hg in advanced stage of preexpulsion.

182

eventually terminates in expulsion of the fetus after partial effacement and dilatation of the cervix. The contractility pattern, particularly the intensity of the contractions, is very high, as one would expect from a uterus of small volume and small radius. At the same time, the tonus increases regularly until it stabilizes at a value considered too high in term uteri. The response of the pregnant uterus to intraamniotic $PGF_2\alpha$ does not seem to change much, and at 20 weeks gestation responds as rapidly as in earlier stages (Figure 9-35). Only with intrauterine fetal demises has it been used in more advanced stages of pregnancy.

The *intravenous route* has been applied particularly in advanced gestation for induction of labor. The human uterus responds to continuous infusions of 4 µg/min or more; the labor-like activity usually being triggered by infusion rates of 10 to 40 µg/min (Anderson et al, 1972; Spellacy and Gall, 1972). The majority of investigators who have worked with these drugs claim that they are very safe for mother and fetus but, at the same time, they report on the unpredictable episodes of *hypertonus* (Figure 9-36), which may occur at any time and at any infusion rate, and which often cause severe changes in FHR. The incidence of hypertonus occurring with these "physiologic" doses has been reported to have been observed in up to 25% of the cases.

After the infusion is discontinued, $PGF_2\alpha$ disappears from the bloodstream rapidly because its half-life is less than 2 min. Nevertheless, the uterine effects are maintained for a much longer time, although a "decreasing" activity as for oxytocin has not been worked out for these substances. It disappears much more slowly from the amniotic cavity, where the half-life has been estimated at between 6 and 20 hours after the standard injection of 25 to 50 mg to induce abortion.

The oral administration of $PGF_2\alpha$ triggers similar response from the myometrium (Barr, 1972) but much higher doses are required (on the order of 30 to 100 mg) to complete an induction of labor. The main disadvantage of this route,

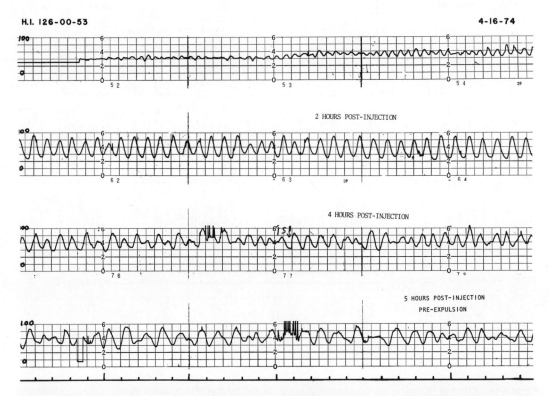

Figure 9-35 Effect of $PGF_2\alpha$ on uterine contractility in a 20-week multiparous pregnant uterus. *(Top)* The intraamniotic injection of 40 mg triggered a rise in tonus and small, rapid contractions. Two hours later the tonus was very high and the contractions were of relatively low intensity. This pattern continued until explusion time.

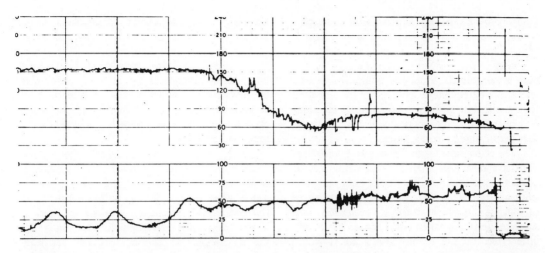

Figure 9-36 Intrauterine pressure and FHR tracings in a term labor induced with PGF$_2\alpha$. Severe episode of hypercontractility recorded during infusion and characterized by marked hypertonus, which triggered a prolonged fetal bradycardia. Reprinted from Spellacy WN, Gall SA: *J Reprod Med* 9:300, 1972.

other than the side effects, is the unpredictable rate of absorption and therefore changeable uterine responses.

PGE$_2$ has been used *intravenously* and has been demonstrated to be several times more potent than PGF$_2\alpha$. At infusion rates of 2 to 5 μg/min labor-like contractility patterns were obtained (Anderson et al, 1972; Elias, 1972), but again the investigators reported episodes of hypertonus that did not seem quite related to the amount being given.

The oral administration of PGE$_2$ has been more extensively studied (Karim and Sharma, 1972); it is reported as effective in interrupted doses of 0.5 to 2 mg and up to a total of 10 mg (Elias, 1972; Barr, 1972). Again the problems of absorption and hypercontractility should prompt serious reservations of its use with a viable fetus in utero.

Administered in vaginal suppositories, PGF$_2\alpha$ and PGE$_2$ have been demonstrated to trigger uterine activity comparable to that produced by the other routes, but required larger doses. Of course, the side effects are proportional to the amount gives.

Precautions Like the very potent oxytocics, the PGs should be used with caution in patients with scarred uteri because of the unpredictable intensity of response, especially when PGs are used to interrupt pregnancies in early second trimester. Very strong induced contractions have

produced *ruptures* of apparently healthy uteri. The lacerations usually occur between the *lower segment* and the corpus; however, ruptures along the insertion of the broad ligament are known to have occurred with relatively high frequency. Another relatively common consequence of uncontrollable hypercontractility is *laceration of the cervix,* which can vary in extension and importance — from small longitudinal tears, to complete circumferential separation of the cervix. The difficulty in preventing these accidents is the unpredictability of the uterine response; after the drug has been injected into the amniotic cavity, its effects are beyond control.

In term uteri the major problem is erratic episodes of hypercontractility with increased tonus. These episodes have been seen to occur when the drug was given either intravenously or orally, and, as with intraamniotic injections, responses cannot be predicted. The numerous *side effects* of the PGs may limit, on many occasions, their use in clinical obstetrics. Some clinical conditions constitute contraindications to their use; PGs may trigger acute attacks in patients with history of asthma, severe hypertension, cardiovascular diseases, or epilepsy.

Less dramatic, but frequently occurring undesirable *side effects,* are pain in the area of injection, nausea, vomiting, diarrhea, headaches, dizziness, hyperventilation, paresthesias, drowsiness, sensation of flushing, chest and epigastric pains, profuse sweating, hypertension and tachy-cardia, bronchiolar spasm, and hyperthermia. Most of these symptoms are dose dependent, and they tend to diminish soon after the infusion has been discontinued. A delayed complication seen with relative frequency is phlebitis of the vein used for the infusion. Some of these adverse reactions may be treated symptomatically with other drugs, thus permitting the continuation of the infusion.

The effects of PGs on the uterus at *midgestation* have been well studied. Within minutes of intraamniotic injection, the tonus rises and contractions start. This predictable effect, the degree of which is impossible to foresee accurately, in a stage of gestation when other drugs have only little effect on the uterine contractility, is the reason for the preferential use of the PGs for evacuation of the uterus in midtrimester.

On the other hand, in *term pregnancy* side effects and unpredictable response to PGs make them the second-choice drugs to stimulate the uterus physiologically. It seems that, in spite of the well-intentioned claims, oxytocin is still a more easily manageable drug with lesser undesirable reactions in mother and fetus.

Hypertonic Solutions

Aburel in 1934 postulated the intraamniotic administration of *oversaturated* (35%) *saline solutions* for the *induction of labor at term*. He demonstrated the possibility of triggering the process of labor by this means; however, the number and severity of complications observed with this technique precluded its widespread use as the method of choice for induction of labor. It was completely discarded with the introduction of intravenous administration of physiologic amounts of oxytocin by Theobald (1948).

Much later its use was revived for application in midtrimester gestations, when elective abortions were legalized in several countries. A change in concentration to 20% was an important variant from the original Aburel technique. It is a significant difference to inject only 20 gm NaCl instead of 35 gm, which is going to be rapidly taken up by the maternal organism, to the circulating blood, and the interstitial space.

The mechanism of action is unknown, although some hypotheses have been offered to explain the way the contractions are stimulated and maintained. Several hours pass after the intraamniotic administration of 20 gm NaCl before the uterus begins to contract in a slow, increasing manner (Figure 9-37). The contractions continus to progress, the intrauterine pressure reaching high values because of the relatively small size of the uterus. Changes occur in the cervix, and expulsion of the products of conception is the eventual outcome after several hours of very good unterine contractility.

It is impossible to distinguish between the contractions produced, in these midgestation uteri, by either prostaglandins or hypertonic saline, when the activity was well established and the process of evacuation was set in motion. Nevertheless, this observation does not imply that the mechanism of action is similar for both substances.

Precautions   Rigorous care must be taken when using hypertonic saline to avoid severe complications. The *intravascular* injection of the heavily hypertonic preparation has caused sudden death, probably by spasm of the pulmonary artery (shown in experimental animals). This accident should be preventable, provided the operator takes care to ascertain that the needle is in free amniotic cavity before or during the injection of the solution.

A less preventable condition is the syndrome of *disseminated intravascular coagulation* (DIC) observed to occur a few hours after the injection of hypertonic saline in the amniotic cavity. The mechanism of production is not well understood, but within 4 hours of the injection, the platelet count and fibrinogen level tend to drop drastically, with an increase in the partial thromboplastin time (PTT). If these alterations reach the threshold to cause bleeding, there will be clinical manifestation of the syndrome, but in general they go unnoticed because they do not reach this point. Usually, after 4 hours of the injection, when they reach the lowest values, clotting factors slowly recover to satisfactory levels by the time the products of conception are expelled.

The hypercontractility triggered by this solution may be as violent as that induced by PGs, and as a consquence *cervical lacerations and ruptures* of the lower part of uteri have been observed in midtrimester gestations. There does not seem to be any relationship between the total amount injected or the age of gestation with the occurrence of this accident.

Urea and glucose   Hypertonic solutions of urea and glucose have also been used to stimulate

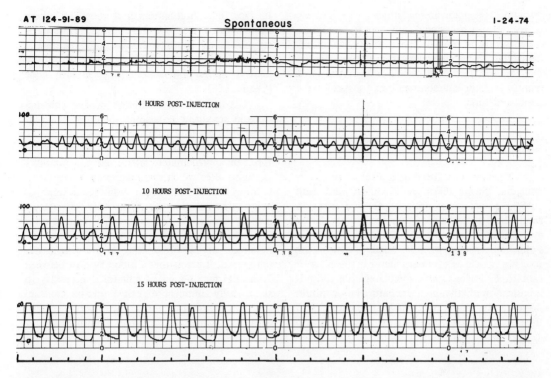

Figure 9-37 Effect of intraamniotic injection of hypertonic saline on the uterine contractility at 16 weeks gestation. *(Top)* Spontaneous activity. *(Second tracing)* Four fours after injection of 20 gm NaCl, slight rise in tonus, small rapid contractions, and some incoordination. *(Third tracing)* Ten hours after injection shows a well-established contractility. *(Bottom)* Shortly before explusion, very strong, regular contractions and moderately high tonus. Compare with the cases in which PG was used.

uterine contractions in early second trimester of pregnancy with the aim of evacuating the cavity of the products of conception. Both are also effective oxytocics, comparable to hypertonic saline, although experience with them is less extensive. Nevertheless, they may be used for the same indications and, in general, one may expect comparable results. The known exception is that hypertonic glucose is contraindicated in cases of intrauterine fetal death because many cases of severe infection (amnionitis) have been reported when this preparation was used to evacuate those uteri. As for hypertonic saline, the mechnism of action of these preparations is not understood.

UTERINE RELAXANTS

The control of excessive or undesirable uterine contractility has been one of the most pressing needs in obstetrics. Premature delivery is

the outcome of untimely onset of labor and the greatest challenge to modern obstetrics. In spite of the significance of the problem and the amount of effort directed at understanding the process of premature labor, relatively little progress has been made regarding the mechanisms that trigger abnormal contractions. On the other hand, notwithstanding the better knowledge of the elements converging to initiate normal labor (Chapter 8) the clinical application of uterine relaxants remains largely empirical. Some of the substances used are directed ostensibly at blocking some of the steps in the cascade of reactions terminating in myometrial contraction. However, the mechanism of action of the more effective ones does not quite interfere with the sequential action determining a normal contraction: they act by actively promoting relaxation rather than by preventing contractions. Some of these agents are used not only in attempting to arrest premature labors but also to correct intrapartum hypercontractility, the

186

"irritable" pregnant uterus subjected to surgery, or to perform occasional intrauterine manipulations during second or third stage. Therefore, depending on the clinical need, a uterine relaxant may be used for a brief period or in a protracted manner to prevent contractions for prolonged periods of time.

Ethanol

Originally introduced in clinical obstetrics as analgesic during labor by Belinkoff and Hall (1950), it was soon noticed that the infusion resulted in a decrease of uterine activity. However, the mechanism of action remained obscure. Following the work of A.R. Fuchs (1964) on the role of oxytocin as a primary factor in the labor of rabbits, F. Fuchs (1965) postulated that the administration of ethanol in premature labor should decrease uterine contractions by interfering with the release of oxytocin by the posterior pituitary.

In fact, his observations and those of others demonstrated that the intravenous infusion of ethanol at appropriate dosages and maintained for a sufficient period of time can practically abolish uterine contractions of premature labor (Figure 9-38).

To diminish or obliterate uterine contractions in advanced gestation, ethanol must be infused intravenously with a specific technique to be successful: a loading dose of 100 gm must be infused in approximately 90 to 120 min (about 1 gm/min) after which the maintenance dose, one-tenth of that (0.1 gm/min), should be infused for at least 6 hours, or longer if necessary. The uterine activity diminishes within 15 to 25 minutes after the onset of the infusion and usually remains low or almost absent for as long as the drug is administered. It seems that a blood level of between 70 to 180 mg/100 ml of ethanol is necessary to successfully diminish excessive uterine contractions of premature labor. The blood level can easily be estimated by using the Breathalyzer,

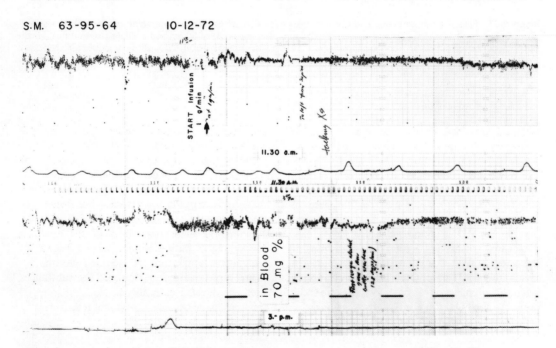

Figure 9-38 Continuous uterine activity and FHR tracings obtained by external methods in the premature labor of a 34-week pregnant class C diabetic patient. *(Above)* Ethanol infusion was started at 1 gm/min, and uterine activity promptly diminished. *(Below)* Three hours later, with an alcohol blood level at 70 mg/100 ml, infusion rate was diminished to 0.1 gm/min. Tracing shows an almost quiescent uterus and FHR with good baseline oscillations. Reprinted from Cibils LA: The management of impending labor prior to the thirty-fifth week, in Reid DE, Christian CD (eds): *Controversy in Obstetrics and Gynecology II.* Philadelphia, Saunders, 1974, pp 88–102.

which measures the ethanol concentration in the expired air; there is a good correlation between this reading and the concentration in blood.

It is speculated that the *mechanism of action* is by suppression of the release of oxytocin from the posterior pituitary. This hypothesis has been postulated by the group of investigators who think that labor (or premature labor) is triggered by increased sensitivity of the myometrium to a normal, stable level of oxytocin. It finds support in animal experiments, but extrapolation to the human remains to be demonstrated.

It has been observed in clinical investigation that discontinuing the infusion of the maintenance dose will rarely be followed by resumption of uterine activity: probably the feedback mechanism that maintains labor could be interrupted by this medication.

The undesirable side effects more frequently observed have been intoxication (drunkenness), nausea and vomiting, and restlessness in some patients while others rest very quietly. There is a slight tachycardia, but the blood pressure is maintained within normal values. The FHR remains within normal limits and with good baseline characteristics in spite of some metabolic changes observed in the mother, particularly diminution of gluconeogenesis and thus potential hypoglycemia. The significant changes in fetal acid–base balance observed in sheep and monkeys have not been observed in the human fetuses studied: the blood levels are similar to those of the mother, and the metabolic state is usually within the range seen in medicated fetuses.

Progesterone

Called the "hormone of pregnancy" and for a long time considered the substance responsible for the "quiescence" of the uterus during pregnancy, its effect on the pregnant human uterus has been studied after administration by several routes and dosage schedules. From studies in rabbits, Csapo (1961) postulated that it "blocks the myometrium" and prevents the propagation of contractile stimuli until a "progesterone withdrawal" facilitates the coordinated action of the myometrium to permit effective contraction and the progress of labor.

The *intramuscular* administration of large doses of crystalline progesterone (1400 mg) to term pregnant patients by Pose and Fielitz (1961) failed to affect the expected onset of labor, uterine work to dilate the cervix, uterine response to oxytocin, or duration of labor.

Likewise, the oral administration, studied by Brenner and Hendricks (1962), of high doses of medroxyprogesterone in advanced gestation did not affect either the expected date of onset or the normal characteristics of the labors studied.

The *intramyometrial* route was studied by Bengtsson (1962), who injected from 250 to 400 mg medroxyprogesterone into the wall of the uterus in premature labor. It is claimed that this preparation is, weight by weight, up to 40 times more potent than progesterone, but nevertheless in those cases where the cervical dilatation was "two fingers" the uterine activity was not affected. Only when the cervix was unchanged was uterine contractility suppressed.

When given *intravenously* in relatively large doses (up to 2 gm) by Kumar et al, (1963) crystalline progesterone did not arrest the progress of early labor even though blood levels 10 to 20 times higher than those observed in term pregnancy were maintained for several hours (Figure 9-39). The administration of intravenous pregnenolone was likewise unable to produce more than a transient diminution of uterine contractions of spontaneous labor.

More recently, Johnson et al (1975) reported that the *long-term oral administration* of hydroxyprogesterone prevented premature labor in a significant number of patients at risk. This study renewed the possibility of using progesterone in the control of premature uterine contractions, and thus also its clinical usefulness.

Antiprostaglandins

The pivotal role assigned by recent studies to PGs in the control of myometrial contractions has promoted the study of some drugs that interfere with PG synthesis as possible pharmacologic agents to block undesired uterine contractions. Several substances commonly used as analgesics have been shown to prevent the synthesis of PGs by acting on the group of prostaglandin synthetases. A number of retrospective studies of moderately large groups of patients taking long-term analgesic medication suggested that perhaps interference with PG action could explain the abnormalities observed in those labors.

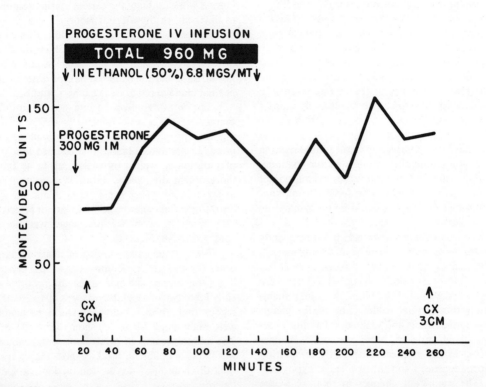

Figure 9-39 Uterine activity (Montevideo Units) plotted against time in a case of premature labor at 34 weeks. Continuous infusion of crystalline progesterone dissolved in ethanol was given for 130 min (total 690 mg), after a dose of 300 mg IM. The fluctuations of the unaffected uterine activity are similar to those seen in normal spontaneous labor. Reprinted from Kumar D, et al: In vivo effects of intravenous progesterone infusion on human gravid uterine contractility. *Bull Johns Hopkins Hosp* 113:53, 1963. The Johns Hopkins University Press, © 1963.

Aspirin Indirect evidence suggests that aspirin administered simultaneously with either PG precursors or hypertonic solutions to the amniotic cavity significantly prolongs the so-called instillation-abortion time or even prevents the abortion in some cases. The *mechanism* of action would be by inactivating some of the enzymes of the PG synthetase group and thereby preventing the stimulation of myometrium. There are no observations in humans of aspirin alone used to arrest uterine contractions; therefore, it is impossible to know the administration response time, dose–response relationship, or duration of action. It has minimal *side effects* on the mother when taken long-term in large doses; a slight increase in postpartum hemorrhage has been reported, presumably due to decreased uterine stimulation. Although some have suggested that aspirin may cause congenital malformations, there is no evidence that this occurs in humans.

Indomethacin Probably the best studied anti-PG, indomethacin has a *mechanism* of action that, like aspirin, interferes with PG synthetase. Its use in subhuman primates delayed onset of normal labor. The application to humans proved that large doses administered during premature labor may diminish and arrest uterine contractions (Figure 9-40). The intrarectal dose of 100 mg will decrease uterine contractions within 30 to 60 min, and the effect may last for several hours or need to be reinforced by supplemental doses by mouth. No known *immediate side effects* on the mother or fetus have been reported. However, long-term use of the preparation may cause serious complications to the fetus (see Chapter 11).

Beta-Adrenergics

The depressant effect of adrenaline on contractions of the uterus in labor was observed more than 50 years ago by Rucker (1925) who added it to anesthetics to prolong their action. Further studies by other investigators confirmed his observations but, at the same time, revealed that the effects vary depending on the dose and duration of infusion. It was later seen that adrenaline is a mixture of epinephrine and norepinephrine, and

that these two amines have opposite effects on myometrium. The availability of pure preparations facilitated the clarification of their pharmacologic effect and their mechanism of action. The natural amines differ minimally in their structure (Figure 9-41), and some synthetic preparations are similar to epinephrine with minor substitutions in the aromatic ring and the terminal amino group.

Alquist (1948) defined the presence of α and β receptors by the pharmacologic response of target organs: the stimulation of α receptors produced contraction of smooth muscles and that of β receptors relaxation of smooth muscles and stimulation of the cardiac muscle. The observation that there were substances producing different effects when theoretically they should have

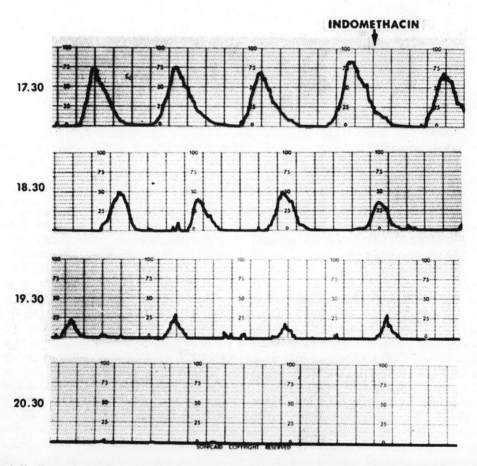

Figure 9-40 External recording of uterine activity in a 31-week gestation, premature labor. Rectal 100 mg indomethacin given (arrow) rapidly diminished the uterine contractility, particularly the intensity of contractions. Note quiescence after 3 hours. Reprinted from Zuckerman H, et al: Inhibition of human premature labor by indomethacin. *Obstet Gynecol* 44:787, 1974.

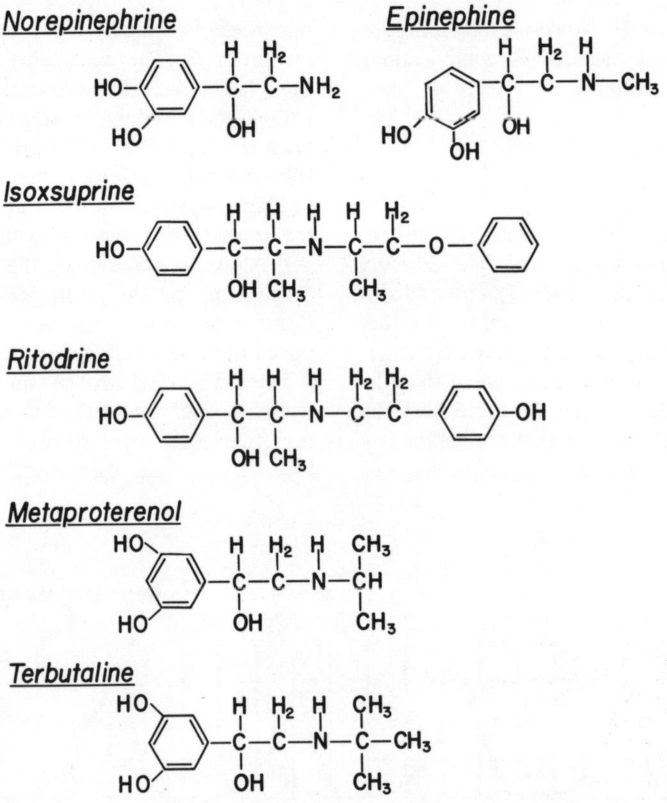

Norepinephrine

Epinephine

Isoxsuprine

Ritodrine

Metaproterenol

Terbutaline

Figure 9-41 Structural formulas of natural and synthetic adrenergic substances. Note similarities among the new β-mimetic preparations.

had similar actions led to the subdivision of β receptors in two types (Lands et al, 1956): β_1 receptor stimulation would cause cardiac acceleration and stimulation, and β_2 activation would cause smooth muscle relaxation (bronchi, vessels, uterus).

The β-mimetic amines are thus substances which cause active uterine relaxation by direct action on the muscle cell receptors. The *mechanism of action* seems to be through activation of adenylcyclase and inhibition of phosphodiesterase (Figure 9-42). They would stimulate the production of cAMP, which in turn promotes the binding of calcium ions in the sarcoplasmic reticulum and mitochondria. The unavailability of free calcium ions prevents the activation of actomyosin, which results in uterine relaxation. Also, the free calcium ion probably acts on the cell membrane and intracellular ionic concentration, affecting the resting membrane potential and the transmembrane movement of sodium and potassium ions.

Epinephrine The first natural substance known to relax uterine contractions, epinephrine, as the predominant compound of adrenaline, was used by Rucker (1925) with that specific purpose after he observed that it decreased uterine activity when it was added to anesthetic agents with the aim of prolonging their action. Subsequent studies confirmed his observation but they also revealed a biphasic response coupled to a very short lasting effect.

When *infused* at 2 to 5 μg/min and up to 10 μg/min to patients undergoing *induced labors,* it predictably decreases uterine contractility mainly at the expense of the intensity of the contractions (Figure 9-43), but there is also a diminution in their frequency. If the infusion is maintained at the same rate, the contractility starts to recover slowly after approximately 30 min as if it were "adapting" to the drug effect (Figure 9-44).

The *mechanism of action* is through the β

RELAXATION MECHANISM IN MYOMETRIUM

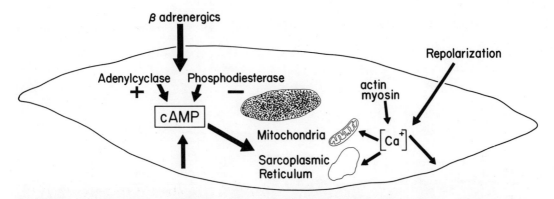

Figure 9-42 Schematic drawing to illustrate the most relevant elements involved in the process of active relaxation of the myometrium when exposed to β-mimetic substances. These act by increasing the activity of adenylcyclase and diminishing that of phosphodiesterase, which results in an increase in cAMP. The effect of this is an active binding of calcium ion in mitochondria and sarcoplasmic reticulum. The diminution of free calcium ion facilitates repolarization of the membrane and relaxation of actomyosin.

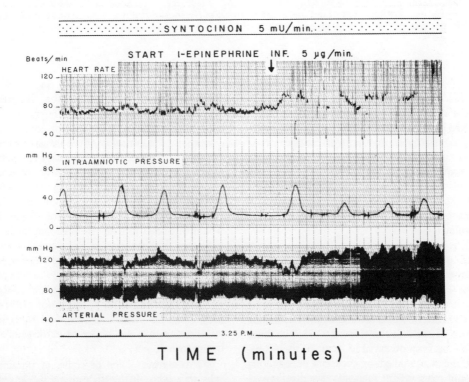

Figure 9-43 Start of an epinephrine infusion on a term *labor induced* with 5 mU/min oxytocin. The top tracing is maternal heart rate. *(Center)* Intrauterine pressure. *(Below)* Intraarterial pressure. Note the rapid decrease of intensity of contractions, the rapid transient hypotension, and rebound hypertension. Reprinted from Pose SV, et al: Effect of *l*-epinephrine infusion on uterine contractility and cardiovascular system. *Am J Obstet Gynecol* 84:297, 1962.

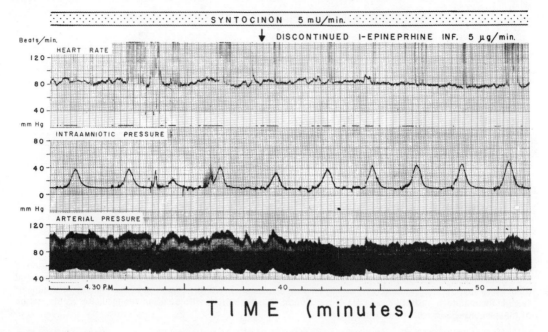

Figure 9-44 Same case as in Figure 9-43. After slightly over one hour of continuous infusion, uterine activity remains low. The blood pressure is lower than at preinfusion and the pulse rate higher. After the infusion was discontinued, blood pressure continued to fall smoothly, with very slow recovery. The uterine activity started to recover in a steady, regular manner. Reprinted from Pose SV, et al: Effect of *l*-epinephrine infusion on uterine contractility and cardiovascular system. *Am J Obstet Gynecol* 84:297, 1962.

receptors, but the adaptation may be due to a dual effect of epinephrine stimulating also the α receptors. The latter effect is usually overridden by the β action but after enough time of exposure, or if used in high doses, the α effect will predominate with recovery of the contractility. The probable mechanism of this apparently paradoxical effect is better observed with a mixture of both amines in the proportion they are assumed to be in natural adrenaline (Figure 9-45).

The delayed, or longer, α effect is more consistently observed when the infusion is given during *spontaneous labor* with very impressive immediate effects (Figure 9-46), but recovery slowly takes place, and complete recovery followed by a rebound phenomenon occurs immediately following cessation of the infusion (Figure 9-47). The latter reaction has been observed to occur in about one-half of the cases studied, on occasions necessitating the use of other uterine relaxants to control a worrisome hypercontractility (see Figure 9-64).

The *cardiovascular effects* of epinephrine are well known in the nonpregnant individual: tachy-

cardia and hypertension. However, the pregnant woman at term responds in a different manner to the low infusion rates used for these studies. Essentially the initiation of the infusion produces a transient hypotension followed by recovery, rebound hypertension, and slowly progressing hypotension, stabilized during the infusion (Figure 9-48). The action is produced by *active vasodilatation* of the arteriolar tree (Figure 9-49), which indicates that in the pregnant state the β receptors predominate in the vessels where no adaptation, recovery, or rebound were observed with the low infusion rates. The pulse rate mirror images the blood pressure changes, indicating that the cardiac stimulating effect is not affected by pregnancy; in fact, with infusion rates of 20 $\mu g/min$ one may see bursts of extrasystoles and hypertension.

Isoxsuprine The objective of obtaining a substance without the undesirable side effects of epinephrine but still conserving its uterine relaxant properties culminated in the synthesis of isoxsuprine, which demonstrated excellent effects on

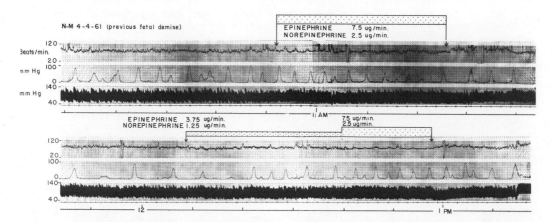

Figure 9-45 Continuous three hours of intrauterine, blood pressure, and maternal pulse rate recordings in term *spontaneous labor.* *(Above)* Infusion of a mixture of 75% epinephrine and 25% norepinephrine slowly decreased the uterine activity, with minimal effect on blood pressure and pulse rate. Infusion was discontinued after 35 min, and a slight fall in blood pressure with tachycardia may be observed while uterine contractility recovered minimally by increasing the intensity of the contractions. *(Below)* Infusion was resumed, and the uterine activity was very slowly stimulated, more so when the infusion rate was increased. Discontinuing infusion of amines elicited a transient episode of hypotension with tachycardia and a small decrease in uterine activity.

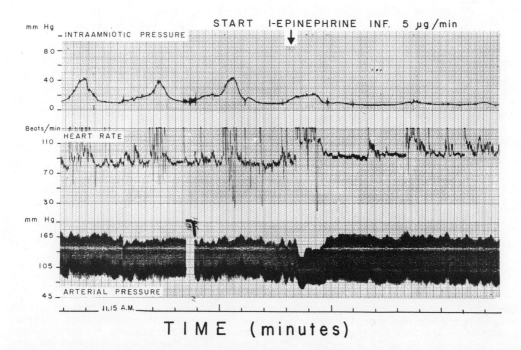

Figure 9-46 Start of an epinephrine infusion in a term *spontaneous labor.* The infusion triggers a rapid decrease in uterine contractility and a transient episode of hypotension followed by rebound hypertension and moderate tachycardia. Reprinted from Pose SV, et al: Effect of *l*-epinephrine infusion on uterine contractility and cardiovascular system. *Am J Obstet Gynecol* 84:297, 1962.

194

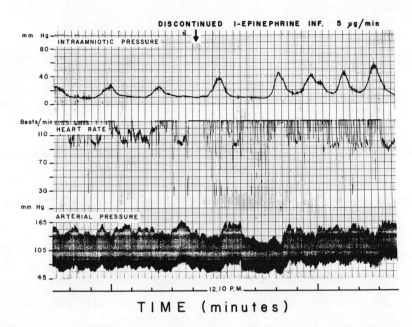

TIME (minutes)

Figure 9-47 Same case as in Figure 9-46. After 45 minutes of continuous infusion, the uterine activity had *partially recovered,* the blood pressure was lower, and pulse rate higher than before infusion. Discontinuing it triggered further hypotension with tachycardia. The uterine activity recovered rapidly with *rebound hypertonus* and polysystoly. Reprinted from Pose SV, et al: Effect of *l*-epinephrine infusion on uterine contractility and cardiovascular system. *Am J Obstet Gynecol* 84:297, 1962.

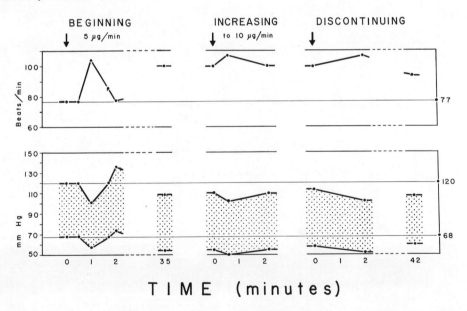

TIME (minutes)

Figure 9-48 Average values of blood pressure and pulse rate in patients infused with epinephrine. Preinfusion control figures on ordinates, right; scales, left. Time in the abscissa. Thirty seconds after starting the infusion the systolic and diastolic pressures drop, with recovery and rebound at 2 min. After 35 min of infusion the blood pressure is steady and lower than control. An increase in the infusion rate triggers a further fall in blood pressure with partial recovery but without rebound. On discontinuing the infusion there is still a fall in systolic and diastolic followed by slow recovery, which is still incomplete 40 min later. The pulse rate "mirror images" the changes in blood pressure. Reprinted from Pose SV, et al: Effect of *l*-epinephrine infusion on uterine contractility and cardiovascular system. *Am J Obstet Gynecol* 84:297, 1962.

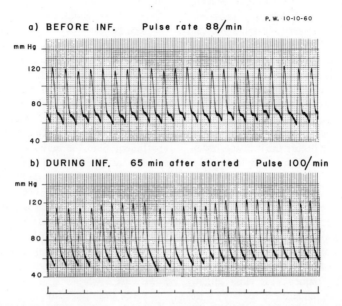

Figure 9-49 Intraarterial pressure tracings recorded at high paper speed to observe the pulse wave and effect of a 5 μg/min epinephrine infusion sustained for over one hour. *(Above)* Preinfusion record clearly shows dicrotic notch. *(Below)* Dicrotic notch has disappeared, the systolic and diastolic pressures are lower, and the pulse rate is much higher. Reprinted from Pose SV, et al: Effect *l*-epinephrine infusion on uterine contractility and cardiovascular system. *Am J Obstet Gynecol* 84:297, 1962.

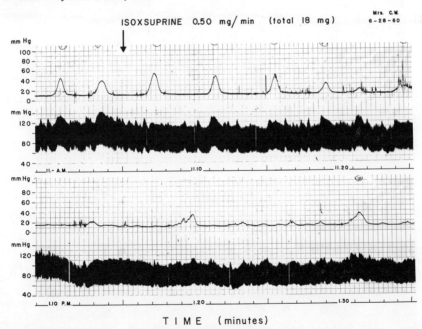

Figure 9-50 Effect of isoxsuprine on spontaneous contractility of term uterus. Intrauterine and arterial pressure recordings. Infusion started at 500 μg/min (arrow) and induced a gradual decrease in *uterine activity. (Below)* Two hours later, the total dose (18 mg given in 36 min) produced an almost complete suppression of uterine contractions. *Blood pressure* dropped slightly at the start of infusion and stabilized at lower values, including in the postinfusion tracings. Reprinted from Hendricks CH, et al: Pharmacologic control of excessive uterine activity with isoxsuprine. *Am J Obstet Gynecol* 82:1064, 1961.

in vitro specimens. The in vivo human observations confirmed the exclusive β-mimetic properties of the drug and the powerful uterine relaxant action.

The *intravenous infusion* of 500 to 750 µg/min within 15 min decreases the uterine contractility of *spontaneous labor* (Figure 9-50) with a combined effect on intensity and, more markedly, on frequency of the contractions. This effect is usually prolonged unless the contractility was exaggeratedly high before the infusion began. Term pregnant uteri may need to be stimulated to resume labor-like activity (Figure 9-51) after the drug has been discontinued for a few hours.

Likewise, *induced uterine contractility* at term can be diminished within a short time to very low levels with an infusion of isoxsuprine at 500 to 1000 µg/min (Figure 9-52). In these cases the contractility is diminished mainly by a diminution of intensity, while frequency is only slightly affected. However, no tendency to recovery is obvious in spite of maintaining the oxytocin infusion at rates that, before isoxsuprine, triggered good activity (Figure 9-53). Nevertheless, the reactivity

to increased infusion rates of oxytocin is maintained intact, enabling one to stimulate the uterus if need be.

The contractility of *premature labor* may be diminished within 10 to 15 min provided an infusion rate of sufficient concentration is given (Figure 9-54). The effect is produced by a dramatic decrease in frequency and a somewhat less impressive decrease in intensity of the contractions. When the infusion is maintained for a sufficient time the activity of the uterus should remain at a level insufficient to induce cervical changes and premature delivery.

Intramuscular and *oral* isoxsuprine are also effective in reducing uterine activity, but have less predictable response than the intravenous route. The effects are often evident within a short time, but they do not last long enough to be clinically effective unless large amounts or reinforcing doses are used.

The duration of the effect on spontaneous or induced uterine activity depends on rate and duration of the infusion. Insufficient medication may transiently reduce the contractility, which will

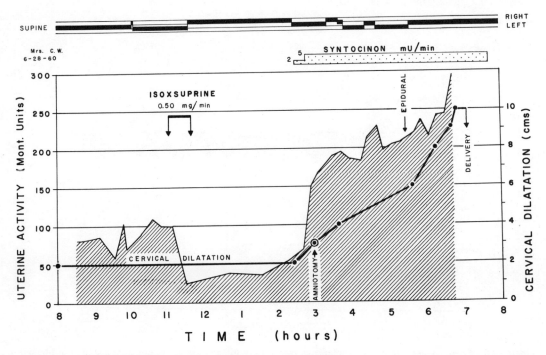

Figure 9-51 Summary of clinical events, same patient as in Figure 9-50. The initial spontaneous activity (striped area) was almost 100 Montevideo Units, characteristic of normal prelabor. Uterine activity was significantly decreased by isoxsuprine and stayed down until 3 hours later when amniotomy and oxytocin at physiologic rates brought the patient into active labor. Reprinted from Hendricks CH, et al: Pharmacologic control of excessive uterine activity with isoxsuprine. *Am J Obstet Gynecol* 82:1064, 1961.

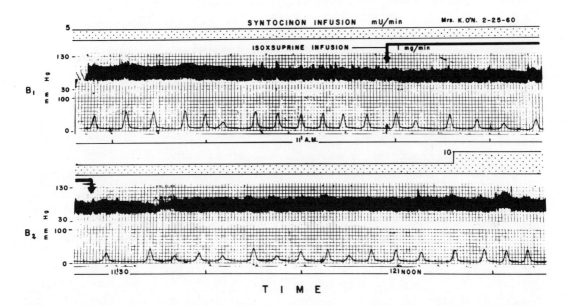

Figure 9-52 Effect of isoxsuprine on the induced uterine contractility in term labor. Continuous 110-min tracing. *(Above)* Stable activity diminished by 1000 μg/min isoxsuprine. Lower activity was well maintained until oxytocin infusion was increased. Lower tracing *(right)* with the expected recovery of uterine activity. The blood pressure fell slightly and was well stabilized throughout the total infusion of 20 mg medication. Reprinted from Hendricks CH, et al: Pharmacologic control of excessive uterine activity with isoxsuprine. *Am J Obstet Gynecol* 82:1064, 1961.

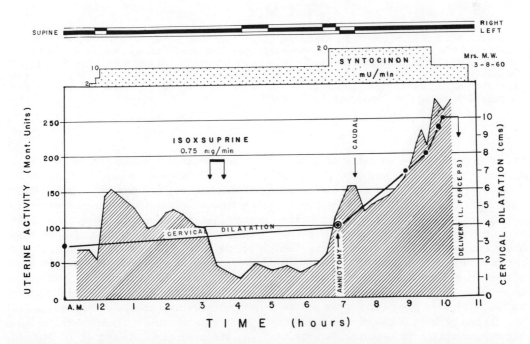

Figure 9-53 The labor-like *uterine activity* (striped area) *induced* with oxytocin in early first stage was sharply curtailed by 20 mg isoxsuprine infused at 750 μg/min. Activity remained low for 3 hours in spite of the oxytocin infusion at 10 mU/min. Amniotomy and rise of oxytocin infusion reactivated labor, and dilation progressed uneventfully. Reprinted from Hendricks CH, et al: The pharmacologic control of excessive uterine activity with isoxsuprine. *Am J Obstet Gynecol* 82:1064, 1961.

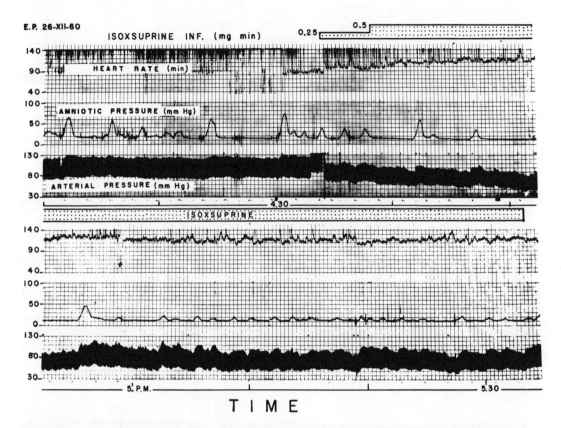

Figure 9-54 Effect of isoxsuprine on the contractility of premature labor. Continuous 1.25-hour recording of intrauterine and arterial pressures and pulse rate. *(Above, left)* Spontaneous uterine activity. Dotted area indicates isoxsuprine infused at 250 μg/min and increased to 500 μg/min because it had no noticeable effect. The higher infusion rate produced a marked decrease in uterine contractility, which was maintained for several hours. Blood pressure fell from 120/65 mm Hg, and the pulse rate rose from 80 to 115 beats/min. Reprinted from Cibils LA, Zuspan FP: Pharmacology of the uterus. *Clin Obstet Gynecol* 11:34, 1968.

recover spontaneously within a short time. Sufficient drug sustained for a long enough time will reduce uterine activity to low levels from which spontaneous recovery is very unlikely (Figure 9-55).

The *cardiovascular effects* of isoxsuprine have been carefully studied bycause they may hinder the ·clinical application of the drug. The systolic and diastolic *blood pressures* are generally affected by the intravenous infusion of doses above 200 μg/min (Figures 9-50, 9-52, 9-54), and their fall tends to be proportional to the infusion rate, the average being 20 mm Hg systolic and 15 mm Hg diastolic. At the same time the stimulatory effect of the heart is manifested by a significant rise in *pulse rate* of 20 to 30 beats/min. The maximum effects are usually seen within 10 min for the intravenous route, and within 15 min

for intramuscular injections. The action is by active vasodilatation of the arterioles (Figure 9-56). Occasionally one may deal with a patient whose cardiovascular system is either hypersensitive to β-adrenergic stimulation or is actively constricted to compensate for a relatively diminished blood volume. In either circumstance, the infusion of an active vasodilator will produce a dramatic *hypotension* (Figure 9-57), which is very difficult to control with the standard medications. Recovery will probably occur because of the metabolism of the drug rather than for any other reason.

Metaproterenol Another of the β-mimetic agents, metaproterenol has been used for a long time as bronchodilator. The uterine relaxant properties have been studied and found to be highly predictable. Infusion rates of 10 to 40

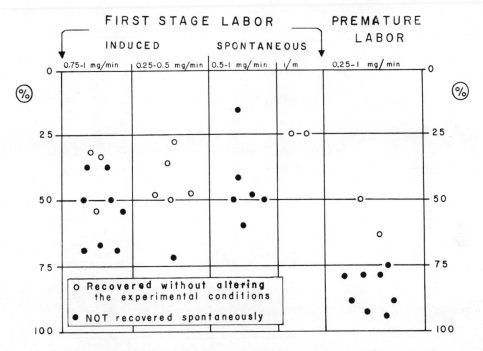

Figure 9-55 Percentile decrease of uterine activity under isoxsuprine administration. The zero on top represents 100% of uterine activity (Montevideo Units) recorded during the control preinfusion period. Each point represents the relative decrease in uterine activity after full effect had stabilized. Reprinted from Cibils LA: Inhibitory effect of isoxsuprine on uterine contractility. *Am J Obstet Gynecol* 94:762, 1966.

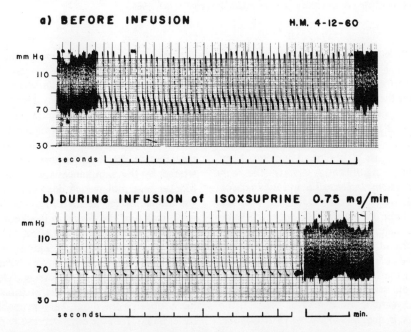

Figure 9-56 Effect of isoxsuprine on the arterial pressure, wave recorded in the femoral artery. *(Above)* Before infusion. Dicrotic notch is clear in slow- and high-speed recordings. *(Below)* During isoxsuprine infusion, dicrotic notch is no longer present. Note also the higher pulse frequency. Reprinted from Hendricks CH, et al: The pharmacologic control of excessive uterine activity with isoxsuprine. *Am J Obstet Gynecol* 82:1064, 1961.

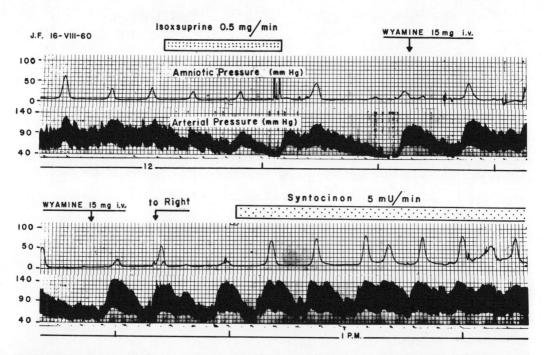

Figure 9-57 Continuous 86 min of intrauterine and arterial pressure recordings in term spontaneous labor. *(Above)* Infusion of isoxsuprine, 500 μg/min, produced a marked hypertension, which became severe and did not quite respond to Wyamine, 30 mg IV in divided doses, or change of position *(below)*. Oxytocin infusion was started to increase the contractility and thus maintain a good pressure between contractions. Probably borderline compensated hypovolemia or extreme cardiovascular sensitivity caused this reaction. Reprinted from Cibils LA: Inhibitory effect of isoxsuprine on uterine contractility. *Am J Obstet Gynecol* 94:762, 1966.

μg/min produce significant diminution of uterine activity at any stage of labor (Figure 9-58). However, after an infusion has been maintained for some time the uterine activity tends to recover, or "escape," necessitating an increase in rate to maintain the effect, much like that seen with epinephrine.

Because it is a potent β-mimetic agent metaproterenol significantly affects the *cardiovascular system;* tachycardia and hypotension may be relatively tolerable, particularly at the lower doses, but the tachycardia can reach levels that might endanger a patient's well-being (Figure 9-59). On the other hand, *arrhythmias* directly related to the use of the drug have been described by some observers. In addition, the transplacental passage of the drug affects the fetus with a predictable tachycardia, which may be severe if the infusion rate is maintained for some reasonable period of time.

Terbutaline Among the more recently synthetized β-mimetic agents, some, claimed to have a selective β_2 effect, have been studied in the past

few years. Terbutaline is one of those, derived from metaproterenol and with effective uterine depressant properties. The *infusion* of 10 to 15 μg/min triggered almost complete obliteration of the uterine contractility (Figure 9-60) at the expense of both intensity and frequency of contractions. The mechanism of action through the β_2 receptors of the myometrium has been demonstrated by the simultaneous injection of the β_1 blocker practolol, which does not interfere with the uterine effect of the drug, whereas the administration of the β_1 and β_2 blocker propranolol prevents the uterine relaxant effect of terbutaline. When both are injected simultaneously, the uterine contractility fully recovers during the infusion of terbutaline. The time required for the uterine activity to resume its preinfusion values has not been worked out, but it probably does not differ much from the other substances of the same family.

The *cardiovascular effects* are particularly manifested in the pulse rate, which rises markedly even when the specific β_1 blocker practolol was

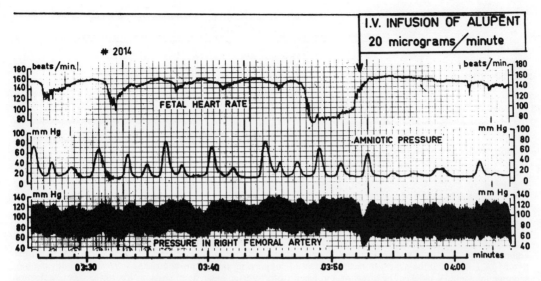

Figure 9-58 Forty minutes of FHR, intrauterine, and blood pressure recordings in advanced first stage, showing episodes of fetal hypoxia triggered by contractions, and a period of severe bradycardia at 3:50. The intravenous infusion of metaproterenol at 20 µg/min (arrow) dramatically decreased the uterine activity with only a modest fall in blood pressure. FHR stabilized because the contractions became mild. Reprinted from Caldeyro-Barcia R, et al: Pan American Health Organization Scientific Publication 185, 1969.

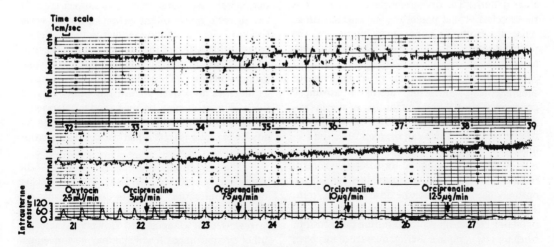

Figure 9-59 Continuous 75-min recording of fetal and maternal heart rates and intrauterine pressure, from a term, oxytocin-stimulated labor. Intravenous infusion of metaproterenol at increasing rates from 5 to 12.5 µg/min produced an almost complete obliteration of uterine contractility *(bottom)* and a significant increase in maternal pulse rate from 105 to 160 beats/min. FHR had a modest rise from 150 to 160 beats/min. Reprinted from Tyack AJ, et al: In-vivo response of human uterus to orciprenaline in early labour. *Br Med J* 2:741, 1971.

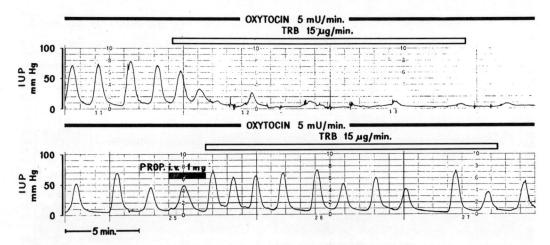

Figure 9-60 Effect of terbutaline infusion on oxytocin-induced contractility of term pregnant uterus. *(Above)* Infusion of 15 μg/min had the almost immediate effect of suppressing the uterine contractions. *(Below)* Preinjection of propranolol 1 mg IV blocked the effect of another infusion started again at 15 μg/min. Reprinted from Andersson KE, et al (1975).

given. Often such a rise may create the need to discontinue an infusion given as a therapeutic measure. On the other hand, the effect on the blood pressure seems minimal with slight fall in diastolic and practically no change in systolic.

Ritodrine Probably the most extensively studied derivative of isoxsuprine, ritodrine has rather selective and potent uterine relaxant properties. It affects the nonpregnant uterus and the pregnant uterus at all stages. The *intravenous* administration of 50 to 200 μg/min induces significant uterine relaxation of an induced or spontaneously contracting uterus in advanced gestation (Figure 9-61). Diminution of uterine activity is achieved mainly at the expense of intensity of contractions, which fall dramatically; the frequency is minimally affected. Infusion rates of over 40 μg/min are required for successful control of clinically good uterine contractions, and often one may need to increase the dose to 100 μg/min. The duration of the effect depends on the degree of uterine relaxation achieved during the infusion: when almost complete uterine quescence has been obtained (Figure 9-62), the effect should last a long time, and it may be sustained by either *intramuscular* or *oral* administration of smaller doses.

The *cardiovascular effects* are tolerable by the patients: a minimal change in systolic pressure, usually a small rise, and no change or a small drop in the diastolic with the net consequence of a clear increase in the pulse pressure (Figure 9-61). The action seems to be affected by peripheral vasodilatation with disappearance of the dicrotic notch of the arterial pressure wave (Figure 9-62). This action, added to the moderate tachycardiac effect of the drug, produces a significant increase in cardiac output, which is usually proportional to the infusion rate and may increase as much as 50% over preinfusion values (Figure 9-63). The fetus may become moderately tachycardic but acid–base studies have failed to reveal any deleterious effects when ritodrine is used in therapeutic regimens.

The potential therapeutic use of the β-mimetic agents is extensive — whenever excessive uterine contractility needs to be diminished or arrested. The specific problem of premature labor is reviewed in Chapter 11. However, there are other circumstances in which it may be convenient to arrest uterine contractions in labor. Caldeyro-Barcia has proposed the administration of β-mimetic substances in cases of intrapartum fetal distress aggravated by uterine contractions. The

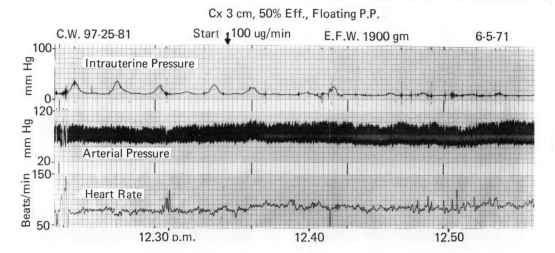

Figure 9-61 Intrauterine and arterial pressures and maternal heart rate recordings at 32 weeks gestation, *premature labor.* The good uterine activity began to decrease very shortly after ritodrine infusion was started at 100 μg/min (arrow). Blood pressure tracing shows progressive widening of the pulse pressure, mainly at the expense of a small rise in systolic. The pulse rate increased from 75 to 95 beats/min. Reprinted from Cibils LA: The management of impending labor prior to the thirty-fifth week, in Reid DE, Christian CD (eds): *Controversy in Obstetrics and Gynecology II.* Philadelphia, Saunders, 1974, pp 88–102.

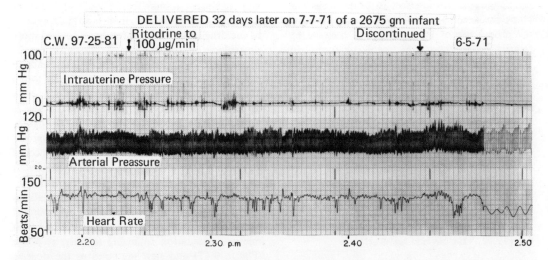

Figure 9-62 Same case as in Figure 9-61, 2 hours later. Note the completely quiescent uterus before and after cessation of ritodrine infusion. The pulse pressure is still higher than control, but there is a small fall in diastolic. The pulse rate increased to 120 beats/min. Reprinted from Cibils LA: The management of impending labor prior to the thirty-fifth week, in Reid DE, Christian CD (eds): *Controversy in Obstetrics and Gynecology II.* Philadelphia, Saunders, 1974, pp 88–102.

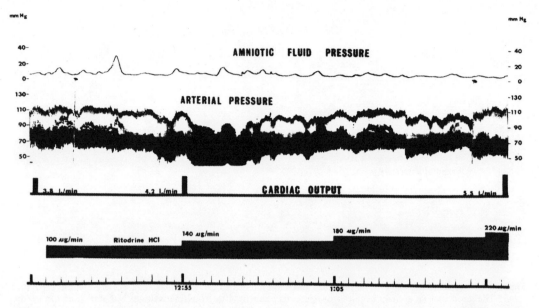

Figure 9-63 Intrauterine and arterial pressure tracings obtained in premature labor at 33 weeks. Ritodrine infusion at rates increasing from 100 to 220 µg/min (shown at bottom) produced a transient drop in blood pressure with recovery. The cardiac output (small bars) increased progressively from 3.8 to 5.5 liters/min. Reprinted from Bieniarz, et al: Cardiac output during ritodrine treatment in premature labor. *Am J Obstet Gynecol* 118:910, 1974.

aim would be to promote an intrauterine oxygenation and improvement of the fetal acidosis before the fetus is exposed to extrauterine life and needs to sustain his own homeostasis. Episodes of transient hypercontractility have been controlled by infusion of these drugs. Occasionally, the unexpected pharmacologic effect of other drugs may create the need to administer a uterine relaxant; the proper use of β-mimetics may then be extremely useful (Figure 9-64, see also Figure 11-6).

It appears that the new group of β-mimetic agents with minimal effect on blood pressure and diminished chronotropic action on the heart have a most promising therapeutic potential in obstetrics. Their use may be rewarding, provided clinicians observe the contraindications and remember that all these preparations markedly increase cardiac output and thus the workload of the heart, which may be compromised in certain clinical syndromes.

OTHER NEUROHORMONES

Norepinephrine

As a selective α-mimetic amine, norepinephrine is a strong oxytocic. It has been studied in re-

cent years as a pure substance, but in the past its effect was overlapped with that of epinephrine because both are components of the natural adrenal extract (adrenaline).

The *intravenous infusion* of small doses triggers quickly very strong and frequent contractions with increased tonus (Figure 9-65) and incoordinated pattern; however, there is an "adaptation" to the drug, after the first response, toward more physiologic looking tracings. At the same time the uterine activity decreases, and the tonus tends to come down toward normal values (Figure 9-66). When the infusion rate is increased a similar cycle of rapid hypertonic response and adaptation is repeated, with response in proportion to the infusion rate. Cessation of the infusion is rapidly followed by disappearance of any evidence of stimulation: there is no rebound as observed with epinephrine.

The *cardiovascular* response is as dramatic as that of the uterus and, also, in direct proportion to the rate of infusion: there is hypertension with minimal adaptation following the first response (Figure 9-67) and new increases as the dose is augmented. All these responses occur simultaneously with mirror image changes in the pulse rate. Discontinuing the infusion is followed by a rapid fall in blood pressure to values slightly lower than

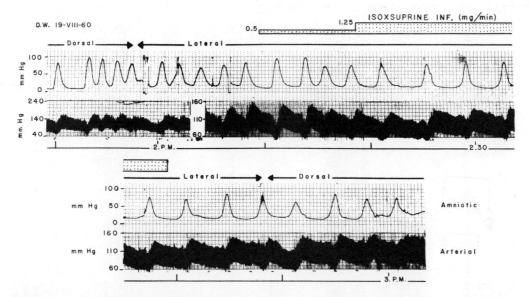

Figure 9-64 Continuous 75 min of intrauterine and arterial pressure recordings of term labor in patient with mild preeclampsia. (Note change in scale in upper part of arterial pressure scale.) *(Above, left)* Hypercontractility with hypertonus following cessation of epinephrine infusion. Turning the patient from supine to lateral decreased frequency of contractions but not enough to correct the hypercontractility. An infusion of isoxsuprine started at 500 μg/min and increased to 1250 μg/min succeeded in reducing the excessive uterine activity to normal values with normal progress of dilatation to completion. Reprinted from Cibils LA: Inhibitory effect of isoxsuprine on uterine contractility. *Am J Obstet Gynecol* 94:762, 1966.

those observed before the drug was begun and a tachycardia above control levels.

Acetylcholine

In its physiologic mechanism of action this substance acts on the autonomic effector cells and fibers of ganglion cells and the adrenal, as well as on motor nerves of skeletal muscles. Exogenous administration has minimal penetration into CNS sites because of its structure.

Intravenous infusion of acetylcholine in a pregnant patient demonstrates that it is an excellent oxytocic. Uterine response is characterized by increasing contractility (Figure 9-68), which reaches a steady activity after about 20 min. The pattern looks somewhat incoordinated, and slightly exaggerated fluctuations are normally observed. The *mechanism* of action has not been clarified: it may be a direct effect on the myometrium, by stimulation of either the short axon ganglion cells of the paracervical plexus or catecholamines released by the adrenals. Never-

theless, the postinfusion effect is relatively long lasting. The response may be completely blocked by the administration of atropine.

ANALGESICS, SEDATIVES, ATARACTICS

Classic obstetric teaching has perpetuated the concept that many sedatives used in daily practice are so-called antispasmodic and therefore relax the uterus. In addition, some have successfully postulated that certain compounds have specific properties to act selectively on different areas of the uterus and relax some but not affect others. The introduction of intrauterine recordings enabled us to evaluate objectively those claims and to establish the clinical pharmacology of the uterus on more scientific grounds. The uterus is a unique organ, constantly contracting, and, unlike the central nervous system it does not "go to sleep" or become tranquilized by drugs. It can be stimulated or relaxed by specific drugs; some of the

206

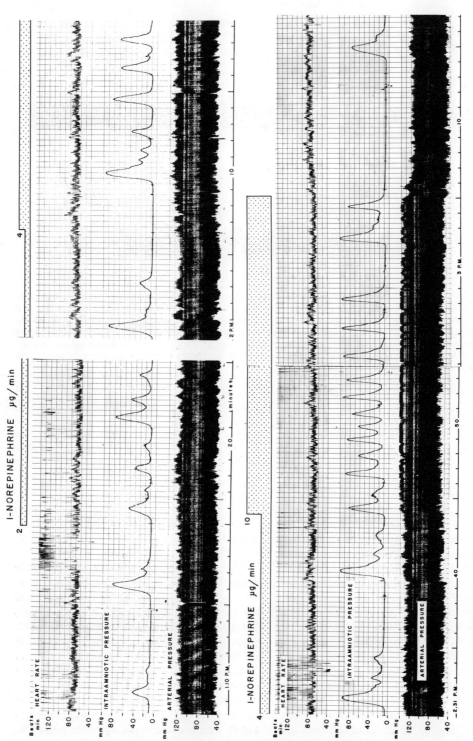

Figure 9-65 Arterial and intraamniotic pressures and maternal pulse rate recordings in term pregnant patient carrying a dead fetus. (*Above*) Spontaneous uterine contractility is rapidly increased by an infusion of 2 µg/min norepinephrine (dotted bar). After some slowdown, the infusion was raised to 4 µg/min with, again, a rapid increase in uterine activity. This pattern was again followed by partial decrease of activity without change of the infusion rate, but a further increase on infusion to 10 µg/min (*bottom*) produced polysystoly and hypertonus, and again a slowdown. Cessation of norepinephrine infusion was followed by immediate marked diminution of uterine activity. There was mild increase in blood pressure with 2 and 4 µg/min infusions but a significant one at 10 µg/min. The pulse rate dropped slightly with each increment of infusion. Reprinted from Cibils LA, et al: Effect of *l*-norepinephrine infusion on uterine contractility and cardiovascular system.

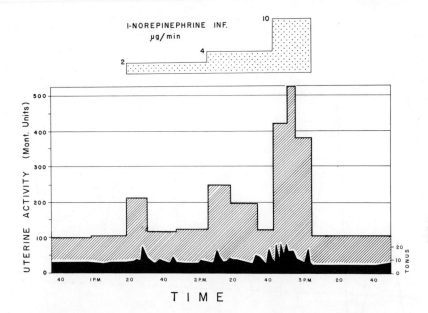

Figure 9-66 Three-hour recording obtained in patient shown in Figure 9-65 analyzed and calculated to illustrate the uterine response to increasing doses of norepinephrine infusion. Increase in uterine activity (stripped area) and tonus (black area) and their adaptation following each change in infusion rate. The immediate drop of uterine activity to preinfusion levels following cessation of infusion is clear. Reprinted from Cibils LA, et al: Effect of *l*-norepinephrine infusion on uterine contractility and cardiovascular system. *Am J Obstet Gynecol* 84:307, 1962.

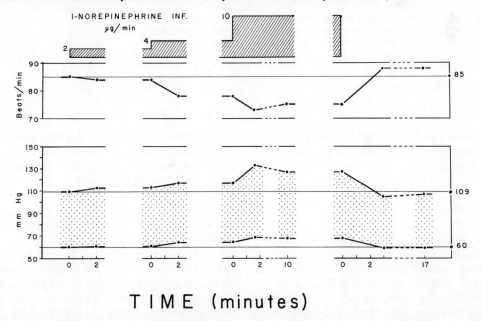

Figure 9-67 Averaged results of cardiovascular response to increasing rates of norepinephrine infusion. (Control preinfusion values in ordinates, right). The infusion of 2 μg/min produces a mild increase in blood pressure stabilized at 2 min. A still moderate increase is the result of raising the norepinephrine to 4 μg/min with a drop in pulse rate. A further increase in blood pressure peaking at 2 min followed by slight fall stabilized at 10 min follows the infusion of 10 μg/min. Interruption of the infusion is followed by a rapid fall in blood pressure stabilized after 3 min below the preinfusion levels and lasting more than 17 min. The pulse rate mirror images all these changes. Reprinted from Cibils LA, et al: Effect of *l*-norepinephrine infusion on uterine contractility and cardiovascular system. *Am J Obstet Gynecol* 84:307, 1962.

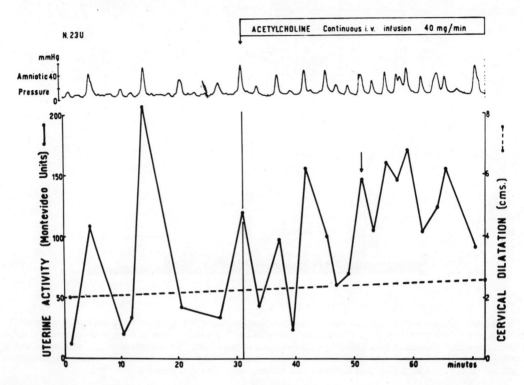

Figure 9-68 Effect of acetylcholine infusion on term pregnant uterine contractility. Upper part of figure, the intrauterine pressure tracing and below the uterine activity (Montevideo Units) calculated for each contraction. The broken horizontal line indicates cervical dilatation. The settling time is from the start of infusion until the small arrow, when activity seems to have stabilized with the normal fluctuations. Reprinted from Sala NL, Fish L: Effect of acetylcholine and atropine upon uterine contractility in pregnant women. *Am J Obstet Gynecol* 91:1069, 1965.

substances used for the control of systemic symptoms may affect the uterus but not necessarily by "sedating" it.

Morphine

A proven analgesic, morphine was for many decades the analgesic of choice in obstetrics when there was need for strong sedation. In addition to its good analgesic effects, it was used for its uterine relaxing properties in cases of uterine inertia and long labor when "both mother and uterus needed a rest" to regain their ability to carry on with a normal labor. This erroneous concept is still widely accepted and taught in modern obstetrics, in spite of the number of well-documented clinical studies, which have shown the lack of response of the term pregnant uterus to the administration of morphine. The *intramuscular*

administration of a large therapeutic dose does not interfere with induced uterine activity (Figure 9-69). Likewise, the *intravenous* injection of a therapeutic dose does not alter oxytocin-*induced uterine activity* (Figure 9-70). The same response is systematically observed when the drug is given, even intravenously, to patients with *spontaneous* uterine activity in prelabor (Figure 9-71) or in advanced first stage. The ultimate demonstration that morphine does not affect uterine contractions may be observed when the drug is administered intramyometrically, which gives a very high local concentration of the drug (Figure 9-72). The injection seems totally inert regarding uterine contractility, which is neither increased nor decreased by it.

The *cardiovascular* effects are negligible because neither blood pressure nor heart rate is influenced by the drug. Only the respirations become deeper and more regular. It, therefore,

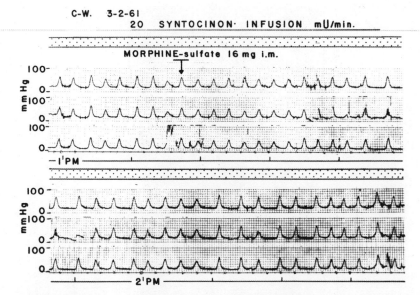

Figure 9-69 Continuous 100 minutes of intrauterine *(C)* and intramyometrial pressure recordings *(A,B)* in term induced labor of patient receiving 20 mU/min oxytocin. At the arrow morphine sulfate 16 mg IM given. Note that uterine contractility is unaffected throughout the long tracing. Reprinted from Cibils LA, Zuspan FP: Pharmacology of the uterus. *Clin Obstet Gynecol* 11:34, 1968.

seems an ideal drug to use as systemic analgesic when the delivery of the infant is not expected within 4 hours of its administration.

Meperidine

The most frequently used synthetic analgesic in obstetrics is meperidine (Demerol), which was originally thought to be an "antispasmodic" for the cervix and lower segment. However, clinical studies have demonstrated that it does not have the property of relaxing the lower areas of the uterus, or any part of it, when given by the *intramuscular* route. Thus its use as an intrapartum analgesic became widespread, in doses ranging from 50 to 100 mg IM. However, other studies have demonstrated that the exposure of the pregnant myometrium to high concentrations of meperidine is followed by contractions. Shortly thereafter it was shown that the *intravenous* administration of the substance in rapid injection triggers an enhancement of existing uterine activity in either prelabor or labor. Even at low total doses it increased contractility in mid-first stage (Figures 9-73 and 9-74). The response to higher single injections is of relatively short duration

(Figure 9-75) but may endanger the condition of a fetus with precarious intrauterine reserves; it also may suffice to trigger an impending labor. The action is related to the concentration of the drug injected as a bolus and reaching the myometrium sufficiently undiluted to exert its oxytocic effect. It is well known that the slow infusion of meperidine alone or in combination with other drugs does not have an oxytocic effect.

The systemic effects are almost negligible. The cardiovascular system is not directly influenced. Nausea and vomiting are the most consistent and predictable untoward effects of the rapid intravenous injection. Effects on the fetus will be discussed in Chapter 18.

Pentazocine

A potent synthetic analgesic, pentazocine (Talwin) has been in use in the United States for several years, and claims have been made that it is as strong as morphine, has minimal side effects, and is not habit forming. Few studies have been carried out in obstetrics but some have demonstrated a strong oxytocic effect when pentazocine is injected intravenously (Figure 9-76) in rapid,

210

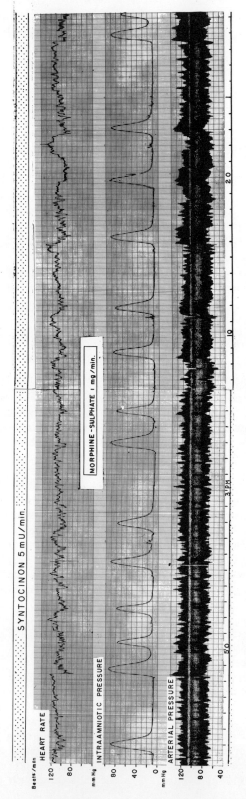

Figure 9-70 Arterial and intrauterine pressures, and maternal heart rate recordings from *term induced labor* with 5 mU/min oxytocin. Intravenous infusion of morphine at 1 mg/min for 8 min did not change the characteristics observed in any of the three channels. Reprinted from Eskes TKAB: Effect of morphine upon uterine contractility in late pregnancy. *Am J Obstet Gynecol* 84:281, 1962.

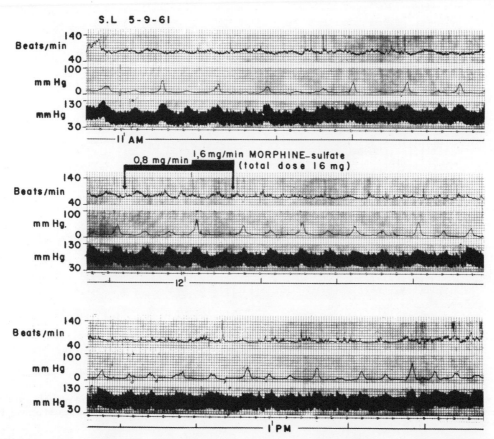

Figure 9-71 Continuous 150 min of arterial and intrauterine pressures and maternal heart rate recordings in *term spontaneous advanced prelabor. (Center)* Intravenous infusion of morphine up to 16 mg did not induce any noticeable change in either uterine contractility or cardiovascular parameters. Reprinted from Eskes TKAB: Effect of morphine upon uterine contractility in late pregnancy. *Am J Obstet Gynecol* 84:281, 1962.

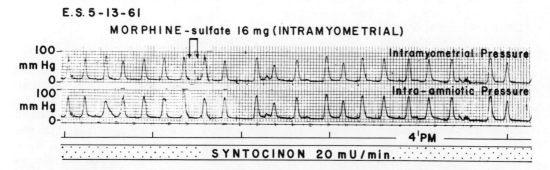

Figure 9-72 Intramyometrial and intrauterine pressure tracings in *term induced labor* with 20 mU/min oxytocin. The intramyometrial injection of 16 mg morphine did not affect the uterine contractility of either the local area of injection or the total uterus.

212

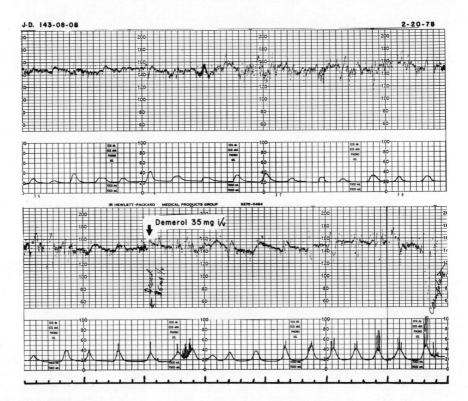

Figure 9-73 Last 70 min of recordings in *spontaneous labor* of multipara at term. Intrauterine pressure and FHR tracings. The *rapid intravenous* injection of 35 mg meperidine triggered a period of transient increased activity followed by rapid completion of dilatation.

single doses of 40 to 45 mg. It produces a sharp increase in the frequency of the contractions and, occasionally, hypertonus of considerable duration. The overall uterine activity is thus significantly increased, and therefore the cervical dilatation seems to be accelerated.

It appears to have a negligible influence on the cardiovascular system of the patient. Likewise, no clinical effects have been observed on FHR or condition of the infant at birth.

Fentanyl

One of the newest synthetic analgesics, fentanyl (Sublimaze) is by weight several hundred times more potent than meperidine. Another previously unknown similarity to Demerol is its *potent oxytocic effect* when given intravenously. It may produce marked hypotonus and polysystoly when used as premedication in obstetrics and, depending on the clinical case, it may cause

counterproductive effects because of the oxytocic action (see Figure 11-6). Intravenous use should probably be contraindicated in obstetric cases when the objective is other than to terminate a nonviable gestation. Used alone in the standard dose of 0.1 mg, it is equivalent to 75 mg Demerol; in the combination form (Innovar) it is equally effective as analgesic and as oxytocic.

Phenothiazines

The family of phenothiazines has an extraordinarily extended use in modern medicine, and particularly in obstetrics, where its potentiating and mild sedative effects are much appreciated by clinicians. Promazine, chlorpromazine, promethazine, prochlorperazine, and trifluoperazine are the preparations commonly available and the ones used in pregnant patients. A number of claims about their effect on the uterine contractility have found their way into some books or monographs

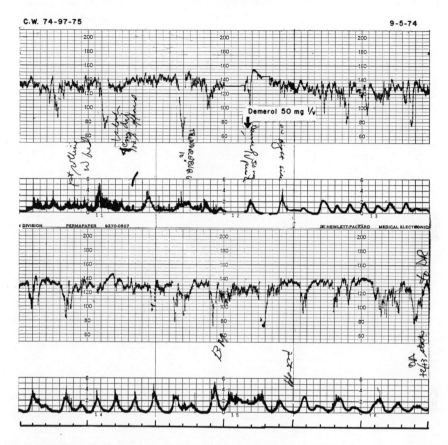

Figure 9-74 Last 60 min of intrauterine and FHR recordings in term *enhanced labor*. At 4 cm cervical dilatation, a *rapid intravenous* injection of 50 mg meperidine triggered marked hypercontractility with polysystoly and some irregular pattern. Dilatation was completed rapidly, 42 min later.

on general pharmacology, not all of them substantiated by well-conducted studies. The *intravenous* administration of 50 mg *chlorpromazine* during labor in normal patients produces no noticeable changes in uterine contractility: the tonus, frequency, and intensity of contractions are not affected (Figure 9-77) nor is uterine activity. However, Zourlas (1964) reported that the intramuscular administration of Phenergan and Sparine markedly decreased uterine activity mainly at the expense of the intensity of the contractions. Chlorpromazine combined with Phenergan and Demerol in intravenous infusion does not affect uterine activity, even when given at reasonably rapid rates (Figure 9-78).

The cardiovascular effects of these drugs administered intravenously are interesting because they have only a mild hypotensive effect, if any, when given to normal patients, but they produce a beneficial hypotensive response when administered to hypertensive preeclamptic patients (Figure 9-78). In fact, the infusion of high doses of a mixture of Demerol with Phenergan and chlorpromazine may lead to clinical hypotension during labor. It seems that they have no discernible effect on the fetus.

Magnesium Sulfate

Introduced by Stroganoff in the 1920s as part of a multidrug treatment of eclampsia, magnesium sulfate had periods of acceptance and rejection depending on the type and claims made about new drugs with anticonvulsant properties introduced to clinical use. In the last decade, with a better approach for evaluation of its effects on preeclamptic patients, it has been accepted as standard in the

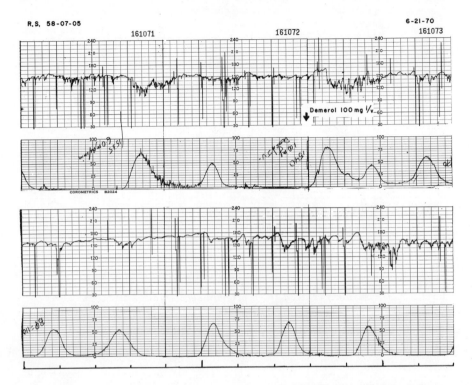

Figure 9-75 Continuous 24 minutes of intrauterine pressure and FHR tracings, obtained at paper speed of 3 cm/min, in term multipara with *enhanced labor*. The rapid intravenous injection of 100 mg meperidine increased the frequency of contractions from 2 in 8 min to 8 in 16 min. The FHR does not seem affected.

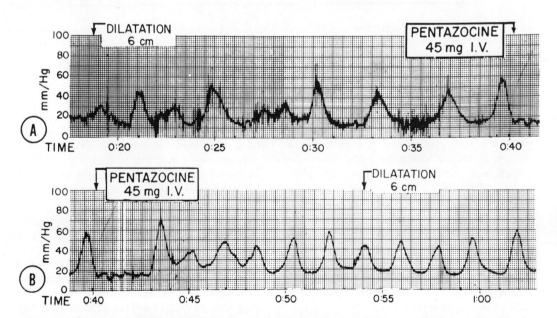

Figure 9-76 Continuous uterine pressure tracing in term pregnant patient in *spontaneous labor*. The rapid intravenous injection of 45 mg pentazocine triggered a marked hypercontractility with polysystoly and hypertonus. Reprinted from Filler WN, Filler NW: Effect of a potent non-narcotic analgesic agent (pentazocine) in uterine contractility and fetal heart rate. *Obstet Gynecol* 28:224, 1966.

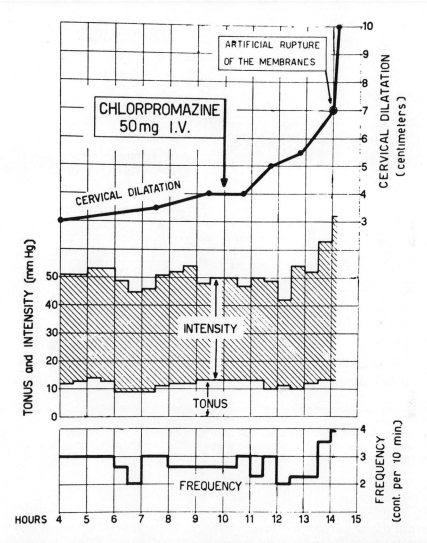

Figure 9-77 Intensity, frequency, and tonus of contractions calculated for 10 hours in a *normal term spontaneous labor*. The rapid intravenous injection of 50 mg chlorpromazine did not affect any of the parameters analyzed. Cervical dilatation was not influenced either, until amniotomy facilitated dilatation. Reprinted from Caldeyro-Barcia R, et al: The action of chlorpromazine on uterine contractility and arterial pressure in normal and toxemic pregnant women. *Am J Obstet Gynecol* 75:1088, 1958.

management of severe preeclamptic and eclamptic patients. However, apart from the anticonvulsant properties, there is no clear understanding of its influence on uterine contractility, the cardiovascular system, or renal function.

 As an anticonvulsant its pharmacologic effect is exerted at the neuromuscular plate where it inhibits the transmission of the nerve impulse by blocking the release of the neurotransmitter acetylcholine. By preventing the muscle stimulation in this way, magnesium effectively impedes

the occurrence of the grand mal type of seizures characteristic of the eclamptic convulsion. On the other hand, the magnesium ion may also block the contraction of smooth muscle by interfering with the excitation–contraction coupling, which normally follows the firing of the action potential. However, this effect is obtained in vitro with high concentrations of magnesium in the water bath, 2.5 mg/100 ml added to the already present 2.5 mg/100 ml in the Ringer-Tyrode solution. The *rapid intravenous* infusion of 4 gm at a rate of

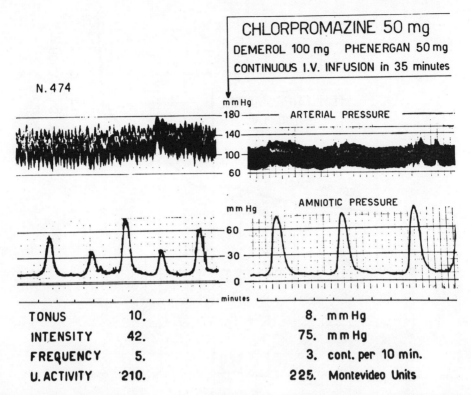

CHLORPROMAZINE 50 mg

DEMEROL 100 mg   PHENERGAN 50 mg

CONTINUOUS I.V. INFUSION in 35 minutes

N. 474

TONUS	10.		8.	mm Hg
INTENSITY	42.		75.	mm Hg
FREQUENCY	5.		3.	cont. per 10 min.
U. ACTIVITY	210.		225.	Montevideo Units

Figure 9-78 Arterial and intrauterine pressures recorded in a *preterm eclamptic* patient. The continuous infusion of 50 mg chlorpromazine with meperidine and promethazine did not affect uterine activity (values of analysis given at the bottom). However, the hypertension was reduced to normal blood pressure readings. Reprinted from Caldeyro-Barcia R, et al: The action of chlorpromazine on uterine contractility and arterial pressure in normal and toxemic pregnant women. *Am J Obstet Gynecol* 75:1088, 1958.

0.50 gm/min (Figure 9-79) has a transient effect on the uterine contractility, either spontaneous or induced with oxytocin. Very shortly after the rapid injection is completed, the contractions regain and continue their previous pattern unless other interfering maneuvers take place. When the rapid injection is given at doses of less than 0.50 gm/min, the uterine effects are almost negligible even with large amounts (Figure 9-80).

Intramuscular administration has no noticeable effect upon the uterine contractility, perhaps because the absorption is relatively slow and therefore the blood levels never reach the concentrations attained by the bolus of a rapid intravenous injection.

The *intramyometrial* injection of concentrated magnesium sulfate transiently depresses the rhythmic pattern of contractions, but generally for one contraction, and without influence on other areas of the uterus (see Figure 5-51), lower tracing).

It is clear then that magnesium sulfate given in high loading doses and maintained by continuous infusion for several hours does not depress induced or spontaneous contractions of established labor—this in spite of the recent observations by Steer and Petrie (1977), who suggest that it is a good drug to arrest premature labor. This observation, if corroborated, may well indicate that there may be subtle differences in the mechanism of term labor and premature labor contractions.

The *cardiovascular effects* of the intravenous injection of magnesium sulfate have been misunderstood for a very long time. In fact, it is still accepted by the great majority of obstetricians as a good antihypertensive drug, to be used for that purpose in severe preeclamptic patients.

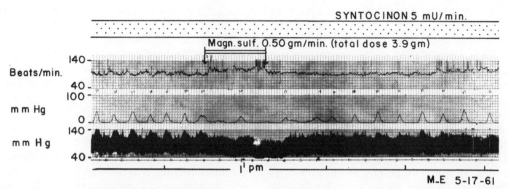

Figure 9-79 Continuous blood and intrauterine pressures and maternal heart rate tracings obtained in *term labor induced* with 5 mU/min oxytocin. The infusion of 4 gm magnesium sulfate at 0.50 gm/min produced a transient episode of hypotension with a subjective sensation of warmth, palpitations, and flushing. There was transient tachycardia. At the same time the uterine contractility diminished. All parameters recovered, and the subjective symptoms disappeared when the infusion was completed.

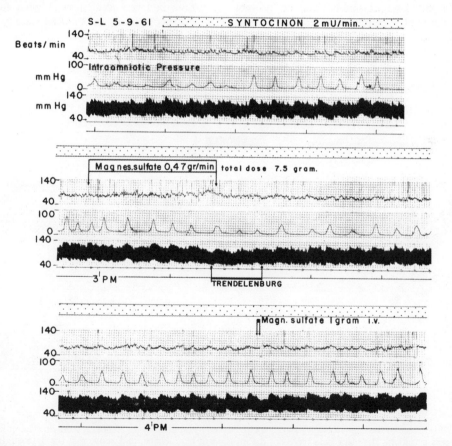

Figure 9-80 Continuous 150 min of intrauterine and blood pressures and maternal heart rate recordings obtained in *term induced labor. (Center)* Infusion of 7.5 gm magnesium sulfate at 0.5 gm/min produced some diminution of uterine activity at 10 min with minimal hypotension. At 15 min the hypotension was more marked (95/50) with subjective symptoms of palpitations, warmth, and flushing, moderate tachycardia, and depression of uterine contractility. About 10 min after cessation of the infusion all parameters had returned to control values. *(Below)* An additional gram of magnesium sulfate IV produced no effect. Reprinted from Cibils LA, Zuspan FP: Pharmacology of the uterus. *Clin Obstet Gynecol* 11:34, 1968.

218

In fact, *it is not hypotensive* at the therapeutic blood concentrations of 4 to 8 mg/100 ml even when these levels are maintained for several hours. Its relaxing effect on the vascular smooth muscles is manifested only when very high concentrations are locally attained, as by the head of the bolus during rapid injections at 0.50 gm/min or more (Figures 9-79 and 9-80). This response is accompanied by subjective sensations of warmth, palpitations, dizziness, anxiety, and clinical signs of vasodilatation as flushing. The pulse rate does not change except during the short episodes of hypotension triggered by the very high infusion rates. When the need arises to decrease a dangerous hypertension, it is necessary to add an antihypertensive medication to the magnesium sulfate infusion, which is not only inadequate to diminish the blood pressure but may not prevent severe bouts of hypertension (Figure 9-81). The

treatment of hyperreflexia is thus separate from treatment of hypertension, but both may have to be conducted simultaneously. From these observations, it is hard to understand the claims, previously published, that magnesium sulfate is such an excellent antihypertensive in preeclampsia. The hyperreflexia of severe preeclampsia is rapidly controlled, and the effect sustained, when the blood concentrations are maintained within the therapeutic levels of 4 to 8 mg/100 ml.

The *urinary output* of the preeclamptic or eclamptic patients is usually very low, less than 60 to 80 ml/hour and very concentrated. The high blood concentration of magnesium seems to facilitate the renal function because within a few hours of the loading dose the kidneys appear to "open up" with a sustained diuresis of 150 to 300 ml/hour and very clear urine (Figures 9-81 and 9-82). This high output is not necessarily related

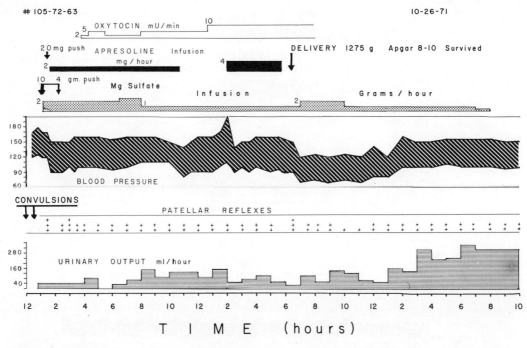

Figure 9-81 Some of the most relevant parameters of flow chart tabulated over 30 hours, from an eclamptic patient at 32 weeks gestation. The black bars represent the infusion of hydralazine, and above that the oxytocin infusion. After three convulsions, the patient was given 14 gm push magnesium sulfate in the first hour to control the hyperreflexia, and a 2 gm/hr maintenance dose was instituted. At the same time, 20 mg push and *2 mg/hr hydralazine* were given for severe hypertension. Shortly thereafter induction of labor started with 2 to 10 mU/min oxytocin, and it was completed 18 hours after initiation of treatment with the birth of an infant in good condition. Note the need of additional hydralazine after it had been discontinued. It is noticeable that the urinary output markedly improved at 8 hours. The magnesium sulfate was maintained for 12 hours after delivery for a total of 58 gm in 31 hours. In spite of a negative fluid balance of 1550 ml, the urinary output was 300 ml/hour for the last 4 hours shown.

to increased fluid intake, usually tightly controlled in eclamptic or severe preeclamptic patients. In fact, it is often observed that there is a negative intake–output fluid balance in these patients during labor and immediately postpartum.

Precautions The pharmacologic action of the magnesium ion is preferentially exerted on the neuromuscular plate of the striated muscles. There is a gradation of effect, in proportion to blood concentration, from peripheral striated muscles to more centrally located muscles. The first ones to be blocked are the muscles of the extremities where the tendon reflexes (patellar, Achilles tendon, biceps) are first diminished and then obliterated. This has been observed to occur with blood levels above 12 mg/100 ml. The next striated muscles to be blocked are the respiratory muscles when the blood level reaches or surpasses 15 mg/100 ml, with respiratory arrest as a conse-

quence. Finally, if the infusion continues and the heart does not fibrillate because of the hypoxia, the myocardium will be paralyzed when the blood levels are above 25 mg/100 ml. There is then a perfectly established gradation of response, which facilitates the dosification of the ion without the need to resort to laboratory tests of doubtful accuracy. If the patient has patellar or biceps reflexes, it is highly unlikely that she will have a respiratory or cardiac arrest.

The elimination of the exogenously administered magnesium ion takes place almost exclusively by the kidneys. For that reason, the maintenance dose of the infusion must be geared against the urinary output of the patient. When urinary excretion is low, it is probable that the magnesium therapeutic blood level will be rapidly reached and only a small amount per hour will be necessary to maintain it. On the other hand, a

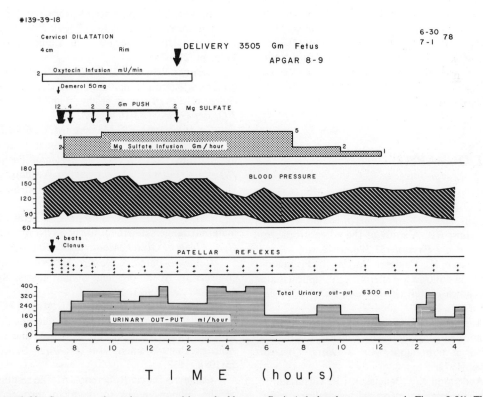

Figure 9-82 Severe preeclampsia at term with marked hyperreflexia (tabulated parameters as in Figure 9-81). The patient required *16 gm push magnesium sulfate* in the first hour to control the severe hyperreflexia. Urinary output increased rapidly and mandated a high maintenance dose of 5 gm/hour magnesium sulfate to prevent the return of hyperreflexia. Blood pressure and uterine contractility were not affected by the very high magnesium doses; 2 mU/min oxytocin was enough to induce labor. The urinary output continued to be high; a negative fluid balance of 3300 ml was recorded by the end of the tabulation. Total magnesium given: 82 gm in 17 hours.

high urinary output attests to a rapid elimination of the infused magnesium, and high maintenance doses will be required to prevent hyperreflexia and convulsions (Figure 9-82).

The loading dose of intravenous magnesium sulfate has been established at about 4 gm to be rapidly injected, and approximately 1 gm/hour as a maintenance dose—in general, probably the minimum effective dose in the great majority of severe preeclamptic hyperreflexic patients requiring treatment. Actually, the loading dose should be specifically titrated in each case by close follow-up of the patellar reflexes, which should be maintained between one and two plus. Often, one may need much more to attain the therapeutic objective of controlling hyperreflexia: the two cases illustrated in Figures 9-81 and 9-82 required significantly more in spite of low urinary output at the beginning of treatment. Frequent examination of the reflexes after completing an intravenous injection of 2 to 4 gm should determine whether more medication is required. From the description of the cardiovascular side effects it is clear that the loading dose should be injected at less than 0.50 gm/min, preferably at about 0.25 to 0.30 gm/min. Because of its lack of effect upon the myometrium, postpartum hemorrhages are not to be expected when the medication is continued after delivery.

BIBLIOGRAPHY

Adair FL, Davis ME, Kharasch MS, et al: A study of a new and potent ergot derivative, ergotocin. *Am J Obstet Gynecol* 30:466, 1935.

Alquist RP: A study of the adrenotropic receptors. *Am J Physiol* 153:586, 1948.

Alvarez H, Caldeyro-Barcia R: Fisiopatologia de la contraccion uterina y sus aplicaciones en la clinica obstetrica. *II Cong Lat-Am Obstet Ginecol* 1:1, 1954.

Anderson GG, Hobbins JC, Speroff L: Intravenous prostaglandins E_2 and $F_2\alpha$ for the induction of term labor. *Am J Obstet Gynecol* 112:382, 1972.

Andersson KE, Bengtsson LP, Gustafson I, et al: The relaxing effect of terbutaline on the human uterus during term labor. *Am J Obstet Gynecol* 121:602, 1975.

Andersson KE, Ingemarsson I, Persson CGA: Effects of terbutaline on human uterine

motility at term. *Acta Obstet Gynecol Scand* 54:165, 1975.

Barr W: Induction of labor with prostaglandin E_2. *J Reprod Med* 9:353, 1972.

Belinkoff S, Hall J: Intravenous alcohol during labor. *Am J Obstet Gynecol* 59:429, 1950.

Bengtsson LP: Experiments on the suppressive effect of a synthetic gestagen on the activity of the pregnant human uterus. *Acta Obstet Gynecol Scand* 41:124, 1962.

Bieniarz J: Cardiovascular effects of high doses of oxytocin, in Caldeyro-Barcia R, Heller H (eds): *Oxytocin*. NY, Pergamon, 1961, pp 80–83.

Bieniarz J, Ivankovich A, Scommegna A: Cardiac output during ritodrine treatment in premature labor. *Am J Obstet Gynecol* 118:910, 1974.

Branda LA, Ferrier BM: Chemistry of neurohypophyseal hormones and their synthetic analogues, in Heller H, Pickering BT (eds): *The neurohypophysis*. New York, Pergamon, 1970, pp 19–58.

Brenner WE: The place of prostaglandins in modern obstetrics, in Aladjem S (ed): *Risks in the Practice of Modern Obstetrics*. St. Louis, Mosby, 1975, pp 210–244.

Brenner WE, Hendricks CH: Effect of medroxyprogesterone acetate upon the duration and characteristics of human gestation and labor. *Am J Obstet Gynecol* 83:1094, 1962.

Caldeyro-Barcia R, Magana JM, Castillo JB, et al: A new approach to the treatment of acute intrapartum fetal distress, in *Perinatal Factors Affecting Human Development*. Washington, DC, Pan American Health Organization Scientific Publication 185, 1969, pp 248–253.

Caldeyro-Barcia R, Poseiro JJ: Fetal and maternal dangers due to misuse of oxytocin. *II Int Cong Gynecol Obstet (Montreal)* 2:450, 1958.

Caldeyro-Barcia R, Poseiro JJ: Oxytocin and contractility of the pregnant human uterus. *Ann NY Acad Sci* 75:813, 1959.

Caldeyro-Barcia R, Poseiro JJ, Alvarez H, et al: The action of chlorpromazine on uterine contractility and arterial pressure in normal and toxemic pregnant women. *Am J Obstet Gynecol* 75:1088, 1958.

Caldeyro-Barcia R, Sereno JA: The response of the human uterus to oxytocin throughout pregnancy, in Caldeyro-Barcia R, Heller H (eds): *Oxytocin*. NY, Pergamon, 1961, pp 177–200.

Caldeyro-Barcia R, Sica-Blanco Y, Poseiro JJ, et al: A quantitative study of the action of synthetic oxytocin on the pregnant human uterus. *J Pharmacol Exp Ther* 121:18, 1957.

Carsten ME: Prostaglandin's part in regulating uterine contraction by transport of calcium. *J Reprod Med* 9:277, 1972.

Chesley L: Parenteral magnesium sulfate and the distribution, plasma levels and excretion of magnesium. *Am J Obstet Gynecol* 133:1, 1979.

Cibils LA: Inhibitory effect of isoxsuprine on uterine contractility. *Am J Obstet Gynecol* 94:762, 1966.

Cibils LA: Effect of mesuprine hydrochloride upon non-pregnant uterine contractility and cardiovascular system. *Am J Obstet Gynecol* 111:91, 1971.

Cibils LA: Clinical significance of fetal heart rate patterns during labor. II. Late decelerations. *Am J Obstet Gynecol* 123:473, 1975.

Cibils LA: The management of impending labor prior to the thirty-fifth week, in Reid DE, Christian CD (eds): *Controversy in Obstetrics & Gynecology II*. Philadelphia, Saunders, 1974, pp 88–102.

Cibils LA, Caldeyro-Barcia R: Accion de la ocitocina sobre el tono uterino. *Res Reun Lat-Am Cienc Fisiol* 53, 1957.

Cibils LA, Hendricks CH: Efecto de la isoxsuprina sobre la contracilidad del utero humano gravido. *Mem X Reun Ginecol Obstet (Mexico)* 1:418, 1961.

Cibils LA, Hendricks CH: Effect of ergot derivatives and sparteine sulfate upon the human uterus. *J Reprod Med* 2:147, 1969.

Cibils LA, Pose SV, Zuspan FP: Effect of *l*-norepinephrine infusion on uterine contractility and cardiovascular system. *Am J Obstet Gynecol* 84:307, 1962.

Cibils LA, Poseiro JJ, Noriega-Guerra L: Comparison of the effects on the pregnant human uterus of highly purified natural oxytocin, Pitocin, synthetic oxytocin (Syntocinon), valyl-3-oxytocin and arginine vasopression, in Caldeyro-Barcia R, Heller H (eds): *Oxytocin*. NY, Pergamon, 1961, pp 266–275.

Cibils LA, Santonja-Lucas JJ: Clinical significance of fetal heart rate patterns during labor. III. Effect of paracervical block anesthesia. *Am J Obstet Gynecol* 130:73, 1978.

Cibils LA, Zuspan FP: Pharmacology of the uterus. *Clin Obstet Gynecol* 11:34, 1968.

Cobo E, Quintero CA, Estrada G, et al: Uterine behavior in abruptio placentae. *Am J Obstet Gynecol* 93:1151, 1965.

Csapo AI: The onset of labor. *Lancet* 2:277, 1961.

Dudley HW, Moir JC: The substance responsible for the traditional clinical effect of ergot. *Br Med J* 1:520, 1935.

DuVigneaud V, Ressler C, Swan JM, et al: The synthesis of oxytocin. *J Am Chem Soc* 76:3115, 1954.

DuVigneaud V, Ressler C, Trippett S: The sequence of amino acids in oxytocin with a proposal for the structure of oxytocin. *J Biol Chem* 205:949, 1953.

Elias JA: Experience with prostaglandins E_2 and $F_2\alpha$ for induction of labor. *J Reprod Med* 9:307, 1972.

Eskes TKAB: Effect of morphine upon uterine contractility in late pregnancy. *Am J Obstet Gynecol* 84:281, 1962.

Eskes TKAB, Stolte L, Seelen J, et al: Epinephrine derivatives and the activity of the human uterus. *Am J Obstet Gynecol* 92:871, 1965.

Filler WN, Filler NW: Effect of a potent non-narcotic analgesic agent (pentazocine) in uterine contractility and fetal heart rate. *Obstet Gynecol* 28:224, 1966.

Flowers CE: Magnesium sulfate in obstetrics. *Am J Obstet Gynecol* 91:763, 1965.

Freeman DW, Barno A: Maternal deaths associated with the use of pituitary substances. *Obstet Gynecol* 18:729, 1961.

Fuchs AR: Oxytocin and the onset of labor in rabbits. *J Endocrinol* 31:217, 1964.

Fuchs F: Treatment of threatened premature labor with alcohol. *J Obstet Gynaecol Br Comwlth* 72:1011, 1965.

Gonzalez-Panizza VH, Sica-Blanco Y: Estimacion de la ocitocinemia durante el parto inducido por infusion intravenosa de ocitocina. *II Cong Uruguayo Ginecotocol* 2:330, 1957.

Gonzalez-Panizza VH, Sica-Blanco Y, Mendex-Bauer C: The fate of injected oxytocin in the pregnant woman near term, in Caldeyro-Barcia R, Heller H (eds): *Oxytocin*. NY, Pergamon, 1961, pp 347–357.

Hendricks CH: Efectos cardiovasculares de la ocitocina. *II Cong Uruguayo Ginecotocol* 2:1957.

Hendricks CH, Brenner WE: Cardiovascular effects of oxytocin drugs used post partum. *Am J Obstet Gynecol* 108:751, 1970.

222

Hendricks CH, Cibils LA, Pose SV, et al: The pharmacologic control of excessive uterine activity with isoxsuprine. *Am J Obstet Gynecol* 82:1064, 1961.

Hendricks CH, Gabel RA: Use of intranasal oxytocin in obstetrics. *Am J Obstet Gynecol* 79:780, 1960.

Hendricks CH, Pose SV: Intranasal oxytocin in obstetrics. *JAMA* 175:384, 1961.

Hiller K: Prostaglandins and thromboxanes: Pharmacologic and biosynthetic aspects. *Semin Perinatol* 2:197, 1978.

Horiguchi T, Suzuki K, Comas-Urrutia AC, et al: Effect of ethanol upon uterine activity and fetal acid–base state of the rhesus monkey. *Am J Obstet Gynecol* 109:910, 1971.

Hutchinson HT, Nichols MM, Kuhn CR, et al: Effects of magnesium sulfate on uterine contractility, intrauterine fetus, and infant. *Am J Obstet Gynecol* 88:747, 1964.

Johnson JWC, Austin KL, Jones GS, et al: Efficacy of 17 α hydroxyprogesterone caproate in the premature labor. *N Engl J Med* 293:675, 1975.

Karim SMM, Sharma WW: Oral administration of prostaglandin E_2 for the induction and acceleration of labor. *J Reprod Med* 9:346, 1972.

Karim SM, Trussell RR, Patel RC, et al: Reponse of pregnant human uterus to prostaglandin $F_2\alpha$-induction of labor. *Br Med J* 4:621, 1968.

Kumar D, Goodno JA, Barnes AC: In vivo effects of intravenous progesterone infusion on gravid uterine contractility. *Bull Johns Hopkins Hosp* 113:53, 1963.

Kumar D, Zourlas PA, Barnes AC: In vitro and in vivo effects of magnesium sulfate on human uterine contractility. *Am J Obstet Gynecol* 86:1036, 1963.

Lands AM, Arnold A, McAuliff JP, et al: Differentiation of receptor systems activated by sympathomimetic amines. *Nature* 214:597, 1967.

Lewis RB, Schulman JD: Influence of acetylsalicylic acid, an inhibitor of prostaglandin synthesis, on the duration of human gestation and labor. *Lancet* 2:1159, 1973.

Lipton B, Hershey SG, Baez S: Compatibility of oxytocics with anesthetic agents. *JAMA* 179:410, 1962.

MacDonlad PC, Porter JC, Schwarz BE, et al: Initiation of parturition in the human female. *Semin Perinatol* 2:273, 1978.

Munsick RA: Renal hemodynamic effects of oxytocin in antepartal and postpartal woman. *Am J Obstet Gynecol* 108:729, 1970.

Niebyl JR, Blake DA, Burnett LS, et al: The influence of aspirin on the course of induced midtrimester abortion. *Am J Obstet Gynecol* 124:607, 1976.

Noriega-Guerra L, Sereno JA, Cobo E, et al: Reactividad del utero humano gravido a la ocitocina en el polihidramnios, la gran multiparidad y el feto muerto y retenido. *Arch Ginecol Obstet (Uruguay)* 18:3, 1960.

Novy MJ, Cook MJ, Manaugh L: Indomethacin block of normal onset of parturition in primates. *Am J Obstet Gynecol* 118:412, 1974.

Pike JE: Prostaglandin chemistry. *J Reprod Med* 9:258, 1972.

Pinto RM, Lerner U, Mazzocco N, et al: The oxytocic action of intraamniotic estradiol-17β on the pregnant human uterus. *Am J Obstet Gynecol* 94:876, 1966.

Pinto RM, Votta RA, Montuori E, et al: Action of estradiol-17β on the activity of the pregnant human uterus. *Am J Obstet Gynecol* 88:759, 1964.

Plentl AA, Friedman EA, Gray MJ: Sparteine sulfate. A clinical evaluation of its use in the management of labor. *Am J Obstet Gynecol* 82:132, 1961.

Pose SV, Cibils LA, Zuspan FP: Effect of *l*-epinephrine infusion on uterine contractility and cardiovascular system. *Am J Obstet Gynecol* 84:297, 1962.

Pose SV, Fielitz C: The effects of progesterone on the response of the pregnant human uterus to oxytocin, in Caldeyro-Barcia R, Heller H (eds): *Oxytocin*. NY, Pergamon, 1961, pp 229–239.

Poseiro JJ: Investigaciones sobre la farmacologia uterina en la toxemia. *III Cong Uruguayo Ginecotocol* 1:223, 1960.

Poseiro JJ, Noriega-Guerra L: Dose-response relationships in uterine effects of oxytocin infusions, in Caldeyro-Barcia R, Heller H (eds): *Oxytocin*. NY, Pergamon, 1961, pp 158–174.

Roberts G, Turnbull AC: Uterine hypertonus during labour induced by prostaglandins. *Br Med J* 1:702, 1971.

Rucker JP: The action of adrenalin on the pregnant human uterus. *South Med J* 18:412, 1925.

Sala NL, Fisch L: Effect of acetylcholine and atropine upon uterine contractility in pregnant women. *Am J Obstet Gynecol* 91:1069, 1965.

Scommegna A, Burd L, Goodman C, et al: The effect of pregnenolone sulfate on uterine contractility. *Am J Obstet Gynecol* 108:1023, 1970.

Sica-Blanco Y, Rozada H, Remedio MR: Effect of meperidine on uterine contractility during pregnancy and pre-labor. *Am J Obstet Gynecol* 97:1096, 1967.

Sica-Blanco Y, Sala NL: Uterine contractility at the beginning and end of an oxytocin infusion, in Caldeyro-Barcia, Heller H (eds): *Oxytocin*. NY, Pergamon, 1961, pp 127–136.

Silva P, Allan MS: Water intoxication due to high doses of synthetic oxytocin. *Obstet Gynecol* 27:517, 1966.

Spellacy WN, Gall SA: Prostaglandin $F_2\alpha$ and oxytocin for term labor induction. *J Reprod Med* 9:300, 1972.

Stander RW, Thompson JF, Stanley JR: Continuous intrauterine pressure recordings in the evaluation of sparteine sulfate. *Am J Obstet Gynecol* 86:281, 1963.

Steer CM, Petrie RH: A comparison of magnesium sulfate and alcohol for the prevention of premature labor. *Am J Obstet Gynecol* 129:1, 1977.

Theobald GW: Clinical pharmacology: Oxytocin, in Heller H, Pickering BT (eds): *The Neurophypophysis*. New York, Pergamon, 1970, pp 399–422.

Theobald GW, Graham A, Campbell J, et al: The use of post-pituitary extract in physiological amounts in obstetrics. *Br Med J* 2:123, 1948.

Theobald GW, Lundborg RA: Changes in myometrial sensitivity to oxytocin provoked in different ways. *J Obstet Gynaecol Br Comwlth* 69:417, 1962.

Turner G, Collins E: Fetal effects of regular salicylate ingestion in pregnancy. *Lancet* 2:338, 1975.

Tyack AJ, Baillie P, Meehan FP: In-vivo response of human uterus to orciprenaline in early labour. *Br Med J* 2:741, 1971.

Witting WC, Work BA, Laros RK: Uterine activity response to constant infusion of prostaglandin F_2 in term human pregnancy. *J Reprod Med* 9:283, 1972.

Zilianti M: Action of orciprenaline on uterine contractility during labor, maternal cardiovascular system, fetal heart rate and acid-base balance. *Am J Obstet Gynecol* 109:1073, 1971.

Zourlas PA: In-vitro and in-vivo effects of Sparine (promazine hydrochloride) on human uterine contractility. *Am J Obstet Gynecol* 88:770, 1964.

Zourlas PA: In-vitro and in-vivo effects of promethazine hydrochloride on human uterine contractility. *Am J Obstet Gynecol* 90:115, 1964.

Zuckerman H, Reiss U, Rubinstein I: Inhibition of human premature labor by indomethacin. *Obstet Gynecol* 44:787, 1974.

CHAPTER 10
Induction of Labor

Induction of labor is the deliberate initiation of labor by artificial means (either mechanic or pharmacologic) *in advanced pregnancy, before labor starts spontaneously.* Induction of labor has been practiced for a long time, and the list of the means and techniques used for that purpose is long and varied. Many of these have become obsolete and are now part of medical history because of the advances over the last two decades in understanding the physiology of late pregnancy and labor. Thanks to this better knowledge, proper uterine stimulation in late pregnancy and labor has become one of the most important skills of a competent obstetrician. Labor, properly induced, is of extraordinary help to obstetrician and patient, but when improperly used, it may be so dangerous as to be catastrophic. The number of cases of obstetric misadventures reported in maternal mortality statistics, and severe complication seminars attest to the importance of the proper training and experience required to use this technique safely and successfully. It is, therefore, fundamental that the clinicians who practice stimulation of uterine contractions become thoroughly familiar with the concepts that govern the response of the uterus to oxytocics, the physiology of these uterine contractions, and the pharmacologic action on the pregnant uterus at term. The benefits of proper stimulation of the uterus are too numerous and obvious to elaborate on. Suffice it to say that the physiologic concepts and good clinical judgment for correct management of cases are as indispensible in the training of an obstetrician as exposure to other fundamental aspects of obstetrics and gynecology.

Among the classical components of the complex phenomenon of labor—the passages, the passenger, and the powers—emphasis will be especially put on the importance of the physiology of the last because understanding of its proper function has been very late to come about,

whereas the first two are basically governed by mechanical and physical laws well understood and explained for a long time in classic obstetrics.

It was only after Alvarez and Caldeyro-Barcia described their method of continuous intrauterine pressure recording that meaningful observations were made of the changes produced by uterine contractions in late pregnancy. Among the important facts demonstrated by the observations carried out with intrauterine pressure recordings, the most pertinent are that 1) the uterus is never quiescent throughout pregnancy, 2) it is contracting constantly in an ever-accelerating manner, and 3) this acceleration process reaches its maximum during second stage. Thereafter, a deceleration begins as uterine activity regresses toward its slow pace during uterine involution in the puerperium (see Chapter 5).

The concept of *cervical readiness* is of paramount importance when contemplating an induction of labor. The assessment of the cervix should determine the probable duration of the process because, as it has been seen in Chapter 5, more than 75% to 80% of the total uterine contractions and time are spent in ripening the cervix when inductions are started with unripe cervices. Unless this fact is clearly understood, an induction of labor may be labeled a failure prematurely, and probably the patient will be submitted to an unnecessary or premature cesarean section.

To avoid unnecessary interference, the progress in cervical changes must be accurately assessed; these changes occur slowly and very gradually when induction starts with an unripe cervix. An assessment of the clinical condition and an estimation of total duration of induction should be made before action is undertaken. On the average, inductions with unripe cervices may require *more than 24 hours of good uterine contractions* before the cervix begins to ripen and is ready for first stage. If the contractions are not good, regular, and satisfactory, the time may be much longer. In other words, prelabor is by far the longest period in the process of parturition, and the duration of an induction depends on how much prelabor has already been accomplished when the clinician starts the stimulation of the uterus (see Figure 5-18).

Recapitulating, during active dilatation, the contractions tend to improve in coordination and become more regular in intensity and frequency as labor progresses (see Figures 5-19 and 5-27). The factors that influence the efficiency of the contractions to dilate the cervix are state of the membranes, variety of position of the head, and, of course, parity. The contractility pattern, as ascertained from the recorded intrauterine pressure changes, is not influenced by these factors. Familiarity with the effects of drugs on the uterus is mandatory before any attempt at stimulating the uterus is undertaken (see Chapter 9). Only mastery in handling drugs will facilitate a safe and smooth induction or stimulation of labor.

Induction of labor may be *elective,* when the obstetrician deliberately starts labor without a compelling reason to do so, or *therapeutic* (mandatory), when clinical condition, either maternal or fetal, indicates that the pregnancy should be terminated within a reasonably short time.

The importance of induction of labor in modern obstetrics is reflected in its high incidence in the statistics of maternity hospitals. However, it is still a controversial procedure because at some large institutions it is used so infrequently that it is considered forbidden. The list of surgical catastrophes ascribed to induction of labor is almost endless, but a careful review of most case reports reveals that they had occurred at the hands of incompetent, careless, or untrained individuals. Probably, as a consequence to those unfavorable reports, the list of contraindications to induction and/or enhancement of labor is very long, and the list of indications very short. The current (in 1980) furor against induction of labor and the national campaign to outlaw the use of oxytocin may well be based on the accidents that occurred because of inadequate training of those applying the procedure or insufficient supervision during its execution.

INDICATIONS

Induction of labor may be undertaken as an elective procedure, but in a vast number of clinical circumstances initiation of labor by the obstetrician constitutes the most important therapeutic step in solving a problem or preventing the appearance of other problems that may be life threatening to the mother or her infant. Only the more frequent indications are reviewed here.

Elective

Ideally, a patient to be induced electively should be near term, in good health, have an adequate pelvis, and have a *ripe cervix.* When these circumstances are present, the presenting part is usually well applied against the lower uterine segment and "dipping" into the pelvis. Foremost among the prerequisites, the patient must understand the steps and evolution of the procedure, and accept it without any afterthoughts. This group of patients should give the best results in any study or statistical evaluation because the absence of pathologic conditions indicates that this population is the one at lowest risk to go through the process of labor. When *elective induction* is properly conducted, it should very closely imitate the evolution of spontaneous labor.

Prolonged Pregnancy

A syndrome almost ignored in the United States until the last few years, *prolonged gestation (beyond the 42nd week of amenorrhea)* has been shown to be an important contributor of perinatal death in studies done in Britain and continental Europe. The British obstetricians should be given credit for calling attention to this problem when they demonstrated the sharply rising perinatal mortality after the end of the 41st week of gestation. In fact, this syndrome is the leading indication for induction of labor in the British Isles. Its importance should be emphasized in this country because the *postterm pregnancy* constitutes about 10% of all deliveries conducted in maternity hospitals.

Premature Rupture of Membranes

The high risk of intrauterine infection (amnionitis), along with the improvements in the technique of induction and conduction of labor, have contributed to make of this condition the leading indication for induction of labor at the Chicago Lying-In Hospital. The reasons for this approach are based on sound clinical studies: a high percentage of infants born after 24 hours of ruptured membranes have bacteremia. As high as 25% of those born 40 hours after the membranes were ruptured had positive blood cultures (Tyler and Albers, 1966), and definitely a higher percentage must have bacteriologic contamination of the amniotic fluid. The old policy of waiting 24 hours for spontaneous labor to start has been gradually changed; now, as soon as the diagnosis has been established and the infant estimated to be viable with good probability of survival (2000 gm or more), induction of labor is undertaken. It is critical to remember that the majority of these patients have an unripe cervix and therefore will require many hours of good contractility to bring about the necessary cervical changes before dilatation progresses rapidly.

Hypertensive Conditions

High blood pressure, from whatever cause, is a most serious complication of gestation and one that endangers equally the lives of the mother and her fetus. Anyone with hypertension is a potential candidate for therapeutic induction of labor. In fact, hypertension represents the second most frequent indication for induction at the Chicago Lying-In Hospital, and the leading one for when the membranes are intact. *Preeclamptic* patients who do not respond satisfactorily to conservative treatment of hospitalization, bed rest, and low-sodium diet should be seriously considered for induction of labor even when the state of the cervix is unfavorable. Other hypertensive conditions that precede pregnancy, and are often aggravated by it, are a serious threat to patient health and cause a high rate of perinatal mortality if the pregnancies are left to evolve on their own. Interference in the form of induction of labor, properly timed and conducted, may be the only safe way to obtain a live infant in these cases.

Diabetes

Among diabetic mothers, the high incidence of intrauterine fetal death occurring when the pregnancies are allowed to reach term has been one of the major concerns in the last few decades, when improvement in the treatment of young diabetics enabled more people to conceive and carry their pregnancies to term. In spite of good control, the incidence of perinatal mortality among diabetics has been about 10% to 12% until the last few years, in the best series. Intrauterine fetal death around, or before, term contributed about one-half of those cases. Until recently, induction of labor at 37 weeks gestation seemed to be the best management for class B or C diabetic mothers. However, more recently, refinements in the assessment of the fetal condition in utero (estrogen determination in maternal serum or urine; nonstress test, and/or contraction stress test of the fetal heart, phospholipids in amniotic fluid) make it possible to individualize the treatment of each case and to choose more accurately the date of delivery. It has been by these means that class A diabetics are now usually allowed to reach term before termination of pregnancy with excellent perinatal survival figures obtained in that group.

Intrauterine Growth Retardation

This syndrome, adequately recognized only in the last few years, was originally described by Gruenwald (1966) in a review of autopsy material when he observed the discrepancy between gestational age and somatic growth of the fetus. The accurate assessment of fetal size and growth, now possible with ultrasound measurements of the fetal head and trunk, has brought to the fore the so-called small-for-date fetus or growth-retarded infant. Close follow-up of pregnancy often determines the need to induce labor before term when signs of fetal deterioration are observed. As the awareness of the syndrome is disseminated, the diagnosis is made more often and the need to interfere increases in proportion—particularly in tertiary care centers where obstetrics pathologic conditions are concentrated.

Rh Isoimmunization

Rh isoimmunization is still an important cause of perinatal mortality, but the treatment has been significantly improved since Liley introduced his therapeutic approach of amniocentesis and intrauterine transfusion. Also, the prophylaxis with specific anti-D gamma globulin antibodies has sharply curtailed the number of cases. Early delivery is necessary when the baby is severely affected and as soon as viability is estimated to be satisfactory (that is after the 36th week of pregnancy). Induction of labor should surely be considered as an alternative mode of termination of pregnancy, even though many cases have an unfavorable (unripe) cervix.

Placental Insufficiency

The inability of the placenta to continue to *satisfy adequately* the needs of the growing fetus has been associated with some of the pathologic conditions just described. In other cases, there seems to be no explanation for a slow growing fundus or small-for-date fetus. Placental insufficiency seems to be present in a great number of the so-called high-risk pregnancies. With the variety of laboratory techniques now at our disposal to make the diagnosis of fetal maturity and fetal well-being in utero, it is possible to assess the possibilities of the infant for survival after delivery and, therefore, plan carefully an induction of labor and choose the best date for it.

Intrauterine Fetal Death

It is a matter of concern for the obstetrician when labor does not start soon after fetal death. Relatively often a tertiary referral center receives a patient whose infant died before spontaneous onset of labor. These patients are at risk of developing the slow defibrination syndrome a few weeks after the infant's death. Therefore, the best prophylaxis is induction of labor before it develops, in general a procedure without incident.

CONTRAINDICATIONS

There are few contraindications to induction of labor, and they must be strictly observed if one is to avoid serious problems. The first and most important contraindication is the refusal of the patient to accept it as a means to deliver the infant. A patient's conviction that the induction of labor is the best means at the time for termination of her pregnancy is so important that the procedure should never be undertaken without it.

The conviction must be genuine, without reservations, and not the result of a hard-sell push by the obstetrician or someone close to the patient.

From the obstetrics standpoint, *only contraindications to vaginal delivery are absolute contraindications to induction* of labor. It follows therefore that if grand multiparity, twin gestation, breech presentation, or a distended uterus are not contraindications to spontaneous labor and vaginal delivery, they should not be contraindications to careful induction of labor.

An unripe cervix, in an obstetric situation requiring a relatively rapid delivery of the infant, would constitute a contraindication at attempting induction of labor, if one remembers that the process of ripening of the cervix is long and protracted, needing more than 24 hours of good uterine contractions to be completed and then followed by first stage. Any attempt at induction of labor without considering this circumstance will therefore be misguided, a waste of time, and will only prove the lack of clinical judgment by the person who made the decision to go ahead with the induction.

The last absolute contraindication is the inability of the obstetrician, or someone with experience in conducting stimulated labors, to continuously supervise the evolution of the process.

REQUIREMENTS

A thorough understanding by the obstetrician of the pharmacologic effects of the many drugs to be used (oxytocics, sedatives, anesthetics) is mandatory. Induction of labor is an action planned and started by the obstetrician, in agreement with the patient, and therefore the obstetrician should be responsible throughout its evolution for every detail in the management of the process.

In the last few years, with the widespread marketing of equipment for monitoring uterine contractions and FHR, now available even at small hospitals in the country, continuous monitoring until successful completion should be considered indispensable to good practice.

This approach seems to be accepted by most obstetricians wherever monitoring equipment is available. Unfortunately, because the patient is being hooked to a recording machine, the assumption is often made that miraculously everything will go all right. The lack of understanding that a monitoring record should be constantly reviewed, supervised, and maintained free from artifacts is, in all probability, a very important contributing factor in creating obstetric catastrophes. This problem goes hand in hand with the improper or wrong interpretation of the recordings, if they are accurate and free from distortions. The marketing and widespread use of monitoring devices has not been accompanied by a massive training program for practicing obstetricians. The handouts and selected bibliography distributed by the manufacturers of the equipment have been aimed not at teaching the methods and difficulties in using their monitors, but at making the potential customers buy the hardware. This gap in the technical competence of the practicing obstetrician is certainly one of the important factors facilitating the occurrence of severe complications. If this deficiency is not promptly corrected, it will continue to be the cause of a number of completely preventable catastrophes.

METHODS

Induction of labor has been attempted since medical history has been recorded, and the techniques and methods, quite naturally, have been limited only by the boundaries of human imagination. In modern medicine there are just a few used with live infants in utero, and few additional reserved for the cases of intrauterine fetal demise.

Surgical

These methods are called surgical because they require the insertion of instruments or maneuvers with them into the uterine cavity.

Artificial rupture of membranes It has been said that "amniotomy is the most potent single means of inducing labor" (Theobald, 1963) after the observation that about 80% of patients at term will go into active labor within 24 hours after amniotomy. The remainder go into labor in decreasing proportion, and about 2% require several days before the onset of spontaneous contractions. This experience, gathered mostly in Great Britain, has been substantiated by the few studies that have been conducted in the United States.

This relatively high success rate will be obtained only when the strict conditions outlined to attempt the use of this method are followed. The cervix must be ripe or favorable, and the head well applied against the lower segment and dipping into the inlet. The membranes should be ruptured, allowing a slow flow of as much amniotic fluid as possible, and then the patient must remain in bed.

The mechanism of action whereby amniotomy stimulates labor is unknown. There have been several hypotheses postulated to explain this effect but none has demonstrated by what specific mechanism rupturing the membranes triggers contractions. The more ripe the cervix, the more likely that labor follows amniotomy; therefore, ripeness of the cervix is the single most important clinical factor for the prediction of success or failure in the induction of labor within a reasonable period of time.

The possibility, or almost certainty, of intrauterine bacterial contamination after the membranes have been ruptured should caution the clinician against the surgical technique for the induction of labor. The possibility of infection rules out amniotomy as the method of choice for induction of labor at the Chicago Lying-In Hospital. The prophylactic use of antibiotics after the membranes have been ruptured gives some obstetricians a sense of security, and they wait for the spontaneous onset of contractions. That "feeling" should not preclude the early stimulation of the uterus, perhaps even before amniotomy. As Theobald stated, he "would start oxytocin drip immediately after amniotomy" if he were to postulate a new method of induction.

The introduction of *extraovular* sounds, catheters, or semirigid stems (method of Krause) into the uterus is known to stimulate contractions and is still used by some, but should not be recommended in the practice of modern obstetrics. The insertion of small balloons for recording contractions may have the same stimulating effect on uterine contractility.

Medical

The stimulation of the contractions by means of pharmacologic agents given to the patient by any route (intravenous, intramuscular, subcutaneous, intranasal, oral, vaginal, rectal) with the objective of stimulating uterine contractions, constitutes the technique of medical induction of labor. There is an extraordinary number of substances with oxytocic properties, but only those used in modern obstetrics to induce labor will be discussed. The action of some of the others has been reviewed in Chapter 9.

Sparteine sulfate Sparteine sulfate has an unpredictable effect on the uterus, particularly in prelabor. In addition, its long-lasting effect, seen to occur even where no immediate uterine response could be observed, predisposes the patient to abnormal uterine activity in advanced first stage. Incoordination, hypertonus, polysystoly, and tumultuous labor have been observed to develop after the intramuscular administration of 150 mg, the standard recommended dose. Of course, this type of uterine response leads to fetal distress, in addition to the high incidence of cervical lacerations reported in some series where this drug was exclusively used. For these reasons, sparteine sulfate is no longer used at the Chicago Lying-In Hospital, and it probably should never be used in obstetrics when the fetus is viable.

Prostaglandins As discussed in Chapter 9, PGE_2 and $PGF_2\alpha$ are the two prostaglandins used in clinical obstetrics to induce labor at term. Karim, Embrey, and Anderson have the most extensive experience with PGs, and they think that the effects of the PGs are comparable to those of oxytocin. However, numerous other authors have tried both PGs by the intravenous, oral, and intravaginal routes and reported a variety of side effects, particularly nausea, vomiting, diarrhea, and hyperthermia, as well as unpredictable episodes of hypertonus occurring under the strictest control in the administration of the drug. It seems, then, that PGE_2 and $PGF_2\alpha$ are not the ideal oxytocics to stimulate labor in late gestation with a live fetus. Prostaglandin $F_2\alpha$, given by the *intraamniotic* route to initiate labor in a patient carrying a dead fetus, is most effective. Labor starts promptly and, because excessive contractility does not concern the obstetrician (unless having to stimulate a scarred uterus), progress is the rule in bringing about rapid expulsion of a stillborn fetus. Probably PGE_2 by the intravaginal route should have the same satisfactory effect.

Oxytocin The use of oxytocin as the drug of choice for stimulation of the uterus in advanced gestation has been well established after Caldeyro-Barcia and co-workers published in 1957 their classic work on the progressive response of the pregnant human uterus to increasing doses of oxytocin. The detailed studies on the pharmacology of oxytocin have been reviewed in Chapter 9. Oxytocin could be administered by several routes, but the only one over which the clinician may have total control is intravenous. *The intravenous use of very dilute oxytocin solutions is the safest way to physiologically stimulate a pregnant uterus.* Rarely the intranasal way could be the route of choice for minimal requirements, because of relatively uncertain absorption and particularly a very bothersome nasal congestion. The intramuscular route should be considered obsolete in modern obstetrics because of the large dose injected and the uncertain rate of absorption.

Ideally, an infusion of oxytocin should be given by a continuous infusion pump, but if one is not available, the drip method would be acceptable provided continuous observation is assured. A small intravenous catheter should be inserted in a brachial vein and used only for the purpose of infusing oxytocin. Before the administration of the hormone, the catheter should be kept open with an infusion of standard intravenous fluids. Once the infusion is started, it should be given at a rate of no more than 1 to 2 mU/min (2 to 4 drops of a solution from one ampule of oxytocin in 1000 ml) with the clinician in constant attendance to observe the uterine contractions and evaluate the fetal heart tones — relatively easily done when a continuous monitoring device has been applied and contractions and fetal heart tones are being recorded. If monitoring equipment is not available, the hand of an experienced obstetrician and a fetoscope should substitute. A uterus close to term, or at term, will probably start responding to the infusion rate of 1 mU/min within 10 min, and the response will increase steadily until it reaches a plateau between 50 and 60 min later. If at this time and activity of the uterus is not yet satisfactory (that is, the contractions are not strong enough or frequent enough), the infusion rate should be doubled to 2 mU/min. Again, observation should be close, as a safeguard against undesirable excessive effects, which occur much more often with the drip method because of the difficulties in calibrating the droppers. As with the lower rate, after at least 45 to 50 min has elapsed, it is necessary to assess the uterine contractility and increase the infusion rate if the activity is not yet satisfactory by again doubling the infusion rate to 4 or 5 mU/min. This step of doubling the infusion rate at preestablished times should always be observed when uterine activity does not reach a satisfactory level, keeping in

230

mind that the lower the infusion rate, the longer it takes to reach a level of steady activity. Most pregnancies close to term respond well to 2 to 4 mU/min; some necessitate 10 mU/min; and very rarely will any pregnancy at term require 20 mU/min to develop a satisfactory uterine activity. These infusion rates apply to *term or close-to-term pregnancies only*. Not infrequently, at 32 or 33 weeks gestation, a patient necessitates 20, 30, or even 40 mU/min to have a labor-like contractility pattern (see Chapter 9).

Another fundamental concept in induction of labor is related to physiologic variations in uterine response to oxytocin infusion. The aim of inducing labor is to obtain good, steady uterine contractions. One should not judge by the number of hours a given patient has been "pitted" or the number of "bottles" she received. If she does not have good, relatively frequent contractions, there should be little expectation that she will make any significant progress toward delivery. Under normal conditions, only good contractions help to achieve cervical dilatation.

Frequently, when an induced labor is progressing satisfactorily under a steady oxytocin infusion rate, it may become necessary to decrease the infusion progressively, also by halves, and even discontinue it altogether because the feedback mechanism for spontaneous labor is working at its maximum and is sufficient to maintain a good labor pattern (Figure 10-1). In other circumstances, after discontinuing the oxytocin infu-

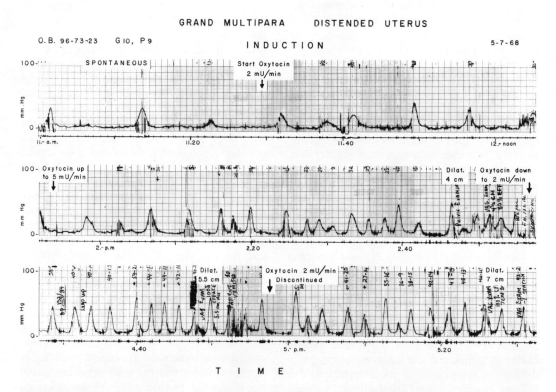

Figure 10-1 Partial records of three different stages in the evolution of an induction of labor in a grand multipara (premature rupture of membranes). *(Above)* Low spontaneous activity and beginning of an oxytocin infusion at 2 mU/min (arrow), with minimal increasing response. Still only moderate contractility obtained after 2½ hours at 2 mU/min. *(Center)* Progressively increasing response to 5 mU/min. When the frequency seemed too high, the infusion rate was decreased to 2 mU/min. *(Below)* Contractility 2 hours later, still on 2 mU/min oxytocin. When the frequency of contractions was considered high, the oxytocin was discontinued (arrow), and labor continued with a normal pattern until completion (the infant weighed 4240 gm). This case underscores the importance of continuous recording to assess the slow, progressive effects of oxytocin and how it can be used effectively to maintain a safe and satisfactory contractility pattern. Reprinted from Cibils LA: Enhancement and induction of labor, in Aladjem S (ed): *Risks in the Practice of Modern Obstetrics II.* St. Louis, Mosby, 1975, pp 182–210.

sion, it may be necessary to restart it, but at lower rates because the sensitivity is already increased (Figure 10-2).

The excessive use of oxytocin will produce polysystoly and hypertonic conditions that will endanger not only fetal life but also the maternal life if rupture of the uterus occurs.

The evolution of a well-conducted induction should not be different from a normal, spontaneous labor. The same factors of adequate feto–pelvic proportion, state of membranes, and position of the fetal head are of paramount importance in determining the efficiency of the contractions to dilate the cervix, and therefore the

rate of progress of first stage. Frequently forgotten is that *induction of labor is not a contest against time*. What is important is how well the obstetrician may conduct it and how good his judgment is.

As already stressed when discussing physiology, the prognosis of an induction depends on the obstetric conditions of the case. A thorough evaluation of the cervix is a prerequisite for predicting the total evolution of induced labor.

The stage of dilatation (first stage) evolves in the same, smooth manner as it does in spontaneous labor, being influenced by the same factors: state of the membranes, variety of position

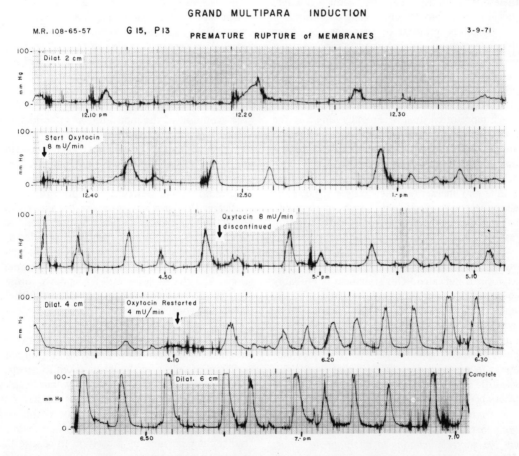

Figure 10-2 Three different stages of the contractility pattern of the labor induced in a grand multipara for premature rupture of membranes, at 36 weeks gestation. *(A, B)* Continuous recording of the spontaneous contractility and the slow response to 8 mU/min oxytocin infusion. *(C)* After 4 hours of good activity oxytocin was discontinued and contractility diminished rapidly. *(D, E)* Response to a restarted oxytocin infusion at 4 mU/min 1 hour later. The rapid response, stabilized about 40 min after the onset of infusion, produced strong contractions with smoothly progressing cervical dilatation and the eventual delivery of a 2425 gm infant in good condition. Reprinted from Cibils LA: Enhancement and induction of labor, in Aladjem S (ed): *Risks in the Practice of Modern Obstetrics II.* St. Louis, Mosby, 1975, pp 182–210.

of the presenting part, parity, and position of the patient. The total amount of *uterine work* required to accomplish the *stage of dilatation* during induction is higher than in spontaneous labor for all variables considered (see Tables 5-2, 5-3, 5-4, and 5-5). The uterine work required to complete prelabor is roughly similar in spontaneous as well as induced labors.

The manner in which the uterine work of prelabor is completed is not important: it may be done in one long uninterrupted session, or it may be accomplished in daily sessions of several hours each. The uninterrupted session is a practical possibility because the contractions of prelabor are painless even when they are strong, and therefore the patient may sleep with a minimal sedation as the process of ripening continues.

When the progress of first stage is slower than expected, in spite of good uterine contractions, a clinical reevaluation should be carried out, entailing an assessment of the pelvis and precise diagnosis of the presenting part: height, position, variety of position, flexion, synclitism. Much more often than is generally taught in the textbooks, minor abnormalities of these factors are responsible for slow progress of labor (dilatation and/or descent) and create borderline fetopelvic disproportions. Correction of some of these factors may markedly hasten progress; however, when there is no significant change, there should be no hesitation in deciding on a cesarean section (as would be done with a spontaneous labor).

Indications In all conditions in which induction of labor is recommended, intravenous oxytocin is indicated. This statement is probably controversial, particularly in the United States, where the textbooks carry longer lists of contraindications than indications for the use of intravenous oxytocin. Nevertheless, the study of the pharmacologic response of the term pregnant uterus to oxytocin demonstrates that there is no scientific evidence to withhold its proper use in cases where spontaneous labor would be permitted.

Contraindications *The only contraindications to the proper use of intravenous oxytocin are the contraindications to spontaneous labor.* This is also likely to be a controversial statement if one judges the teaching in current textbooks, some of which list "commandments for the use of oxytocin," and long lists of contraindications. However, the paradoxical position is evident on perusal of chapters dealing with the listed contraindications: implicitly spontaneous labor and

vaginal delivery are permitted in cases of grand multiparity, twins, breech presentation, distended uteri, or primiparas with fetal floating head. No satisfactory reasons are given to deny the patients with these conditions the potential benefit of a carefully controlled uterine stimulation with intravenous oxytocin.

FAILURES

As Hendricks has said, "Strictly speaking, there is no such thing as a failed induction." This axiom represents the analysis of a physiologist with regard to our ability to trigger good uterine contractions or to induce changes in the lower segment and cervical canal. However, because the aim of the clinician is to attempt to obtain a vaginal delivery, his inability to accomplish it, and the need to resort to a cesarean section, define a failure of induction of labor. This decision may be the consequence of either fetal or maternal indications and may present itself at any time during the evolution of the induction, as often happens during spontaneous labor.

The arrest of progress for a reasonable period of time, in spite of good uterine contractions (defining progress as advance of effacement, dilatation and/or descent of the presenting part) indicates the need to reevaluate the mechanical conditions involved in labor. There could be several reasons for a less than satisfactory progress, the more common being minor fetal malpositions, borderline cephalopelvic disproportions, and the negative effect of poorly formed bag of water ("flat membranes syndrome"). There is general consensus that the membranes should be ruptured for some time before speaking of "failure to progress." If the diagnosis of mechanical difficulties is made, after thorough evaluation, measures should be taken to proceed with a cesarean section, as ordinarily done in cases of poorly progressing spontaneous labors. The only thing at stake is the well-being of mother and infant; the obstetrician's honor may be enhanced rather than smeared by a decision to change the original plan of action.

An exceedingly large number of so-called failed inductions are diagnosed *before the period of prelabor has been completed,* that is before advanced effacement or dilatation of less than 3 cm. Often the real cause can be traced to an improper or inadequate evaluation of cervical readiness and thus inaccurate projection of the events to follow. Because an unripe cervix does not dilate in a few hours as expected, due to a faulty evaluation, it will be diagnosed as "lack of progress" and failed induction.

Another rather common "etiology" of failed inductions is unrecognized *insufficient stimulation of the uterus.* Total time of oxytocin infusion (or "pitting") is not the same as total time of adequate uterine stimulation, which should be evaluated accurately by the quality of contractions recurring with physiologic frequency (about 150 Montevideo Units, or 1000 mm Hg uterine work per hour). The uterus may be, and often is, understimulated for many hours, with little progress to show for all the time elapsed, because of inadequacy of the contractions. (Of course, progress will be lacking when good contractions are required to develop the lower segment and efface the cervix, but they are not obtained.)

A third factor often responsible for the diagnosis of failed induction, in prelabor, is the very popular concept that the *induction must "take"* in a few "sessions" of oxytocin infusion. Most likely, in these cases, there is inadequate assessment of cervical readiness usually superimposed on insufficient stimulation. Probably there is no such thing as true failure to induce progress in prelabor by proper oxytocin stimulation. Even in cases of moderate cephalopelvic disproportion there is progress made because engagement is not necessary for the progress of cervical ripening; only good application against the lower segment and/or cervix is required.

Particularly in therapeutic inductions started with unengaged presenting parts, one often may observe the slow progress of dilatation and total stagnation of descent. A complete evaluation of physiologic and mechanical conditions will likely reveal that the presenting part does not apply against the cervix because of *faulty position of the patient.* For not very clear reasons, the complete lateral position of the laboring patient is generally advised, and with an unengaged presenting part this has the same effect as that of a moderate Trendelenburg position; in other words, the fetus "hangs away" from the inlet instead of tending to engage into it. Correction of the patient's lie to a semi-Fowler's position usually produces amazing results. The *semi-Fowler's position is ideal* for a patient in labor with an unengaged presenting part, regardless of the state of the membranes.

Exceptionally, one may face a true failure to trigger contractions by what seems to be and feels like a term pregnant uterus. A systematic review of all possible causes of error may be negative, but the uterus would not respond to the physiologic rates of oxytocin for the estimated stage of gestation. This is the time to suspect the unusual, the extraordinary. With intrauterine catheters, the author has observed two full-term gestations requiring 50 mU/min oxytocin to respond with good labor-like contractions. The tubal gestation with intraamniotic catheter (Figure 10-3) is one of those extraordinary cases and the other was a tubo-ovarian abdominal gestation attached to the fundus observed with an external tokometer applied below the umbilicus which recorded contractions of the unoccupied uterus in advanced premature labor (author's observation). These anecdotal cases emphasize that a documented term pregnant uterus responds to physiologic infusions of oxytocin (1 to 20 mU/min), and that when it does not do so the clinician must look for an explanation rather than call it failure to respond to oxytocin.

ENHANCEMENT OF LABOR

Stimulating a labor that started spontaneously but does not progress satisfactorily due to poor or ineffective contractions is called enhancement of labor.

Indications

Many conditions lead to slow progress of labor. When uterine contractility is implicated two of the most common are hypotonic and hypertonic inertia, either primary or secondary. These two syndromes are generally assumed to be the result of cephalopelvic disproportion, fetal malposition, transverse or posterior positions, distension of the uterus, twinning, "exhaustion" of the uterus, and drug-induced hypocontractility.

Primary hypotonic inertia is generally accepted as an indication for enhancement of labor, provided there are no unrelated conditions to contraindicate uterine stimulation. Usually, it appears as a labor in which contractions of low intensity and frequency are barely perceived by the patient.

Hypertonic inertia is considered in the current textbooks an absolute contraindication to the

234

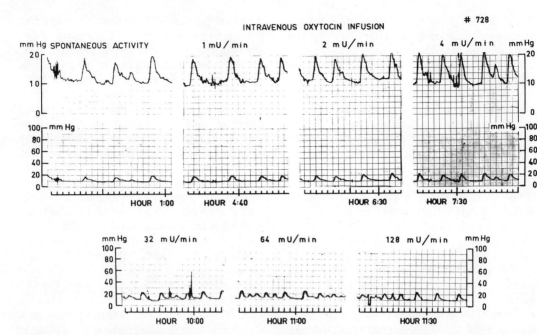

Figure 10-3 Intraovular pressure of patient carrying a dead fetus at 42 weeks. The upper part shows pressure changes recorded with two sensitivity ranges: above 0 to 20 mm Hg and below the standard 0 to 100 mm Hg on paper running at a slow speed (marks indicate minutes). Segments of spontaneous contractility and responses to increasing infusion rates of oxytocin. *(Below)* Tracings obtained with the standard sensitivity range, and segments of contractility during oxytocin infusion at supraphysiologic rates. Complete inability of the organ to increase intensity of contractions while frequency was increasing regularly. Due to failure to obtain a response, this patient was sectioned after a clinical diagnosis of ectopic gestation. An intact tubal pregnancy with a term size, moderately macerated fetus was found. The adnexa was easily removed. Record obtained by H. Alvarez, R. Caldeyro-Barcia, S.V. Pose, J.J. Poseiro, Y. Sica-Blanco, L.A. Cibils, and C. Mendez-Bauer. Courtesy R. Caldeyro-Barcia.

use of oxytocic substances. However, an intrauterine recording of a case diagnosed clinically reveals that in fact these cases are the most typical expressions of incoordinated uterine contractility (see Chapter 5) evolving with an increased resting pressure due to uneven relaxation. Patients are usually restless, in state of continuous discomfort, they have a hard uterus by palpation, and dilatation does not progress in spite of this seemingly effective (because it is painful) labor. Caldeyro-Barcia has shown the very satisfactory response of this syndrome to oxytocin, but the traditional teaching still prevails: "resting the uterus" with sedatives is supposed to be the treatment of choice. This general point of view notwithstanding, hypertonic inertia is an excellent indication to enhance labor either mechanically or pharmacologically.

So-called *"secondary inertia"* occurs under varied clinical circumstances. If obstructed labor

or cephalopelvic disproportion is not present, these cases are almost ideal for pharmacologic enhancement of labor.

Contraindications

As for induction of labor, only contraindications to vaginal delivery should preclude enhancement of labor. This is stated in spite of the number of contraindications listed in the textbooks, generally the same as those prohibiting induction of labor.

Methods

Artificial rupture of membranes A time-honored means to improve labor is to rupture the membranes artificially, following which the uterine contractions increase a great deal in their efficiency as dilating forces. This change takes place without appreciable alteration in the contractility pattern when the pattern is normal. However, when the pattern is abnormal, it may change but usually not immediately. Nevertheless, the improved efficiency of the contractions is the most relevant effect of the maneuver. If, in spite of the amniotomy, proper patient positioning, and good application of the presenting part against the lower segment, there is no satisfactory improvement of pattern, active uterine stimulation with oxytocics should be contemplated.

Oxytocin infusion Intravenous infusion of physiologic amounts of oxytocin to enhance abnormal labor exerts the same effect as when it is used to induce labor in term gestation: it will progressively increase the uterine contractility. However, the response will be conditioned by the preexisting pattern of contractions and uterine activity. The sensitivity of the uterus to oxytocin is more uniform among the labors to be enhanced, as a group compared to those to be induced. This uniformity is in the low rate range. The need for infusion rates above 2 to 5 mU/min is unlikely, and therefore great care should be exercised in the delivery of very diluted amounts of oxytocin if undesirable excessive contractility is to be prevented. The response of the uterus is similar to that described for induction: prelabor like pattern of contractions increasing slowly in frequency and/or intensity and reaching maximum response in about 50 to 60 min (Figure 10-4). When a satisfactory response has been obtained, the evolution of that labor should be similar to the progress of a normal spontaneous labor, but it might require slightly more uterine work to complete dilatation (see Tables 5-4 and 5-5). When the contractions are good and strong, but of low frequency, this parameter will be the more clearly stimulated as the response to oxytocin takes effect (Figure 10-5).

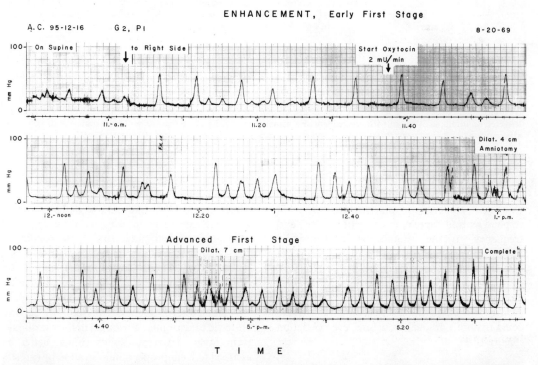

Figure 10-4 Partial recordings of *labor enhancement* in a secundipara at term. *(Above and center)* Continuous recordings illustrate the spontaneous contractility with good contractions but low frequency, and the progressive response to 2 mU/min oxytocin (arrow). *(Below)* Then, 3½ hours later, the contractility pattern of advanced first stage—increased frequency but still moderately irregular as dilatation approaches completion. Labor was enhanced with 2 mU/min oxytocin throughout until delivery of a 3075 gm infant. Reprinted from Cibils LA: Enhancement and induction of labor, in Aladjem S (ed): *Risks in the Practice of Modern Obstetrics II.* St. Louis, Mosby, 1975, pp 182–210.

236

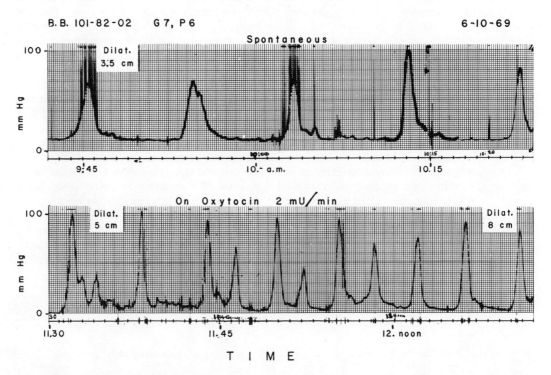

Figure 10-5 Partial tracings of labor enhancement in a grand multipara at term. *(Above)* Spontaneous contractions of 60 mm Hg and stronger, recurring every 8 to 10 min. *(Below)* Uterine contractility after 1 hour of oxytocin infusion at 2 mU/min: the same strong contractions but recurring every 2 to 3 minutes with still some normal irregularities in intensity and frequency. Dilatation completed 20 min after the end of this record and the patient delivered an infant of 3075 gm without incident. Reprinted from Cibils LA: Enhancement and induction of labor, in Aladjem S (ed): *Risks in the Practice of Modern Obstetrics II.* St. Louis, Mosby, 1975, pp 182–210.

As occurs with the other syndromes of inadequate contractility, *hypertonic uterine inertia* will respond with an improved pattern of intensity and frequency to the stimulation triggered by physiologic amounts of oxytocin (Figure 10-6). As is the case with inductions of labor, the evolution of these labors should be facilitated by amniotomy and it may be expected that with the progress of dilatation, the infusion rate of oxytocin could require a gradual reduction, even cessation (Figure 10-1).

RISKS WITH THE USE OF OXYTOCIN

As with any potent medication, there are predictable, particularly dangerous, conditions

produced by the administration of oxytocin, which should all be preventable if the physician has some experience in using the drug and exercises good clinical judgment. These conditions can be diagnosed only if the obstetrician has observed his patient continuously, and if he has a good, clean, artifact-free tracing of uterine contractions.

The obstetric literature periodically reports obstetric catastrophes attributed to the use of oxytocin, when the responsibility should better be ascribed to its improper administration by careless or negligent physicians. The two most common obstetric complications due to excessive oxytocin stimulation are 1) intrauterine fetal death or fetal distress due to prolonged hypercontractility and 2) rupture of the uterus because of overstimulation. Scrutiny of a bad accident attributed to oxytocin

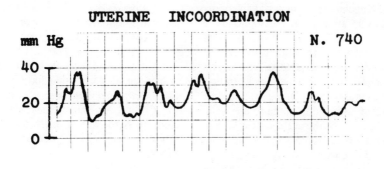

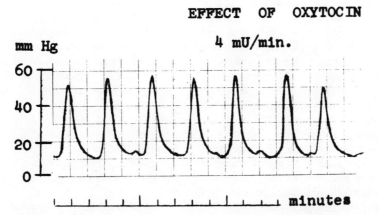

Figure 10-6 Two segments of intrauterine pressure tracings from a patient in spontaneous, protracted labor. *(Above)* A characteristic incoordinated pattern of contractions with hypertonus seen in *hypertonic inertia. (Below)* Stabilized activity and excellent contractility pattern obtained with 4 mU/min oxytocin infusion. Reprinted from Caldeyro-Barcia (1958).

will invariably reveal its misuse or inadequate supervision. The incidence of obstetric accidents, when intravenous oxytocin is properly used, should not be greater than for spontaneous labors. In fact, such accidents should be less frequent because a competent physician should always be in attendance for induced or enhanced labor, whereas a spontaneous labor often has an unsupervised evolution. (A more detailed discussion may be found in Chapter 9.)

The use of oxytocin, being such a powerful hormone, should be understood as well as any other potent medication. If this care is taken, and its use is properly supervised, catastrophes should not occur. Obstetricians who have had no good experience or exposure in the use of this drug and use it carelessly will be directly responsible for some serious and undesirable complications. In such cases, the drug should not be blamed for the

misadventures; the responsibility should be laid down where it belongs—with the obstetrician.

In the past 12 years the method described here has been followed in the majority of the over 6000 cases of induction or enhancement of labor at the Chicago Lying-In Hospital. As stated, the contraindications to vaginal delivery hold as contraindications to enhancement or induction of labor; cases of multiple gestation (twins, triplets), breech position, elderly or young primiparas, hypertonic inertia, secondary arrest, chronic hypertension, eclampsia and severe preeclampsia, grand multiparas, etc, have received oxytocin stimulation at various stages of labor.

The only maternal accident occurred in 1971, when the oxytocin tube was inadvertently opened by the anesthesiologist in the delivery room; consequently a large dose passed, and instant hypercontractility followed. Because the patient was fully dilated, immediate spontaneous delivery occurred, but at exploration a tear was found in the lower uterine segment. This case points out two serious breaks of the rules that should govern the safe use of oxytocin: 1) the oxytocin was "piggy-backed" through the same vein used for hydration and other medications; and 2) use of the drip method instead of an infusion pump to inject the medication. The trap for the accident was set up: when there was need for rapid administration of intravenous fluid to correct the hypotension triggered by the spinal anesthesia, the tube supplying the dextrose in water was opened to run fast, and excessive amounts of oxytocin were infused. Having a separate vein for the oxytocin and, still better, an infusion pump for the injection, should be double insurance against such an accident.

Other less severe episodes of hypercontractility have occurred, all of them due to failure to rigorously follow the recommendations described here. Some of them have served to illustrate in the respective chapters the possible consequences of such breaks in technique. Oxytocin is a safe medication indicated to stimulate the uterus whenever vaginal delivery is advisable as long as the appropriate steps are followed, based on an understanding of the pharmacologic effect of this drug.

BIBLIOGRAPHY

Alvarez H, Caldeyro-Barcia R: Fisiopatologia de la contraccion uterina y sus aplicaciones en la clinica obstetrica. *II Lat-Am Cong Obstet Gynecol* 1:5, 1954.

Alvarez H, Cibils LA, Gonzalez-Panizza VH: Cervical dilatation and uterine "work" in labor induced by oxytocin infusion, in Caldeyro-Barcia R, Heller H (eds): *Oxytocin.* NY, Pergamon, 1961, pp 203–211.

Anderson G, Hobbins J, Cordero L, et al: Clinical use of prostaglandins as oxytocic substances. *Ann NY Acad Sci* 180:499, 1971.

Caldeyro-Barcia R: Uterine contractility in obstetrics. *II Int Cong Gynecol Obstet* 1:65, 1958.

Caldeyro-Barcia R, Heller H (eds): *Oxytocin.* NY, Pergamon, 1961.

Caldeyro-Barcia R, Sereno JA: The response of the human uterus to oxytocin throughout pregnancy, in Caldeyro-Barcia R, Heller H (eds): *Oxytocin.* NY, Pergamon, 1961, pp 177–202.

Caldeyro-Barcia R, Sica-Blanco Y, Poseiro JJ, et al: A quantitative study of the action of synthetic oxytocin on the pregnant human uterus. *J Pharmacol Exp Ther* 121:18, 1957.

Cibils LA: Efecto de la rotura de las membranas en el parto inducido con ocitocina. *II Cong Uruguayo Ginecotocol* 2:346, 1957.

Cibils LA: Enhancement and induction of labor, in Aladjem S (ed): *Risks in the Practice of Modern Obstetrics II.* St. Louis, Mosby, 1975, pp 182–210.

Cibils LA, Caldeyro-Barcia R: Efectos de la ocitocina sobre el tono uterino. *Res Reun Lat Am Cien Fisiol* (Punta del Este), p 53, 1957.

Cibils LA, Caldeyro-Barcia R, Carballo MA, et al: Uterine work during labor. *Proc XXI Internat Cong Physiol* (Buenos Aires) 1959, p 65.

Cibils LA, Hendricks CH: Normal labor in vertex presentation. *Am J Obstet Gynecol* 89:1049, 1964.

Dilts PV, Greene RR: Effects of increasing parity on the myometrium. *Am J Obstet Gynecol* 89:1049, 1964.

Friedman EA, Sachtleben MR: Amniotomy and the course of labor. *Obstet Gynecol* 22:755, 1963.

Gruenwald P: Growth of the human fetus. II. Abnormal growth in twins, and infants of mothers with diabetes, hypertension, or isoimmunization. *Am J Obstet Gynecol* 94:1120, 1966.

Karim SM, Trussell RR, Patel RC, et al: Response of pregnant human uterus to prostaglandin $F_2\alpha$-induction of labour. *Br Med J* 4:621, 1968.

Lipton B, Hershey SG, Baez S: Compatibility of oxytocics with anesthetic agents. *JAMA* 179:410, 1962.

Poseiro JJ, Noriega-Guerra L: Dose-response relationships in uterine effects of oxytocin infusions, in Caldeyro-Barcia R, Heller H (eds): *Oxytocin.* NY, Pergamon, 1961, pp 158–176.

Reycraft JL: Induction of labor. *Am J Obstet Gynecol* 61:801, 1951.

Sica-Blanco Y, Sala NL: Uterine contractility at the beginning and end of oxytocin infusion, in Caldeyro-Barcia R, Heller H (eds): *Oxytocin.* NY, 1961, Pergamon, pp 127–136.

Tennet RA, Black MD: Surgical induction of labor in modern obstetric practice. *Br Med J* 2:833, 1954.

Theobald GW: Induction of labor and of premature labor, in Claye E (ed): *British Obstetric Practice*. London, Heinemann, 1963, pp 1055–1088.

Theobald GW: Oxytocin reassessed. *Obstet Gynecol Surv* 23:109, 1968.

Theobald GW, Graham A, Campbell J, et al: The use of post-pituitary extract in physiological amounts in obstetrics. *Br Med J* 123, 1948.

Tyler CW, Albers WH: Obstetric factors related to bacteremia in the newborn infant. *Am J Obstet Gynecol* 94:970, 1966.

CHAPTER 11
Premature Labor

Premature labor evolves when, in a pregnant patient, the process of labor, ending in delivery, starts between the 20th and the 36th week of amenorrhea. It may occur with a fetus before it is capable of survival (premature labor with nonviable fetus), or with a product of conception in a sufficient state of development to enable it to survive under favorable circumstances (premature labor with viable fetus). The latter occurs in general after about 28 weeks of gestation and only exceptionally before that. The viability of premature fetuses at earlier gestational ages is the result of admirable improvements made in the last decade in the care of these infants. The general incidence of premature deliveries in the United States is on the order of 10%, with higher incidences in subgroups of the population reaching as much as 20%. These figures refer to gestational age (before the 37th week), and no longer to fetal weight (less than 2500 gm). With better understanding of the many factors controlling fetal growth and more refined physical neurologic examination of the newborn, the old classification based on fetal weight has become obsolete in the centers caring for patients at high risk for premature delivery. Among these patients it is frequent to observe fetuses of chronologic age about term but underweight (intrauterine growth retardation), as well as fetuses chronologically premature but weighing above the arbitrary 2500 gm limit. Thus one must attempt to define with precision the chronologic age of a given pregnancy resorting, if necessary, to all available means of evaluation.

Premature delivery is the cause of a disproportionately high number of *neonatal deaths* in the United States in spite of the relatively low (10%) incidence of total births. The toll is particularly high among the infants born at 32 weeks of gestation or less. Furthermore, the number and incidence of the *physically and men-*

tally handicapped among the survivors is of staggering proportions, creating a most serious social and economic problem for the community. Premature delivery is, therefore, one of the most critical conditions in modern obstetrics, the reduction of its incidence being one of the major objectives of current epidemiologic and clinical investigations. The causes of premature delivery, the outcome of premature labor, are varied, from socioeconomic and nutritional predisposing conditions, to systemic diseases, iatrogenic factors, or "essential" causes. The common element among all of them is the *initiation of labor-like contractions* with progressive changes in the cervix and lower segment characteristic of term labor.

Preventive measures applied during prenatal care often succeed in reducing the incidence of premature deliveries. Among the *socioeconomic factors* implicated in epidemiologic studies have been poor nutrition and poor general hygiene, young age, unmarried status, pharmacodependency of habit-forming drugs, tobacco smoking, and race.

Systemic disease, such as chronic renal disease, hypertension, preeclampsia, heart disease, anemias, diabetes mellitus, generalized acute infections (viral or bacterial), pyelonephritis, have all been associated with the premature initiation of labor.

Mechanical factors, such as uterine malformations, abnormal distension of the uterus from multiple gestation or polyhydramnios, uterine tumors, incompetent cervical os, are invariably found among the conditions present in large series of premature labors. A relatively small proportion of miscellaneous conditions also trigger premature labor: abruptio placentae, placenta previa.

All these factors have been associated with premature labor in approximately 25% of the cases, but it is possible to reduce their effect by early prenatal care and close follow-up. However, a large proportion (about 50%) of premature labors are triggered by no apparent cause, often associated only with a history of previous premature labors. Both groups should be amenable to pharmacologic treatment to arrest labor when there are no medical contraindications. Nevertheless, some theoretically good candidates cannot have their labor arrested because it may be already too advanced. However, between 20% and 30% of premature labors are triggered by premature rupture of the membranes, a well-known uterine stimulating factor. Therefore, a realistic estimation would be to consider that about one-half of all preterm deliveries are the result of premature uterine contractions triggered by unknown causes or factors which, if controlled, would allow the pregnancy to continue without undue risk for mother or fetus. Currently there are few means at the disposal of the obstetrician to attempt to reverse the effect of these labor-triggering factors. The possibilities of success are better if the selection of patients fulfills some essential requirements.

INDICATIONS FOR ARRESTING LABOR

When selecting the patients to be treated for premature labor it is important to remember that, by convention, this definition applies only to those cases which *chronologically occur before the 37th week of amenorrhea.* Fetal weight is not a consideration, although, of course in the majority of cases, there is a general correlation between fetal weight and age of gestation.

The first requisite in considering the need to arrest a premature labor is to ascertain that the patient is having labor-like contractions—those recurring with certain regularity (every 3 to 8 min, abnormal for the stage of gestation) and with an intensity equivalent to that observed in early labor. This determination may be accomplished by 1) estimating it by abdominal palpation, 2) external recording and abdominal palpatation (to assess the true intensity), or 3) a transabdominal intrauterine catheter recording the actual intensity of the contractions.

In addition, *the cervical changes must not be so advanced* as to make all attempts futile.

Experience has demonstrated that when the dilatation is over 4 cm the likelihood of success is remote. Likewise, when effacement is too advanced (complete in nulliparas, over 70% in multiparas) the contractions tend to return even after having been successfully stopped for some time. The cervix must be effaced less than 70% in multiparas, may be complete but not too thin in nulliparas, and dilated 4 cm or less.

Usually in premature labor the presenting part is not deeply engaged. Most important, the *membranes must be intact*—a requirement critical for two reasons: 1) The chances of successfully arresting a premature labor with ruptured membranes are extremely limited because, as a matter of observation, labor starts and progresses rapidly after spontaneous or artificial amniotomy; and 2) in addition, there is a significant risk of chorioamnionitis after the inevitable contamination following the break of the barrier at the internal os. (This last point may be controverted because in some limited series a few cases have been carried successfully after documented premature labor.) However, the likelihood of an infection is always great, and at least passive noninterference should be advisable.

Of course, the labor process must be triggered by factors known to produce and sustain uterine contractions, and the progressive changes in the cervix and lower segment must mimic those observed in term spontaneous or induced labors. Operative procedures directly on the uterus such as insertion of a cervical cerclage or myometry can stimulate labor in a similar manner as other operations that produce peritoneal irritation.

A most important prerequisite when attempting to arrest a premature labor is the *patient's willingness* to undergo the necessary treatments, and her understanding of what is involved from the moment the physician intervenes until she is delivered, prematurely or at term.

CONTRAINDICATIONS

The contraindications to attempt the arrest of a premature labor are dictated, by and large, by pathologic conditions affecting the mother. However, in a few circumstances it may be to the advantage of the fetus that the physician abstain from intervention and let the premature delivery occur.

Hypertension

In severe *preeclampsia and eclampsia,* the undelivered products of conception are the cause of the syndrome; effective, definitive treatment can be carried out only after delivery. Likewise, when there are *acute episodes of hypertension* unaccompanied by the other signs or symptoms of preeclampsia, premature labor should be allowed to continue until completion; the presence of the fetus in the uterus constitutes a hindrance to adequate management of the excessive blood pressure. In chronic *severe renal disease and hypertension,* the management of the high blood pressure is facilitated by termination of the pregnancy. Evacuation of the fetus removes an important contributing factor to the severity of the hypertension.

Bleeding Syndromes

Hypercontractility produced by the retroplacental clots, in either concealed or bleeding *abruptio placentae,* should not be arrested because relaxation of the uterus will allow better blood supply into the IVS and thus facilitate the further growth of the clot and diminution of effective circulating blood volume. On the few occasions where uterine relaxants were used for this syndrome, results were catastrophic. The bleeding caused by placenta previa in the second half of pregnancy is usually the result of premature uterine contractions, which may or may not be felt by the patient. Nevertheless, the separation of a small area of placental implantation from the lower segment opens some of the vessels, which may continue to bleed. On the other hand, because the lower segment is formed predominantly by connective tissue and little smooth muscle, hemostasis tends to be promoted by the pressure of the presenting part against the lower segment, a condition favored by the contractions. The antagonic effects of the contractions make it impossible to predict either the amount and duration of the bleeding episode or the possible consequence of arresting the contractions. In view of the dilemma, abstention from active intervention is probably wise.

Amnionitis

Infection of the amniotic sac is usually the corollary to rupture of the membranes. Timing varies, but contamination of the amniotic cavity evolves into a clinically well-defined infection with systemic signs and symptoms. Onset of uterine contractions is one of the earliest indicators of a developing infection. A prolonged infection of this type is curable only after evacuation of the uterus; therefore any attempt at suppressing the contractions is absolutely contraindicated because of the danger to mother and child.

Other

A number of clinical conditions may cause or accompany premature labor and would contraindicate attempts at arresting it. Systemic infections, severe heart disease, markedly unbalanced endocrine disorders, and collagen diseases or autoimmune diseases may all flare up (and perhaps cause loss of the fetus) if premature labors are arrested.

Premature Rupture of the Membranes

By an as yet unexplained mechanism, the rupture of membranes is usually shortly followed by labor. To attempt to arrest labor when the fetal weight ranges between 1000 and 1500 gm or when the fetus is between 28th and 32nd weeks gestation is controversial. There seems to be general agreement that no benefit may be obtained by arresting a premature labor beyond the 34th week of gestation. The controversy revolves around the ability of the clinician to postpone the delivery sufficiently to allow him to stimulate the maturation of fetal lungs and thus prevent the very high incidence of respiratory distress syndrome observed between the 28th and 32nd weeks. For this purpose, corticosteroids would be administered to the mother at the same time as the uterine relaxant medication is given. Opponents of this procedure believe that even if the medication worked, which they doubt, the risk of infection is increased by the use of the steroid; thus it should not be used. A group of electics suggests that prolongation of gestation for about 48 hours (without steroids) would alone suffice as an endogenous stimulus to promote lung maturation of the fetus. However, the ever-present danger of amnionitis (or serious postpartum infections), or even prolapse of the umbilical cord, have been used as arguments against the arrest of premature labor with rupture of the membranes. At the Chicago Lying-In Hospital no woman in premature labor with ruptured membranes is given any drug aimed at preventing prompt spontaneous delivery.

METHODS OF ARRESTING PREMATURE LABOR

Ideally to arrest unwanted uterine contractions, one should aim at preventing the action of the specific triggering mechanism producing the contractions. In the case of premature labor, a number of *hypotheses* postulate that the mechanism is identical to that of term labor, only occurring before it is due to start its normal action. As discussed in Chapter 8, the several hypotheses advanced to explain the normal mechanism for the onset of labor would all suggest the possibility of a direct attack on the primary cause to arrest labor. However, none of the specific treatments based on those hypotheses is consistently successful to arrest premature labor, as it is the nonspecific technique of operating directly on the myometrium. Only the few practical techniques will be discussed in this chapter.

Ethanol

In a systematic series of experiments, A.R. Fuchs and Wagner (1963, 1964, 1966) demonstrated the primary role of oxytocin in the process of labor in rabbits. They further demonstrated that the release of oxytocin, essential for labor in that species, may be blocked by the administration of ethanol. Ethanol had been transiently used earlier as an analgesic in labor when administered by the intravenous route, and significant slowdown and even arrest of labors were observed to occur by an unknown mechanism. Several years later Fuchs (1965) proposed the use of ethyl alcohol administered intravenously to arrest

uterine contractions. He further demonstrated the possibility of arresting premature labor with a controlled infusion of this substance. A number of investigators have reproduced his observations while others, using slightly different techniques of administration, failed to obtain the same encouraging results. However, the majority of those who have followed the original schedule of administration have reproduced the results first reported by Fuchs, that is, a success rate between 65% and 80% — success defined as prolongation of gestation beyond 3 days of starting the treatment in patients fulfilling the requirements listed as indications.

Technique The ethanol must be infused intravenously in diluted form (about 10% strength in 5% dextrose or saline), starting with a *loading dose* of 100 gm to be administered in approximately 2 hours (around 0.7 to 1 gm/min). This amount will, on the average, establish a blood level ranging between 80 and 150 mg/100 ml, depending on the subject's ability to metabolize alcohol. After the loading dose has been completed, the *maintenance dose* should be infused at about one-tenth of the original rate, that is 0.07 to 0.10 gm/min for a patient weighing 70 kg. This dose should be maintained for at least 6 hours to be sure that the uterine activity does not recover after having been stopped. With this schedule, the ethanol blood level in the patient rises steadily to reach stable therapeutic levels between 100 and 120 mg/100 ml (Figure 11-1), a level subsequently sustained by the lower maintenance infusion. The uterine response to this medication is usually predictable and rapid (see Figure 9-38) particularly when the membranes are still intact. As a matter of fact, it has been observed that even patients with ruptured membranes will respond favorable to the initial infusion of ethanol and have a sustained quiescent uterus for 24 hours or more. The contractions tend to recur after that time in a number of cases. When recurrence is observed, a new course of treatment may be instituted, and a satisfactory response could be expected if the cervical changes have not progressed beyond 4 cm as maximum acceptable to interfere (Figure 11-2). With appropriate patient selection and close observation, it is possible to expect a continuation of pregnancy in 65% to 80% of cases (Fuchs, 1967; Zlatnick and Fuchs, 1972; Lauersen et al, 1977) even though others who used

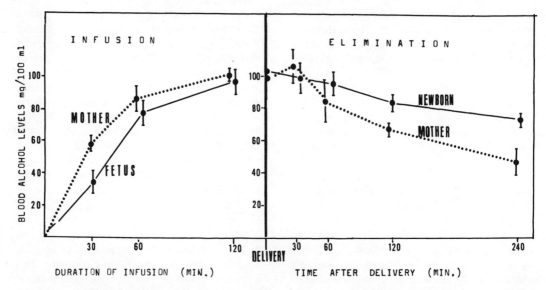

Figure 11-1 *(Left)* Blood ethanol levels determined in *mother and fetus* at the beginning of an infusion at the rate of 0.5 gm/min. The elimination (or metabolism) by the same subjects is demonstrated on the right side. The neonates dispose of the alcohol less well than their mothers. Reprinted from Idänpään-Heikkilä J, et al: Elimination and metabolic effects of ethanol in mother, fetus, and newborn infant. *Am J Obstet Gynecol* 112:387, 1972.

different, shorter schedules had less favorable results (Graff, 1971; Watring et al, 1976).

Side effects Like all drugs with systemic action, ethanol has a number of undesirable side effects that should be well understood by the clinician before it is given to a patient in labor. The *mother* experiences a state of alcoholic intoxication usually accompanied by excitation or depression, crying, laughter, aggressiveness, or marked quietness. Furthermore, there may be a very moderate tachycardia but without changes in blood pressure. Vomiting is relatively common, as well as profound sleep, the former potentially dangerous because of the possibility of aspiration. The *fetus* experiences very minimal effects, even though the blood level seems to equilibrate with that of the mother rather rapidly and the metabolism is significantly slower in the early neonatal period (Figure 11-1). The sometimes impressive metabolic changes that a number of authors have described in lambs and monkeys have not been observed in humans although the fetal blood levels are as high as those in the mother and that after birth metabolism of ethanol is much slower. Potential problems may develop if the already depressed CNS of the neonate is subjected to the effect of other depressant drugs commonly used around delivery time: diminished

muscular tone, sleepiness, unsatisfactory respiratory efforts, vomiting—all requiring special attention by the pediatrician. When adequately treated, they do not present significant problems.

When given in the manner here recommended, ethanol is a good choice to use in arresting premature labors particularly when it is difficult to supervise vital signs closely. The absence of cardiovascular effects is a significant asset in this regard. Our experience with it has been satisfactory, but at the Chicago Lying-In Hospital it is not the drug of choice.

Contraindications In a few clinical circumstances ethanol should not be used to arrest premature labor. The only real contraindications are severe liver insufficiency, and a former, currently abstinent, alcoholic patient. It is wise not to use general anesthesia in these patients for the additive effects of the depressant drugs on maternal, and particularly the fetal, CNS.

Beta-Mimetic Drugs

The mechanism of action and the pharmacology of the β-mimetic drugs has been described in some detail in Chapter 9. The

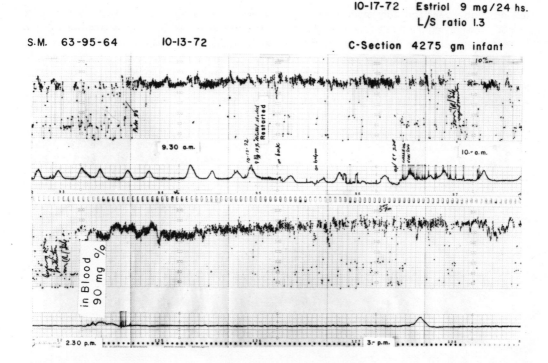

Figure 11-2 External tracings of uterine contractions and FHR obtained at 34 weeks gestation, from class C diabetic patient G4, P3 (all C-sections) in premature labor. Labor had to be arrested the day before with intravenous ethanol (see Figure 9-38) because of the L/S ratio of only 1:2 and good urinary estriol excretion. *(Above)* Spontaneous activity and the early effect of a reloading dose of ethanol 1 gm/min. *(Below)* Five hours later uterine activity, under 0.1 gm/min infusion rate, was almost nil with an ethanol blood level of 90 mg/100 ml. The drug had to be given continuously for 4½ days because the uterine activity resumed as soon as the ethanol was discontinued. Finally, the pregnancy had to be terminated because of a sharp fall in urinary estriol level from 22 mg to 9 mg in 24 hours. The cesarean section produced a large infant in heart failure which responsed to therapy. Both left the hospital on the seventh postoperative day. Reprinted from Cibils LA: The management of impending labor prior to the thirty-fifth week, in Reid, DE, Christian, CD (eds): *Controversies in Obstetrics and Gynecology II.* Philadelphia, Saunders, 1974, pp 88–102.

desirable action, in case of premature labor, would be exclusive uterine relaxation, which should be produced by a β_2-mimetic substance. However, the peripheral arterioles are also provided with the same type of receptors and therefore respond, simultaneously with the uterus, to the infusion of the active drugs. The one characteristic that allows certain latitude in the clinical use of the β-mimetic substances is the probable different sensitivities of the various systems to their stimulating action and thus the ability to obtain uterine relaxation without excessive or intolerable cardiovascular effects. The few drugs with acceptable effect, and with which there is sufficient reproducible clinical experience, are described in the following paragraphs.

Isoxsuprine Isoxsuprine, the first synthetic β-mimetic preparation to be assayed in humans, was predicted, on theoretical grounds, that it would produce less tachycardia than epinephrine and that it would be effective if given orally. Both of these predictions were confirmed, but some clear cardiovascular effects still remained, necessitating close supervision when the drug is administered intravenously. It has β_1 and β_2 effects but, fortunately, the action on the uterine contractility seems to predominate in the majority of the patients studied.

Technique For a rapid response, the drug must be administered by continuous intravenous infusion. It is reasonable to start with a dose of 500 μg/min, with which one may expect clear effect on contractions and only moderate effect on blood pressure and pulse rate (Figure 11-3). If the uterine response is not satisfactory within 15 min, the infusion rate should be doubled (see Figure 9-54), and this process may continue up to amounts as high as the patient's cardiovascular system will safely tolerate (Figure 11-4) (see also Figure 9-64). The infusion should be maintained at the effective rate for a minimum of 2 hours, following which it could be tapered down (if high doses were used) or discontinued. To maintain the quiescent condition of the uterus, *intramuscular* doses of 20 mg could be given every 4 to 6 hours for about 24 hours before switching to the *oral form*. This regimen effectively decreases the undesired activity, which tends to recur (Figure 11-5), and it should be administered every 4 to 6 hours while the patient is hospitalized. The dose most frequently given the Chicago Lying-In Hospital patients on discharge is 20 mg every 6 hours, maintained until, in the obstetrician's judgment, the patient is ready for safe delivery.

Side effects Undesirable effects on the mother are reviewed in Chapter 9. The hypotension may be controlled with rapid administration of intravenous fluids and positioning the patient on her side. The effects on the fetus consist mainly of moderate tachycardia. Those infants who were studied during term labor, or delivered because of failure to arrest premature labor, have

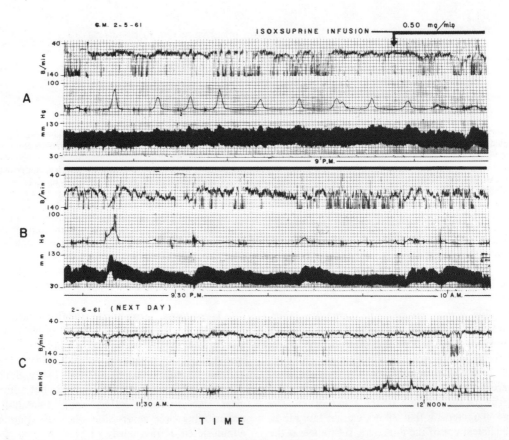

Figure 11-3 Maternal heart rate *(top)*, intrauterine pressure *(middle)*, and arterial blood pressure *(bottom)* recorded in a multipara admitted at 29½ weeks in *premature labor* with cervix dilated 4 cm, 50% effaced, and intact membranes. *(A)* and *(B)* Continuous recordings of the preinfusion values, and the response to isoxsuprine infusion (arrow) given in 500 µg/min. Note the prompt decrease of uterine activity, moderate fall in blood pressure, and mild tachycardia. *(C)* After discontinuing the infusion and an overnight dose of 100 mg IM, the uterine contractility remained low with a stable pulse rate. The patient was discharged, took 80 mg/day by mouth, and was readmitted 24 days later. Allowed to labor, she delivered a 1950 gm infant who did well. Reprinted from Hendricks CH, et al: The pharmacologic control of excessive uterine activity with isoxsuprine. *Am J Obstet Gynecol* 82:1064, 1961.

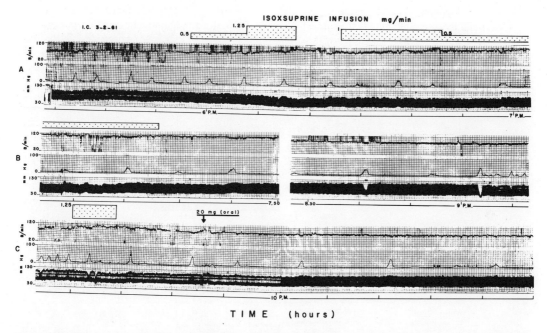

Figure 11-4 Four hours and 40 min of almost continuous recordings of maternal heart rate *(top)*, intrauterine pressure *(middle)*, and arterial pressure *(bottom)* in a multipara (three previous premature infants) admitted at 29 weeks gestation in premature labor, with the cervix dilated 2 cm, 30% effaced, and intact membranes. *(A)* Spontaneous activity, a poor response to 500 µg/min infusion (dotted area). *(B)* It was necessary to maintain the infusion at 100 µg/min and taper it to 500 µg/min to sustain the desired effect. *(C)* A burst of activity was controlled with another short intravenous infusion at 1250 µg/min, and 20 mg by mouth. Note only a mild drop in blood pressure and tachycardia, in spite of the very high doses infused. Both may be seen recovering in *(C)*. Reprinted from Hendricks CH, et al: The pharmacologic control of excessive uterine activity with isoxsuprine. *Am J Obstet Gynecol* 82:1064, 1961.

not shown any metabolic alterations that would preclude the short-term use of the drug. Because the β-mimetic substances have a glycogenolytic effect on the liver, they tend to induce a moderate hyperglycemia. This metabolic action, when maintained for several weeks, is responsible for excessive fetal growth (moderate macrosomia) manifested as heavier infants at term.

Ritodrine The structure of ritodrine is similar to that of isoxsuprine from which it is derived (Figure 9-41). However, it is a much more selective uterine depressant drug than the parent compound, but it still maintains significant β_1 effect. On a weight basis, it is also more potent when given parenterally.

Technique An *intravenous infusion* should be started at a rate of 50 to 100 µg/min, and the response should be quick and clear (see Figures 9-61 and 9-62). If the uterine response is not satisfactory, the dose should be doubled to 200

µg/min, which is reasonably high. Rarely will it be necessary to increase the infusion rate to 400 µg/min, which may produce too much tachycardia and perhaps the necessity to discontinue the infusion. As with isoxsuprine, the effective rate should be maintained for at least 2 hours and then tapered down as the *intramuscular* route is used to inject 10 mg to be given up to every 4 hours. The *oral* route should be used for ambulatory treatment at doses ranging from 10 mg every 4 to 6 hours, depending on the irritability of the uterus.

Premature labor caused by uterine or cervical surgical trauma should also be amenable to treatment with β-mimetic substances. The direct stimulation of the uterus by manipulations on the lower segment and cervical area produced during a cervical cerclage (Shirodkar's or McDonald's procedure) trigger uterine contractions immediately on grasping of the cervix. However, hypercontractility may start before the surgical

248

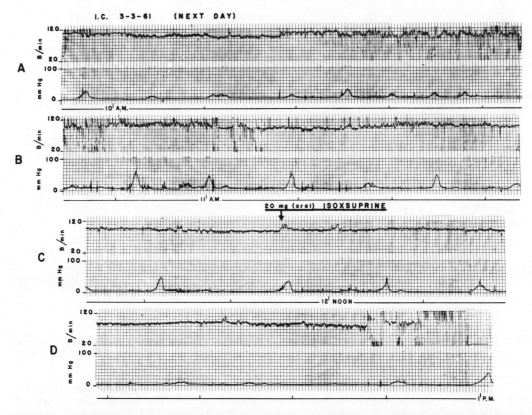

Figure 11-5 Continuous 3 hours and 10 min of maternal heart rate *(top)* and intrauterine pressure tracings *(bottom)* on same patient as in Figure 11-4, the following day. *(A, B)* Mildly increased uterine activity. *(C, D)* Response to 20 mg oral medication. Patient was discharged, took 80 mg/day by mouth, ruptured membranes 11 days later, and delivered a 1950 gm infant (her largest) who did very well. Reprinted from Hendricks CH, et al: The pharmacologic control of excessive uterine activity with isoxsuprine. *Am J Obstet Gynecol* 82:1064, 1961.

maneuver if the patient is inadvertently (or unknowingly) given oxytocic medications (Figure 11-6). This emergency is usually the preamble to the expected hypercontractility produced by the surgical procedure, which should be treated as a true premature labor (Figure 11-7). The systematic documentation of abnormal uterine activity during operations for cervical incompetence should prompt the obstetrician to use these compounds *prophylactically,* anticipating that the circumstance triggers premature labor. If used in this manner, their effectiveness should be increased, requiring lower infusion rates than those used to arrest an already established hypercontractility. Along this line, it is now routine at the Chicago Lying-In Hospital to use 20 mg intramuscular

isoxsuprine prophylactically before the operation, followed by the same dose every 4 to 6 hours depending on the uterine activity. Only rarely will the intravenous route be required. Oral doses are used when the patient tolerates the ingestion of fluids, at 20 mg by mouth every 6 hours, for several days.

Extensive clinical experience with ritodrine has been accumulated in Europe and South America. The results are encouraging—up to 80% successful prolongation of gestation in spontaneous premature labors with intact membranes.

Side effects Ritodrine has a mild effect on blood pressure, increasing the pulse pressure and causing moderate tachycardia, both of which are responsible for a significant increase in cardiac

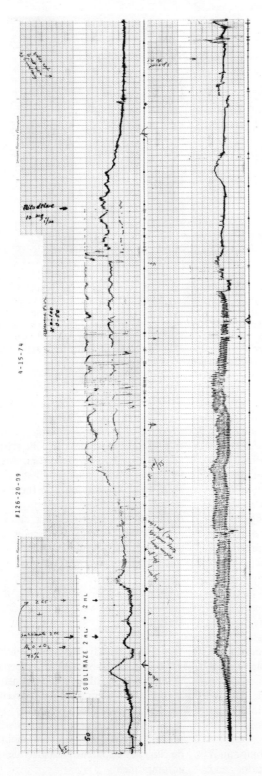

Figure 11-6 Continuous 45-min recording of transabdominal intrauterine pressure in secundigravida with incompetent cervical os, to undergo a Shirodkar operation at 24 weeks gestation. *(Above, left)* The moment of induction of general anesthesia with nitrous oxide and oxygen, and the consecutive intravenous administration of 0.1 mg fentanyl, repeated within 2 min (arrows). Less than 30 sec after the second dose the uterus started a contraction which continued with a state of severe hypercontractility and hypertonus, lasting until after a dose of 10 mg ritodrine was given intramuscularly (arrow). The hypercontractility was sustained for 10 min and produced a marked bulging of the membranes that protruded to the vulva. The degree of hypertonus reached almost 50 mm Hg. After the contractility was controlled, the operation was started. *(Below)* Quiescent uterus during manipulations on the cervix, the deep oscillations of intrauterine pressure representing respiratory movements of the patient. Penthrane was substituted for nitrous oxide at this point. (The markers in the abscissa indicate time in minutes, paper speed, 3 cm/min; the intrauterine pressure range 0 to 50 mm Hg, and during hypertonus simultaneous recording with 0 to 100 mm Hg range.)

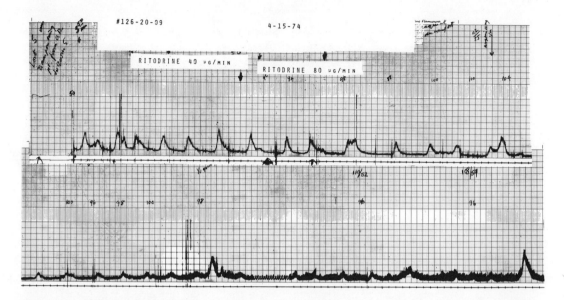

Figure 11-7 Same patient as in Figure 11-6. Fifteen minutes after completion of operation and recovery from Penthrane anesthesia. Continuous 140 min of intrauterine pressure recording. Recording range 0 to 50 mm Hg. *(Above)* Pattern of abnormally high uterine activity. Ritodrine infused at 40 μg/min (first arrow). In view of its modest effect on the contractions, the infusion rate was increased to 80 μg/min. *(Below)* Better response and eventual quiescence. The infusion rate was maintained for 60 hours before switching to intramuscular, then oral medication, and final discharge. She was readmitted 30 days later and delivered a surviving infant. (Time in minutes, paper speed, 0.5 cm/min, no significant change in pressure, and only moderate tachycardia.)

output. In addition, it has the same metabolic effects as β-mimetic substances discussed for isoxsuprine. Ritodrine is easier to handle than isoxsuprine, and, when available, it is preferred in clinical practice.

Contraindications Because of their significant effect on cardiac output, these drugs should never be used on patients with *cardiac disease* or borderline heart function as they may precipitate immediate heart failure. *Preeclamptic patients* should be treated with extreme caution, if at all, because the characteristic peripheral arteriolar constriction and hemoconcentration make their cardiovascular responses extremely labile. *Chronic hypertension* and hypertensive *renal disease* are also contraindications to the use of these compounds; peripheral vascular disease predisposes to unpredictable reactions, and the heart is usually affected by the chronic disease. The most absolute of all contraindications is the *inability to closely supervise* the intravenous administration of the drug.

Other beta-mimetics Other compounds with basic effects similar to isoxsuprine and ritodrine are currently being tested to evaluate their clinical usefulness and the claims of specific action upon the β₂ receptors. Metaproterenol, terbutaline, and salbutamol have had limited use by a few investigators, and their effects do not seem substantially different from those of ritodrine. As a matter of fact, some of them produce more marked cardiovascular effects without better control of uterine action.

Failures

Unfortunately, a relatively high proportion of premature labors cannot be arrested with administration of ethanol or β-mimetic substances, even under seemingly ideal circumstances. The failure rates may range from 13% to 23% depending on the agent used. Some of the causes for failures can be anticipated, while others may not be clinically apparent until after delivery has been accomplished.

Rupture of the membranes When a patient is admitted in premature labor with the membranes already ruptured, it is our policy not to attempt to arrest the contractions because of the likelihood of amniotic infection. Further, in cases of ruptured membranes, uterine contractions tend to resume shortly after the intravenous infusion has been discontinued. This accident may occur even during the infusion period of the drug (Figures 11-8 and 11-9) and very rapid delivery will follow as soon as the administration of the drug is interrupted. We are still completely ignorant of the mechanism involved in this well known clinical condition. This response follows systematically, regardless of the compound used to arrest labor, be it alcohol, β-mimetic or antiprostaglandins.

Retroplacental clots The classically described clinical picture of premature separation of a normally implanted placenta (abruptio placentae) with a "board-like uterus" and hypertonus with polysystoly in the intrauterine tracing, is clearly a contraindication to any attempt at arresting that labor. However, only some of those cases present the textbook syndrome, while a significant number of others have neither board-like uterus nor hypercontractility (see Chapter 6). They may clinically resemble any idiopathic premature labor and therefore they are treated as such (Figures 11-10, 11-11, and 11-12). Retrospective review of these cases shows that they are destined to end in premature delivery, even though such a pessimistic outlook is not at all foreseeable when the treatment is started.

Amnionitis It is not unusual to observe intrauterine infections develop while membranes are still intact. When these cases are seen, invariably the uterus contracts with a labor-like pattern as a response to the irritation of the acutely inflamed chorio-amnion. The myometrium may transiently respond to uterine relaxants, but activity will resume shortly after discontinuing the medication or even during the infusion of the maintenance dose of the drug.

It seems unavoidable that a number of similar cases will be treated in large clinical series, but our inability to diagnose these conditions precisely should not deter any attempt to prolong gestation in a significant proportion of fetuses, which should benefit from a few more days or weeks of intrauterine life and the consequent chronologic maturation. What these cases prove, along with those with far advanced cervical dilata-tion, is that when the mechanism of labor has been triggered and has progressed beyond a certain stage there is no return, and then all methods are destined to fail.

Miscellaneous Drugs

Progesterone For a long time this steroid constituted the hope of obstetricians to control excessive uterine contractility because of its presumed quiescent effect on the myometrium — Csapo's widely known hypothesis of maintenance of pregnancy. However, all hopes and years of research had to yield to the irrefutable fact that even very large quantities of progesterone given by all possible routes are unable to arrest established premature labor. Nevertheless, recent new studies (Johnson et al, 1975) suggest that it may be valuable for the prophylactic treatment of premature labor in patients who have a history of premature labor or are prone to it.

Diazoxide A potent antihypertensive medication with a chemical structure resembling the thiazide diuretics, diazoxide is not a diuretic but has been shown to have dramatic uterine relaxant properties. Very few investigators have used it in humans, but they report encouraging results in their efforts to arrest premature labor. The great disadvantage is the requirement of intravenous injection of doses that have a drastic effect on blood pressure and corresponding exaggerated tachycardia. Until it is adequately tested it seems reasonable to resort to other substances with less impressive or less dangerous side effects.

Magnesium sulfate It has been claimed for a long time that magnesium sulfate is a uterine relaxant drug. However, studies aimed at observing that specific action have been unable to demonstrate that time-honored postulate (see Chapter 9). Nevertheless, that concept has been revived (Steer and Petrie, 1977) as one possible means to arrest premature labor. The blood levels required to produce a uterine relaxant are said to be the same (4 to 8 mg/100 ml) as those usually attained in the treatment of hyperreflexic pre-eclampsia. But even the direct intramyometrial administration of magnesium sulfate at high concentration does not significantly affect the contractility pattern of the postpartum uterus (Figures 11-13 and 11-14). Only highly concentrated solutions directly injected in the

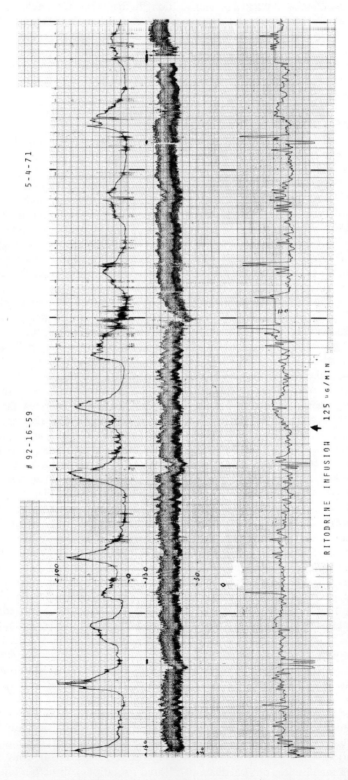

Figure 11-8 Primipara at 34 weeks gestation in premature labor; cervix dilated 4 cm. Intrauterine and intraarterial pressures and maternal heart rate recordings for 32 min. The infusion of ritodrine, started at 125 μg/min (arrow), rapidly decreased uterine activity without complete suppression. The pulse pressure increased at the expense of a mild rise in systolic. There is also a moderate increase in pulse rate. The pressure ranges are shown on the ordinates. The range for pulse rate is from 50 to 150 beats/min (paper speed, 1.5 cm [3 lines]/min).

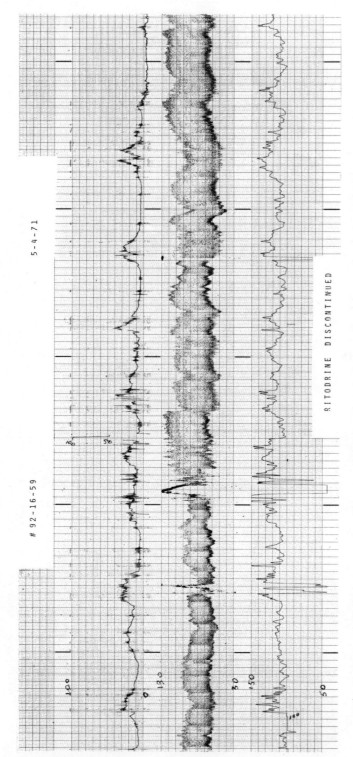

Figure 11-9 Same patient as Figure 11-8, 15 min later. Incomplete control of uterine activity shown during 32 min of recording, in the middle of which clear amniotic fluid started to leak. Ritodrine infusion had to be discontinued. At this point the effects of blood pressure and heart rate were more marked, with tachycardia reaching peaks of 130 beats/min. One hour and 20 min after discontinuing the tracing, a 2450 gm normal infant was born and did well (paper speed, 1.5 cm/min).

254

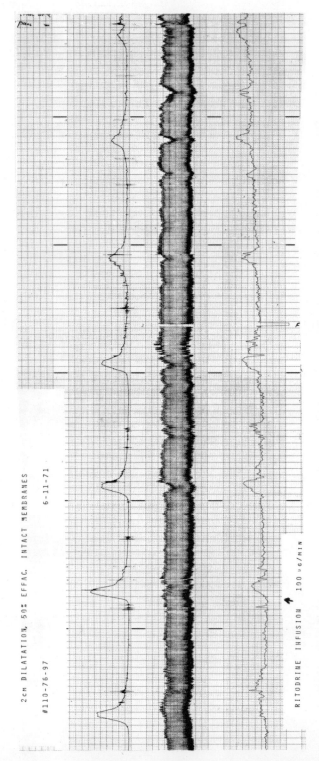

Figure 11-10 Continuous 37 min of intrauterine and intraarterial pressures and maternal heart rate of a multipara in premature labor at 24 weeks gestation. Ritodrine was started at 100 μg/min (arrow) followed by clear decrease in intensity of contractions, a slight decrease in diastolic pressure, unchanged systolic (increased pulse pressure), and moderate tachycardia (paper speed, 1.5 cm/min). (In this and the following two figures the uterine contraction record scale is 0 to 100 mm Hg, arterial pressure scale 20 to 120 mm Hg, and heart rate 50 to 150 beats/min.)

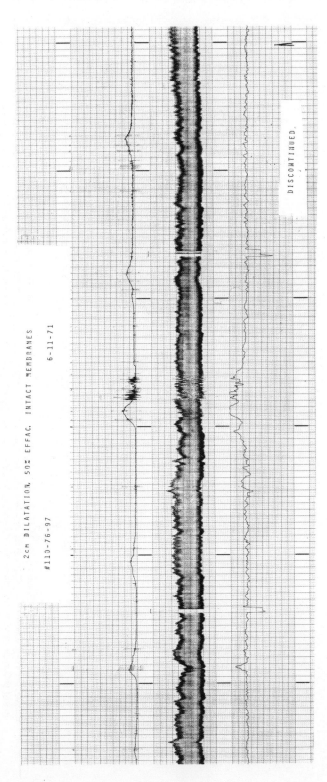

Figure 11-11 Same patient as in Figure 11-10, two hours later, showing 37 min of same parameters, with uterine activity not completely controlled. By this time, the moderate low blood pressure coupled with a tachycardia of 120 to 130 beats/min precluded increasing the infusion rate and, in fact, dictated the need to discontinue the drug. Because of rapid recovery of uterine activity, the infusion was restarted 1 hour later but there was minimal response at that time.

256

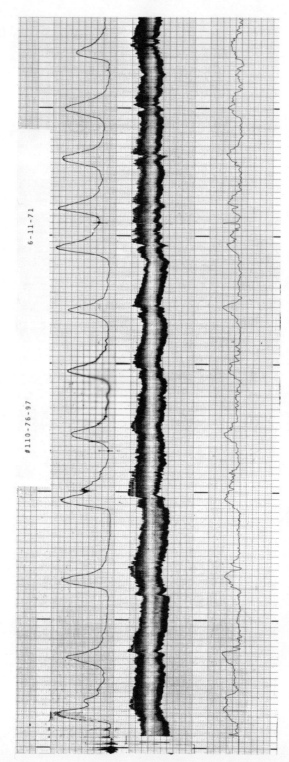

Figure 11-12 Same patient as in Figure 11-11. Thirty-six minutes of tracings after ritodrine had been discontinued for 3 hours. High uterine activity, which produced a rapid progress in dilatation, terminated in the expulsion of a 250 gm fetus 15 min after end of tracing. Behind a 170 gm placenta came well-formed blood clots, indicating that this patient had a concealed abruptio placentae. Note the return to normal values of blood pressure and pulse rate compared to Figures 11-10 and 11-11.

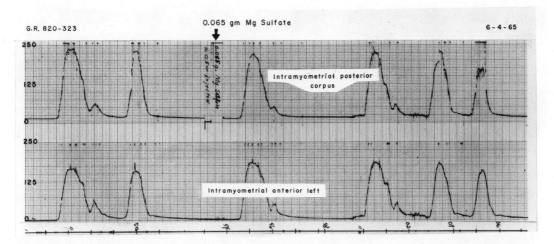

Figure 11-13 Intramyometrial pressures obtained immediately after term repeat cesarean section. *(Above)* Recorded from posterior aspect of midcorpus, right side. *(Below)* From the left side, both deep into myometrium. There is good coordination of very strong spontaneous contractions. Magnesium sulfate, 0.065 gm, injected via catheter (arrow) did not affect the pattern of contraction that followed 1 min later or the overall contractility. (Pressure ranges on ordinates in mm Hg; time markers in minutes.)

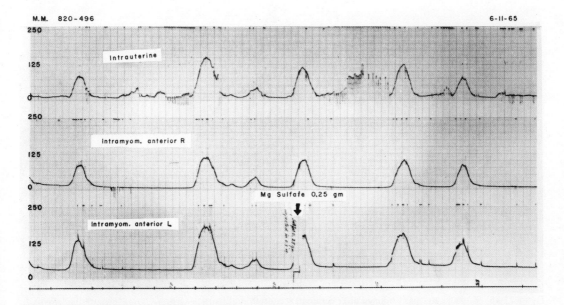

Figure 11-14 Pressure tracings obtained after cesarean section in multipara at term. *(A)* Intrauterine. *(B)* Intramyometrial anterior right. *(C)* Left. The spontaneous, strong contractions that seem to start closer to the right side catheter failed to change their pattern or intensity when magnesium sulfate 0.25 gm (in 0.5 ml) was injected deep in the left anterior aspect of the myometrium. (Pressure ranges on ordinates in mm Hg; time in minutes.)

myometrium have transiently decreased the intensity of localized contractions (Figure 11-15). In fact, there seems to be a dose-related response at these high doses (Figure 11-16). The calculated concentration of the drug in these instances is hundreds of times above the one obtained with the intravenous therapeutic infusion. Thus it seems reasonable to wait until more experience is acquired with magnesium sulfate as a drug to arrest premature labor before one may advise it for that purpose.

Over the past few years, magnesium sulfate has been the treatment of choice in cases of hyperreflexic preeclampsia, providing a large experience from which to observe its effects on the fetus. A few authors claim that it depresses the infant to a dangerous point—unsubstantiated by the great majority of investigators working with the drug. The concentration of magnesium in fetal blood is not higher than in the mother's, and Apgar scores at birth are related to neither the amount of magnesium infused per hour nor to duration of infusion before delivery.

Antiprostaglandins The mechanism of action of these substances has been reviewed in Chapter 9. The only ones accessible for clinical use are aspirin and indomethacin. *Aspirin* administered over the long term seems to have postponed the onset of labor in a significant number of patients. As medication to arrest premature labor, it is used only as adjuvant to other procedures that have a more dramatic action on the uterus. On the other hand, *indomethacin* has given good results in the treatment of premature labor when used by a few authors (Zuckerman et al, 1974). Nevertheless, serious reservations exist with regard to possible deleterious effects on the fetal circulation and its adaptation to neonatal life.

Fetal side effects include the possible premature closure of the ductus arteriosus and pulmonary hypertension or "persistent fetal circulation," particularly when the fetus is subjected to episodes of transient hypoxia.

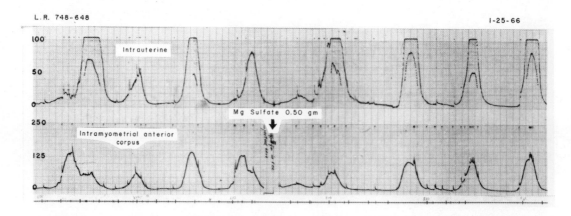

Figure 11-15 Pressure tracings obtained after cesarean section in multipara at term. *(Above)* Intrauterine. *(Below)* Intramyometrial, moderately deep in middle corpus. The strong, regular intrauterine contractions are not affected by the injection of 0.50 gm (in 1 ml) magnesium sulfate given in the myometrium through the lower catheter. The local strength of one contraction within 2½ min of injection seems of lesser intensity. There was immediate full recovery without change in pattern. (Pressure ranges in mm Hg on ordinates; time in minutes.)

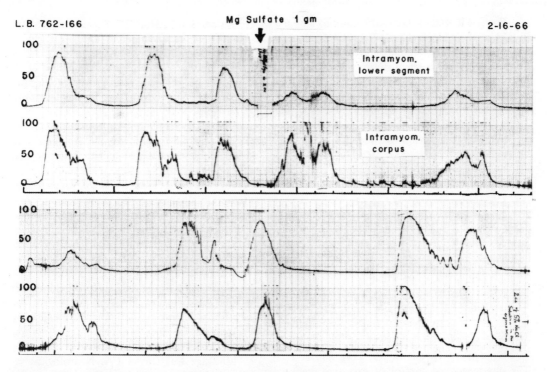

L.B. 762-166   Mg Sulfate 1 gm   2-16-66

Figure 11-16   Continuous 56 min of recordings of intramyometrial lower segment and corpus tracings obtained in postterm delivery, multipara. The local injection of 1 gm magnesium sulfate (in 2 ml) (arrow) decreased the intensity of the contractions in that spot for about 15 min while the other area of the myometrium did not seem affected. The frequency pattern was not changed, and recovery was full after 20 min.

BIBLIOGRAPHY

Abramowicz M, Kass EH: Pathogenesis and prognosis of prematurity. *N Engl J Med* 275:878, 1966.

Barden RP: Effect of ritodrine on human uterine motility and cardiovascular responses in term labor and the early postpartum state. *Am J Obstet Gynecol* 112:645–652, 1972.

Bieniarz J, Motew M, Scommegna A: Uterine and cardiovascular effects of ritodrine in premature labor. *Obstet Gynecol* 40:65–73, 1972.

Belinkoff S, Hall J: Intravenous alcohol during labor. *Am J Obstet Gynecol* 59:429–432, 1950.

Cibils LA: Inhibitory effects of isoxsuprine on uterine contractility. *Am J Obstet Gynecol* 94:762–764, 1966.

Cibils LA: The mangement of impending labor prior to the thirty-fifth week, in Reid DE, Christian CD (eds): *Controversies in Obstetrics and Gynecology II*. Philadelphia, Saunders, 1974, pp 88–102.

Cibils LA, Hendricks CH: Effecto de la isoxsuprina sobre la contractilidad del utero humano gravido. *Mem X Reun Gin Obstet (Mexico)* 1:418–437, 1961.

Chapman ER, Williams PT: Intravenous alcohol as an obstetrical analgesic. *Am J Obstet Gynecol* 61:676–679, 1951.

Csapo AI, Herzog J: Arrest of premature labor by isoxsuprine. *Am J Obstet Gynecol* 129:482, 1977.

Donnelly JF, Flowers, CE, Credick RN, et al: Maternal fetal and environmental factors in prematurity. *Am J Obstet Gynecol* 88:918, 1964.

Fedrick J, Anderson ABM: Factors associated with spontaneous pre-term birth. *Br J Obstet Gynaecol* 83:342, 1976.

260

Fuchs AR: Oxytocin and the onset of labour in rabbits. *J Endocrinol* 30:217, 1964.

Fuchs AR: The inhibitory effect of ethanol on the release of oxytocin during parturition in the rabbit. *J Endocrinol* 35:125, 1966.

Fuchs F: Treatment of threatened premature labour with alcohol. *J Obstet Gynaecol Br Comwlth* 72:1011-1013, 1965.

Fuchs F: Prevention of prematurity. *Am J Obstet Gynecol* 126:809-817, 1976.

Fuchs F, Fuchs AR, Poblete VF, Jr, et al: Effect of alcohol on threatened premature labor. *Am J Obstet Gynecol* 99:627, 1967.

Fuchs AR, Wagner C: The effect of ethyl alcohol on the release of oxytocin in rabbits. *Acta Endocrinol* 44:593-605, 1963.

Graff G: Failure to prevent premature labor with ethanol. *Am J Obstet Gynecol* 110:878, 1971.

Harbert GM, Cornell GW, Thornton WN, Jr: Effect of toxemia therapy on uterine dynamics. *Am J Obstet Gynecol* 105:94, 1969.

Hendricks CH, Cibils LA, Pose SV, et al: The pharmacologic control of excessive uterine activity with isoxsuprine. *Am J Obstet Gynecol* 82:1064, 1961.

Heymann MA, Rudolph AM: Effects of acetylsalicylic acid on the ductus arteriosus and circulation in fetal lambs in utero. *Circ Res* 38:418, 1976.

Horiguchi T, Suzuki K, Comas-Urrutia AC, et al: Effect of ethanol upon uterine activity and fetal acid-base state of the rhesus monkey. *Am J Obstet Gynecol* 109:910, 1971.

Hutchinson HT, Nichols MM, Kuhn CR, et al: Effects of magnesium sulfate on uterine contractility, intrauterine fetus, and infant. *Am J Obstet Gynecol* 88:747, 1964.

Idanpään-Heikkilä J, Jouppila P, Akerblom HK, et al: Elimination and metabolic effects of ethanol in mother, fetus and newborn infant. *Am J Obstet Gynecol* 112:387, 1972.

Ingemarsson I: Effect of terbutaline on premature labor. *Am J Obstet Gynecol* 125:520, 1976.

Johnson JWC, Austin KL, Jones GS, et al: Efficacy of 17α hydroxyprogesterone caproate in the prevention of premature labor. *N Engl J Med* 293:675, 1975.

Koh KS: Premature labour. *Can Med Assoc J* 114:700, 1976.

Kumaresan P, Han GS, Anandarangam PB, et al: Oxytocin in maternal and fetal blood. *Obstet Gynecol* 46:272, 1975.

Lauersen NH, Merkatz IR, Tejani N, et al: Inhibition of premature labor: A multicenter comparison of ritodrine and ethanol. *Am J Obstet Gynecol* 127:837, 1977.

Lewis RB, Schulman JD: Influence of acetylsalicylic acid, an inhibitor of prostaglandin synthesis, on the duration of human gestation and labour. *Lancet* 2:1159, 1973.

Liggons GC, Howie RN: A controlled trial of antepartum glucocorticoid treatment for prevention of the respiratory distress syndrome in premature infants. *Pediatrics* 50:515, 1972.

Lipsitz PJ: The clinical and biochemical effects of excess magnesium in the newborn. *Pediatrics* 47:501, 1971.

Manchester D, Margolis HS, Sheldon RE: Possible association between maternal indomethacin therapy and primary pulmonary hypertension of the newborn. *Am J Obstet Gynecol* 126:467, 1976.

Marriage KJ, Davies PA: Neurological sequelae in children surviving mechanical ventilation in the neonatal period. *Arch Dis Child* 52:176, 1977.

Mehra P, Raghvan KS, Devi PK, et al: Effect of intravenous alcohol on premature labour. *Int J Gynecol Obstet* 8:160, 1970.

Miller JM, Pupkin MJ, Crenshaw C: Premature labor and premature rupture of the membranes. *Am J Obstet Gynecol* 132:1, 1978.

Stander RW, Barden TP, Thompson JF, et al: Fetal cardiac effects of maternal isoxsuprine infusion. *Am J Obstet Gynecol* 89:792, 1964.

Steer CM, Petrie RH: A comparison of magnesium sulfate and alcohol for the prevention of premature labor. *Am J Obstet Gynecol* 129:1, 1977.

Stone SR, Pritchard JA: Effect of maternally administered magnesium sulfate on the neonate. *Obstet Gynecol* 35:574, 1970.

Wallace RL, Caldwell DL, Ansbacher R, et al: Inhibition of premature labor by terbutaline. *Obstet Gynecol* 51:387, 1978.

Wagner G, Fuchs AR: Effect of ethanol on uterine activity during suckling in post-partum women. *Acta Endocrinol* 58:133, 1968.

Watring WG, Benson WL, Wiebe RA, et al: Intravenous alcohol—a single blind study in the prevention of premature delivery: A preliminary report. *J Reprod Med* 16:35, 1976.

Wesslius-de Casparis A, Thiery M, Yo Le Sian, et al: Results of double-blind multicentre study with ritodrine in premature labour. *Br Med J* 3:144, 1971.

Wynn M, Wynn A: *The Prevention of Preterm Birth*. London, Foundation for Education and Research in Child-Bearing, 1977.

Zlatnick FJ: The applicability of labor inhibition to the problem of premature labor. *Am J Obstet Gynecol* 113:704, 1972.

Zlatnick FJ, Fuchs R: A controlled study of ethanol in threatened premature labor. *Am J Obstet Gynecol* 112:610, 1972.

Zuckerman H, Reiss U, Rubinstein I: Inhibition of human premature labor by indomethacin. *Obstet Gynecol* 44:787, 1974.

CHAPTER 12
Fetal Heart Rate Baseline Patterns

The widespread use of continuous FHR monitoring has brought to the fore the relevance of continuous observation and has revealed a variety of changing patterns and phenomena, the interpretation of which is still not completely clear. The appropriate interpretation of what is known of FHR changes has facilitated better care and judgment of pathologic clinical conditions, thereby improving overall neonatal outcome of selected populations managed by well-trained personnel. However, most monitored patients have not had full benefit from the potential advantages of continuous recording of intrapartum FHR and uterine contractions because of lack of in-depth education and training of personnel. The consequence has been an increase in the incidence of operative deliveries, without improvement in the neonatal outcome, when compared to nonmonitored groups of patients. This fact has evoked the feeling that fetal monitoring is not only not beneficial but may even be deleterious to the mother's or infant's well-being. Meticulous study and analysis of the normal tracings and careful evaluation of the mechanisms involved in the FHR alterations observed during labor may help to dispel this fallacy and, at the same time, promote the understanding so necessary for accurate interpretation of the tracings, an absolute prerequisite for correct judgment of the various clinical situations.

NORMAL PATTERNS

Baseline Rate

Normal rate A rate between 120 and 150 beats/min was considered normal by the clinicians before continuous monitoring was available. It is probably still a good measure of what should be considered normal because the fetuses of the majority of uncomplicated pregnancies have an FHR within that range. Within the general context of clinical observation, it seems that the 160 beats/min proposed by Hon as upper limit for normal may be considered too high. This appears valid even for preterm fetuses, which maintain a frequency close to the upper range, but usually near 150 beats/min frequency. This *baseline rate must be read between contractions* when these cause changes and after complete recovery if there are alterations triggered by contractions (Figure 12-1).

Tachycardia is present when the baseline between contractions is more than *150 beats/min;* under severe conditions it may reach values close to 200 beats/min (Figure 12-2). This alteration of FHR tracing may be triggered by a great variety of clinical conditions, which will be discussed at the appropriate moment. Furthermore, it may also represent the pharmacologic response of the FHR to drugs administered to the mother or directly to the fetus.

Bradycardia is observed when the rate between contractions is less than 120 beats/min. Rarely one may see a sustained bradycardia rate not associated with a pathologic condition (Figure 12-3). Almost always it represents the fetal cardiovascular response to severe distress complicated by hypoxia and/or metabolic alterations of fetal homeostasis. In these circumstances, it may represent what Caldeyro-Barcia called "overlapping" late decelerations.

Rapid oscillations of the baseline are fluctuations that take place under normal circumstances within a range of 5 and 20 beats/min and cycling

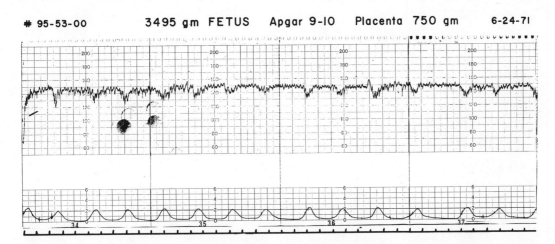

 # 95-53-00   **3495 gm FETUS**   **Apgar 9-10**   **Placenta 750 gm**   **6-24-71**

Figure 12-1 Forty minutes of direct intrauterine pressure and FHR recordings of spontaneous labor at term. The small rapid oscillations of the FHR baseline occur 4 to 5/min and fluctuate within a range of 4 to 10 beats. The small decelerations coinciding with the contractions of moderate intensity are of the early type. Average rate *between these early decelerations* is about 145 to 150 beats/min. A normal infant and placenta were delivered. Reprinted from Cibils LA: Clinical significance of fetal heart rate patterns during labor. I. Baseline patterns. *Am J Obstet Gynecol* 125:290, 1976.

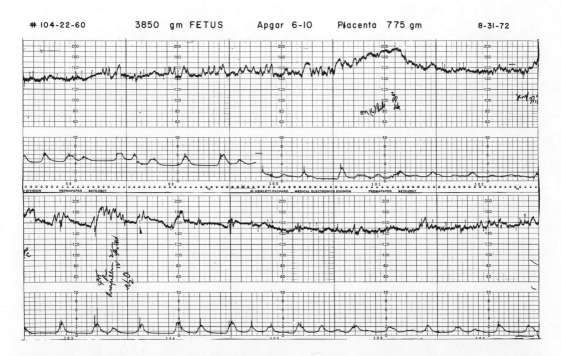

 # 104-22-60   **3850 gm FETUS**   **Apgar 6-10**   **Placenta 775 gm**   **8-31-72**

Figure 12-2 One hundred minutes of continuous recording of UC (external) and FHR (direct) of term labor enhanced with oxytocin, 5 mU/min. Note the rising baseline, which after 20 min is greater than 150/min and reaches 195 at the 36th minute, to drop slowly thereafter to a steady rate of less than 150 at the 75th minute (in lower tracing). There is associated decrease of the baseline oscillations in spite of some sporadic accelerations. There was no apparent cause for the sudden high FHR (mother's temperature 37 C). Subsequently, a mildly depressed infant and normal placenta were delivered.

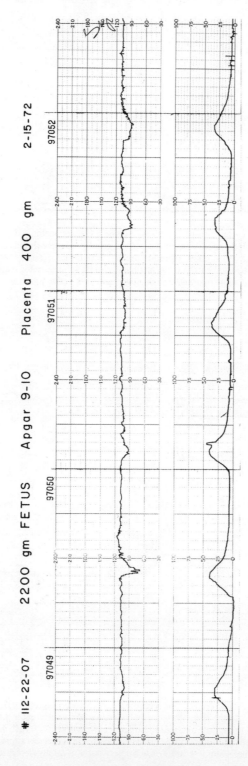

Figure 12-3 Sixteen minutes of direct UC and FHR recordings of induced labor for premature rupture of membranes. In advanced first stage the baseline of the *FHR is bradycardic* and fluctuates between 106 and 110 with minimal or no rapid oscillations (fixed). The only pathologic finding was that the fetus appeared growth-retarded, a condition not necessarily associated with persistent bradycardia. Apgar scores were normal, size of placenta was normal for the size of the infant. Note four early decelerations. Reprinted form Cibils LA: Clinical significance of fetal heart rate patterns during labor. I. Baseline patterns. *Am J Obstet Gynecol* 125:290, 1976.

at a frequency of 2 to 6/min (Figure 12-1). There is a normal tendency to slight irregularity of these fluctuations, usually within the range of 5 to 10 beats, the most frequently observed pattern. However, one may see larger oscillations of great regularity bordering the limit of what has been defined here as normal (Figure 12-4) and without pathologic significance. It is most critical for the proper reading of a tracing to pay close attention to the speed at which the recording paper is running, and to the scale in which the frequency has been recorded (Figure 12-5). Errors may be easily made when interpreting recordings made with different makes of monitors if one pays attention to only the visual aspect of a tracing, because they may run at different paper speeds and have recording ranges of unequal value. The rapid oscillations are the same as those described by Hon as normal beat-to-beat variations and correspond to types I and II oscillations described by Hammacher. They are the consequence of variations in the frequency of each heart contraction (so called short-term variability by Hon), and cyclic alterations recurring 2 to 6 times/min (long-term variability by Hon). In fact, both of these phenomena are interdependent, one not occurring without the other, for which reason they are considered and analyzed as a single characteristic: the rapid oscillations of the normal fetal heart rate.

Accelerations   These are transient increases of FHR, greater than 10 beats and lasting usually between 20 and 60 sec before returning to the baseline level. They often coincide with the uterine contractions, as if triggered by them (Figure 12-6), and may be up to 40 beats above the baseline. More rarely, they may occur without any relationship to uterine contractions or other discernable phenomena (Figure 12-7). The incidence of accelerations during first stage of labor ranges between 10% and 15% in large hospital series of patients. Often the clean profile of an acceleration may be interrupted by a rapid deceleration that recovers quickly, giving the impression of having a "blunting" effect on the acceleration (Figure 12-8). On occasion, this response may appear in advanced first stage, and it may then be difficult to distinguish it from the classic *early* decelerations more often seen at this stage of labor (Figure 12-9). In the series at the Chicago Lying-In Hospital, this response has been seen to occur in coincidence with cord problems, including cord around the neck in about one-half of the cases, strongly suggesting a cause-and-effect

relationship. This finding has been so consistent that it is now considered an early sign of potential cord problem, and the patient is observed as such. For a discussion on the mechanism, see Chapter 15.

Regulation of FHR

As briefly mentioned in Chapter 3, the fetal cardiac muscle has an intrinsic rhythmicity set at variable rates depending on the anatomic area of the heart. The sinoatrial node seems to have the highest frequency of firing depolarization spikes: on the order of 140/min; the atrioventricular node is set at a lower frequency, and the myocardium at still an even lower rhythm. The rapid propagation over the entire heart of the excitation wave originated in the sinoatrial node predominates and sets the pace for the FHR. Moreover, there are numerous other factors that may influence the frequency with which the heart contracts; the most important of these are the sympathetic and parasympathetic nerves, which exert a direct *tonic effect* on the node, or serve as mediators of autonomic reflexes originated in distant parts of the fetal anatomy. From observations made in a variety of mammals, it seems irrefutable that by the middle of gestation some cardiovascular reflexes are already developed, making it possible to obtain responses with the administration of sympathomimetic and parasympathomimetic substances as well as their blockers.

The stimulation of the *sympathetic system* accelerates the heart rate and improves the force of the contraction by its chronotropic and bathmotropic effects. This activity may be effected continuously or in an intermittent or sporadic fashion. The continuous or tonic effect is demonstrated when blocking substances are injected and relative diminution of FHR frequency is obtained. Transient or *sporadic action* may be observed by stimulation of the adrenals or the direct injection of small amounts of epinephrine, which triggers tachycardia by its predominantly β-mimetic effect (Figure 12-10). A variety of baroreceptor- and chemoreceptor-mediated reflexes exert their influence via the sympathetic system (release of epinephrine and norepinephrine) and thereby affect the frequency of the heart rate.

The *parasympathetic system* stimulation tends to slow down the frequency of the heart rate

266

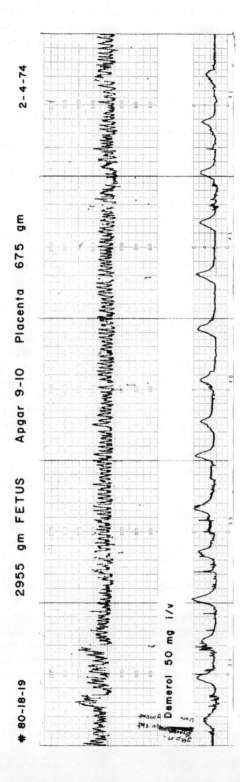

Figure 12-4 Fifty minutes of UC (external) and FHR (direct) recordings of elective induction at term. In early first stage the *rapid oscillations* of the FHR fluctuate within a *wide range of 12 to 20 beats* and recur at a rate of 2 to 4/min. They are not affected by the contractions, and the average baseline rate is 125 to 130. Incidentally, 50 mg meperidine IV to the mother did not affect the pattern of FHR for at least 45 min. An infant in good condition and a normal placenta were delivered. Reprinted from Cibils LA: Clinical significance of fetal heart rate patterns during labor. I. Baseline patterns. *Am J Obstet Gynecol* 125:290, 1976.

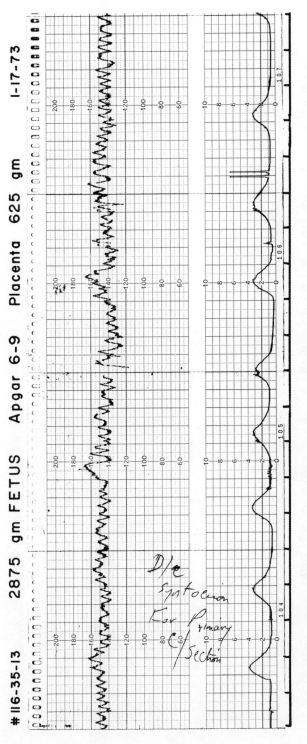

Figure 12-5 Twenty minutes of direct UC and FHR recordings of induced labor in term preeclamptic patient. The *normal rapid oscillations* look different because the paper speed is double (2 cm/min), the standard in the majority of tracings. However, they still recur 4 to 5 times/min and fluctuate within a range of 8 to 15 beats. Note that the UC curves also are more wide open because of the increased paper speed. A mildly depressed infant and normal placenta were delivered by cesarean section. Reprinted from Cibils LA: Clinical significance of fetal heart rate patterns during labor. I. Baseline patterns. *Am J Obstet Gynecol* 125:290, 1976.

268

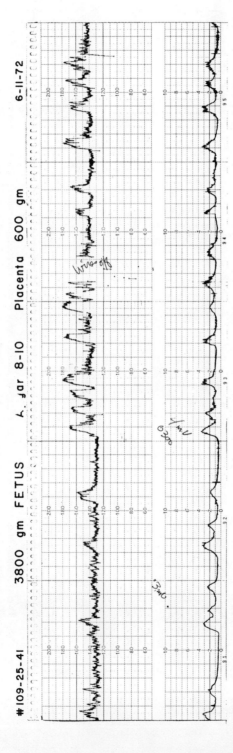

Figure 12-6 Fifty minutes of direct UC and FHR recordings of enhanced labor in primipara at term. Marked transient *accelerations of the FHR* start shortly before the strongest contractions reach their peak. The accelerations range from 18 to 45 beats and last between 25 and 45 sec. There are no other alterations of either the pattern or rate of baseline. A normal infant and placenta, without obvious cord problems, were subsequently delivered. Reprinted from Cibils LA: Clinical significance of fetal heart rate patterns during labor. I. Baseline patterns. *Am J Obstet Gynecol* 125:290, 1976.

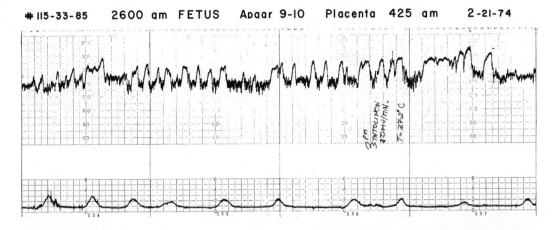

Figure 12-7 Forty minutes of direct UC and FHR recordings of induced labor in moderate preeclampsia at 37 weeks. Note the repetitive *transient accelerations* of the FHR on a normal baseline, completely unrelated to uterine contractions or fetal movements. They range from 15 to 35 beats and last 25 to 55 sec. A normal fetus and placenta were delivered vaginally. Reprinted from Cibils LA: Clinical significance of fetal heart rate patterns during labor. I. Baseline patterns. *Am J Obstet Gynecol* 125:290, 1976.

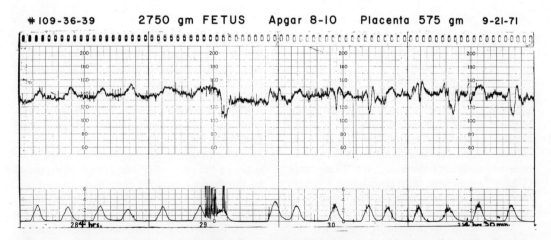

Figure 12-8 Forty minutes of direct UC and FHR recordings of enhanced labor in term normal pregnancy. *Transient accelerations* with the contractions are seen on the left one-third of the figure. On the right half, the *accelerations are interrupted* (or blunted) by rapid, sharp decelerations, which recover soon enough to meet the descending leg of the original acceleration. There are no changes in baseline pattern. A normal infant and placenta were eventually delivered vaginally. Reprinted from Cibils LA: Clinical significance of fetal heart rate patterns during labor. I. Baseline patterns. *Am J Obstet Gynecol* 125:290, 1976.

270

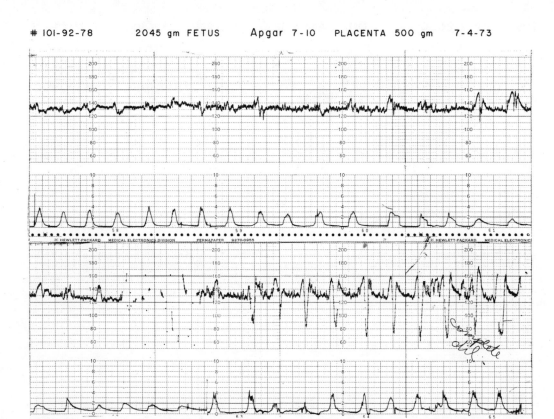

Figure 12-9 Continuous 80 min of direct UC and FHR recordings of induced labor in 35-week pregnancy with premature rupture of membranes. The small transient accelerations *(top)* increase in size as labor advances; when dilatation is almost complete, increasing, large decelerations blunt the accelerations *(bottom)*. Shortly after the end of the tracing a vigorous premature infant with one loop of cord around the neck was delivered. Reprinted from Cibils LA: Clinical significance of fetal heart rate patterns during labor. I. Baseline patterns. *Am J Obstet Gynecol* 125:290, 1976.

in the fetus, as it does in the adult. The *tonic effect* is clearly manifested when blocking its action by the administration of atropine which triggers a marked tachycardia (Figure 12-11). Likewise, its *sporadic action* is evidenced by the response to the injection of acetylcholine (the mediator when the vagus is stimulated) as an episode of rapid bradycardia. Due to the rapid action of acetylcholinesterase, the bradycardic effect of intermittent vagal stimulation is usually short, with a recovery as fast as the induction of the FHR deceleration.

The tonic action of both the sympathetic and parasympathetic systems has been studied in human fetuses by Hon and collaborators, and by Caldeyro-Barcia and co-workers. Both groups of investigators propose the concept that the FHR in pregnancy is the result of the interplay of the tonic

action of both autonomic systems, but exerted in a constantly "pulsating" action, the consequence being the rapid oscillations of the baseline observed in the last trimester of pregnancy—their presence has been taken as an indication of autonomic nervous system integrity and indirect evidence of good fetal condition.

The transient discharge of stimulation by either of the two autonomic systems is expressed by the predominance of their respective effects, which then override the tonic action of the other: bradycardia by the vagus, and tachycardia by the sympathetic. These circumstances may be precipitated by a variety of conditions, the most common ones being hypoxia, acidosis, hyperthermia, and fetal movements, which, in their turn, may stem from different situations: placental insufficiency, hypercontractility, hypotension, cord

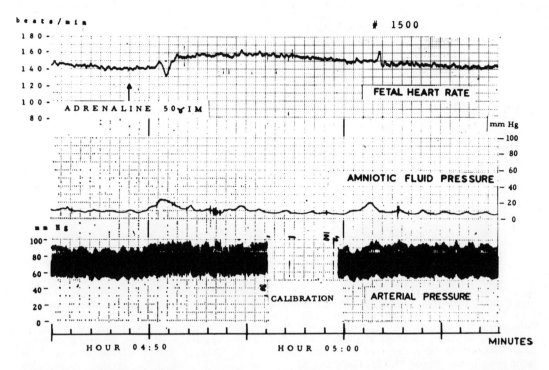

Figure 12-10 Fetal heart rate, intrauterine pressure, and maternal blood pressure recorded in prelabor of multipara at term. The direct *intrafetal* administration of 50 μg intramuscular adrenaline (arrow) was followed within 2 minutes of sustained tachycardia, which slowly subsided. The response was similar to that of an adult given an equivalent dose of adrenaline. Reprinted from Caldeyro-Barcia R, et al: Control of human fetal heart rate during labor, in Cassels, DE (ed): *The Heart and Circulation in the Newborn Infant*. New York, Grune & Stratton, 1966, pp 7–36. By permission.

compression, systemic infection, amnionitis, dehydration, prolonged maternal fasting and ketosis, or reflex movements. Only under particular situations of chronic or severe distress (see Chapter 16) will be autonomic nervous system not respond to stimuli that normally would cause rapid changes in FHR.

A number of pharmacologic preparations, without a specific action on the autonomic systems, have been reported to induce changes on the FHR pattern and its response to stimuli—presumed to be by their action on the CNS or the nuclei in the lower and midbrain. These substances would interfere with the normal reflex mechanisms that influence the effects of both tonic and transient action of the autonomic nervous system on the FHR and its baseline oscillations. The stimuli carried by the two systems most likely originate in the cardiovascular system (baroreceptors and chemoreceptors), the respiratory system (trachea, alveoli, pleura), the senses (auditory and tactile in particular), or the musculoskeletal system (sudden movements); they are integrated in the CNS before the effector component acts upon the sinoatrial node.

The myocardium is directly affected by the availability of oxygen as demonstrated by persistent episodes of bradycardia during periods of hypoxia, even on strongly atropinized fetuses (which obliterates the vagal influence). Likewise, carbon dioxide and other metabolites capable of affecting the hydrogen ion concentration of the blood may significantly influence the pattern of heart rate because of the effect of pH on the contractile properties of the myocardium. (For more details of FHR regulation, see Chapters 13, 14, and 15.)

ABNORMAL PATTERNS

Variations from the previously described FHR patterns must be considered abnormal until

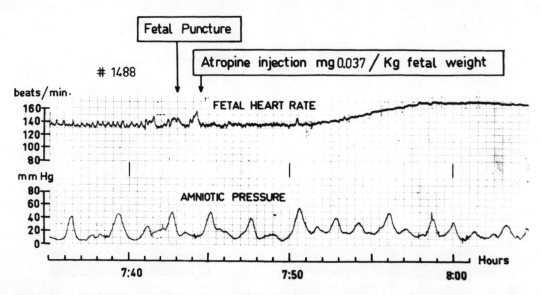

Figure 12-11 Fetal heart rate and intrauterine pressure recordings of multipara at term in spontaneous early first stage. The normal FHR baseline, with good rapid oscillations, was clearly altered by the *intrafetal injection* of atropine 9.15 mg. A progressively rising baseline, with disappearance of the rapid oscillations (fixed baseline) about 7 min after the administration of the drug, may be seen. An infant in very good condition was delivered 6 hours later, after enhancement of labor. Reprinted from Mendez-Bauer C, et al: Effects of atropine on human heart rate during labor. *Am J Obstet Gynecol* 85:1033, 1963.

proved otherwise. A good number are already known to be serious aberrations, indicating fetal distress of variable severity. The abnormalities may be observed on the *baseline* only, or may occur in conjunction with, or as a consequence of, *uterine contractions.* The last are slowings of the FHR and have been variously called *decelerations, dips,* or *periodic FHR changes.* The word deceleration will be adopted because of its graphically descriptive meaning without prejudging about the cause or pathophysiology of the change. Three distinctive patterns have been characterized as *early, late,* and *variable* decelerations, and each will be discussed in subsequent chapters. Their incidence during first stage among the total population of monitored patients with the fetus in the cephalic presentation is on the order of 20% for early decelerations, about 25% for variable decelerations, and slightly over 12% for late decelerations. About 45% of cases would progress through first stage without any deceleration. However, these incidences vary sharply if one groups the patients according to age of gestation: preterm fetuses having a disproportionate incidence of variable decelerations, almost 50% compared to the more advanced stages of gesta-

tion (Figure 12-12). Alterations of the baseline pattern and frequency may affect the rate or the oscillating fluctuations described in normal cases.

Baseline Changes

Any one, independently, or several of the characteristic elements of the normal FHR baseline pattern may change because of pathologic conditions or the effect of medications.

Fixed baseline Fixed baseline is characterized by the *absence of the normal rapid oscillations* or, if these are present, their fluctuation within a range of 4 beats or less (Figures 12-3 and 12-13). This alteration may be seen at the beginning of labor, or it may develop as signs of fetal distress appear in the tracing. On the other hand, it may appear as a transient observation during part of labor, or it may become a premanent pattern of the FHR tracing until labor has been completed. It has been called "absence of beat-to-beat variability" by Hon, and Hammacher labeled it "silent" baseline pattern. The cause of this change has not been clearly explained, but it has been observed that it frequently follows episodes of

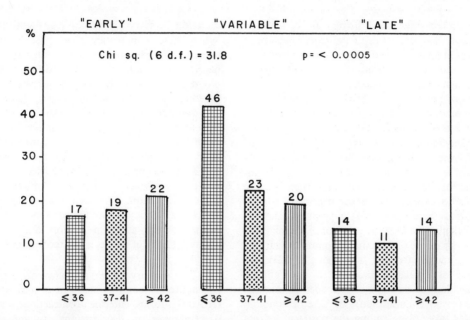

Figure 12-12 Incidence of *FHR decelerations* in the monitored high-risk population at the Chicago Lying-In Hospital, grouped according to age of gestation (preterm, term, and postterm). The proportion of preterm infants with variable decelerations predominates as the deceleration most often recorded. Reprinted from Cibils LA: Clinical significance of fetal heart rate patterns during labor. I. Baseline patterns. *Am J Obstet Gynecol* 125:290, 1976.

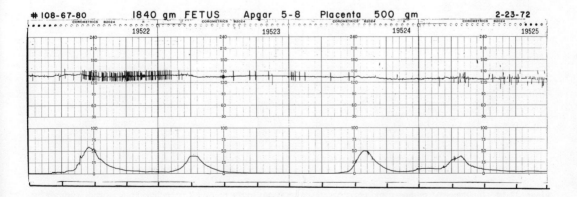

Figure 12-13 Sixteen minutes of direct UC and FHR recordings of enhanced labor in preeclamptic patient at 36 weeks gestation. A completely *fixed baseline* at 135 beats/min is not affected by the contractions. Less than 1 hour later, a mildly depressed, growth-retarded infant was delivered spontaneously. Reprinted from Cibils LA: Clinical significance of fetal heart rate patterns during labor. I. Baseline patterns. 125:290, 1976.

more or less severe fetal distress. In the Chicago Lying-In Hospital series of patients, it has been present in almost 40% of all postterm pregnancies at the start of monitoring (Figure 12-14), and it persists in a sustained manner in 35% of the same group of patients. It is clearly much more infrequent among the preterm fetuses, and rare within the group of chronological term infants.

The *mechanism* whereby this alteration of FHR baseline is triggered has not been clearly worked out. Nevertheless, knowledge of the influence of the autonomic nervous system over the regulation of the FHR makes it possible to surmise that there must be 1) a preponderance of sympathetic tone over the vagus or 2) a diminished sensitivity of the centers that integrate the various stimuli and control the fine tuning of FHR expressed as oscillating baseline. It may not be strange that the chronologic or sequential maturation (or overmaturation) of the autonomic reflexes takes place among the postterm infants who contribute a large proportion of those showing this pattern. Furthermore, a fixed baseline has been associated with a variety of abnormalities of FHR tracings, and it has been found in a very high proportion of infants born with some degree of moderate or severe depression (see Figure 14-36). When there is persistent fixed baseline in late labor, the Apgar scores are lower, suggesting fetal depression, a finding corroborated by lower cord blood pH in the same group of infants as compared to those with good baseline oscillations.

Saltatory pattern A saltatory pattern is present when the range of *rapid oscillations is more than 20 beats,* reaching on occasion up to 70 beats, although more often they range between 20 and 30. It was originally so called by Hammcher, and it is equivalent to the "marked variability" described by Hon. The rapid, sharp fluctuations are characteristic because the wide range that the tracing has to cover in a short time imposes pointed, clear-cut breaks in the recordings (Figure 12-15).

The saltatory pattern appears more often between uterine contractions, but it may also be recorded during uterine contractions, or be superimposed on decelerations. As far as the cause is concerned, some authors have ascribed the appearance of this pattern to episodes of transient hypoxia (Martin, 1978) or to partial cord compression (Hammacher, 1966, 1968). However, in the series at the Chicago Lying-In

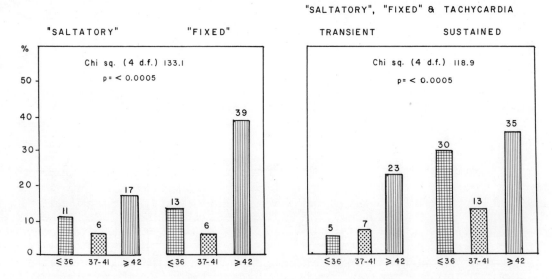

Figure 12-14 Incidence of *saltatory* and *fixed baseline* alterations in the high-risk population monitored, grouped by gestational age. *(Left)* Fixed and saltatory patterns are common among postterm patients. *(Right)* Incidence of three alterations occurring independently or simultaneously in the same groups. Incidence of transient changes and those that were sustained for the remainder of the recording. The latter were very high among preterm and postterm fetuses. Reprinted from Cibils LA: Clinical significance of fetal heart rate patterns during labor. I. Baseline patterns. *Am J Obstet Gynecol* 125:290, 1976.

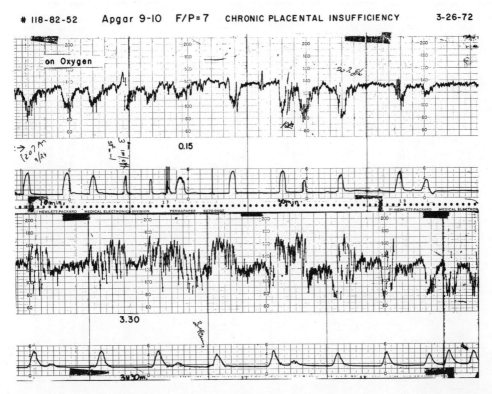

Figure 12-15 *(Above)* Forty minutes of direct UC and FHR recordings of spontaneous early labor at term with meconium-stained amniotic fluid during oxygen administration by mask. Normal oscillating baseline is interrupted by variable decelerations triggered by contractions. *(Below)* Three hours later, good contractions every 5 min and FHR with *prominent saltatory pattern* superimposed on a general pattern of decelerations with contractions. For moderate fetal distress of unknown cause early in first stage, cesarean section was performed, with delivery of a slightly growth-retarded infant in good condition, and small placenta. The F/P ratio of 7 suggests chronic placental insufficiency, a probable explanation for the FHR alterations. Reprinted from Cibils LA: Clinical significance of fetal heart rate patterns during labor. II. Late decelerations. *Am J Obstet Gynecol* 123:473, 1975.

Hospital, the pattern has been observed in a variety of circumstances, some with hypoxia or partial cord compression but more often when there was no evidence of either. A striking observation was the high incidence of almost 20% among the postterm pregnancies, and the lesser incidence among the fetuses of younger age (Figure 12-14). It was observed, in association with a fixed baseline and other alterations, in over 50% of those postterm infants either transiently or in a sustained manner. Surprisingly, it was observed to occur in the same patients in whom a fixed baseline was recorded, even alternating from one to the other in a pendular fashion (Figure 12-16).

The *mechanism* responsible for this alteration is not clear. Nevertheless, it may be reasonable to assume that a strong *pulsating vagal effect* must be triggering it in part. The rapid oscillations would speak for a predominantly vagal action, suggesting that the sympathetic system may be secondary. Furthermore, as seen for the fixed baseline, it is *predominantly observed among the postterm fetuses* (and almost absent among the preterms) allowing one to postulate the probability that chronologic maturation of the nervous system and/or enzymatic mechanisms may be preconditions for this type of FHR response to be triggered by certain stressful situations.

It is important to pay close attention to the ranges within which the FHR is recorded, and to the paper speed of the tracing, to make an

276

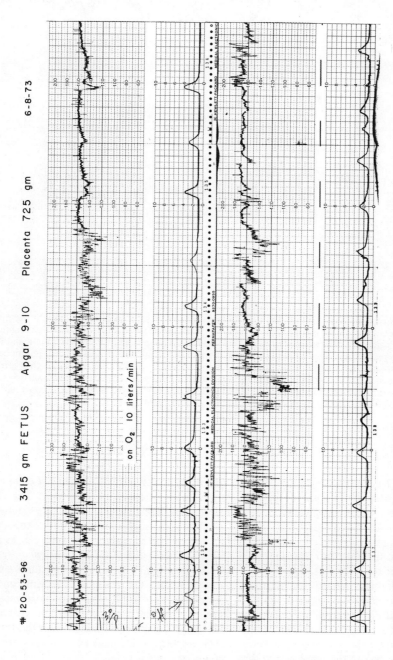

Figure 12-16 Continuous 100 minutes of direct UC and FHR recordings of enhanced labor in middle first stage of 42-week pregnancy. *(Above)* Continuous oxygen administration by mask and short *bursts of saltatory pattern* coinciding with the peak of the contractions. Suddenly, the baseline became fixed *(right)* with minimal decelerations. *(Below)* Baseline was interrupted by a burst of marked saltatory pattern and late decelerations. This again suddenly changed to *fixed baseline* with late decelerations and short episodes of saltatory patterns. By cesarean section a vigorous infant and normal placenta were obtained. Reprinted from Cibils LA: Clinical significance of fetal heart rate patterns during labor. I. Baseline patterns. *Am J Obstet Gynecol* 125:290, 1976.

accurate reading and diagnosis. Figure 12-17 illustrates the *unequal visual aspects of the baseline patterns,* recorded by different monitors, which would cause misinterpretation unless carefully analyzed.

Tachycardia

A regular FHR frequency over 150 beats/min between contractions constitutes tachycardia. Although it is often taught that the normal FHR in preterm gestations is above 150, this statement has not been the observation at the Chicago Lying-In Hospital. In fact, an FHR above 150 is a rarity in the absence of pathologic circumstances, either maternal or fetal. In the total high-risk population studied, it was present at the begin-

ning of monitoring in a significantly higher proportion among preterm fetuses than among the group of term or postterm, but not nearly in so predominant a proportion (Figure 12-18).

The *etiology* of fetal tachycardia is observed in a great variety of circumstances, and it may occur as a transient episode or in a sustained manner, depending on the severity or continuous action of the cause. Tachycardia usually develops as labor progresses in the group of pathologic pregnancies, significantly increasing its incidence among gestations of all ages (Figure 12-18). It is particularly frequent among preterm and postterm gestations, in which cases it may be associated with late decelerations and other baseline alterations (Figure 12-16). Rarely, it may not be possible to ascertain an associated pathologic condition, in which case it must be labeled idiopathic

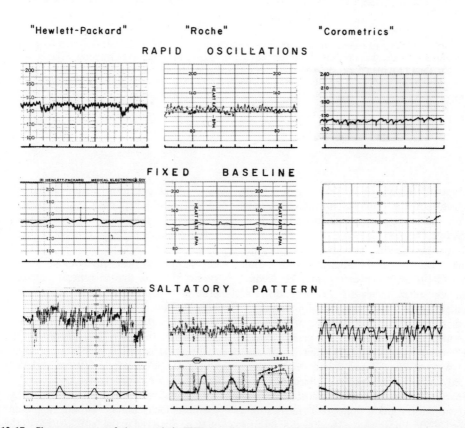

Figure 12-17 Short segments of characteristic FHR baseline patterns obtained with three makes of monitors to illustrate the variable aspects of the same pattern, depending on the range of recordings and the speed at which the paper is run. All have the same range of UC. The Hewlett-Packard and Roche models have the same speed but the FHR range is much more compressed in the latter, giving smaller looking deflections for equivalent changes. Roche and Corometrics models have the same ranges, but the faster paper speed in the latter opens up the tracings, changing the visual image.

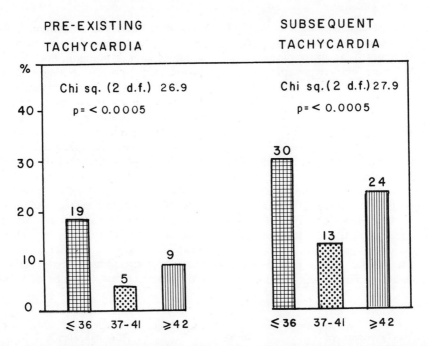

PRE-EXISTING
TACHYCARDIA

SUBSEQUENT
TACHYCARDIA

Figure 12-18 Incidence of baseline tachycardia in the high-risk population monitored, grouped by gestational age. *(Left)* Tachycardia present at the time of starting the record. *(Right)* Incidence of tachycardia as labor progressed indicates that the postterm fetuses developed it proportionally in highest numbers. The preterms, although more numerous at the beginning, did develop subsequent tachycardia in lesser proportion. Reprinted from Cibils LA: Clinical significance of fetal heart rate patterns during labor. I. Baseline patterns. *Am J Obstet Gynecol* 125:290, 1976.

or "essential" (Figure 12-2). Very often, a transient tachycardia is observed following episodes of hypercontractility that trigger periods of fetal distress (see Chapter 14).

Hyperthermia must be considered among the common causes of intrapartum tachycardia (Figure 12-19), in which case it may be accompanied by other indicators of fetal distress, particularly when there are signs of amniotic infection. Nevertheless, hyperthermia of unknown source may trigger relatively long periods of extremely severe tachycardia (Figures 12-20 and 12-21) without superimposed late decelerations and only transient moments of fixed baseline. Moreover, these cases respond satisfactorily to treatment with routine antipyretic medications (Figure 12-22) with which the baseline rate returns to normal values and the pattern of baseline alterations disappears. On other occasions the hyperthermia may induce tachycardia of extraordinary proportions and still the fetus may be born

in excellent condition (Figure 12-23) after rapid intervention. These cases indicate that, unlike in animals (Morishima, 1975) maternal hyperthermia alone does not appear to lead to fetal distress and acidosis.

In spite of these observations, there seems to be no question that in general tachycardia constitutes a sign of fetal distress. From clinical observations in the premonitoring era to current studies undertaken with continuous monitors, the association of acute fetal distress episodes and tachycardia has been well established. Likewise, states of chronic fetal distress and tachycardia have been well documented.

These well-recognized facts notwithstanding, extreme tachycardias without apparent causes may be observed in the fetus in utero as they are in the adult. *Paroxysmal atrial tachycardia* has been recorded and reported in humans (Figure 12-24) and of course may create a difficult dilemma for the clinician observing this unusual condition.

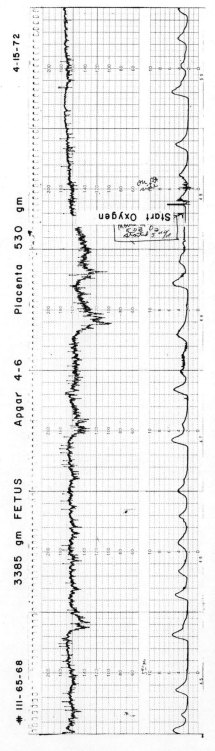

Figure 12-19 Sixty minutes of direct UC and FHR recordings of enhanced labor at 42 weeks gestation, patient with premature rupture of membranes. Advanced first stage, 39 C *temperature*. *Tachycardia* and a *few late decelerations*. The administration of oxygen by mask was followed by disappearance of the late decelerations and persistence of fixed baseline. A depressed infant was born by low forceps 2 hours later.

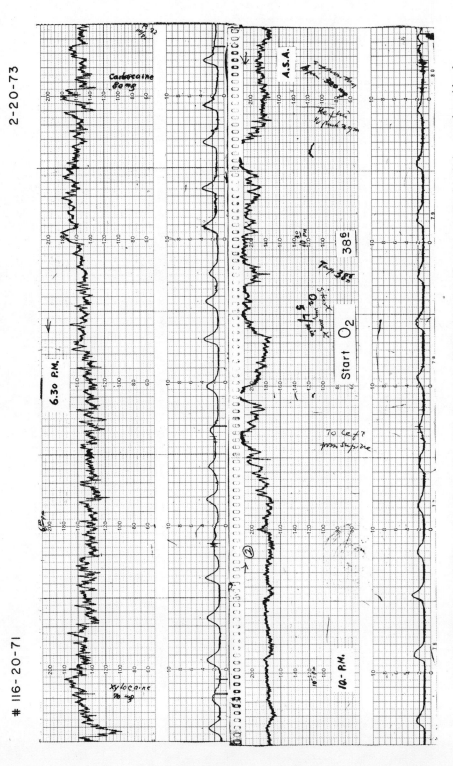

Figure 12-20 Direct UC and FHR tracings obtained in middle first stage of induced labor at 42 weeks gestation in primipara under epidural anesthesia. *(Above)* Fifty minutes recording of normal tachycardia with rapid oscillations and a brief period of transient tachycardia. *(Below)* Three hours later, an established *tachycardia with fixed baseline*, with brief periods above 200 beats/min. Because there was no obvious reason for her hyperthermia of 38.6 C, the patient was given continuous oxygen by mask and acetylsalicylic acid 300 mg.

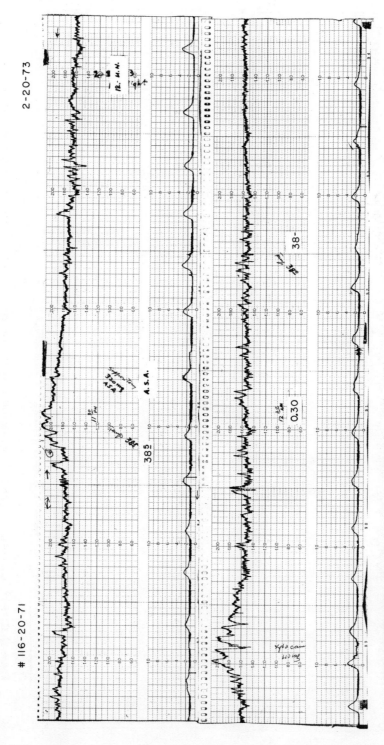

Figure 12-21 Same case as Figure 12-20, 30 min later. Two hours of continuous tracing illustrating the effect of an additional dose of 320 mg acetylsalicylic acid. The temperature decreases slowly and, parallel with it, the heart rate slowed down to around upper limits of normal and *regained some oscillation of the baseline,* lost during periods of severe tachycardia.

282

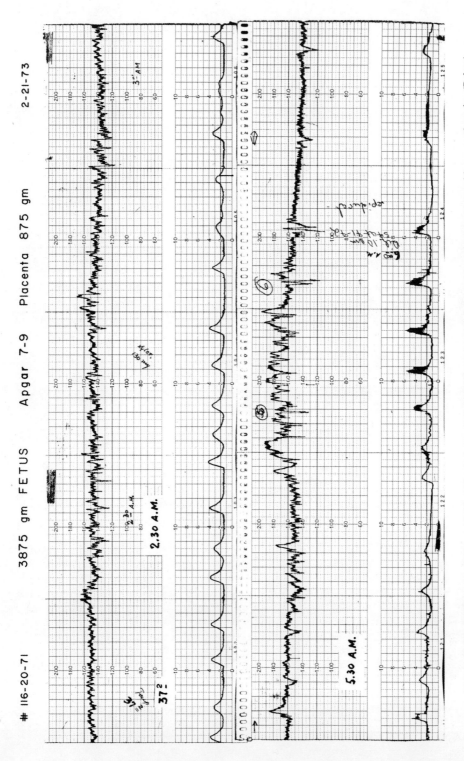

Figure 12-22 Same case as Figure 12-21, 150 min later. *(Above)* Fifty minutes of normal heart rate pattern with normothermia. *(Below)* With complete dilation 2½ hours later, FHR was normal, altered only by the patient's bearing down efforts (tachycardia and saltatory pattern). An infant in good condition was delivered by low forceps 30 min later.

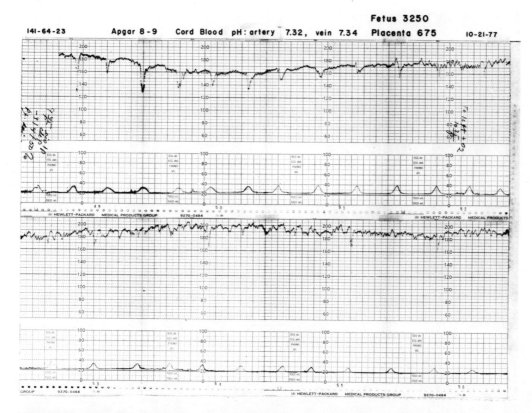

Figure 12-23 Direct UC and FHR tracings from term multipara in early induced labor for premature rupture of membranes. Moderate *hyperthermia* of 38.2 C and *severe tachycardia* steadily rising up to over 200 beats/min. In spite of it, the baseline oscillations were still present. Because the patient did not respond to antipyretics, she had a cesarean section 90 min later, with delivery of a 3250 gm infant, Apgar 8-9. The umbilical cord blood pH was 7.32 in the artery and 7.34 in the vein.

The *mechanism* of production seems to be the preponderance of the tonic sympathetic stimulation over the vagus, triggered by a series of homeostatic alterations affecting the baroreceptors and chemoreceptors. The release of epinephrine would then be ultimately responsible for the increased heart rate. This same set of circumstances may explain the higher proportion of preterm cases having tachycardia because it is believed that they have a lower vagal tonus than at term or past term. However, the proportion of cases becoming tachycardic during labor is higher in the postterm group, suggesting either mediation by a different mechanism in this group, or a diminished ability to withstand the action of those extraneous factors without significant change (Figure 12-18).

Bradycardia

The sustained *FHR under 120 beats/min* has been defined, by general agreement, as below the normal, and thus accepted as the threshold of bradycardia. Some authors have defined degrees of severity according to specific lower ranges: below 100 beats/min or below 80 beats/min. It probably represents a good way to study the pathophysiology of what controls it. However, it is difficult to assess the various elements that may trigger it in the human because too few cases are allowed to have sustained bradycardias without active intervention from the observers to correct it. Unlike tachycardias, the number of sustained bradycardias studied for any length of time is very limited.

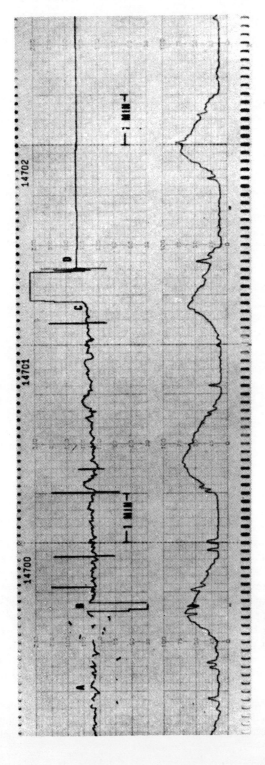

Figure 12-24 External UC recording of term primipara early in labor. *(A)* Indirect FHR tracing. *(B)* Direct electrode was applied and a good normal pattern was obtained. *(C)* An abrupt, *extreme tachycardia* started. *(D)* Because of the electronic setup, the monitor recorded alternate fetal heartbeats, ascertained by auscultation done by three separate observers. After several maneuvers and continuous oxygen by mask without improvement, the patient underwent cesarean section. A 2660 gm infant (Apgar 9–10) and normal placenta were obtained; there was fresh meconium in the amniotic fluid. The neonate had several episodes of abrupt supraventricular tachycardia (to 240 beats/min) which ceased spontaneously. Final diagnosis was paroxysmal atrial tachycardia. Reprinted from Hughey M, Elesh R: Profound atrial tachycardia. *Am J Obstet Gynecol* 128:463, 1977.

The *etiology* of this alteration has been identified, by convention and clinical observations, with circumstances leading to severe fetal distress. Exceptionally a nonaffected fetus will have a heart rate of less than 120 beats/min, and reveal no congenital malformation at birth (see Figure 12-3). When these rates are recorded, they are never in the severe bradycardia range of less than 100 beats/min. The most frequent cause of sustained bradycardia has been observed to be triggered by episodes of *hypercontractility, either spontaneous or induced,* and in both situations it may be preceded and/or followed by other abnormalities of the FHR tracing. The hypercontractility may be sudden and acute, triggered at the start of an oxytocin infusion by the injection of an ex-

cessive amount of the hormone (Figure 12-25; see also Figure 9-12). The recovery is usually complete and rapid as soon as the excessive uterine activity has been corrected.

The general rule is that those relatively short episodes of bradycardia are followed by an FHR higher than that which preceded it (thus called *rebound tachycardia)* and late decelerations of decreasing severity. Not uncommonly, during improperly supervised induction or stimulations of labor, the oxytocin infusion, satisfactory for middle of first stage, becomes exaggerated as dilatation progresses, and with it a *slowly* established iatrogenic hypercontractility. One may then observe alterations of the FHR pattern and progressively worsening bradycardia (Figure

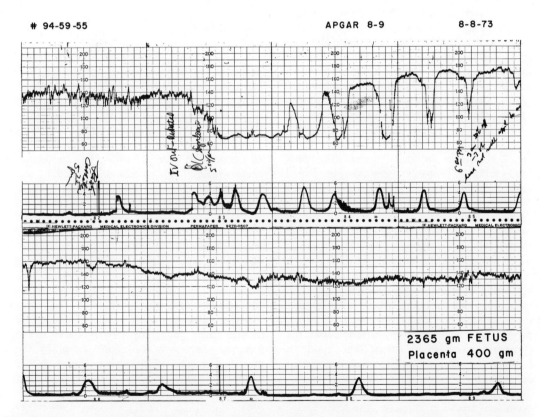

Figure 12-25 Continuous 80 min of direct UC and FHR recordings in early part of induced labor at 34 weeks gestation for premature rupture of membranes. *(Above)* Oxytocin infusion, interrupted, was restarted, at unspecified rate. The brief but marked *hypercontractility with hypertonus* that was triggered produced a short, *sudden bradycardia* lasting over 5 min followed by severe *late decelerations* and slowly rising baseline. This became *fixed with rebound tachycardia. (Below)* Abnormalities slowly subsided as the contractions spaced and reached normal values 40 min after the original insult. A normal infant and placenta with small abruptio were delivered 5 hours later. Reprinted from Cibils LA: Clinical significance of fetal heart rate patterns during labor. II. Late decelerations. *Am J Obstet Gynecol* 123:473, 1975.

12-26). A similar effect, although probably due to another pathophysiologic mechanism, may be seen *after the administration of a paracervical block* (Figure 12-27), also compounded by associated alterations of the FHR. Less often the excessive uterine activity is *apparently spontaneous,* that is without extraneous intervention, but the explanation for the subsequent bradycardia may not only be the increased contractility but other associated pathologic conditions such as *abruptio placentae* (see Figure 6-9). A predictable sudden increase in uterine activity is, almost always, triggered by an *eclamptic seizure;* the oxytocic effect of large amounts of norepinephrine released into the bloodstream produce polysystoly and hypertonus, and with these a sustained fetal bradycardia is usually observed (Figure 12-28). The recovery period is followed by rebound tachycardia.

However, on other occasions the hypercontractility may be genuinely without identifiable cause, thus *idiopathic,* but nonetheless the fetal reaction is very real (see Figure 6-14). Unrelated to uterine contractility changes, episodes of *hypotension* predictably lead to fetal bradycardia. Usually these are consequences of either sudden blood loss or, more often, of exaggerated reaction to conduction or general anesthesia (see Chapter 18).

The *mechanism* that controls the fetal bradycardia is probably complex. The strong vagal effect (baroreceptor reflex), triggered by the fetal hypertension that follows the *hypoxic episodes* produced by hypercontractility and/or maternal hypotension, overshadows the sympathetic (chemoreceptor reflex) response to hypoxia, which would tend to induce tachycardia as it releases epinephrine. This hormone in small amounts will produce only tachycardia, but in large quantities it triggers hypertension because then its α-mimetic vasoconstrictive effect predominates on the peripheral arterioles over the β-mimetic vasodilating action. The result is hypertension and bradycardia, which may persist as long as the triggering causes are not corrected. When these are adequately treated, and better oxygenation tends to diminish the epinephrine release, the β-mimetic effect then predominates with a rebound tachycardia followed by a slow return to normal baseline frequency (Figure 12-25). On the other hand, hypoxia of severe degree affects the myocardium, contributing to further bradycardia suggesting a direct effect on the heart. When one observes this situation, it is quite probable that the fetal cardiovascular adaptation deteriorates, with hypotension as a result of a weakened myocardial function. The persistence of the insult inevitably leads to progressive alteration of fetal homeostasis and acidosis.

Alterations of the FHR baseline are rarely seen as isolated phenomena. They are usually associated, and as a matter of fact, are superimposed on decelerations triggered by the contractions. The association of the baseline alterations in the Chicago Lying-In Hospital high-risk population has been shown to be exceedingly high among the preterm and postterm fetuses in labor (see Figure 12-14) who showed these changes to appear and persist until delivery in one-third of them.

Sinusoidal Pattern

A distinct pattern of baseline oscillations was described by Manseau and co-workers (1972) as being observed predominantly among severely affected erythroblastotic infants in the third trimester of gestation, shortly before death. It consists of an *extremely regular undulating trace* fluctuating within a range of 5 to 15 beats recurring every 15 to 30 seconds (Figure 12-29). The outstanding characteristic of this pattern is its regularity and smooth, rounded profile lacking the sharp break so typical of the normal baseline oscillations. It has also been recorded in late second, as well as early third, trimester of pregnancy in erythroblastotic fetuses (Figure 12-30). A similar pattern has been observed by other investigators in fetuses free from Rh disease but in situations of extreme distress, suggesting that it may not be peculiar to erythroblastosis-affected fetuses.

The *cause,* as mentioned, was originally thought to be characteristically produced in the preterm, *severe erythroblastotic infant* by the preagonal changes which must take place before intrauterine death. However, others have recorded comparable tracings in *postterm fetuses shortly before death* (Figure 12-31), an observation subsequently confirmed by others (see Figures 16-1 and 16-12). There is a difference, however, between these two groups of tracings: the range of undulation is much wider (15 to 30 beats) and the duration of the cycle longer (25 to 50 sec) than in erythroblastotic infants, overall similar to the one

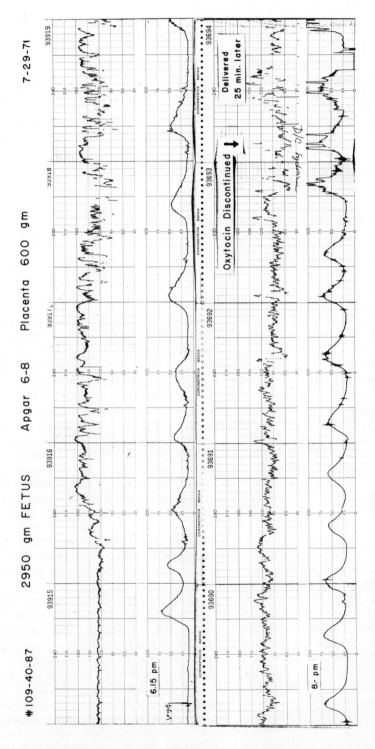

Figure 12-26 Direct UC and FHR recordings of term enhanced labor for uterine inertia. *(Above)* Twenty minutes of borderline high uterine contractility obtained with 2 mU/min oxytocin and the following alterations of FHR: the normal pattern changed to tachycardia and saltatory pattern. *(Below)* Obtained 90 min later with 5 mU/min oxytocin illustrates *uterine polysystoly, fetal bradycardia,* and small decelerations ending in saltatory pattern in advanced first stage (paper speed, 3 cm/min). A mildly depressed fetus was delivered 25 min later. Reprinted from Cibils LA: Clinical significance of fetal heart rate patterns during labor. II. Late decelerations. *Am J Obstet Gynecol* 123:473, 1975.

288

FETUS 2875 gm   PLACENTA 525 gm   APGAR 6-9

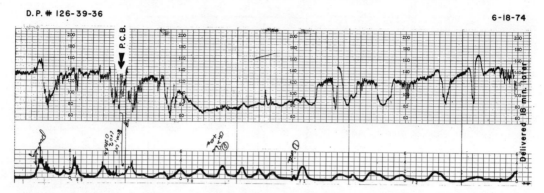

Figure 12-27 Forty-five minutes of direct UC and FHR recordings of advanced spontaneous labor in term primipara. Three and one half minutes after a paracervical block the normal FHR dropped rapidly and a *bradycardia* lasting 12 min was recorded. Simultaneously there was *fixed baseline,* and with slow recovery *late decelerations* were recorded. The slightly increased contractility pattern started 5 min after the bradycardia. A mildly depressed infant was delivered 18 min after the end of the tracing.

case observed by Manseau and collaborators in the only fetus free from Rh disease in their original description.

As far as the *mechanism* of production is concerned, one may not even speculate because there are very few good observations made, and these only in preterminal fetuses. It has not been recorded from laboratory animals commonly used to study the fetus at term and during labor. The only positive thing that may be said is that when it is observed in fetuses, either erythroblastotic or postterm, it has very serious prognostic significance in spite of the few survivals observed after recording this pattern (Figure 12-30).

Arrhythmias

Some very irregular baseline patterns may be exact replicas of the arrhythmias observed in the adult and, theoretically, they may cover the complete range of them. In fact, prenatal arrhythmias are extremely rare indeed, and, unlike the adult arrhythmias, they almost always are devoid of severe pathologic implications. They have been recorded intermittently during labor, to disappear rapidly in the neonatal period. Rarely they may be manifestations of severe disease in which case they are often associated with congenital malformations (Figure 12-32).

A complete *heart block* may be the cause of severe sustained bradycardia that may induce the

clinician to rapid intervention, thinking that he may be dealing with severe fetal distress. When these rare cases are observed, they tend to persist in the neonatal life (Figure 12-33) when the ECG may confirm the conduction defect.

Their causes are as protean as for the adults, and thus the mechanism of production as well. The recording of prenatal arrhythmias requires that the pickup of signals be almost perfect, preferably by ECG either external or direct. Moreover, the processing apparatus needs to have the capability for beat-to-beat recording because those averaging the signals, by their very nature, lose the possibility of discerning between real pathology and artifacts. Ausculation with a stethoscope or a portable Doppler gauge, simultaneously with the signal displayed on the screen of the oscilloscope, should help to make a definitive diagnosis by ruling out the recording of artifacts.

The majority of the baseline alterations described tend to occur in association or alternating with one another, thus indicating that perhaps they may constitute varying degrees of fetal response to stressful conditions either chronic or acute. Also, one must pay special attention to the gestational age of a given pregnancy when making interpretations of FHR tracings. It has been shown that fetuses of disparate ages react in very different ways to seemingly equivalent clinical conditions leading to severe distress or death.

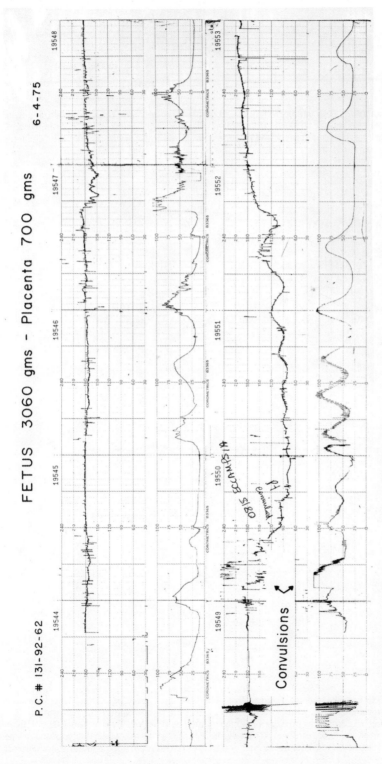

Figure 12-28 Continuous 40 min of direct UC and FHR recording of postterm spontaneous labor in advanced first stage (8 cm). *(Above)* Tachycardia and fixed baseline. *(Below)* An eclamptic convulsion pushed the intrauterine pressure off the scale. This was followed by a severe hypertonus and polysystoly lasting 10 min. Simultaneously the FHR dropped to a sustained *bradycardia* that lasted 10 min, with recovery and *rebound tachycardia*. An infant with Apgar scores 7–9 was delivered by forceps 57 min after the end of the tracings.

290

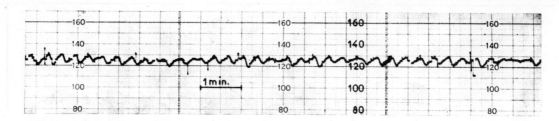

Figure 12-29 Twelve minutes of FHR monitoring obtained with indirect methods from a multipara with severe Rh incompatibility at 33 weeks gestation. The FHR fluctuates regularly within a range of 10 beats in cycles repeating every 20 sec. The smooth rounded profile suggested that the authors call this a *sinusoidal pattern*. The fetus died in utero the following day. Reprinted from Manseau, et al (1972).

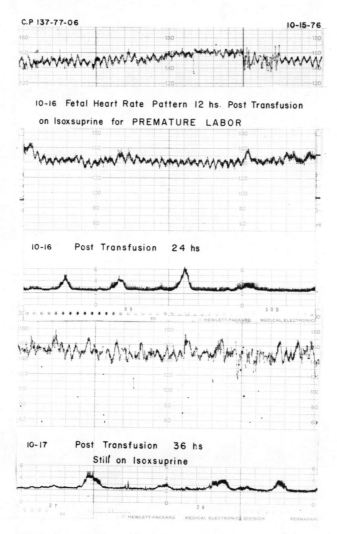

Figure 12-30 External FHR and UC tracings obtained from a severe Rh sensitized patient at 31 weeks gestation *after the fetus was given an intrauterine transfusion. (A)* Sinusoidal pattern 12 hours after the transfusion. Because of premature labor the patient was receiving isoxsuprine 30 μg/min at the time. *(B)* Twelve hours later still *sinusoidal pattern* of 3 cycles/min and about 10 beats range. *(C)* Twelve hours later, somewhat larger cycles of the still persistent sinusoidal pattern. The patient was induced 4 weeks later and an affected infant in good condition, weighing 2840 gm, was delivered.

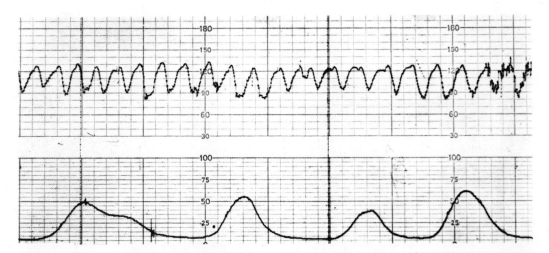

Figure 12-31 Direct UC and FHR tracings obtained from a primipara at 43 weeks in spontaneous labor (meconium-stained amniotic fluid). The regular oscillations cycle, 2.5 times/min within a range of 30 to 35 beats, unaffected by attempts at correction, are a classic *sinusoidal pattern*. Cesarean section produced 25 minutes later a 4080 gm fetus, Apgar 0, who had aspirated thick meconium. Reprinted from Baskett TF, Koh KS: Sinsoidal fetal heart pattern. A sign of fetal hypoxia. *Am J Obstet Gynecol* 44:379, 1974.

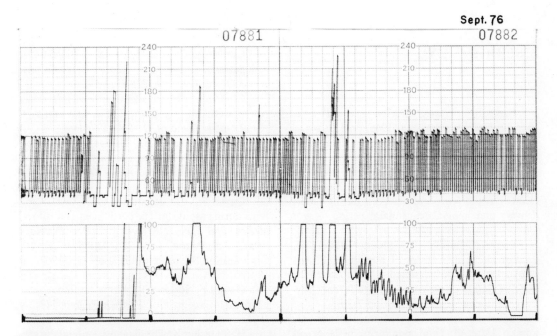

Figure 12-32 Direct FHR and UC recordings obtained in early second stage following premature labor for rupture of the membranes. The regularly alternating FHR tracing, between 45 and 115, indicates an alternating *heart block* that persisted throughout the monitoring. A severely malformed infant with Potter's syndrome was born shortly thereafter and died neonatally (paper speed, 3 cm sec). Courtesy H. Schulman.

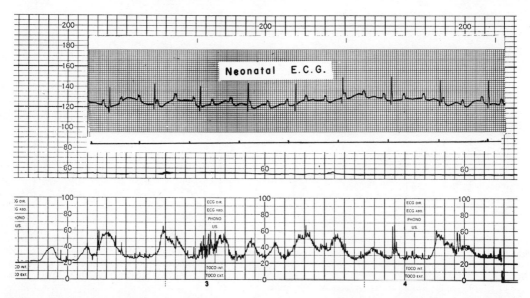

Figure 12-33 External monitoring (25 min) of early spontaneous labor of primipara at term. The advanced prelabor-like contractility *(bottom)* does not explain the severe *bradycardia* of 55 beats/min with completely *fixed baseline* observed in top tracing (regular paper speed, 1 cm/min). The emergency cesarean section produced a grossly normal infant with Apgar 8-9. The neonatal ECG (inset, top) documented complete heart block (marked indicates seconds). Courtesy A. Mejia.

BIBLIOGRAPHY

Barcroft J: *Researches on Prenatal Life,* chap 12. Oxford, Blackwell, 1946, pp 123–144.

Baskett TF, Koh KS: Sinusoidal fetal heart pattern. A sign of fetal hypoxia. *Obstet Gynecol* 44:379, 1974.

Brady JP, James LS, Baker MA: Heart rate changes in the fetus and newborn during labor, delivery and immediate neonatal period. *Am J Obstet Gynecol* 84:1, 1962.

Caldeyro-Barcia R, Mendez-Bauer C, Poseiro JJ, et al: Control of human fetal heart rate during labor, in Cassels DE (ed): *The Heart and Circulation of the Newborn and Infant.* New York, Grune & Stratton, 1966, pp 7–36.

Caldeyro-Barcia R, Mendez-Bauer C, Poseiro JJ, et al: Fetal monitoring in labor, in Wallace HM, Gold EM, Lis EF (eds): *Maternal and Child Health Practices.* Springfield, Ill, Thomas, 1973, pp 332–394.

Cibils LA: Clinical significance of fetal heart rate patterns during labor. II. Late decelerations. *Am J Obstet Gynecol* 123:473, 1975.

Cibils LA: Clinical significance of fetal heart rate patterns during labor. I. Baseline patterns. *Am J Obstet Gynecol* 125:290, 1976.

Cohn HE, Sacks EJ, Heymann AM, et al: Cardiovascular responses to hypoxemia and academia in fetal lambs. *Am J Obstet Gynecol* 120:817, 1974.

Dawes FS: Cardiovascular adjustment of the fetus during asphyxia: The aortic chemoreceptors, in *Perinatal Factors Affecting Human Development.* Washington, DC, Pan American Health Organization Scientific Publication 185, 1969, pp 199–201.

Goupil F, Sureau C: Rythme cardiaque fetal pendant la grossesse. *J Parisien Pediatr* 118:27, 1975.

Hammacher K: The diagnosis of fetal distress with an electronic fetal heart monitor, in *Intrauterine Dangers to the Fetus.* Amsterdam, Excerpta Medica, 1966, pp 228–233.

Hammacher K: The clinical significance of cardiotocography, in Huntingford PJ, Huter KA, Saling E (eds): *Perinatal Medicine*. New York Academic, 1969, pp 80–93.

Hammacher K, Huter KA, Bokelmann J, et al: Foetal heart frequency and perinatal conditions of the fetus and newborn. *Gynecologia* 166:349, 1968.

Hon EH: Electronic evaluation of the fetal heart rate. *Am J Obstet Gynecol* 83:333, 1962.

Hon EH: The classification of fetal heart rate. *Obstet Gynecol* 22:137, 1963.

Hon EH, Quilligan EJ: The classification of fetal heart rate. *Conn Med* 31:779, 1967.

Hughey M, Elesh R: Profound atrial tachycardia. *Am J Obstet Gynecol* 128:463, 1977.

Joelsson I, Westin B: Fetal heart rate during the third trimester of toxemic pregnancy and fetal distress before the onset of labor. *Acta Obstet Gynecol Scand* 43:338, 1964.

Kubli FW, Hon EH, Khazin AF, et al: Observations on the heart rate and pH on the human fetus during labor. *Am J Obstet Gynecol* 104:1190, 1969.

Lee CY, DiLoreto PC, O'Lane JM: A study of fetal heart rate acceleration patterns. *Obstet Gynecol* 45:142, 1975.

Low JA, Boston RW, Pancham SR: The role of fetal heart rate patterns in the recognition of fetal asphyxia with metabolic acidosis. *Am J Obstet Gynecol* 109:922, 1971.

Manseau P, Vaquier J, Chavinie J, et al: Le rythme cardiaque fetal "sinusoidal." *J Gynecol Obstet Biol Reprod (Paris)* 1:343, 1972.

Martin CB: Regulation of the fetal heart rate and genesis of FHR patterns. *Semin Perinatol* 2:131, 1978.

Martin CB, Siassi B, Hon EH: Fetal heart rate patterns and neonatal death in low birth-weight infants. *Obstet Gynecol* 44:503, 1974.

Mendez-Bauer C, Poseiro JJ, Arellano G, et al: Effects of atropine on the human heart rate during labor. *Am J Obstet Gynecol* 85:1033, 1963.

Mendez-Bauer C, Arnt IC, Gulin L, et al: Relationship between blood pH and heart rate in the human fetus during labor. *Am J Obstet Gynecol* 97:530, 1967.

Morishima HO, Glaser B, Niemann WH, et al: Increased uterine activity and fetal deterioration during maternal hyperthermia. *Am J Obstet Gynecol* 121:531, 1975.

Paul RH, Hon EH: Clinical fetal monitoring. V. Effect on perinatal outcome. *Am J Obstet Gynecol* 118:529, 1974.

Paul RH, Suidan AK, Yeh SY, et al: Clinical fetal monitoring. VII. The evaluation and significance of intrapartum baseline FHR variability. *Am J Obstet Gynecol* 123:206, 1975.

Quilligan EJ, Katigbak E, Hofschild J: Correlation of fetal heart rate patterns and blood gas values. II. Bradycardia. *Am J Obstet Gynecol* 91:1123, 1965.

Renou P, Newman NW, Wood C: Autonomic control of fetal heart rate. *Am J Obstet Gynecol* 105:949, 1969.

Saling E, Schneider D: Biochemical supervision of the fetus during labor. *J Obstet Gynecol Br Comwlth* 74:799, 1967.

Schifferli PY, Caldeyro-Barcia R: Effects of atropine and β adrenergic drugs on the heart of the human fetus, in Boreus L (ed): *Fetal Pharmacology*. New York, Raven, 1973, pp 259–278.

Shenker L: Effects of isoxsuprine on fetal heart rate and fetal electrocardiogram. *Obstet Gynecol* 26:104, 1965.

Swartwout JR, Campbell WE, Williams LG: Observations on the fetal heart rate. *Am J Obstet Gynecol* 82:301, 1961.

Vapaavouri EK, Shinebourne EA, Williams RL, et al: Development of cardiovascular responses to autonomic blockade in intact fetal and neonatal lambs. *Biol Neonate* 22:177, 1973.

CHAPTER 13
Early Decelerations

The *rapid slowdown of the FHR tracing* occurring simultaneously with a uterine contraction followed by an equally rapid recovery after an instantaneous low point is called early deceleration of the FHR. It has also been called *dip I* or *cephalic dip*. The time relationship between the intrauterine pressure changes and the fall in FHR is crucial to properly classify an alteration manifested as deceleration below the baseline of an otherwise normal looking tracing. The descending arm of the FHR coincides synchronically with the ascending part of the UC tracing, and its lowest point corresponds with the peak of the contraction (Figure 13-1). Following this moment, as the uterus relaxes and the intrauterine pressure falls, there is a rapid recovery of the FHR toward the baseline. The complete cycle of deceleration acquires the shape of a sharp V when the tracing is run at the standard 1 cm/min paper speed (Figures 13-2 and 13-3), and it is slightly U-shaped when the paper runs at 3 cm/min (Figure 13-4). In either case, the fall in rate is significant, usually between 15 and 30 beats, the total duration of the deceleration fluctuating between 15 and 30 sec. Exceptionally the deceleration is slow in reaching the bottom and again slow in recovering to the baseline (Figure 13-5), in which case it has the shape of a very open V. A slightly increased paper speed may give the false impression that one is observing this type of early deceleration when, in fact, it is typical, short lasting, and recovers rapidly (Figure 13-6). The depth of the deceleration may vary from the arbitrary minimum of 10 beats to very dramatic falls of up to 80 to 100 in some cases, the bottom always being a transient moment coinciding with the maximum intrauterine pressure or apex of the contraction (Figure 13-2). Neither the oscillations of the baseline nor the frequency are affected in cases where there are repeated early decelerations. These seem to occur

with higher frequency as labor progresses and are often seen in second stage, particularly coinciding with maternal bearing down efforts (Figure 13-7).

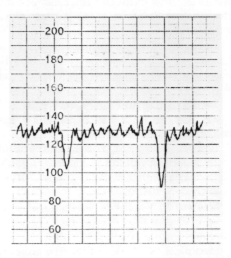

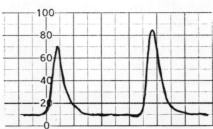

Figure 13-1 Direct FHR and UC tracings on paper running at 1 cm/min. The 7½ min tracing shows a FHR with a baseline about 130 beats/min with normal oscillations. Two sharp *early decelerations* interrupt the baseline: they *start* when the contractions are close to their maximum pressures; their *lowest point* coincides with the apex of the contraction; the recovery is quick to reach the preexisting baseline; the duration of the decelerations is about 20 sec; the stronger contraction produced the larger drop in FHR (40 beats).

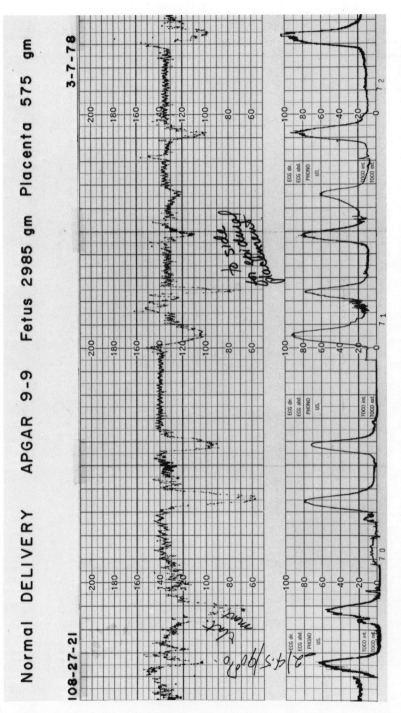

Figure 13-2 Thirty minutes of direct recordings of FHR and UC in mid-first stage of term spontaneous labor. The normal, oscillating baseline of about 140 beats/min is interrupted by sharp early decelerations coinciding with the strong contractions. The FHR drop reaches up to 80 beats in some contractions, but the recovery is rapid and to the baseline. A normal infant with good Apgar scores and normal placenta were delivered with mother under epidural anesthesia.

296

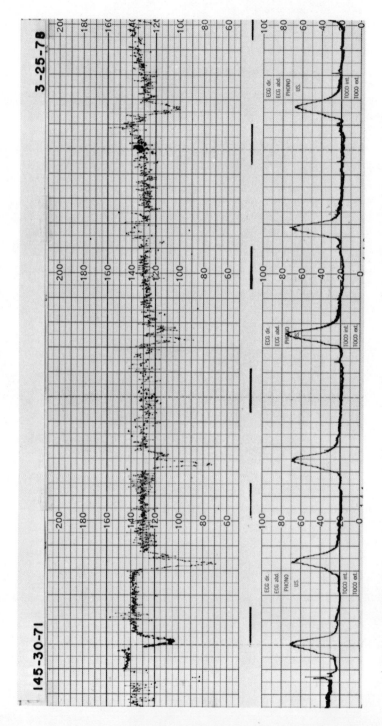

Figure 13-3 Thirty minutes of external FHR and UC tracings obtained in the early stages of labor induced in a hypertensive patient at term. The normal baseline frequency is regularly interrupted by early decelerations, in one of which the FHR fell 70 beats. A normal infant and placenta were obtained.

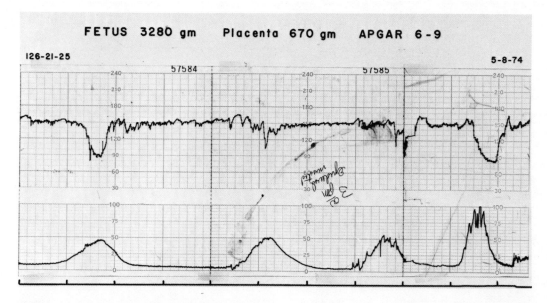

Figure 13-4 Eleven minutes of direct FHR and UC tracings on paper running at 3 cm/min. Advanced spontaneous labor at term. The normal baseline of around 150 beats/min is interrupted by early decelerations of variable amplitude—the first one falling 60 beats with a smooth U shape but lasting only 30 sec from start of the fall to recovery; the last one fell 70 beats, and the duration was 40 sec. The two middle decelerations were of lesser amplitude and duration, but still look like a flat open U. A normal infant and placenta were delivered shortly after the end of the tracing.

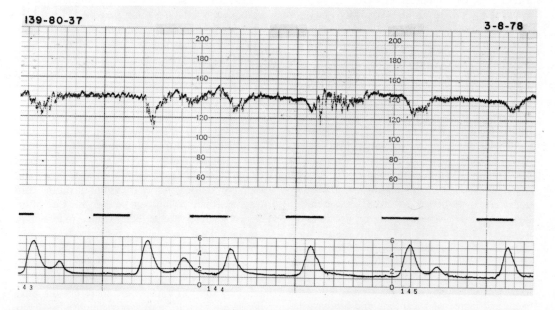

Figure 13-5 Twenty-seven minutes of direct FHR and UC tracings obtained in mid-first stage of term spontaneous labor in primipara. Paper runs at 1 cm/min, and the normal FHR baseline is periodically interrupted by early decelerations of moderate amplitude but lasting over 30 sec. The combination of these two factors gives the impression of wide open U seen more often with paper running at faster speeds.

298

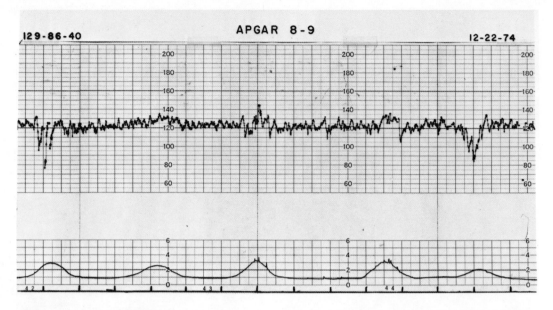

Figure 13-6 Fifteen minutes of direct FHR and UC tracings obtained in mid-first stage of term spontaneous labor in multipara. Paper runs at 2 cm/min, and the normal oscillating baseline is interrupted by two early decelerations of short duration and average amplitude.

PATHOPHYSIOLOGY

The *mechanism* of production has been ascribed to the compression of the fetal head against the cervix or against the birth canal. Hon and Quilligan (1967) postulated that the compression of the fetal head triggers a vagal reflex, which slows down the FHR as the balance of the sympathetic-parasympathetic actions on the heart is broken. They concluded that it does not seem to have any pathologic significance, following their clinical and pharmacologic studies. On the other hand, Caldeyro-Barcia (1973) and Schwarcz (1973) have postulated that they are produced by "uneven compression" of the fetal head and its "deformation," particularly during engagement and following rupture of the membranes. Furthermore, they hypothesized that as a consequence of this suggested mechanism, early decelerations may well be indicators of serious fetal compromise and perhaps derangement of intracranial circulation; thus amniotomy should not be purposely done. The direct physiologic effect of the intracranial changes would be stimulation of the vagus and increased vagal tone and bradycardia. That the deceleration is mediated through the vagus has been repeatedly demonstrated by atropinization of the mother or the fetus or both

with subsequent disappearance of the decelerations (Figure 13-8). The questions remain: which of the many postulated possible mechanisms is directly responsibile for triggering the vagal reflex, and what are the clinical implications of early decelerations? Should they be prevented, or are they innocuous alterations of the FHR? This last question has important practical significance, if one accepts that amniotomy is very often the triggering cause of early decelerations, because it is very frequently performed with the idea of facilitating the progress of labor.

The "uneven compression of the head" is said to be facilitated by the engagement of the cephalic presenting part and by rupture of the membranes. The accommodation of the fetal head would cause "disalignment" of the cranial bones and cephalic "deformation." In addition, during contractions there would be a marked increase of intracephalic pressure with consequent reduction in cerebral blood flow causing early decelerations of low amplitude. All these alterations would be exaggerated after rupture of the membranes when no longer would there be a counter pressure exerted by the forewaters, and therefore the early decelerations will be of larger amplitude. If this hypothesis is correct, practically all labors evolving with ruptured membranes would show early decelerations during the period of dilatation. The

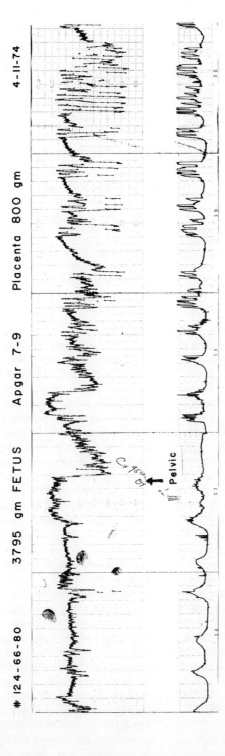

Figure 13-7 Direct 50-min recording of FHR and UC in advanced first stage and early second stage of term spontaneous labor in primipara. In the first 20 min some transient early decelerations and the effect of a pelvic examination on the FHR are seen. In the last half, each *bearing down effort* (indicated in the UC tracing by a transient sharp rise) triggers a marked fall of FHR, which recovers rapidly between maternal pushes. The overall aspect suggests a saltatory pattern, but these changes are actually rapid, large, early decelerations produced by the significant increase pressure on the fetal head. A normal infant and placenta were delivered shortly after the end of the tracing. Reprinted from Cibils LA: Clinical significance of fetal heart rate patterns during labor. I. Baseline patterns. *Am J Obstet Gynecol* 125:290, 1976.

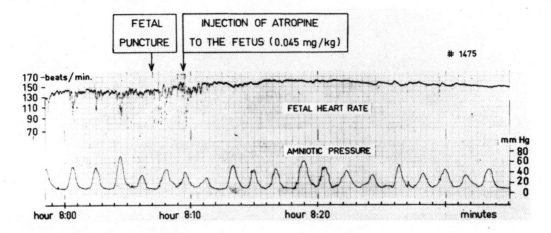

Figure 13-8 Direct 37-min recording of FHR and UC in mid-first stage of term spontaneous labor in multipara. In the first 10 min (extreme left), the strong uterine contractions trigger typical early decelerations, which interrupt a normal, oscillating baseline. The direct intrafetal injection of 0.15 mg atropine is followed by disappearance of the early decelerations, absence of rapid oscillations, and a tachycardia stabilized at 20 beats above the preinjection frequency. A normal infant with Apgar score of 8 and normal placenta were delivered. Reprinted from Mendez-Bauer C, et al: Effects of atropine on the heart rate of the human fetus during labor. *Am J Obstet Gynecol* 85:1033, 1963.

vagal reflexes would be triggered by mechanoreceptors in the head and face, stimulated by the deformation of the bones. Or, the uneven compression of the head would cause a reduction in cerebral blood flow, hypoxia, and hypercapnia. The reduced blood flow would result from "distortion of cerebral vessels" and cranial hypertension greater than the intrauterine or intrafetal pressures, caused by the contractions. The hypoxia and hypercapnia would stimulate the vasomotor center and the resulting hypertension through the baroreceptors would ultimately be the trigger of the vagal stimulation. The inevitable consequence of this mechanism is that the cascade of events leading to early decelerations constitutes a significant hazard to the fetal well-being, and these could result in brain damage (Caldeyro-Barcia et al, 1973). Fortunately, this gloomy outlook has not been demonstrated to occur in clinical practice, as the same propounders of this hypothesis have recognized. In fact, in first stage, the presence of any type of deceleration evolving with ruptured membranes is observed in only slightly over 50% of cases.

CLINICAL OBSERVATIONS

Among the high-risk patients with ruptured membranes monitored at the Chicago Lying-In Hospital, 46% had no decelerations throughout first stage, and only 19% demonstrated early decelerations, the remainder having either late or variable decelerations. This patient population did not respond in the manner suggested by the cephalic deformation hypothesis. As a matter of fact, among the cases that demonstrated early decelerations, these were present in only 20% of the contractions recorded during their labors. No clear relationship exists between stage of dilatation and occurrence of early decelerations. Only in second stage and, particularly during bearing down efforts are these predictable decelerations (Figure 13-9) triggered by the contractions. A comparison among the cases evolving without decelerations and those with early decelerations revealed no differences in baseline patterns, intrapartum distress, or neonatal outcome (Figure 13-10). This finding would indicate that the physical changes postulated to cause the decelerations did not have a damaging effect on the fetuses, at least as evaluated by standard clinical parameters. The frequent observation that large fetuses with a relatively tight cephalopelvic relationship do not have decelerations even during second stage (Figure 13-11) further indicates that either the so-called deformation is relatively unimportant or that it plays less than a peripheral role in producing decelerations.

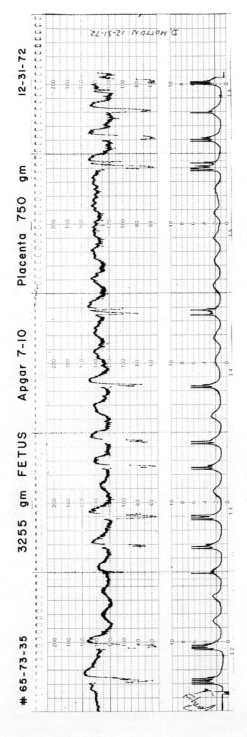

Figure 13-9 Direct 50-min recordings of second stage in induced labor of patient at term with preeclampsia. Note that the contractions with *bearing down efforts* (marked by the sharp rises in the UC tracing) trigger *early decelerations* of very large amplitude, whereas those with which the patient does not push do not alter the FHR tracings. A normal infant and placenta were delivered shortly. Reprinted from Cibils LA: Clinical significance of fetal heart rate patterns during labor. I. Baseline patterns. *Am J Obstet Gynecol* 125:290, 1976.

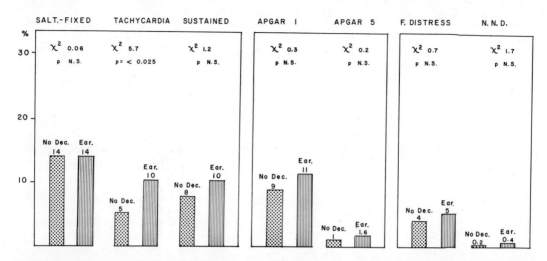

Figure 13-10 Comparison of proportion of fetuses who presented *early decelerations* during first stage and those who had *no decelerations. (Left)* Baseline alterations. Only tachycardia was higher among the early deceleration group. *(Center and right)* Immediate and medium-term neonatal outcome were not different. (Apgar scores of 6 or less at 1 and 5 min, fetal distress, and neonatal death.) Reprinted from Cibils LA: Clinical significance of fetal heart rate patterns during labor. VI. Early decelerations. *Am J Obstet Gynecol* 136:392, 1980.

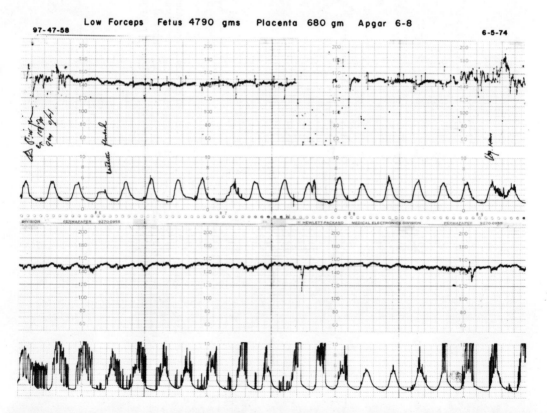

Figure 13-11 *(Above)* Forty minutes of direct recordings of FHR and UC in advanced first stage of spontaneous labor in term multipara. Note *absence of decelerations. (Below)* Forty minutes after the end of the upper tracing, strong bearing down efforts exerted by patient in *second stage* and *absence of decelerations.* A 4790 gm infant, mildly depressed, was delivered by low forceps under pudendal block.

This latter group of patients constitutes a good population within which it is possible to study indirectly the effect of uterine contractions over the unprotected heads of these fetuses. The repetitive action of the contractions should have a cumulative effect, particularly among those cases that required significantly more contractions or those that failed to progress and thus necessitated termination by cesarean section for lack of progress or cephalopelvic disproportion. Curiously, a high number of these cases never had decelerations, in spite of evidence that the contractions produced significant pressure over the head (caput) (Figure 13-12) after receiving a fair trial of labor. In fact, when those fetuses without decelerations that were subjected to prolonged periods of unprotected head against the cervix and required a cesarean section were compared with those who delivered vaginally, no differences

were found among the intrapartum or neonatal parameters, with the exception of Apgar scores at 1 minute (Figure 13-13). These may well have been due to the use of general anesthesia in 82% of the sectioned patients while only 3% of the vaginal deliveries had general anesthesia.

The general anesthetics may depress some of the elements counted to calculate the Apgar score, and therefore they may be a probable cause of the moderate depression observed in the cesarean section infants. Recovery by the fifth minute and the similar outcome indicate that these infants were likely in comparable condition at the end of labor. This clinical observation lends support to the conclusions reached by Lindgren (1960) — that rupture of the membranes does not seem to be of great importance in producing deformation of the fetal head during labor. One may find it difficult to accept the concept that permanent brain

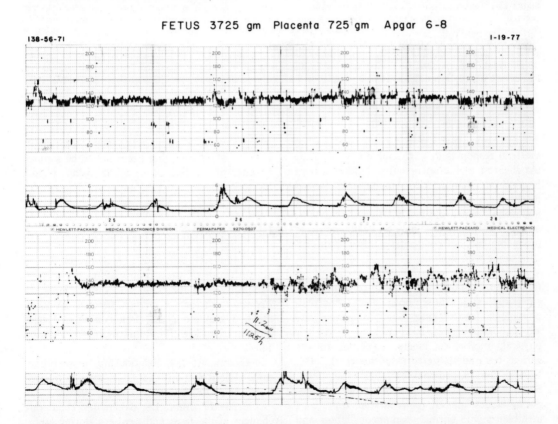

FETUS 3725 gm   Placenta 725 gm   Apgar 6-8

Figure 13-12 *(Above)* Forty minutes of direct FHR and UC recordings of induced labor in first stage, multipara at 42 weeks gestation. Baseline normal, *no decelerations. (Below)* Same pattern 2½ hours later. No progress in labor (5 cm dilatation) and moderate caput succedaneum over the fetal skull; amniotic fluid was meconium stained. Because of *arrest of progress* and physical evidence of *cephalopelvic disproportion,* a cesarean section under epidural anesthesia was performed and a mildly depressed fetus delivered. The caput was over the sinciput, indicating a minor deflection of the fetal head.

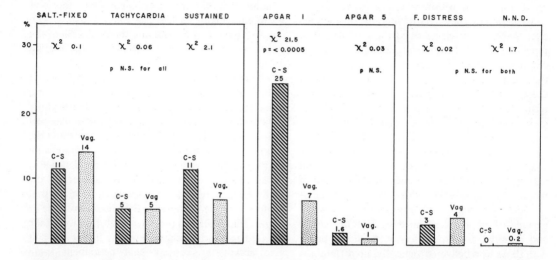

Figure 13-13 Comparison of cases of *labor without decelerations*. *(Left)* The proportion of those who delivered vaginally and had baseline alterations was compared with those who had the same alterations and *delivered by cesarean section*. No differences among the parameters evaluated. *(Center)* Proportion of those having Apgar scores of 6 or less at 1 and 5 minutes were compared; in the cesarean section group (82% general anesthesia) there were 25% at the first minute, and only 7% in the vaginal delivery group (3% general); at 5 min there were no longer differences. *(Right)* No differences observed during labor or in midterm neonatal outcome. Reprinted from Cibils LA: Clinical significance of fetal heart rate patterns during labor. VI. Early decelerations. *Am J Obstet Gynecol* 136:392, 1980.

damage could be the result of amniotomy when the fetal responses during labor do not indicate the slightest alteration of either biochemical or biophysical parameters. Among the fetuses reaching the stage of delivery, either vaginal or abdominal, which did not have decelerations or only had early decelerations, no deaths occurred (excluding cases of congenital malformations incompatible with life).

The few long-term follow-up studies of infants born from labors with ruptured membranes compared with those born from "normal, physiologic labors" have failed to demonstrate any perinatal or long-term differences in their physical, motor, or mental responses to the various tests administered (McBride et al, 1977; Noriega-Guerra, personal communication, 1979). Some of these studies have been conducted comparing labors induced for premature rupture of membranes with normal spontaneous labors and still no differences were observed among the infants.

One can hardly escape the conclusion that early decelerations during labor are innocuous carrying a prognosis as good as that for complete absence of decelerations. Thus, amniotomy seems to be a safe gesture that needs not to be avoided because of the fear of its predisposing to fetal brain damage.

BIBLIOGRAPHY

Althabe O, Aramburu G, Schwarcz RL, et al: Influence of the rupture of membranes on compression of the fetal head during labor, in *Perinatal Factors Affecting Human Development*. Washington, DC, Pan American Health Organization Scientific Publication 185, 1969, pp 143–149.

Bissonnette JM: Relationship between continuous FHR patterns and Apgar score in the new born. *Br J Obstet Gynaecol* 82:24, 1975.

Brady JP, James LS, Baker MA: Heart rate changes in the fetus and newborn during labor, delivery and immediate neonatal period. *Am J Obstet Gynecol* 84:1, 1962.

Caldeyro-Barcia R, Mendez-Bauer C, Poseiro JJ, et al: Control of human fetal heart rate during labor, in Cassels DE (ed): *The Heart and Circulation of the Newborn and Infant.* New York, Grune & Stratton, 1966, pp 7–36.

Caldeyro-Barcia R, Mendez-Bauer C, Poseiro JJ, et al: Fetal monitoring in labor, in Wallace HM, Gold EM, Lis EF (eds): *Maternal and Child Health Practices.* Springfield, Ill, Thomas, 1973, pp 332–394.

Caldeyro-Barcia R, Schwarcz R, Belizan JM, et al: Adverse perinatal effects of early amniotomy during labor, in Gluck L (ed): *Modern Perinatal Medicine.* Chicago, Year Book, 1974, pp 431–449.

Cibils LA: Clinical significance of fetal heart rate patterns during labor. I. Baseline patterns. *Am J Obstet Gynecol* 125:290, 1976.

Cibils LA: Clinical significance of fetal heart rate patterns during labor. VI. Early decelerations. *Am J Obstet Gynecol* 136:392, 1980.

Gabert HA, Stenchever MA: Effect of ruptured membranes on FHR patterns. *Obstet Gynecol* 41:279, 1973.

Gabert HA, Stenchever MA: The results of a five year study of continuous fetal monitoring on an Obstetric Service. *Obstet Gynecol* 50:275, 1977.

Garcia-Austt E: Effects of uterine contractions on the EEG of the human fetus during labor, in *Perinatal Factors Affecting Human Development.* Washington, DC, Pan American Health Organization Scientific Publication 185, 1969, pp 127–136.

Hon EH: The electronic evaluation of the fetal heart rate. *Am J Obstet Gynecol* 75:1215, 1958.

Hon EH, Quilligan EJ: The classification of fetal heart rate. *Conn Med* 31:779, 1967.

Lindgren L: The causes of fetal head moulding in labour. *Acta Obstet Gynecol Scan* 39:46, 1960.

Mann L, Carmichael A, Duchin S: The effect of head compression on FHR, brain metabolism and function. *Obstet Gynecol* 39:721, 1972.

McBride WG, Lyle JG, Black B, et al: A study of five year old children born after elective induction of labor. *Med J Aust* 2:456, 1977.

Mendez-Bauer C, Poseiro JJ, Arellano G, et al: Effects of atropine on the heart rate of the human fetus during labor. *Am J Obstet Gynecol* 85:1033, 1963.

Mendez-Bauer C, Ruiz-Canseco A, Andujar-Ruiz M, et al: Early decelerations of the fetal heart rate from occlusion of the umbilical cord. *J Perinat Med* 6:69, 1978.

Misrahy A, Beran AV, Spradley JF, et al: Fetal brain oxygen. *Am J Physiol* 199:959, 1960.

Mocsary P, Gaal J, Komaromy B, et al: Relationship between fetal intracranial pressure and fetal heart rate during labor. *Am J Obstet Gynecol* 106:407, 1970.

O'Gureck JE, Roux JF, Newman MR: Neonatal depression and FHR patterns during labor *Obstet Gynecol* 40:347, 1972.

Paul RH: Clinical fetal monitoring. *Am J Obstet Gynecol* 113:573, 1972.

Paul RH, Hon EH: Clinical fetal monitoring. V. Effect on perinatal outcome. *Am J Obstet Gynecol* 118:529, 1974.

Schifferli PY, Caldeyro-Barcia R: Effects of atropine and beta-adrenergic drugs on the heart rate of the human fetus, in Boreus L (ed): *Fetal Pharmacology.* New York, Raven, 1972, pp 259–278.

Schwarcz RL, Althabe O, Belitzky R, et al: Fetal heart rate patterns in labors with intact and with ruptured membranes. *J Perinat Med* 1:153, 1973.

Schwarcz RL, Belizan JL, Cifuentes JR, et al: Fetal and maternal monitoring in spontaneous labors and in elective inductions. *Am J Obstet Gynecol* 120:356, 1974.

Schwarcz RL, Diaz AG, Belizan JM, et al: Influence of amniotomy and maternal position on labor. *Proc VIII World Cong Gynecol Obstet (Mexico)* 1:377, 1976.

Schwarcz RL, Strada-Saenz G, Althabe O, et al: Pressure exerted by uterine contraction on the head of the human fetus during labor, in *Perinatal Factors Affecting Human Development.* Washington, DC, Pan American Health Organization Scientific Publication 185, 1969, pp 115–126.

Shenker L: Clinical experiences with heart rate monitoring of one thousand patients in labor. *Am J Obstet Gynecol* 115:1111, 1973.

CHAPTER 14
Late Decelerations

A *late deceleration,* also called *"type II dip"* or *"late dip"* is a typical slowdown of the FHR tracing coinciding with uterine contractions (Figure 14-1). The relationship between the uterine contraction recording and the beginning of the deceleration is the determinant factor to classify the FHR alteration as a late deceleration. Characteristically, the FHR *starts the deceleration after the intrauterine pressure tracing has passed its maximum value.* The FHR slows down smoothly, and reaches its lowest point between 20 and 90 sec after the peak of the uterine contraction tracing. This lag time depends, of course, on the degree of fall in the FHR, which is always slow and regular. The lowest part of the tracing is usually roundish, followed by a slow recovery toward the baseline, which is reached in about 20 to 90 sec, and occasionally longer. The overall aspect of the deceleration (at the standard 1 cm/min paper speed) is that of an open V with a rounded bottom, and a total duration of approximately 1 min. It is not unusual to observe decelerations lasting much longer, particularly when they have a slow recovery arm. When these decelerations occur in repetitive fashion there is, in general, a direct relationship between the intensity of the uterine contractions and the amplitude of the FHR fall (Figure 14-1). The minimum fall, to consider it a deceleration, is the arbitrary number of 10 in the personal observations here reported; however, some authors consider different figures, anywhere from 5 to 20, and others require a fall below a certain threshold to accept the definition of late deceleration. As discussed in previous chapters, the actual aspect of a tracing may vary significantly, depending on the speed at which the recording paper is run and the sensitivity of range within which the heart rate is recorded.

PATHOPHYSIOLOGY

Late decelerations have been observed to occur in about 10% to 12% of all labors monitored in a regular obstetric service, and therefore they constitute an important phenomenon, the significance of which must be clearly understood to manage clinical situations rationally. When the uterus is transiently hyperstimulated, as at the beginning of an oxytocin infusion started at higher than recommended rate, the polysystoly may trigger some late decelerations, particularly the very strong contractions (Figure 14-2). Nevertheless, when the frequency of the contractions diminishes, they may no longer be produced. On the other hand, the association of polysystoly and strong contractions will produce repetitive decelerations of impressive magnitude (Figure 14-3), which disappear when the contractility is normalized. In still other circumstances the uterus may respond to unphysiologic stimulation with episodes of extraordinary hypertonus that trigger late decelerations rapidly following one another without complete recovery between them, giving the impression of observing a state of bradycardia (Figure 14-4); to this pattern of FHR Caldeyro-Barcia gave the name "overlapping type II dips" (or late decelerations), a most fitting and descriptive label for this ominous looking tracing.

Mechanism

Numerous animal studies have been carried out to explore the possible mechanisms involved in the production of late FHR deceleration. Likewise, recordings of human observations analyzed and correlated with the clinical conditions have

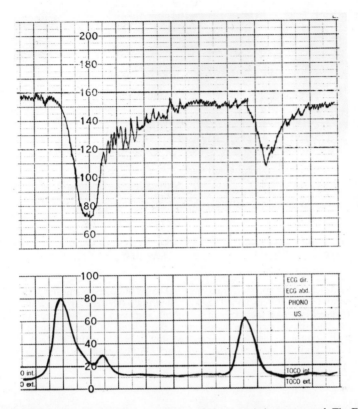

Figure 14-1 FHR and intrauterine pressure and tracings recorded at 1 cm/min paper speed. The FHR baseline of 155 in the first contraction starts a deceleration coinciding with the peak intrauterine pressure and reaches lowest value 60 sec later after a smooth slow fall (lag time, 60 sec). The roundish bottom coincides with the last part of the relaxation phase of the uterus, and the slow recovery takes 3 min before reaching the predeceleration baseline. The total duration of the late deceleration was 4 min and the fall was 80 beats. The second less strong contraction triggered a late deceleration of similar characteristics but with lag time of 55 sec, a duration of 2 min 20 sec, and a fall of 42 beats.

shed some light on understanding this phenomenon. The persistence of the decelerations when they appear for the first time and the worsening of the pattern with the hypercontractility (Figure 14-5) suggest that the triggering mechanism must be related to changes or alterations directly produced by the contractions. As seen in Chapter 7 (Figures 7-1 through 7-4), with each contraction there is a marked diminution in blood supply to IVS and with it a diminution of oxygen available for exchange. This observation has also been made by measuring the blood flow of uterine arteries in pregnant animals, confirming the significant reduction in the flow and thus in oxygen carrying blood (Figure 14-6).

During maximum strength of contraction, and for a period of several seconds, depending on the intensity of the contraction, the blood in the IVS is practically stagnant, whereas the fetal blood continues to circulate rapidly by the placental villi. The oxygen supply available for exchange falls rapidly, and therefore relative fetal hypoxia ensues; simultaneously, exchange of catabolites from the fetus to maternal blood, including carbon dioxide and lactates, is diminished and a tendency toward acidosis is the logical consequence. These homeostatic alterations are maximal at the peak of the contraction, and the hypooxygenated fetal blood will reach its tissues about 20 to 40 sec later (placenta–fetal tissue circulation time). With relaxation of the uterus there is a slow recovery of blood supply to the IVS and regularization of the alterations described above (Figure 14-7).

Obviously, no alterations will occur if the fetal O_2 is sufficiently high to cope with the short

308

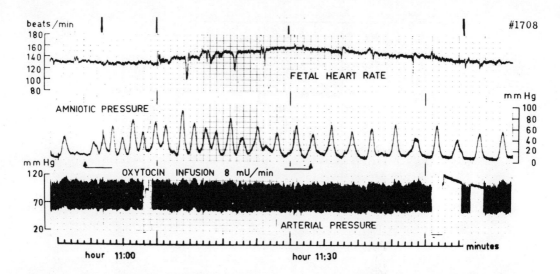

Figure 14-2 Direct FHR, intrauterine pressure, and maternal blood pressure obtained in induced labor at term with an *anencephalic fetus*. Paper speed, 0.5 cm/min. The oxytocin infusion (between arrows), started and maintained at 8 mU/min for 32 min, triggered hypercontractility with polysystoly and hypertonus, which caused *fetal tachycardia* and *three late decelerations*. After the oxytocin was discontinued, the baseline returned to control levels. Reprinted from Caldeyro-Barcia R, et al: Control of human fetal heart rate, in Cassels DE (ed): *The Heart and Circulation of the Newborn and Infant*. New York, Grune & Stratton, 1966, pp 7–36. By permission.

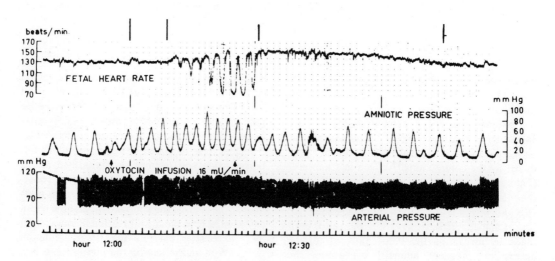

Figure 14-3 Same case as Figure 14-2. Oxytocin infusion was started and maintained at 16 mU/min for 20 min, and the uterine activity responded with marked *hypertonus* and *polysystoly*. After a few minutes the strong contractions triggered impressive late decelerations with a rising baseline. After discontinuing the oxytocin the uterine contractility normalized, the FHR baseline was tachycardic and slowly returned to normal, but no more late decelerations were recorded. Reprinted from Caldeyro-Barcia R, et al: Control of human fetal heart rate, in Casells DE (ed): *The Heart and Circulation of the Newborn and Infant*. New York, Grune & Stratton, 1966, pp 7–36. By permission.

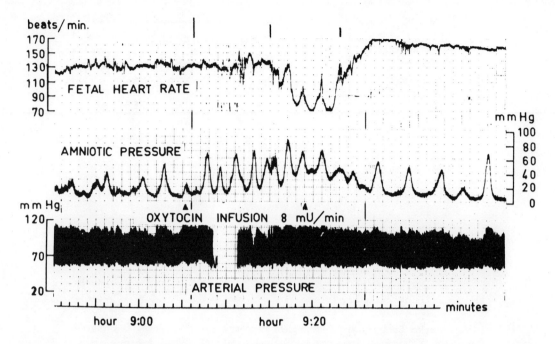

Figure 14-4 Same case as Figure 14-2. The oxytocin infusion started at 8 mU/min and sustained for only 15 min triggered marked hypercontractility with *polysystoly and severe hypertonus*. Coinciding with the latter the strong contraction produced a large late deceleration, followed by another just as its recovery started, and still another again at the start of the recovery. The three overlapped late decelerations occurred with a FHR well below 100 and may be interpreted as bradycardia. When recovery took place the FHR showed a rebound tachycardia and fixed baseline, which started a slow downward trend at the end of the tracing. Reprinted from Caldeyro-Barcia R, et al: Control of human fetal heart rate, in Cassels DE (ed): *The Heart and Circulation of the Newborn and Infant.* New York, Grune & Stratton, 1966, pp 7–36. By permission.

period of diminished exchange seen in a normal contraction, that is, if the "fetal reserve" is satisfactory. However, when either the fetal reserve is below normal, or the uterine contraction is sustained above blood flow level for too long, the fetal O_2 is diminished, and evolution toward acidosis will be inevitable. These two phenomena, occurring simultaneously, are delayed 20 to 40 sec with respect to the acme of the uterine contraction, and thus may be responsible for the fall in FHR which also, by definition, occurs after the maximum intrauterine pressure has occurred.

The question then is, which one of these two is primarily the cause of the fall in FHR? By convention, it has been defined as the threshold of fetal acidosis, a capillary blood pH of 7.25. If acidosis, which develops much more slowly than hypoxia, were responsible, late decelerations should be present whenever the fetal capillary blood pH is below 7.25 during labor. In clinical practice, significant fetal acidosis has been

observed repeatedly without appreciable decelerations (Figure 14-8); decelerations seem to occur only when the oxygen tension of the capillary blood falls below a minimal threshold of 17 or 18 mm Hg.

These observations confirm what has been recorded in subhuman primates under experimental conditions: the direct cause of late decelerations seems to be acute hypoxia, which may occur in the absence of acidosis. Conversely, contractions in states of significant acidosis do not produce late decelerations unless significant hypoxia is present (Figure 14-9). The fall in FHR seems to parallel the changes in oxygen tension, and both are delayed with respect to the maximal intrauterine pressure. The simultaneous changes, as a consequence of the uterine contraction, are a drastic drop in IVS blood flow followed by a drop in fetal blood pO_2, closely followed by the alteration in FHR. All changes revert in the same order as the uterus relaxes and freshly oxygenated blood

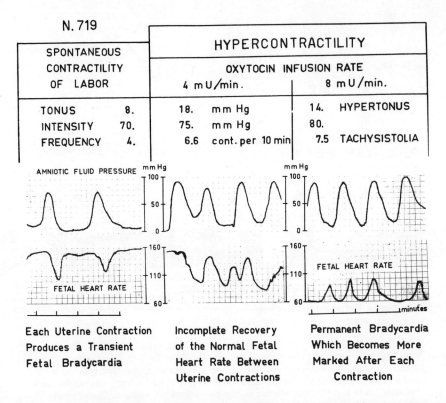

Figure 14-5 Three segments of direct intrauterine pressure and FHR tracings obtained in term pregnancy with an anencephalic fetus. Analysis of the tracings summarized above, and description of FHR alterations below. The fetus having late decelerations with spontaneous normal contractions deteriorates markedly when subjected to oxytocin-induced uterine hyperstimulation with overlapping late decelerations. The pattern worsens when the uterine polysystoly of very strong contractions is produced by further increase of oxytocin infusion. The severe bradycardic pattern preceded fetal death by only several minutes. Courtesy R. Caldeyro-Barcia.

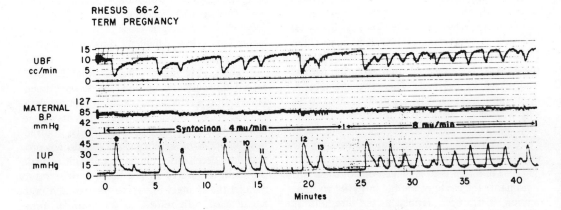

Figure 14-6 Uterine artery blood flow, maternal systemic mean blood pressure, and intrauterine pressure recorded in term labor of Rhesus monkey. The spontaneous uterine activity was stimulated with an oxytocin infusion at 4 and 8 mU/min. With each uterine contraction there is a corresponding fall in uterine blood flow and recovery, a perfect mirror image. The slow blood flow recovery is incomplete until the relaxation phase of the contraction reaches the normal tonus. With polysystoly triggered by 8 mU/min oxytocin, there is incomplete recovery of uterine blood flow as long as the frequency of contractions was too high. Reprinted from Greiss (1968).

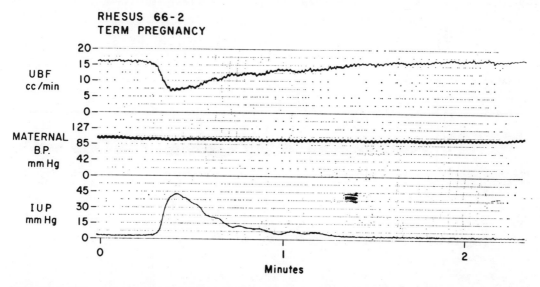

Figure 14-7 Same case as Figure 14-6, recorded at high paper speed to illustrate better the relationship between intrauterine pressure and the complete recovery of uterine blood flow, which is not achieved until the relaxation reaches precontraction tonus. Reprinted from Greiss (1968).

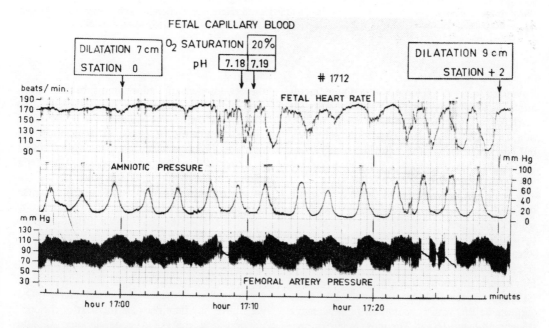

Figure 14-8 Direct FHR, intrauterine pressure, and arterial pressure tracings obtained in induced labor at term. No obvious pathologic condition was found during labor or after delivery. However, there is a clear tachycardia with a normal uterine contractility. In advanced first stage, fetal capillary pH was moderately acidotic. Late decelerations started and at delivery, effected 44 min later, the umbilical vein pH was 7.05 in a very depressed infant (Apgar 1). Reprinted from Mendez-Bauer C, et al: Relationship between blood pH and heart rate in human fetus during labor. *Am J Obstet Gynecol* 97:530, 1967.

312

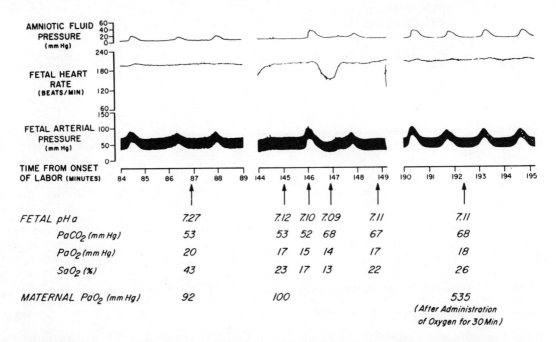

Figure 14-9 Three segments of intrauterine pressure, FHR, and fetal arterial pressure obtained during labor in term pregnant monkey. Fetal blood acid–base status determined (arrows) for each segment. *(Left)* Uterine contractions not affecting FHR, with normal pH and pO$_2$ of 20 mm Hg. *(Center)* Four blood gas determinations on acidotic fetus document that the contraction induces a fall in pO$_2$ from 17 to 14 mm Hg, and a fall in pH as the FHR decelerates. *(Right)* In spite of continuous oxygen to the mother, acidosis is still severe; contraction induces a fall in pO$_2$ to 18 mm Hg, no deceleration recorded. Reprinted from James LS, et al: Mechanism of late deceleration of fetal heart rate. *Am J Obstet Gynecol* 113:578, 1972.

is supplied to the IVS (Figure 14-10). These fluctuations in IVS blood flow, and consequently O$_2$ available to the fetus, occur with every contraction, regardless of the fetal condition or reserve, but late decelerations will be evident only when the fetal capillary oxygen drops below the critical threshold (Figures 14-11 through 14-14).

The transitory episodes of hypoxemia create the need for anaerobic metabolism by the fetus with exaggerated production of lactate and pyruvate and a corresponding fall in pH. Recovery tends to occur during the periods of relaxation with abundant blood flow into the IVS. However, if the contractions recur too frequently (tachysystoly) there will be accumulation of acids (or base deficit) with concomitant fetal acidemia (Figures 14-8 and 14-13). The more severe or prolonged the periods of hypoxia, the faster the accumulation of acids and the deterioration of the fetus (Figures 14-15 and 14-18). This particular aspect of deranged homeostasis has been well studied in humans by Saling (1967) who classified

the development of acidosis into subacute, acute, and superacute depending on the speed with which hydrogen ions accumulate in the fetal blood; superacute development of acidosis, for example, occurred when the pH dropped about 0.01/min (Figure 14-16) in less than 1% of his clinical population, while the slow fall of the subacute group was seen in 11% of his patients.

The start of the deceleration occurs, by definition, after the peak of the uterine contraction, and the fall parallels its relaxation trace. However, there are exceptions to this general rule, which is governed basically by the fetal blood reserve in oxygen. It has been demonstrated experimentally that the lower the fetal reserve (pO$_2$) the shorter the time between the start of the contraction and that of the deceleration (Figure 14-17); when the reserve is very low the deceleration may even start before the contraction reaches its acme (Figure 14-8), thereby creating a potential source of confusion with other deceleration patterns. One needs to reemphasize that for each case

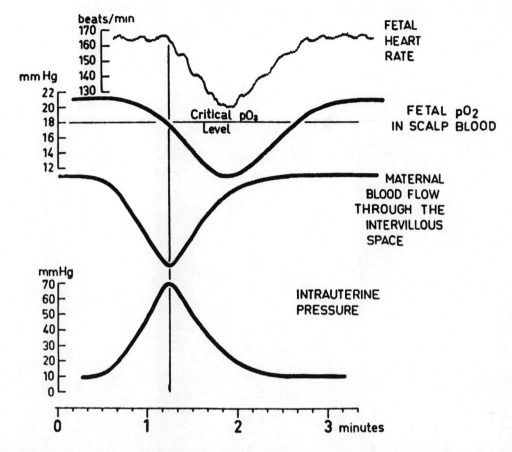

Figure 14-10 Schematic representation of simultaneous changes occurring with uterine contraction. IVS blood flow in mirror image, and fetal capillary blood pO$_2$ decreases slowly from 21 to reach 18 mm Hg at the peak of the contraction; at that moment FHR starts a deceleration parallel to the oxygen pressure curve. The last two reach their lowest points about 45 sec after maximum intrauterine pressure, and then recover slowly. FHR reaches predeceleration level as pO$_2$ of 18 mm Hg is attained. Reprinted from Caldeyro-Barcia R, et al: Fetal monitoring in labor, in Wallace HM, Gold EM, Lis EF (eds): *Maternal and Child Health Practices.* Courtesy of Charles C Thomas, Publisher, Springfield, Ill, 1973, pp 332–394.

there is a direct correlation between the intensity of the contractions and the amplitude of the FHR falls, provided the fetal condition remains approximately the same.

Another question investigated in primates has been how the fetal response to hypoxia is transmitted to the heart. The direct *atropinization* of human (Figure 14-18) as well as monkey fetuses demonstrated that parasympathetic block diminishes the amplitude of the late decelerations, but it does not completely abolish them. Rather, they are still very much in evidence, suggesting that there is a dual mechanism: one mediated by the vagus, and another in all likelihood a direct effect on the myocardium (or its pacemakers). This particular observation may have important thera-peutic consequences.

The hypoxic episode triggers, at the same time, strong sympathetic stimulation (Nakai and Yamada, 1978), and is probably responsible for the increased blood pressure observed in fetuses with good acid–base balance (Figures 14-19 and 14-26); however, a fetus in a state of severe acidosis responds to the episodes of late deceleration with hypotension (Figures 14-9 and 14-27) suggesting that their mechanism of adaptation to stress may be already deranged under these circumstances (Berg et al, 1973; Cohn et al, 1974; Myers, 1972). Thus a *late deceleration is the expression of an episode of transient hypoxia produced by a uterine contraction, which interferes with the blood flow to the IVS.*

314

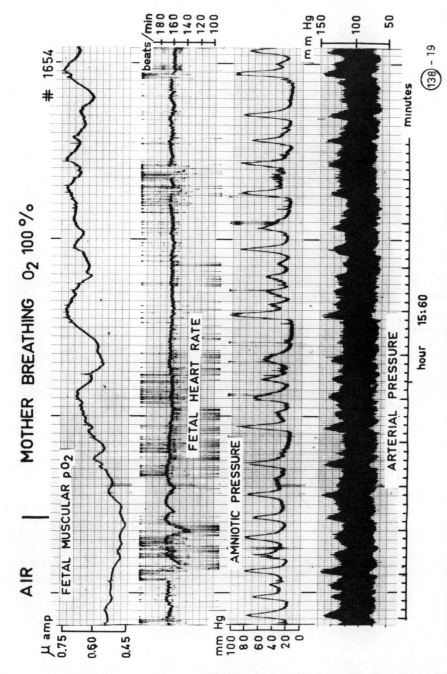

Figure 14-11 Tracings during early stage of induced labor in term primipara. Recordings of the fetal intramuscular pO₂ by transabdominal electrode; paper speed, 0.5 cm/min. During the first 13 min the patient was breathing air, and the strong uterine contractions triggered late decelerations on a tachycardic FHR pattern coinciding with a relatively low fetal muscular pO₂. Administration of 100% oxygen to the mother was followed by a slow and steady rise of fetal pO₂ and disappearance of late decelerations in spite of the contractility pattern, which continued to show strong contractions. Maternal blood pressure was normal. Reprinted from Althabe O, et al: Effect on fetal heart rate and fetal pO₂ of oxygen administration to the mother. *Am J Obstet Gynecol* 98:858, 1967.

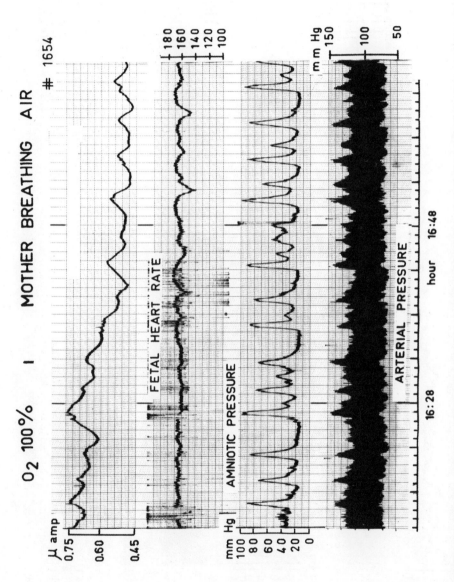

Figure 14-12 Continuation of tracing of Figure 14-11. When oxygen to the mother was discontinued, fetal pO$_2$ came down slowly to previous level. Strong uterine contractions triggered late decelerations only after the fetal pO$_2$ reached the threshold of around 0.5μamp. Each late deceleration (triggered only by the strong contractions) coincides with a fall in fetal pO$_2$ and is followed by a recovery and a slight increase in FHR baseline. Reprinted from Althabe O, et al: Effect on fetal heart rate and fetal pO$_2$ of oxygen administration to the mother. *Am J Obstet Gynecol* 98:858, 1967.

316

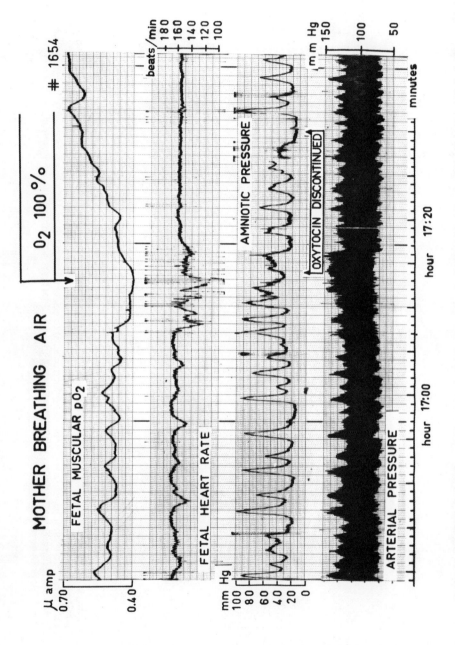

Figure 14-13 Continuation of tracing of Figure 14-12. With the mother breathing air, the strongest uterine contractions triggered late decelerations coinciding with falls in fetal pO₂. Shortly after hour 17.00 an episode of polysystoly and hypertonus triggered overlapping late decelerations, which coincided with a sustained drop in fetal pO₂. Resumption of oxygen administration to the mother caused a steady rise in fetal pO₂ and disappearance of late decelerations. Reprinted from Althabe O, et al: Effect on fetal heart rate and fetal pO₂ of oxygen administration to the mother. *Am J Obstet Gynecol* 98:858, 1967.

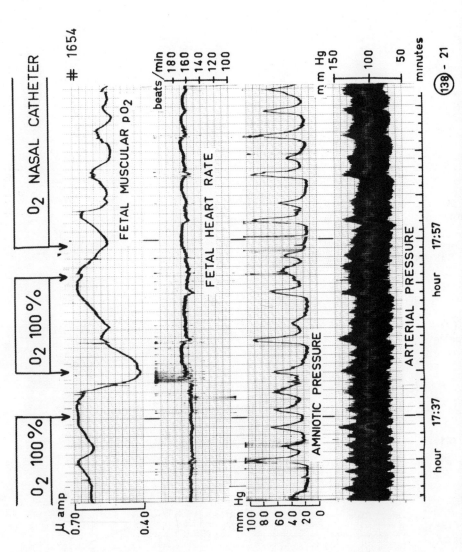

Figure 14-14 Continuation of tracing of Figure 14-13. Five-minute interruption of 100% oxygen to the mother was sufficient to cause a dramatic drop in fetal pO₂, corrected by restoration of oxygen to mother. Note the lower oxygen uptake by the fetus when oxygen was given to the mother by nasal catheter rather than mask. Courtesy R. Caldeyro-Barcia.

318

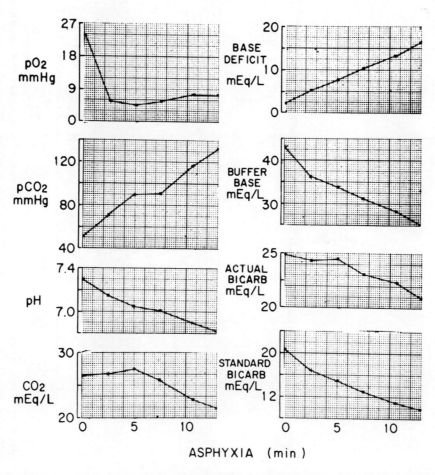

Figure 14-15 Acid–base and respiratory gas changes developing in a term monkey fetus during total asphyxia. Each point corresponds to a blood sample. Note the precipitous drop in pO₂ *(top, left)* compared to the relatively slower changes in the other values. However, these also develop rapidly, the pH falling from 7.30 to 6.80 in 13 min. After 2.5 min there was practically only anerobic metabolism. Reprinted from Myers RE: Two patterns of perinatal brain damage and their condition of occurrence. *Am J Obstet Gynecol* 112:246, 1972.

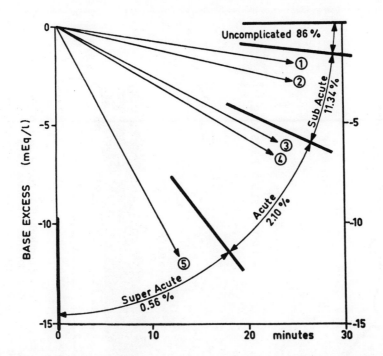

Figure 14-16 Schematic to indicate the relative speed and proportion with which acidosis developed in a patient population. The "superacute group" dropped 15 mEq/liter of base in about 25 min, whereas the uncomplicate. hardly changed at all. Reprinted from Caldeyro-Barcia R, et al: Fetal monitoring in labor, in Wallace HM, Gold EM, Lis EF (eds): *Maternal and Child Health Practices.* Courtesy of Charles C Thomas, Publisher, Springfield, Ill, 1973, pp 332–394.

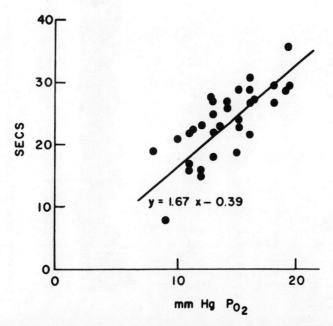

Figure 14-17 Plotting the interval, in seconds, between the onset of a uterine contraction and that of the late deceleration against fetal arterial pO₂ demonstrates a direct relationship: the lower the pO₂ the shorter the time before deceleration starts. Reprinted from Myers RE, et al: Predictability of the state of fetal oxygenation from a quantitative analysis of the components of late deceleration. *Am J Obstet Gynecol* 115:1083, 1973.

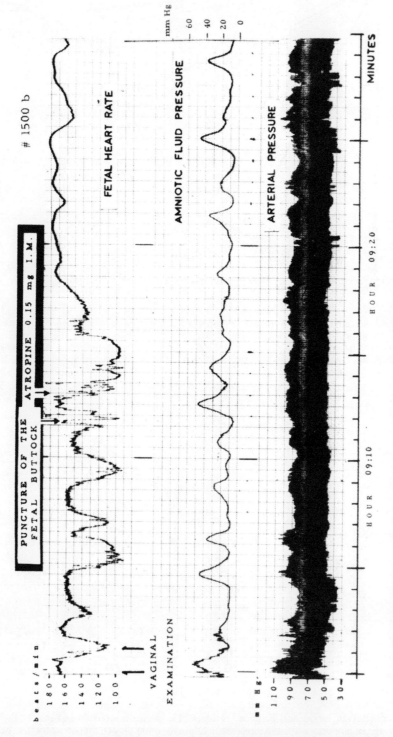

Figure 14-18 Direct FHR, intrauterine, and arterial pressures obtained during early stage of induced labor in term multipara. *(Left)* Moderate uterine contractions trigger marked late decelerations from a tachycardic baseline. Direct injection of atropine 150 μg IM to the fetus induced within 2 min a clear change in the FHR tracing: disappearance of baseline oscillations and further rise of baseline; the amplitude of the late decelerations diminished but the timing of onset and their duration remained unchanged. Reprinted from Mendez-Bauer C, et al: Effects of atropine on the human heart rate during labor. *Am J Obstet Gynecol* 85:1033, 1963.

EFFECTS OF HYPOXIA

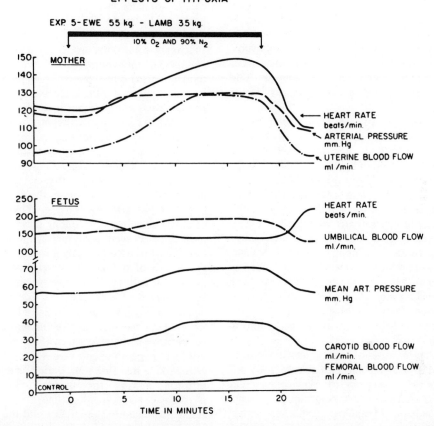

Figure 14-19 *(Lower part)* Effects on the lamb fetus after administration of a gas mixture of 10% O_2 and 90% N_2 to the ewe. FHR falls as the mean arterial pressure, carotid blood flow, and umbilical blood flow rise; slight fall in femoral blood flow. In the ewe *(top)*, heart rate, blood pressure, and uterine blood flow increase. Reprinted from Assali NS, et al: Hemodynamic changes in fetal lamb in utero in response to asphyxia, hypoxia and hypercapnia. *Circ Res* 11:423, 1962. By permission of the American Heart Association Inc.

Causes

Any condition that interferes with either adequate supply of oxygenated blood to the IVS or the available oxygen to reach the fetal tissues (heart, brain) will cause fetal hypoxia and thus late decelerations. They are present in pathologic conditions suffered by the fetus, the mother, or iatrogenically induced by the medical or auxiliary personnel in charge of observing or conducting a given labor.

Fetal Conditions hindering the oxygen carrying capacity of the fetal blood tend to predispose to late decelerations. *Erythroblastosis fetalis* with its severe anemia should be considered among the most frequent causative syndromes. It

may be obvious only in severe cases during the most active part of labor, when the intensity and frequency of the contractions are at their maximum. *Feto-maternal transfusion* syndrome, a less common condition, may also be an etiologic factor because the anemia it produces may at times be significant. A more acute picture is present when a *vasa-previa ruptures* and leads rapidly to acute anemia.

Maternal A great number of pathologic conditions of the mother lead to poor supply of oxygenated blood to the IVS. They may be systemic or localized to the uteroplacental area. Among the systemic conditions, the most prevalent are syndromes in which hypertension is significant: the arteriolar spasm characteristic of these syndromes includes the uteroplacental bed, hindering blood flow. *Chronic* hypertension contributes significantly to hypoxia in this group of patients (Figure 14-20). Severe *preeclampsia* is another leading cause of intrapartum fetal hypoxia; one may see the association of arteriolar spasm to a disproportionately small placenta and thus the syndrome of *placental* insufficiency (Figure 14-21).

The syndrome of *chronic placental insufficiency* may not be so apparent as it is when it is observed in hypertensive diseases; nonetheless it is as significant a cause of hypoxia and dangerous as in hypertensive conditions (Figure 14-22; see also Figure 12-15). It has been speculated that the intimate mechanism causing fetal hypoxia in this condition is insufficient area of exchange to cope with the needs of a relatively large and mature fetus requiring a good supply of oxygen. A somewhat related problem is seen in cases of frank *prolonged gestation* when the fetus may react with the classical signs of late decelerations to the normal stress of uterine contracting (Figure 14-23). See Chapter 16 for some important exceptions to this general rule.

Numerous causes of maternal anemia predispose to this phenomenon, particularly *sickle cell anemia* with its tendency to produce placental alterations. A relatively large group of patients with no apparent pathologic condition, either anatomic or systemic, shows repeated episodes of late decelerations; these must, by necessity, be labeled *"idiopathic cases"* (Figures 14-8, 14-18, and 14-24) and will remain as such until better means of study are devised to understand these complex phenomena.

Localized pathologic disorders are limited mainly to the placenta. The most common and best known syndrome is premature separation of a normally implanted organ (abruptio placentae), constituting what is known as *acute placental insufficiency*. The degree of deceleration is, in general, in direct relationship to the area of placenta separated and to the intensity and frequency of the contractions (Figures 6-9, 6-12, 6-13, and 14-25). The full picture of the classical abruptio placentae with "board-like uterus" characterized by severe hypertonus and continuous pain is rarely present with a live fetus because the association of drastically decreased surface of exchange and severely curtailed blood flow due to the hypertonus constitute a lethal combination that no fetus can survive more than a few minutes.

Not infrequently one may see that the exchange function of the placenta is severely hampered by large areas of infarction (more often white, rarely red), which diminish the number of functional cotyledons and create a condition of *chronic placental insufficiency* even though the total weight ratio between fetus and placenta may be within normal ranges. A bleeding *placenta previa* creates a condition very similar to abruptio placentae, without its hypercontractility. With a decreased area of effective exchange, the stage is set for deficient oxygen supply to the fetus and thus late decelerations with contractions.

Iatrogenic   The most frequent cause of late decelerations in term labors in the United States must be *hypercontractility* triggered by the misuse of *oxytocic substances.* Among these, by far the most common agent is *oxytocin.* This potent hormone must be used correctly if it is to be used for the benefit of the patient. Its effects are highly predictable and therefore excessive responses may be prevented if one exercises adequate care. Hypercontractility may be triggered at various stages: 1) at the *beginning of the infusion* when an excessive amount is given (Figures 9-12 and 9-13) and hypertonus supervenes along with polysystoly; 2) in mid-first stage during *an established infusion* driving the uterus to maximum physiologic activity, which may become exaggerated as dilatation progresses and the intrinsic mechanism of labor pushes the contractility higher (Figures 9-14 and 9-15), triggering polysystoly; and 3) in other cases simply administering *excessive amounts* of oxytocin in a sustained manner is more than enough to exhaust the reserves of a good fetus (Figure 6-8).

The rapid intravenous use of other oxytocic substances, like the *analgesics* meperidine or pentazocine, on uteri with good contractility may trigger sufficient hypercontractility to exhaust fetal reserves and produce transient episodes of hypoxia and late decelerations. The extended use of *conduction anesthesia* when applied indiscriminately (or carelessly) may cause severe diminution of IVS blood flow and fetal hypoxia due to maternal hypotension (see Chapter 18). Like almost all iatrogenic causes of fetal hypoxia, those caused by conduction anesthesia are strictly preventable if proper contraindications are observed and administration is cautious.

The over-enthusiastic use of *antihypertensive drugs* will cause a relative or real hypotension with consequent fall in IVS blood flow and fetal

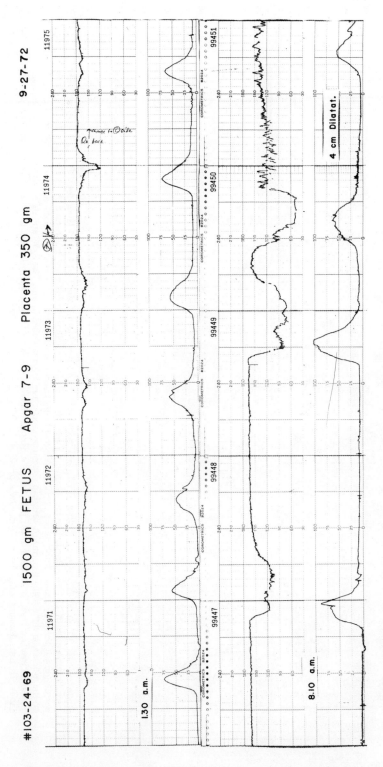

Figure 14-20 Two segments (20 min each) of direct FHR and intrauterine pressure tracings obtained during induced labor in a patient with severe hypertension at 37 weeks gestation. (*Above*) Fixed and tachycardic baseline with small late decelerations induced by a normal uterine contractility pattern (paper speed, 3 cm/min). (*Below*) More than 6 hours later, only sporadic uterine contractions (after discontinuing oxytocin) but marked late decelerations with very slow recovery on a still tachycardic and fixed baseline. A burst of saltatory pattern is seen during the recovery period of the last deceleration. A cesarean section produced a grossly growth-retarded infant in satisfactory condition. Reprinted from Cibils LA: Clinical significance of fetal heart rate patterns during labor. II. Late decelerations. *Am J Obstet Gynecol* 123:473, 1975.

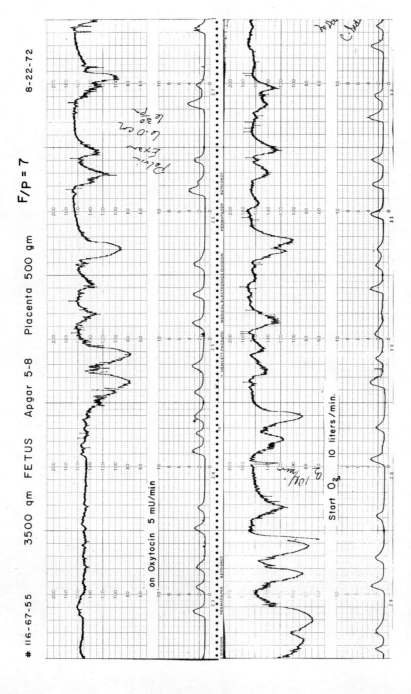

Figure 14-21 Continuous 100 min of direct FHR and intrauterine pressure obtained during induced labor for PRM in a patient with preeclampsia at term. *(Above)* Borderline tachycardic baseline with minimal oscillations suddenly interrupted by marked late decelerations seemingly triggered by a short burst of contractions. *(Below)* Diminution in amplitude of decelerations following administration of oxygen to the mother, and the rising baseline. A cesarean section produced a mildly depressed infant. The F/P ratio of 7 indicates a state of chronic placental insufficiency, in addition to the preeclampsia. Reprinted from Cibils LA: Clinical significance of fetal heart rate patterns during labor. II. Late decelerations. *Am J Obstet Gynecol* 123:473, 1975.

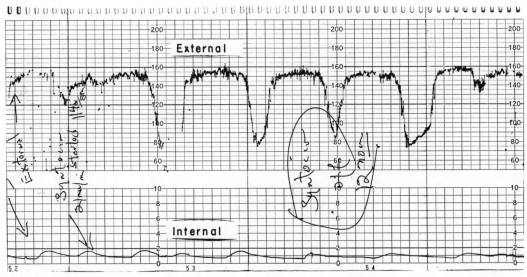

Figure 14-22 Thirty minutes of intrauterine pressure and FHR (external) recording obtained at the beginning of induced labor in term pregnancy. Shortly after amniotomy, a 2 mU/min oxytocin infusion was started, and the mild uterine contractions triggered severe late decelerations, which prompted discontinuing the induction. By cesarean section a mildly depressed term size infant and very small placenta were delivered. The F/P ratio of 8.07 attests to a severe chronic placental insufficiency. Reprinted from Cibils LA: Clinical significance of fetal heart rate patterns during labor. II. Late decelerations. *Am J Obstet Gynecol* 123:473, 1975.

hypoxia. This complication is particularly likely with the multidrug method of treating severe hypertension or preeclampsia still widely used at many centers. It is not widely known that a significant reduction, on the order of 50%, in the IVS blood flow is required before *a well fetus* reacts with a hypoxic deceleration and makes other associated adaptive responses (Figure 14-26); that much of a reduction is easily reached by inducing a fall in the blood pressure. It has been shown in subhuman primates that a small drop in mean blood pressure below a threshold will suffice to induce a fetal hypoxia capable of triggering late decelerations (Figure 14-27). That threshold, however, may already be at the level of severe hypotension when compared to the blood pressure obtained under normal conditions (Figure 14-28), therefore representing significant fall in the relative IVS blood flow. The late decelerations following paracervical blocks seem now to be preventable when a careful technique is

followed and too-deep injections are avoided (see Chapter 18).

CLINICAL SIGNIFICANCE

Late decelerations of the FHR during labor are an ominous sign, which indicates a state of transient hypoxia for the fetus, the cause of which must be immediately determined. Late decelerations are recorded in about 10% to 15% of labors monitored in maternity centers and therefore involve a large group of patients at very high risk. In the experience at the Chicago Lying-In Hospital they have been recorded in 11% of all monitored labors. As judged by the classic criteria for fetal distress, 50% of the cases with late decelerations had those symptoms, and 25% were terminated by cesarean section—a rate much higher than among the cases without FHR alterations (Figure 14-29).

326

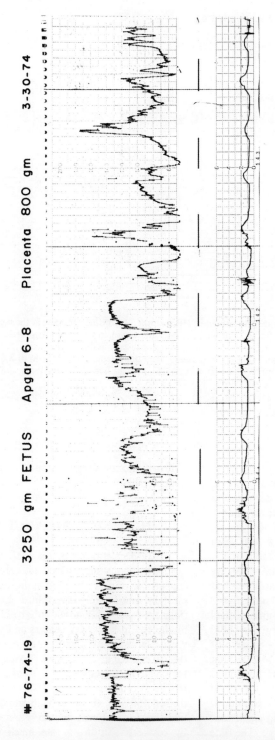

Figure 14-23 Forty-five minutes of direct FHR and UC recordings obtained during early spontaneous labor in prolonged pregnancy (44 weeks). Severe late decelerations are triggered by mild contractions; apparent good oscillation of the normal baseline. Saltatory pattern toward end of tracing. By cesarean section a mildly depressed infant and normal placenta were delivered. Reprinted from Cibils LA: Clinical significance of fetal heart rate patterns during labor. II. Late decelerations. *Am J Obstet Gynecol* 123:473, 1975.

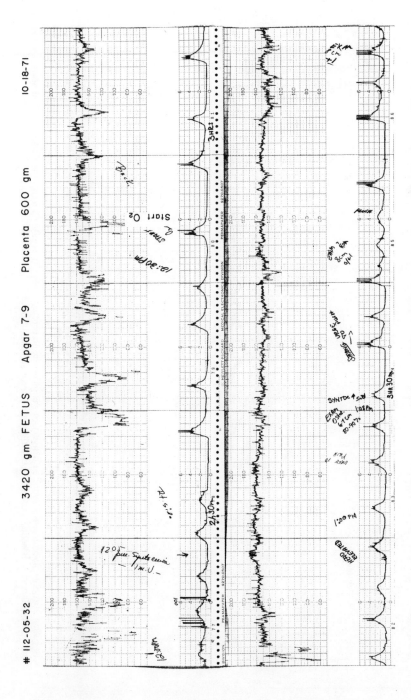

Figure 14-24 Continuous 100 min of direct FHR and UC tracings during enhanced labor in term nonsensitized Rh-negative patient. *(Top)* Moderate tachycardia and late decelerations prompted the administration of oxygen to the mother. After about 15 min the decelerations disappeared and the baseline slowly returned toward normal values. A normal infant was born 2 hours after the end of the recording. Reprinted from Cibils LA: Clinical significance of fetal heart rate patterns during labor. II. Late decelerations. *Am J Obstet Gynecol* 123:473, 1975.

328

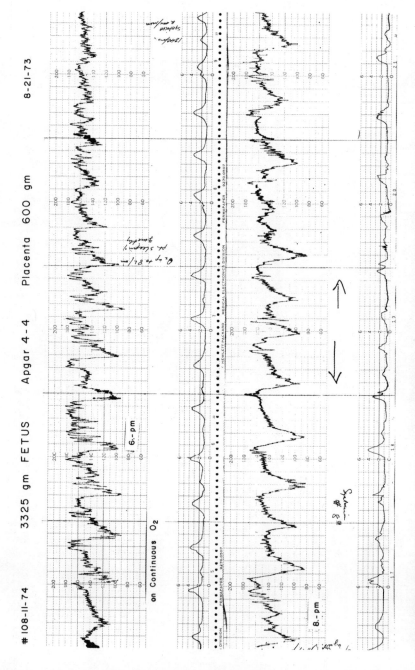

Figure 14-25 Two 50-min segments of continuous direct FHR and intrauterine pressure tracings recorded during term induced labor for PRM. (*Above*) Moderate uterine activity triggering late decelerations and saltatory pattern. Continuous administration of oxygen to the patient was followed by diminution and disappearance of late decelerations. (*Below*) Two hours later, resumed late decelerations, diminishing rapid oscillations, and rising baseline in spite of continuous oxygen. A depressed term infant was delivered by emergency cesarean section. A concealed abruptio placentae was found at delivery of the placenta. Reprinted from Cibils LA: Clinical significance of fetal heart rate patterns during labor. I. Baseline patterns. *Am J Obstet Gynecol* 125:290, 1976.

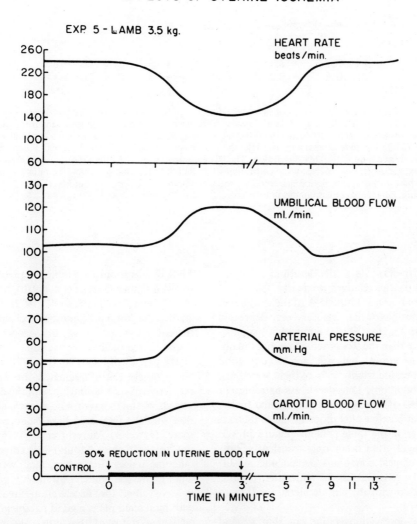

Figure 14-26 Effects on fetus of term pregnant ewe of 90% reduction of uterine blood flow for 3 min. Within 1 min marked FHR deceleration starts, and, in mirror image, an increase in mean blood pressure and carotid and umbilical blood flows. All four parameters start their recovery shortly after uterine blood flow is restored to normal. Reprinted from Assali NS, et al: Hemodynamic changes in fetal lamb in utero in response to asphyxia, hypoxia and hypercapnia. *Circ Res* 11:423, 1962. By permission of the American Heart Association Inc.

330

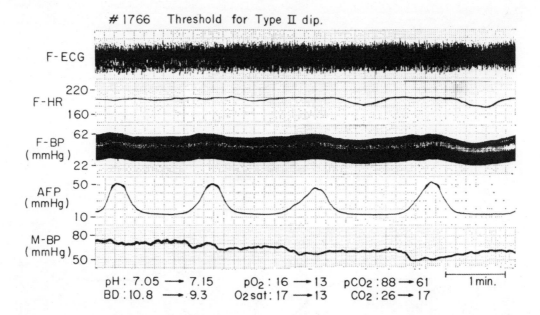

#1766 Threshold for Type II dip.

F-ECG

F-HR 220— 160—

F-BP (mmHg) 62— 22—

AFP (mmHg) 50— 10—

M-BP (mmHg) 80— 50—

pH: 7.05 → 7.15   pO₂: 16 → 13   pCO₂: 88 → 61   1 min.
BD: 10.8 → 9.3   O₂sat: 17 → 13   CO₂: 26 → 17

Figure 14-27 Late decelerations triggered by maternal hypotension. Recording obtained during term induced labor in rhesus monkey. Top three tracings are fetal; lower two are maternal: intrauterine pressure and mean blood pressure below an aortic band capable of reducing the flow and pressure. With the first uterine contraction and a mean blood pressure of 72 mm Hg there is no change in FHR; the second contraction, started with a mean blood pressure of 62 mm Hg, triggered a mild FHR late deceleration. The last contraction, started with a mean blood pressure of 50 mm Hg, triggered a clear fetal late deceleration coinciding with a fall in fetal blood pressure. The fetus had been acidotic before this part of the tracing (blood gas levels shown at the bottom). Reprinted from Myers RE: Two patterns of perinatal brain damage and their condition of occurrence. *Am J Obstet Gynecol* 112:246, 1972.

Nevertheless, late decelerations demonstrated only a relative *predictive value* of the fetal condition at birth: 35% of those who had late decelerations during first stage were depressed at the first minute of life (Figure 14-30) (significantly more than the 9% observed among the no-deceleration group, but still not a very good predictor because wholly 65% of them were born in good condition). Late decelerations represent fetal distress of some degree, as indicated by the finding that baseline alterations of the FHR tracing are seen in the same patients (Figure 14-31); these changes often occur only transiently, but, when the clinical conditions remain unchanged, they may be recorded for the remainder of labor in association with the late decelerations (Figure 14-32).

These observations point out that general predictions are prone to failure unless they are based on extreme and stringent conditions. Several authors have attempted to quantitate the

FHR decelerations to establish a predictive value to given figures. Sureau et al (1970), Sturbois et al (1977), and Tournaire et al (1973, 1976), have studied the "total deceleration area" and fractions thereof expressed as square seconds/hour and found a reasonable correlation with umbilical artery pH. Shelly and Tipton (1971) and Künzel and Cornely (1976) evaluated the dip area, irrespective of its relationship with the contraction, and also claim to have found a reasonably correlation with the fetal acid–base balance and Apgar score. However, Albrecht et al (1975), assessing the "total dip areas," found little correlation with outcome unless "dip parameters" were included among the variables. Lowensohn et al (1975) observed that the deceleration area correlated with fetal scalp pH is a good parameter to predict acid–base status of the fetus. The most recent method offered is the "deceleration index" (Acien et al, 1979), which evaluates several elements of the deceleration: delay to start following onset of

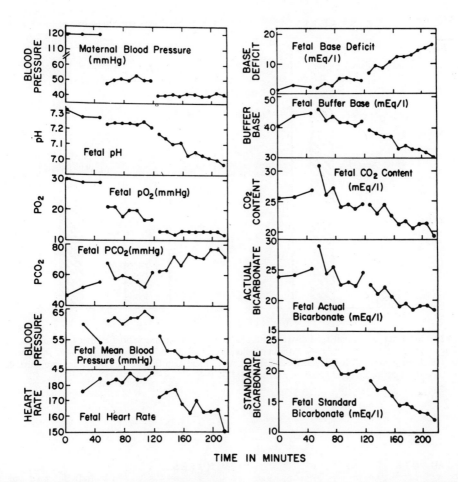

Figure 14-28 Maternal and fetal vital signs, fetal blood gas levels, and acid–base status observed during a period of over 200 minutes. Normal maternal mean blood measure (120 mm Hg), borderline compensated hypotension (50 mm Hg), and decompensated hypotension (40 mm Hg). Each point represents values obtained at the corresponding time. During the first 60 min with normal maternal blood pressure the fetal pO_2 was 30 mm Hg and the pH 7.32. During the period of maternal hypotension at 50 mm Hg the fetal pO_2 dropped to about 20 mm Hg with no significant change in FHR or blood pressure, and the pH stayed around 7.25. When maternal blood pressure dropped to 40 mm Hg, fetal hypoxia supervened followed by fetal bradycardia, hypotension, and progressive fetal acidosis. The threshold for fetal derangement seems to have been just below 50 mm Hg mean maternal pressure in this particular preparation. Reprinted from Myers RE: Two patterns of perinatal brain damage and their condition of occurrence. *Am J Obstet Gynecol* 112:246, 1972.

the contraction, and lag time, duration, and amplitude of the fall. Its proponents claim a good correlation between values calculated in 30 minutes and fetal outcome. All these methods have their merit and are useful research tools, but unless the monitor is hooked to a computer, their application is relative and of limited use in clinical practice. The best predictions, applying any of the described methods, are on the order of 70%, which is not extremely good. Purely clinical

means (careful reading of tracings) should approximate 70% if the observers are adequately trained.

Another way to improve the predictive value of a sign like late decelerations would be to evaluate its incidence in a more specific group of patients rather than a general hospital population and relate findings to fetal outcome, or to determine their ratio with respect to number of contractions and fetal condition at birth. Along these

332

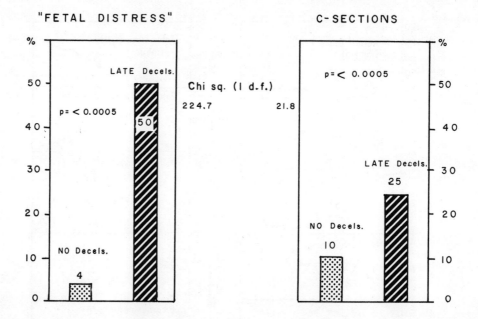

Figure 14-29 Incidence of clinical fetal distress and cesarean section among labors evolving without any decelerations and with late decelerations. Only 4% without decelerations had clinical distress and 10% were sectioned, the majority for "arrest of progress." Reprinted from Cibils LA: Clinical significance of fetal heart rate patterns during labor. II. Late decelerations. *Am J Obstet Gynecol* 123:473, 1975.

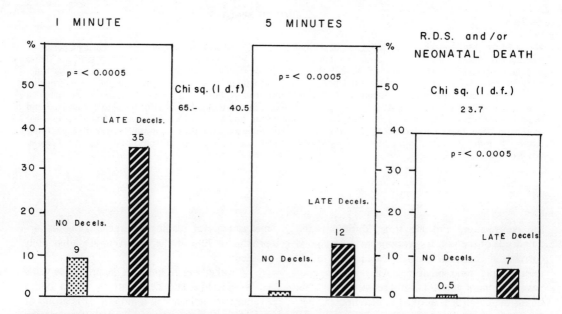

Figure 14-30 Proportion of cases with late decelerations (striped) who at birth had Apgar scores of 6 or less (depressed) at 1 and 5 min, compared with cases evolving without decelerations. Immediate neonatal morbidity and mortality indicates a significant increase among those who had late decelerations. Reprinted from Cibils LA: Clinical significance of fetal heart rate patterns during labor. II. Late decelerations. *Am J Obstet Gynecol* 123:473, 1975.

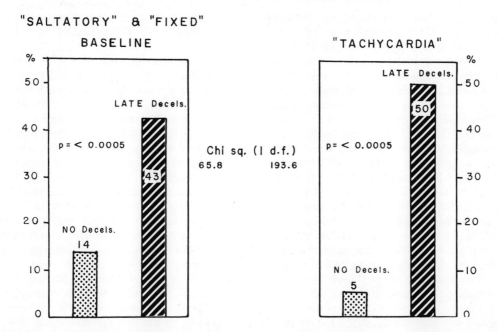

Figure 14-31 Proportion of cases with late decelerations who had associated *transient baseline alterations;* many cases had combination of tachycardia with one or both other changes. When there were no decelerations the incidence of these alterations was relatively very low. Reprinted from Cibils LA: Clinical significance of fetal heart rate patterns during labor. II. Late decelerations. *Am J Obstet Gynecol* 123:473, 1975.

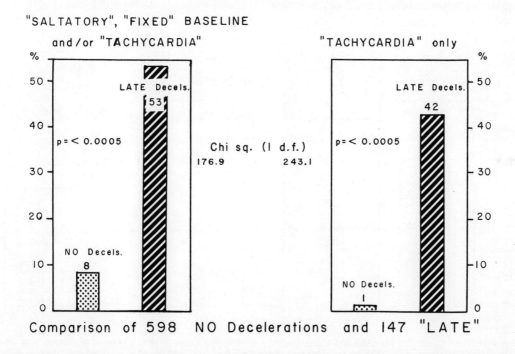

Figure 14-32 Proportion of cases with late decelerations and associated *sustained baseline alterations (Left)* All three abnormalities. *(Right)* Only tachycardias. Very few cases without decelerations had sustained tachycardia. Reprinted from Cibils LA: Clinical significance of fetal heart rate patterns during labor. II. Late decelerations. *Am J Obstet Gynecol* 123:473, 1975.

334

lines, Mendez-Bauer et al (1969) postulated that the recording of "15 contractions is sufficient to detect distress and predict outcome." The experience here reported does not quite agree with that statement because there are too many different potential causes of late decelerations. Also, hypoxia, measured by oxygen saturation at birth, has been found to correlate poorly with fetal vigor (James et al, 1958). The search for specific patient populations has shown that, among the fetuses premature by weight, the finding of late decelerations has a better predictive value (50%) than among the heavier infants (Figure 14-33). The association with baseline alterations indicates that the small infants have high incidences of tachycardia and, curiously, almost total absence of saltatory pattern, a finding that may indicate that chronologic maturity may be an important prerequisite for their occurrence (Figure 14-34). The magnitude of the deceleration does not seem to have a predictive value unless "overlappings" are observed, in which case the tracing has the aspect of persistent bradycardia. Among these small fetuses there is a positive correlation between number of contractions and decelerations; the correlation is negative between number of decelerations and Apgar scores at 1 and 5 min indicating

that, after all, the repetition of hypoxia episodes has an influence on the condition of the infant at birth.

Of course, the prognosis of a given fetus will be poor if late decelerations occur with every contraction and the interval between them is not sufficient to allow for fetal recovery: progressive acidosis will be the inevitable consequence. On the other hand, if the decelerations are triggered only by the very strong contractions and/or there is good interval between them for fetal recovery, it may be possible to observe the patient for some time without drastic intervention. The simultaneous recording of associated baseline alterations constitutes added prognostic, and predictive, elements as they were found to be constantly observed in the overwhelming majority of fetuses born depressed (Figure 14-35). This finding was particularly evident for tachycardia, and, to a lesser degree, for fixed baseline. Furthermore, the same finding held true among the majority of fetuses with clinical fetal distress. Almost 20% of those born depressed and who had late decelerations presented severe neonatal complications or died. The association of these FHR alterations with poor neonatal condition is further demonstrated when one observes that almost all the in-

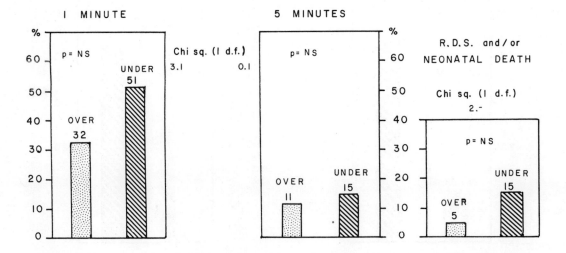

Figure 14-33 Incidence of neonatal depression (Apgar 6 or less) according to weight among all *fetuses with late decelerations* weighing under 2500 gm (striped) and those weighing over 2500 gm (dotted). The small fetuses were depressed in higher proportion and also had a higher incidence of immediate neonatal complications. Reprinted from Cibils LA: Clinical significance of fetal heart rate patterns during labor. II. Late decelerations. *Am J Obstet Gynecol* 123:473, 1975.

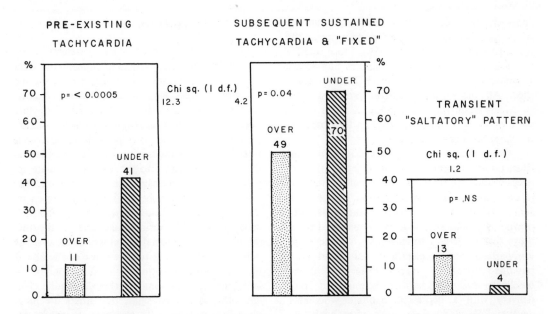

Figure 14-34 Incidence of *baseline alterations among all fetuses with late decelerations*. Those weighing under 2500 gm (striped) had a high incidence of tachycardia from the beginning of the monitoring. An even higher proportion had it sustained and associated with fixed baseline. Of note is the low incidence of saltatory pattern among premature infants. Reprinted from Cibils LA: Clinical significance of fetal heart rate patterns during labor. II. Late decelerations. *Am J Obstet Gynecol* 123:473, 1975.

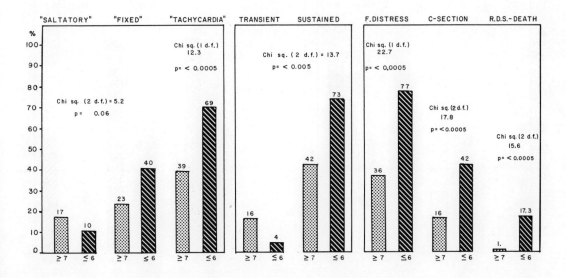

Figure 14-35 *(Left and center)* Incidence of *baseline alterations* and clinical distress, cesarean section rate, and *(right)* neonatal morbidity among *fetuses with late decelerations* born with Apgar scores of 6 or less at *1 min* (striped). All the abnormalities were higher than among those born with good Apgar scores (dotted). Tachycardia and fixed baseline were almost uniformly present.

fants who were still depressed at the fifth minute of life had them in a sustained manner during the latter part of labor (Figure 14-36). Close to 50% of those still depressed at 5 minutes had severe respiratory distress syndrome (RDS) and some died. All the serious neonatal problems were much less frequently seen among the fetuses who were vigorous at birth even though they had late decelerations during labor.

Other clinical characteristics that seem to influence the outcome of the small fetus with late decelerations are maternal pathologic conditions (anemia, heart disease, hypertension, diabetes, Rh sensitization, abruptio placentae, placenta previa). The following sequence—maternal pathology that involves a small fetus which develops intrapartum late decelerations associated with baseline alterations (tachycardia and fixed baseline)—leads the way to termination in a delivery with a depressed neonate who may develop RDS and/or die soon after birth. As pointed out in Chapter 12, age of gestation is a critical variable when one interprets alterations of a FHR tracing (see also Chapter 16).

FETAL DISTRESS

The observation of a late deceleration indicates that at that particular moment the fetus experiences an episode of transient hypoxia and therefore distress. Recurrence is evidence of a persistent hindrance with fetal oxygenation that needs rapid correction if one is to avoid the impending catastrophe. It is possible to refine the interpretation of the tracing and improve the predictive value of this information with ultimate application to the management of each case. The observation of *one late deceleration is not an indication for immediate interference* with labor. It calls for close observation and analysis of the tracing for possible associated changes of the baseline pattern while looking for the cause of the alteration: a maternal factor, a fetal factor, or an iatrogenic factor. Some of these are quite clear and obvious at first sight, but others are more obscure and difficult to elucidate. In either case one must attempt to increase fetal oxygenation by giving oxygen to the mother by mask. Under most circumstances this action will improve the FHR

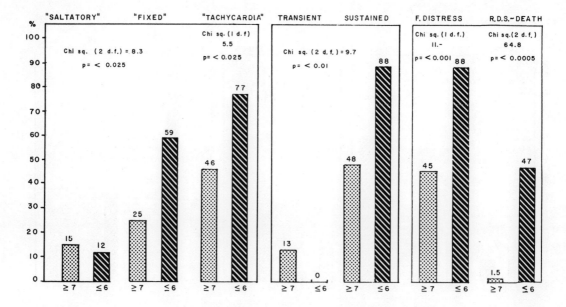

Figure 14-36 Incidence of *baseline alterations* and neonatal outcome among the fetuses with late decelerations who had Apgar scores of 6 or less at *5 min*. Those who were not depressed at the fifth minute had a much lower proportion of baseline abnormalities. Almost all depressed fetuses had sustained abnormalities during labor and almost one-half of them had severe neonatal problems.

even when everything else remains unchanged (Figure 14-11) and no obvious cause can be found. The increased maternal oxygen tension passes on to the fetus and thereby increases the fetal pO$_2$ above the critical threshold (17 to 18 mm Hg) below which the heart decelerates (Figure 14-37). In some cases the extra oxygen thus supplied to the fetus may be enough to allow labor to proceed without fetal deterioration until successful vaginal delivery (Figure 14-24), while in others it may improve the fetal oxygenation but not sufficiently to allow labor to proceed. Then the transient fetal improvement may allow time for adequate preparations for cesarean section (Figure 14-21).

On occasion, the fetal condition may seem to improve with oxygen administration to the mother, but later deteriorate again when the underlying cause continues to exert its negative influence on the IVS circulation (Figure 14-25). The ideal step consists of obtaining a sample of fetal capillary blood to determine the pH, and this sampling may be repeated later depending on the fetal response. When this response is favorable there will be improvement of the fetal acid-base status, while this status may deteriorate rapidly if the decelerations are repeated too frequently (Figure 14-8). The ultimate decision should be based on 1) fetal response to oxygenation; 2) cause of the condition causing poor oxygen uptake by the fetus; 3) speed of the change of fetal acid-base status; and 4) stage of labor when the

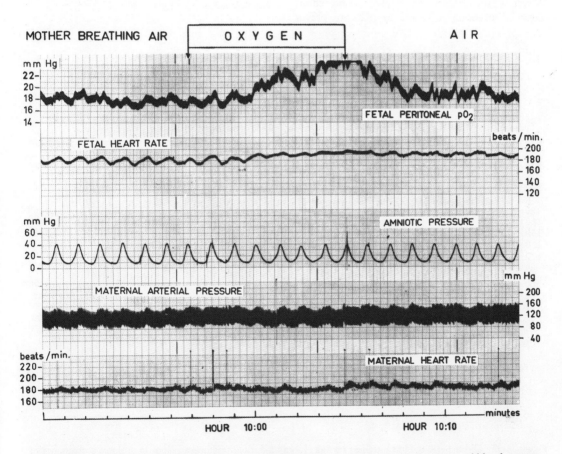

Figure 14-37 Simultaneous recording of fetal peritoneal pO$_2$, FHR, intrauterine pressure, maternal blood pressure, and heart rate during induced labor in term pregnant rhesus monkey. The high induced uterine contractility (1 contraction/min) triggered late decelerations when the fetal peritoneal pO$_2$ was about 18 mm Hg while the mother was breathing room air. The administration of oxygen increased the fetal pO$_2$ to more than 24 mm Hg, and late decelerations were absent, in spite of unchanged uterine activity and maternal BP. The last contraction triggered a deceleration when the fetal pO$_2$ was at 18 mm Hg. Reprinted from Pose, et al (1963).

decelerations are observed. The last is critical because under many conditions a vaginal delivery might be a more rapid procedure than a cesarean section. When the latter is contemplated, and the cause of the fetal distress is normal uterine contractions, Caldeyro-Barcia proposes a most interesting approach: suppression of uterine contractions by the administration of β-mimetic substances to facilitate the intrauterine recovery of an acidotic fetus before the operation (Figure 14-38). This logical way to manage the situation has the same effect as the suppression of oxytocin infusion when the hypercontractility triggered by this hormone is responsible for the fetal distress. However, β-mimetic substances need to be used with great caution because they are hypotensive and may thereby contribute to diminish the IVS blood supply. This move is contraindicated in cases of abruptio placentae or placenta previa for the potential worsening effect on these conditions.

In any event, fetal distress is not diagnosed by one or a few late decelerations observed in a FHR tracing; these are transient episodes of hypoxia that may or may not lead to distress. Before taking any active step to interfere it is critical to watch for the presence of associated FHR alterations: tachycardia, saltatory pattern, fixed baseline, bradycardia, or sinusoidal pattern. Only with these added signs may one strongly suspect fetal compromise, which should be proved by capillary blood pH determination. If this test is not available one must assess the clinical picture, taking into consideration other parameters in addition to FHR changes. Only then will a tentative diagnosis be warranted before one can act accordingly.

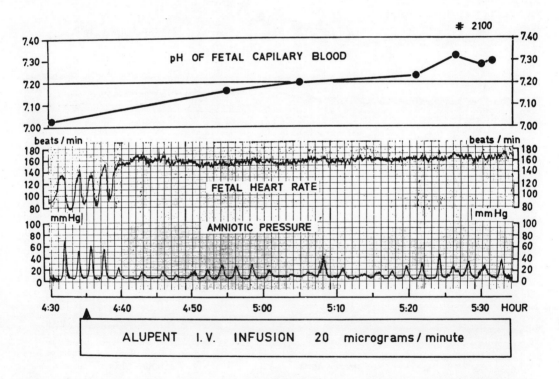

Figure 14-38 Direct FHR and intrauterine pressure recording during spontaneous labor in prolonged pregnancy of primipara. The severe late decelerations triggered by strong contractions of active labor induced a fetal acidosis, pH 7.03 (values above). The intravenous infusion of the β-mimetic metaproterenol at 20 μg/min (arrow) suppressed the very strong contractions. FHR had a rebound tachycardia, and the fetal pH rose steadily to reach normal values at hour 5:25. A vigorous infant was delivered by cesarean section 30 min later, and the placenta had extensive lesions. Reprinted from Caldeyro-Barcia R, et al: Fetal monitoring in labor, in Wallace HM, Gold EM, Lis EF (eds): *Maternal and Child Health Practices.* Courtesy of Charles C Thomas, Publisher, Springfield, Ill, 1973, pp 332–394.

BIBLIOGRAPHY

Acien P, Salvatierra V, Navarrete L: Fetal heart rate deceleration index. Its relation with fetal pH, Apgar score and dips or decelerations. *J Perinat Med* 7:7, 1979.

Albrecht H, Bokelmann J, Morgenstern J, et al: Some remarks concerning the fetal heart rate total dip areas. *J Perinat Med* 3:226, 1975.

Althabe O, Schwarcz RL, Pose SV, et al: Effect on fetal heart rate and fetal pO₂ of oxygen administration to the mother. *Am J Obstet Gynecol* 98:858, 1967.

Assali NS, Holm LW, Sehgal N: Hemodynamic changes in fetal lamb in utero in response to asphyxia, hypoxia and hypercapnia. *Circ Res* 11:423, 1962.

Barcroft J: *Researches on Prenatal Life,* chap 12. Oxford, Blackwell, 1946, pp 123–144.

Beard RW, Morris ED, Clayton SG: Fetal blood sampling in clinical obstetrics. *J Obstet Gynaecol Br Comwlth* 73:562–570, 1966.

Beguin F, Yeh SY, Forsythe A, et al: A study of fetal heart rate deceleration areas. II. Correlation between deceleration areas and fetal pH during labor. *Obstet Gynecol* 45:292, 1975.

Berg D, Schulz J, Wernicke K, et al: The effects of experimental acute decrease of uterine perfusion and maternal hypoxia on the fetus. *J Perinat Med* 1:36, 1973.

Bieniarz J, Fernandez R, Caldeyro-Barcia R: Effects of maternal hypotension on the human fetus. II. FHR in labors associated with cord around neck and toxemia. *Am J Obstet Gynecol* 92:832, 1965.

Brady JP, James LS, Baker MA: Heart rate changes in the fetus and newborn during labor, delivery, and immediate neonatal period. *Am J Obstet Gynecol* 84:1, 1962.

Caldeyro-Barcia R, Mendez-Bauer C, Poseiro JJ, et al: Control of human fetal heart rate during labor, in Cassels DE (ed): *The Heart and Circulation of the Newborn and Infant.* New York, Grune & Stratton, 1966, pp 7–36.

Caldeyro-Barcia R, Casacuberta C, Bustos R, et al: Correlation of intrapartum changes in fetal heart rate with fetal blood oxygen and acid-base state, in Adamsons K (ed): *Diagnosis and Treatment of Fetal Disorders.* New York, Springer-Verlag, 1968, pp 205–225.

Caldeyro-Barcia R, Mendez-Bauer C, Poseiro JJ, et al: Fetal monitoring in labor, in Wallace HM, Gold EM, Lis EF (eds): *Maternal and Child Health Practices.* Springfield, Ill, Thomas, 1973, pp 332–394.

Cibils LA: Clinical significance of fetal heart rate patterns during labor. I. Baseline patterns. *Am J Obstet Gynecol* 125:290, 1976.

Cibils LA: Clinical significance of fetal heart rate patterns during labor. II. Late decelerations. *Am J Obstet Gynecol* 123:473, 1975.

Cohn HE, Sacks EJ, Heymann AM, et al: Cardiovascular responses to hypoxemia and acidemia in fetal lambs. *Am J Obstet Gynecol* 120:817, 1974.

Dawes GS: Cardiovascular adjustment of the fetus during asphyxia: The aortic chemoreceptors, in *Perinatal Factors Affecting Human Development.* Washington, DC, Pan American Health Organization Scientific Publication 185, 1969, pp 199–201.

Gabert HA, Stenchever MA: Continuous electronic monitoring of fetal heart rate during labor. *Am J Obstet Gynecol* 115:919, 1963.

Gabert HA, Stenchever MA: Electronic fetal monitoring as a routine practice in an obstetric service: A progress report. *Am J Obstet Gynecol* 118:534, 1974.

Greiss FC, Anderson SG: Uterine blood flow during labor. *Clin Obstet Gynecol* 11:96, 1968.

Hammacher K, Huter KA, Bokelmann J, et al: Foetal heart frequency and perinatal conditions of the fetus and newborn. *Gynaecologia* 166:349, 1968.

Hon EH: Electronic evaluation of the fetal heart rate. *Am J Obstet Gynecol* 83:333, 1962.

Hon EH: The classification of fetal heart rate. *Obstet Gynecol* 22:137, 1963.

Hon EH: Additional observations on "pathologic" bradycardia. *Am J Obstet Gynecol* 118:428, 1974.

Hon EH, Khazin AF, Paul RH: Biochemical studies of the fetus. II. Fetal pH and Apgar scores. *Obstet Gynecol* 33:237, 1969.

James LS, Weisbrot IM, Prince CE, et al: The acid-base status of human infants in relation to birth asphyxia and the onset of respiration. *J Pediatr* 52:379, 1958.

James LS, Morishima HO, Daniel SS, et al: Mechanism of late deceleration of the fetal heart rate. *Am J Obstet Gynecol* 113:578, 1972.

Kubli FW, Hon EH, Khazin AF, et al: Observations on the heart rate and pH on the human fetus during labor. *Am J Obstet Gynecol* 104, 1190, 1969.

Kunzel W, Cornely M: Dip area in fetal heart rate and its relationship to acid-base observations of fetus and mother during labor. *J Perinat Med* 4:271, 1976.

Lowensohn RI, Yeh SY, Forsythe A, et al: Computer assessed fetal heart rate patterns and fetal scalp pH. *Obstet Gynecol* 46:190, 1975.

Martin CB, Siassi B, Hon EH: Fetal heart rate patterns and neonatal death in low birth weight infants. *Obstet Gynecol* 44:503, 1974.

Mendez-Bauer C, Poseiro JJ, Arellano G, et al: Effects of atropine on the human heart rate during labor. *Am J Obstet Gynecol* 85:1033, 1963.

Mendez-Bauer C, Arnt IC, Gulin L, et al: Relationship between blood pH and heart rate in the human fetus during labor. *Am J Obstet Gynecol* 97:530, 1967.

Mendez-Bauer C, Monleon J, Guevara RG, et al: Changes in fetal heart rate associated with acute intrapartum fetal distress, in *Perinatal Factors Affecting Human Development*. Washington, DC, Pan American Health Organization Scientific Publication 185, 1969, pp 178–187.

Myers RE: Two patterns of perinatal brain damage and their condition of occurrence. *Am J Obstet Gynecol* 112:246, 1972.

Myers RE, Mueller-Heubach E, Adamsons K: Predictability of the state of fetal oxygenation from a quantitative analysis of the components of late deceleration. *Am J Obstet Gynecol* 115:1083, 1973.

Nakai T, Yamada R: The secretion of catecholamines in newborn babies with special reference to fetal distress. *J Perinat Med* 6:39, 1978.

O'Gureck JE, Roux JF, Newman MR: Neonatal depression and fetal heart rate patterns during labor. *Obstet Gynecol* 40:347, 1972.

Paul RH: Clinical fetal monitoring. *Am J Obstet Gynecol* 113:573, 1972.

Pose SV, Escarcena L, Caldeyro-Barcia R: La presion parcial de oxigeno en el feto durante el parto. *IV Cong Mex Ginecol Obstet* 2:41, 1963.

Quilligan EJ, Paul RH: Fetal monitoring: Is it worth it? *Obstet Gynecol* 45:96, 1975.

Saling E, Schneider D: Biochemical supervision of the fetus during labor. *J Obstet Gynaecol Br Comwlth* 74:799, 1967.

Shelly T, Tipton RH: Dip area. A quantitative measure of fetal heart rate patterns. *J Obstet Gynaecol Br Comwlth* 78:694, 1971.

Shenker L: Clinical experience with fetal heart rate monitoring of one thousand patients in labor. *Am J Obstet Gynecol* 115:1111, 1973.

Sturbois G, Tournaire M, Breart G, et al: Evaluation of the fetal state by automatic analysis of the heart rate: Deceleration area and fetal pH. *Eur J Obstet Gynecol Reprod Biol* 7:261, 1977.

Sturbois G, Tournaire M, Ripoche A, et al: Evaluation of the fetal state by automatic analysis of the heart rate. *J Perinat Med* 1:235, 1973.

Sturbois G, Tournaire M, Ripoche A, et al: Calcul automatique des surfaces de ralentissement du rythme cardiaque fetal. *J Gynecol Obstet Biol Reprod (Paris)* 3:955, 1974.

Sureau C, Chavinie J, Cannon M, et al: Recherches sur le rythme cardiaque fetal. Etude d'un integrateur des variations du rythme. *Gen Biol Med* 1:384, 1970.

Sureau C, Chavinie J, Maziou ML, et al: Le rythme cardiaque fetal. *J Gynecol Obstet Biol Reprod (Paris)* 1:249, 1972.

Sureau C, Sturbois G, Tournaire M, et al: Les surfaces de deceleration. *6me J Nation Med Perinat* (Biarritz) 1976, pp 251–263.

Tournaire M, Sturbois G, et al: Evaluation of the fetal state by automatic analysis of the heart rate. II. Deceleration areas and umbilical artery blood pH. *J Perinat Med* 4:118, 1976.

Tournaire M, Yeh SY, Forsythe A, Hon EH: A study of fetal heart rate deceleration areas. I. *Obstet Gynecol* 42:711, 1973.

Wood G: Use of fetal blood sampling and fetal heart rate monitoring, in Adamsons K (ed): *Diagnosis and Treatment of Fetal Disorders*. New York, Springer-Verlag, 1968, pp 163–174.

CHAPTER 15
Variable Decelerations

The decrease in FHR that begins during the ascending phase of the uterine contraction tracing, has a short period of sustained low frequency, and recovers rapidly during the relaxation phase of the contraction has been called *variable deceleration* by Hon and Quilligan (1967). There is no predictable relationship between the amplitude of deceleration and the intensity of the contractions that trigger it; likewise, there is a great *variability* with regard to the timing of their onset, or the ascending phase of those contractions (Figure 15-1). It has been characterized by a U shape because of the sustained slow rate during maximum fall (but of course this shape depends on the speed of the recording paper). Originally Caldeyro-Barcia included this type of deceleration with what he called *type I dip,* but later (1973) subdivided this group and labeled the variable decelerations as *umbilical dips* (calling the remainder *cephalic dips).*

Great variability characterizes this deceleration, but the general common elements are always present: 1) the deceleration *starts* in the ascending phase of the contraction; 2) it *falls* rather rapidly, often precipitously; 3) it *remains* at low frequency for several seconds, frequently prolonged; 4) the *recovery starts* during the relaxation phase of the contraction. These decelerations change because of the variability in moment of onset of FHR fall, the magnitude of this fall, and pattern of the recovery period. These have served as the basis for the subclassification of this FHR pattern into "nonvariables" (when they tend to look generally uniform), moderate or "classic," and "severe variables," depending on the speed of the recovery phase and/or the amplitude of the decelerations. The changing pattern may be an intrinsic variable intimately tied to the mechanisms of production and its consequences on the fetus.

PATHOPHYSIOLOGY

Unlike the "early" and "late" decelerations reviewed in previous chapters, the *direct cause for the production* of the variable decelerations has been accepted, for a number of years, to be a *compression of the umbilical cord.* Barcroft (1946) demonstrated in experimental animals that the interruption of umbilical blood flow would cause a sudden deceleration of FHR, sustained for some time, and rapid recovery after restoring the normal blood circulation (Figure 15-2). These observations have been reproduced in humans under very special conditions (Hon, Goodlin) of prolapsed cords during premature labors with probably nonviable fetuses. However, the reasons for the extraordinary variability in the pattern of decelerations was not clearly understood until much more recently when several groups of investigators made systematic studies in subhuman primates and careful clinical observations.

Among the many interesting associated changes observed in the FHR, in conjunction with variable decelerations, has been the presence of *accelerations* triggered by the contractions (Goodlin, 1974; Lee et al, 1975). These authors observed that when there are transient accelerations produced by contractions in the early stages of labor, variable decelerations are often recorded in more advanced stages of dilatation; in fact, the superposition of a variable deceleration on an acceleration of the FHR has been called "blunted acceleration" (Figures 15-1 and 15-15). These observations were subsequently confirmed by others, who labeled them "mixed cord compression pattern" (Goldkrand, 1975). Studies conducted in baboons and rhesus monkeys (James et al, 1976) demonstrated that partial occlusion of the umbilical vein and/or the intact cord trigger a

342

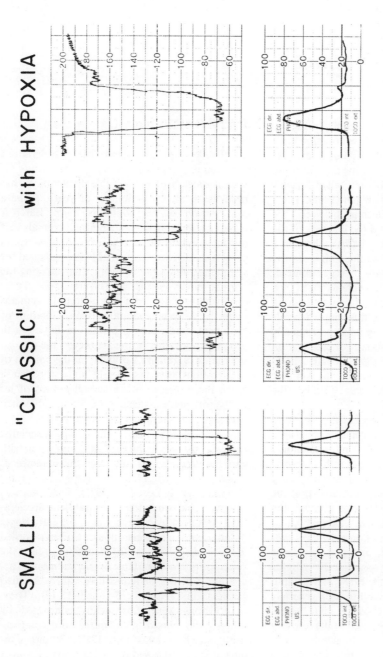

SMALL   "CLASSIC"   with HYPOXIA

Figure 15-1 Most common types of variable decelerations. *(Left) Small:* two sharp looking decelerations starting on the ascending part of the uterine contractions, V shaped with fast recovery to the baseline; the first one seems to start during the beginning of an acceleration, and recovery seems to correspond with descending part of the acceleration. *(Center) Classic:* three decelerations of similar general characteristics, starting during the ascending phase of the contraction a sharp fall of 60 to 100 beats with a low plateau lasting 30 to 45 sec and rapid recovery to the baseline with good rapid oscillations. Duration, 55 to 80 sec. There is no relationship between intensity of contractions and magnitude of fall; the second one seems to start during an acceleration. *(Right)* With hypoxia: a deceleration of large magnitude starting from a tachycardic and fixed baseline at the beginning of the contraction, and with a plateau of 50 sec. Because the recovery phase is slow and curving toward the baseline not quite reached after 150 sec and looks much like the second half of a late deceleration, these decelerations are called *variable with hypoxia* (or variable with late components). Reprinted from Cibils LA: Clinical significance of fetal heart rate patterns during labor. V. Variable decelerations. *Am J Obstet Gynecol* 132:791, 1978.

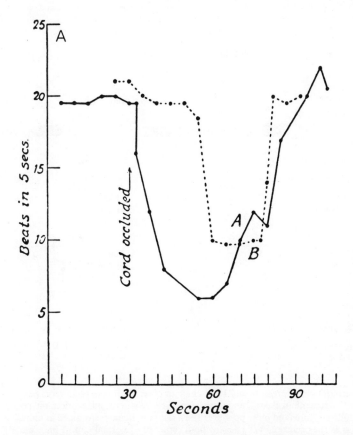

Figure 15-2 Effect on FHR of cord occlusion, in a goat. The heavy line A illustrates the response of the intact animal: immediate dramatic deceleration plateauing after 20 sec; recovery is rapid with slight rebound after circulation restitution. The interrupted line B illustrates the response after bilateral section of the vagus nerves: the FHR deceleration is delayed by 25 sec and the plateau is established at a higher level; the recovery is rapid but without rebound. After Barcroft J: *Researches On Prenatal Life*. Oxford, Blackwell, 1946.

rapid and *sustained acceleration* of the FHR (Figure 15-3) in *well oxygenated fetuses,* thus suggesting that the observations of similar episodes during human labor may well indicate partial compression of the umbilical cord. However, moderately hypoxic fetuses do not respond with acceleration to partial occlusion of the umbilical vessels; on the contrary, they have a sharp deceleration with slow recovery after restoration of the blood flow (Figure 15-4).

The *mechanism* involved in this fetal response was also studied by the same authors. It appears that partial compression of the umbilical vein (and of the whole cord) would decrease blood return to the right side of the heart and set the stage for hypotension; the baroreceptor response would be tachycardia stimulated by the sympathetic system. In fact, the acceleration response

has been blocked using α- and β-mimetic blocking substances; dramatic hypotension occurred when the α-mimetic blockers were used, indicating that release of catecholamines is one of the compensatory mechanisms to maintain homeostasis during partial compression of the cord. The reasons for a different response by the hypoxic, moderately acidotic fetus are less clear but this pattern of response must have very important clinical implications.

The various degrees and types of *decelerations* are clearly the response to more significant interruption of umbilical blood flow such as the severe decelerations observed following partial occlusions of the umbilical cord in the hypoxic fetuses. *Complete occlusion of the umbilical vein* in well oxygenated fetuses triggers a short period of acceleration followed by a rapidly progressing

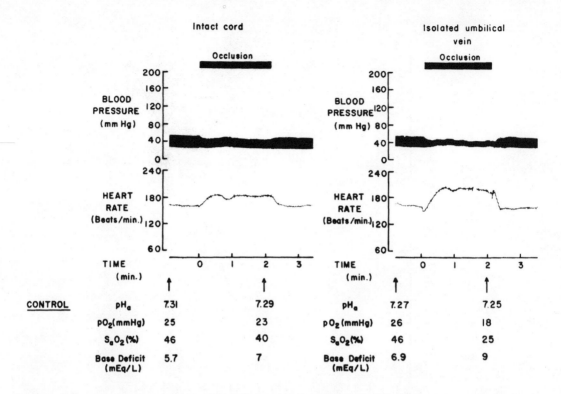

Figure 15-3 Fetal arterial blood pressure and FHR changes observed in a baboon fetus near term following *partial occlusion* in the *(left)* intact umbilical cord, and *(right)* umbilical vein in the intraabdominal portion. In both instances there is a fall of systolic pressure (and pulse pressure) and a rise in pulse rate, sustained as long as partial occlusion was maintained. As soon as the occlusion was released both returned to normal almost immediately. Note the minimal drop in pO_2 and pH, and small rise in base deficit. Reprinted from James LS, et al: Umbilical vein occlusion and transient acceleration of the fetal heart rate. *Am J Obstet Gynecol* 126:276, 1976.

deceleration (Figure 15-5). From the start of the deceleration to the moment of reaching the lowest values 10 to 30 sec usually elapse, depending on the degree of occlusion and amplitude of the deceleration. Simultaneously with the FHR deceleration other alterations occur to compensate for this drastic interference with fetal hemodynamics. If the occlusion is almost complete, two significant changes will suddenly occur in the fetal circulation: 1) severe diminution of venous return to the right heart, leading to hypovolemic hypotension, and 2) release of catecholamines to compensate for this, with increased diastolic pressure and decreased pulse pressure as result of a decreased stroke volume.

Complete occlusion of the umbilical cord, on the other hand, triggers an immediate and pro-gressive bradycardia that reaches the lowest values within 20 sec; at the same time there is a sudden increase in blood pressure followed by slow decline after having reached maximum values within a few seconds of the interference with umbilical circulation (Figure 15-6). The release of the occlusion is followed by a rapid return to normal with a short rebound above preocclusion levels. The hemodynamic effects of total occlusion are different from the isolated venous occlusion because there is an added interruption of the arterial flow to more than 35% to 40% of the fetal vascular tree, resulting in increased peripheral resistance. The sudden increase in blood pressure triggers the baroreceptor reflex and the rapid bradycardia, overcoming the effect of catecholamines probably released at the same time.

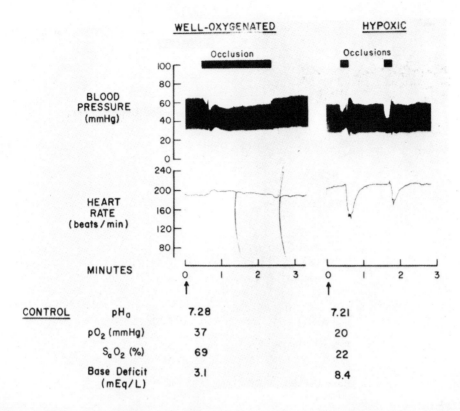

WELL-OXYGENATED   HYPOXIC

Occlusion   Occlusions

BLOOD PRESSURE (mmHg)

HEART RATE (beats/min)

MINUTES

CONTROL		WELL-OXYGENATED	HYPOXIC
	pH_a	7.28	7.21
	pO_2 (mmHg)	37	20
	S_aO_2 (%)	69	22
	Base Deficit (mEq/L)	3.1	8.4

Figure 15-4 Fetal arterial blood pressure and FHR changes observed in a baboon fetus near term following *partial occlusion* of the umbilical cord. The preocclusion values for fetal blood pO_2 and acid–base status are below, sampled at the arrows. The *well-oxygenated* fetus responded with tachycardia and diminished systolic pressure; the *borderline oxygenated* fetus responded with same changes in blood pressure but FHR had a sharp fall and slow recovery following the very short periods of occlusion. Reprinted from James LS, et al: Umbilical vein occlusion and transient acceleration of the fetal heart rate. *Am J Obstet Gynecol* 126:276, 1976.

Mechanisms

The pathways of sudden changes observed after clamping of the cord were originally investigated by Barcroft. The hemodynamic alterations induced by an incomplete cord compression are probably somewhat different from the complete occlusion produced in the laboratory. However, the mechanisms involved must be the same, varying only in degree and intensity. The administration of atropine to a fetus having variable decelerations may reduce or completely obliterate them while inducing other known effects of parasympathetic blockade (Figure 15-7). This response would suggest that the FHR deceleration is exclusively vagus-mediated; however, other observations made under controlled conditions and selected degrees of occlusion suggest that the vagal reflex is only the first component of a complex response (see Figure 15-2). Parasympathetic blockade delays by about 15 to 25 sec the onset of the bradycardia following total occlusion of the cord; furthermore, the mangitude of the deceleration is of lesser degree (Figure 15-8) but tends to continue downward if the occlusion is very prolonged. These are very consistent and predictable findings indicating strong vagal influence on the function of the fetal heart. Nevertheless, the parasympathetic control is less clearly manifested on the blood pressure changes induced by cord occlusion (Figure 15-9).

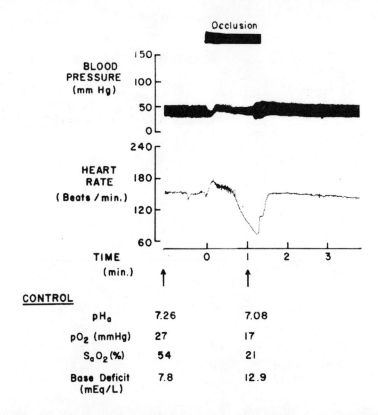

Figure 15-5 Fetal blood pressure and FHR recordings obtained in a baboon fetus near term. Effect of *complete occlusion of the umbilical vein* in well-oxygenated animal (blood gas levels drawn at arrows): a transient acceleration of the heart rate is followed by rapidly progressing bradycardia. At the same time there is a fall in systolic pressure and rise in diastolic with diminished pulse pressure; rapidly progressing acidosis. Recovery takes place immediately following release of occlusion. Reprinted from James LS, et al: Umbilical vein occlusion and transient acceleration of the fetal heart rate. *Am J Obstet Gynecol* 126:276, 1976.

It has been postulated that *myocardial hypoxia* may be, in large part, responsible for the delayed component of the variable FHR decelerations (see Figures 15-2, 15-8, and 15-9) because with sustained occlusion there is rapid development of marked hypoxemia. When the episode of hypoxia is continued for a sustained period of time, the effects on the FHR recovery are manifested, and a pattern similar to the recovery phase of the late deceleration (see Chapter 14) is then recorded (see Figure 15-1); the same phenomenon has been observed under experimental conditions when determinations of pO_2 have been carried out. In Figure 15-9 an average of over 30 sec passed between resumption of umbilical circulation and recovery of preocclusion baseline heart rate frequency. Figure 15-4 illustrates a slow recovery phase in a hypoxic fetus following a very short partial occlusion of the umbilical cord.

Effect on the Fetus

In addition to the described deceleration of the heart rate and changes in blood pressure, the partial or complete interruption of umbilical cord circulation affects other fetal systems, particularly the heart and the acid–base status, as result of the induced hypoxic condition. The strong vagal tone, demonstrated to influence the rate, seems to also affect the *conduction of the impulse* in the myocardium inducing various degrees of atrioventricular *conduction defects* such as second degree blocks (Figure 15-8) or complete AV blocks and

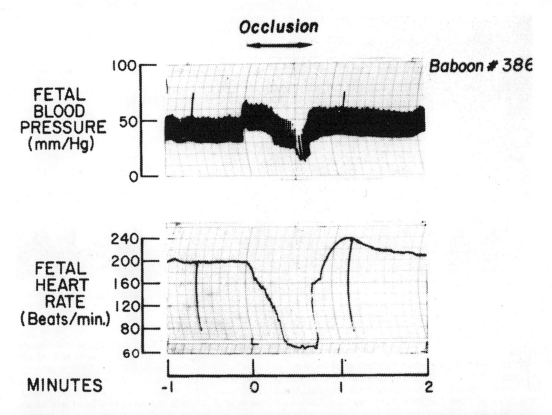

Figure 15-6 Fetal blood pressure and FHR recordings obtained in a baboon fetus near term. Effect of *complete occlusion of the umbilical cord* for 40 sec (arrow). The sudden hypertension followed by slow fall in blood pressure is simultaneous with sharp fall in FHR, which plateaus, after 20 sec, at a slow rate. Recovery is immediate with a *rebound* of both parameters. Reprinted from Yeh M-N, et al: Myocardial conduction defects in association with compression of the umbilical cord. *Am J Obstet Gynecol* 121:951, 1975.

extrasystoles (Figure 15-10), depending on the duration of the occlusion. After about 40 sec of total interruption of blood flow, complete block seems to occur predictably. Disappearance of P waves has not been observed even under the most severe types of induced hypoxia in subhuman primates. The evidence that the vagal tone is responsible for these alterations in the conduction of the impulse is supplied by the response to atropinization (Figure 15-8); following this, even prolonged episodes of occlusion and severe hypoxia were unable to induce AV blocks or extrasystoles. Recovery from conduction defects occurs within 5 sec of restoring umbilical cord circulation and thereby suppressing the vagal impulses that cause them.

The *acid–base status* of the fetus is rapidly affected by complete cord occlusion because after several seconds, when the fetal O_2 reserve has been exhausted, anaerobic metabolism takes place exclusively, with rapid production of the acid catabolites, and the building up of base deficit (Figures 15-4 and 15-8). A similar rapid deterioration of the fetal acid–base status is observed with *complete occlusion* of the *umbilical vein* (Figure 15-5), which leads to the same state of oxygen deprivation and, therefore, rapidly progressing hypoxia. However, the *partial occlusion* of the vein or umbilical cord, in a well-oxygenated fetus, which triggers an acceleration of the FHR, does not significantly alter the fetal oxygenation; therefore, the acid–base status remains stable

348

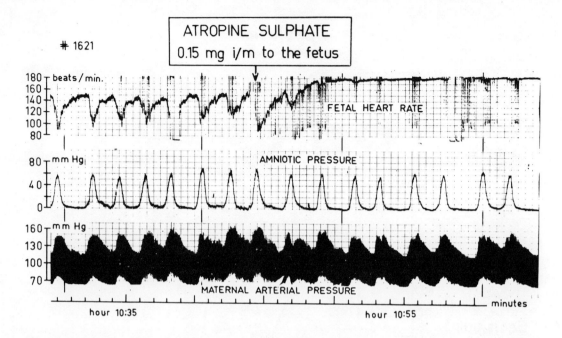

Figure 15-7 Fetal heart rate, intrauterine, and maternal blood pressure tracings obtained in advanced first stage of normal induced labor at term. The regularly occurring variable decelerations (all of similar characteristics) are obliterated 4 min after the fetus had been given an intramuscular injection (by transabdominal tap) of 150 μg atropine (arrow). Note also that there is a significant tachycardia and disappearance of the baseline rapid oscillations. There are no noticeable changes in intrauterine or maternal blood pressures. An infant with a loop of cord around the neck was delivered some time later. Reprinted from Caldeyro-Barcia R, et al: Control of human fetal heart rate during labor, in Cassels DE (ed): *The Heart and Circulation in the Newborn and Infant.* New York, Grune & Stratton, 1966, pp 7–36. By permission.

(Figure 15-3). The ones that are borderline oxygenated will respond with bradycardia and probably metabolic acidosis because the diminished fetal cardiac output, a product of the bradycardia and hypotension, is sufficient to break the unstable threshold of oxygen tension below which there will be hypoxia and anaerobic metabolism.

Causes

The clinical conditions that may predispose to or cause occlusion (or compression) of the umbilical cord are numerous, some more frequent than others. Probably the most common is the presence of one or more *loops of cord around the fetal neck;* when these are loose the chances of significant compression are minimal, but when the loops are tight it is only logical that, as the presenting part decends, the loop will tighten because one of the ends is anchored on the placenta, which does not follow down the fetal head. Descent of the presenting part (head) is probably the direct cause of most of the variable decelerations observed intrapartum, along with stretching of the fetal spine at the peak of the contraction which also tends to pull on the cord and tighten the loop: as this closes, there is lateral compression of the umbilical vein and, with more pressure, of the arteries. Loops of *cord around fetal limbs* or the trunk are also frequently observed among the cases evolving during labor with variable decelerations. The presence of a very *short cord* may create physical difficulties for good circulation with descent of the presenting part—as documented by the recording of variable decelerations (Figure 15-11). Conversely, extremely *long umbilical cords* may loop several times around the

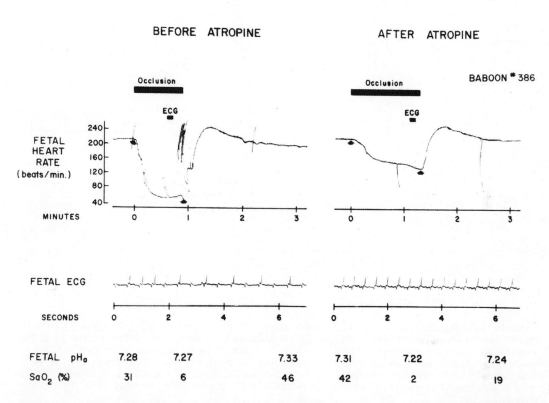

BEFORE ATROPINE   AFTER ATROPINE

BABOON #386

Occlusion   Occlusion

ECG   ECG

FETAL HEART RATE (beats/min.)

240
200
160
120
80
40

MINUTES   0   1   2   3   0   1   2   3

FETAL ECG

SECONDS   0   2   4   6   0   2   4   6

FETAL pH$_a$	7.28	7.27		7.33	7.31	7.22		7.24
SaO$_2$ (%)	31	6		46	42	2		19

Figure 15-8 FHR and ECG recorded from a fetal baboon near term during *complete occlusion of the umbilical cord.* Changes are significantly different *after intravenous atropine.* The bradycardia is established more slowly and is of lesser amplitude after atropinization. The ECG taken (small bars, shortly before restoration of circulation) illustrates heart blocks 50 sec after occlusion before atropine, and no conduction defects after atropinization 80 sec postocclusion in spite of more severe hypoxia and acidosis. The fetal blood gas values sampled at arrows. Reprinted from Yeh M-N, et al: Myocardial conduction defects in association with compression of the umbilical cord. *Am J Obstet Gynecol* 121:951, 1975.

fetal neck and limbs, and still have only moderate decelerations during labor but they may tighten dangerously as the fetus descends in the last stages of labor inducing fetal depression (Figure 15-12).

Prolapse of the cord ahead of the presenting part, with or without ruptured membranes, is a most dangerous situation because it may go unnoticed unless the patient is examined. The first human experimental studies were done on extremely premature fetuses with this condition (Hon, Goodlin); subsequent unplanned observations in advanced gestation have validated those reports and proved how dangerous that complication can be (see Figures 16-6 and 16-7).

The abnormally small amount of amniotic fluid, *olygoamnios,* relatively more frequent in prolonged gestations and/or intrauterine growth-retarded fetuses, creates a condition for an easy compression of the cord during contractions between fetal trunk or parts and the uterus because of the lack of the protective action exerted by normal or excessive amounts of amniotic fluid. Caldeyro-Barcia has repeatedly claimed that amniotomy is a causative factor in the production of variable decelerations; however, that observation has been documented by others only in exceptional circumstances of excessive amounts of amniotic fluid loss at the time, and/or a rapid

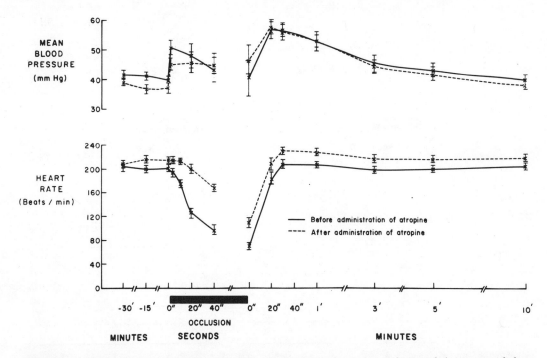

Figure 15-9 Average curves of the *effect of complete cord occlusion* from observations made in near-term baboon fetuses before and after *atropinization*. Cord occlusions ranged from 40 to 360 sec, thus the lines are interrupted. The mean blood pressure rose immediately in both instances and appeared sustained; following release there was clear rebound, also similar in both situations. FHR falls more sharply and deeply before atropinization; recovery is fast in both situations, but the rebound tachycardia is higher and sustained in the atropinized animals. Reprinted from Yeh M-N, et al: Myocardial conduction defects in association with compression of the umbilical cord. *Am J Obstet Gynecol* 121:951, 1975.

descent of the presenting part following that maneuver. In general, the routine amniotomy productive of a moderate amount of amniotic fluid, and with the head already dipping or engaged, does not trigger variable decelerations.

The position of the cord in *breech presentations* favors its compression between the fetal abdomen and thighs, thus inducing variable decelerations—documented repeatedly when those labors are monitored. The syndrome of the so-called "occult prolapse" may be suspected when variable decelerations of significant amplitude are recorded, and fetal deterioration progresses faster than one may justify from the evidence on hand. Occult prolapse is as dangerous as classic prolapse.

All these conditions have been observed to occur during labor, at various stages, so that variable decelerations have been associated only with labor. Nevertheless, recently Mendez-Bauer et al (1978) reported a series of observations made

during *antepartum* testing of a number of high-risk pregnancies. Interestingly, they observed a wide range of variable decelerations recorded while membranes were intact and presenting parts were floating; they subsequently documented (several days later) in labor and at delivery that the umbilical cord was around the fetal neck in the majority of those cases. Among the patterns of FHR alterations recorded, the most frequent was "acceleration blunted by a deceleration." Therefore, sharp decelerations documented during antepartum testing should warn of possible cord problems. From the foregoing one may conclude that *variable decelerations are alterations of the FHR triggered by sudden changes in the umbilical cord blood flow. The great irregularity of the patterns is due to varying conditions and degrees under which the cord blood flow is altered by the many etiologic factors.*

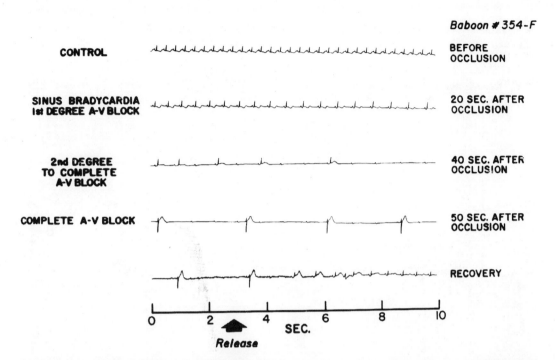

Figure 15-10 Serial ECG obtained in a fetal baboon near term *before* and *after complete occlusion of the umbilical cord* for 1 min. At 20 sec there is a prolongation of the P-R interval, and at 40 sec a 2:1 block rapidly evolves into a complete heart block. At 50 sec the complete block continues and extrasystoles are recorded (compare with Figure 15-8, *right*). Within 5 sec of reestablishing circulation (arrow), the conduction defects disappear. Note the presence of P waves throughout the entire period of recording. Reprinted from Yeh M-N, et al: Myocardial conduction defects in association with compression of the umbilical cord. *Am J Obstet Gynecol* 121:951, 1975.

Classification

Within the almost unlimited variations possible, variable decelerations may be divided into three general catagories (see Figure 15-1):

1. The very minimal type usually takes the shape of a sharp V, indistinguishable from the early decelerations discussed in Chapter 13.
2. The classic U shaped variety is the most frequently recorded (Figure 15-11). The amplitude of the deceleration varies from between 15 to 20 and 80 to 90 beats, the total duration from fall to full recovery lasting 25 to 80 sec, and the baseline between 120 and 150 beats with normal, rapid oscillations.
3. Those with a hypoxic component are characterized by some elements described in late decelerations and known to be produced by significant hypoxia. They are present particularly in the recovery phase of the deceleration, which is slow, often curving above the predeceleration baseline. The duration from fall to full recovery may last as long as 3 to 5 min. Furthermore, alterations of the baseline—tachycardia, and fixed or saltory patterns, or both—are commonly associated findings in these circumstances (Figure 15-13).

As in all cases of this group, the amplitude of the decelerations is extremely variable, and therefore it is not a good guideline for classification. The longer the interruption of blood flow, the faster the development of fetal acidosis due to anaerobic metabolism. In addition, the more frequent these decelerations, the faster the fetal deterioration.

352

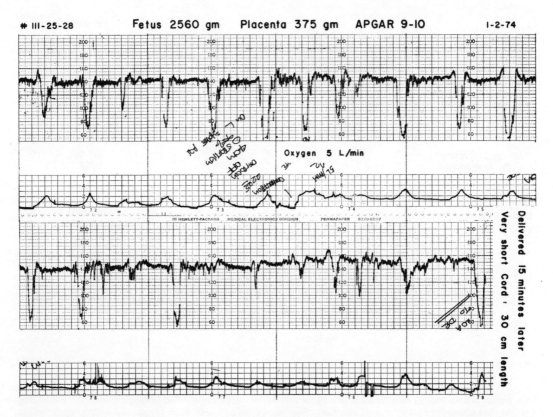

Figure 15-11 Continuous 76-min recording of direct FHR and intrauterine pressure obtained during the last stages of enhanced labor in a multiparous patient at 36 weeks gestation, after PRM. The large variable decelerations (some dropping to below 60 to 70 beats/min) recovered rapidly to the normal baseline with rapid oscillations. Continuous oxygen by mask seemed to improve the decelerations somewhat. A fetus in good condition was born 15 min after the end of the tracing. There was no cord around the neck, but it was only *30 cm long*. Reprinted from Cibils LA: Clinical significance of fetal heart rate patterns during labor. V. Variable decelerations. *Am J Obstet Gynecol* 132:791, 1978.

CLINICAL SIGNIFICANCE

The incidence of so-called cord problems — that is, clinically apparent FHR alterations occurring in conjunction with position of the umbilical cord to interfere with normal easy blood flow — varies according to populations studied. The standard textbooks quote an incidence of 15% to 20% rate of nuchal cords among general obstetric populations, whereas figures from monitored high-risk populations report incidences ranging from 12% to 36%. Because they are so frequent, and because of their pathophysiology, they pose significant intrapartum problems. The incidence among the total high-risk population at the Chicago Lying-In Hospital has been about 26%; however, among the patients carrying small

fetuses (less than 37 weeks gestation), the incidence of cord problems has been 47%, an extraordinarily high incidence.

From a careful review of the pathophysiology of the FHR alterations and the great variability observed, one may rightfully conclude that not all have the same clinical significance. To be assessed for potential value as predictors of fetal outcome, the cases were grouped according to the classification given above and compared. In the first group were included those cases with transient and/or minimal alterations of FHR that had, at delivery, loops of cord around the neck (Figure 15-14). Also in the same group were cases with the more classic type of variable decelerations (Figure 15-15), those who presented impressive looking alterations but alternating with periods without

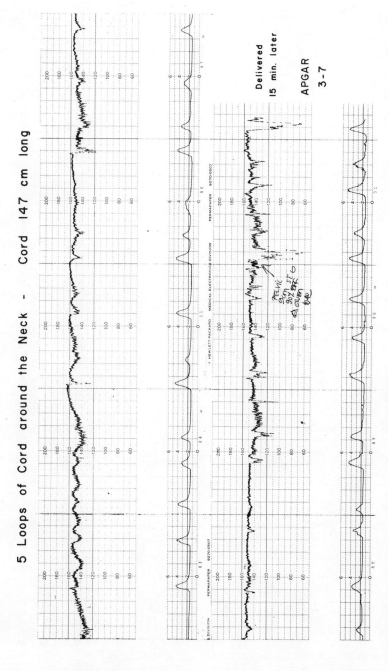

Figure 15-12 Continuous 92 min of direct FHR and intrauterine pressure tracings obtained during the last stages of spontaneous labor in multipara at term. There was meconium-stained amniotic fluid. The slightly tachycardic baseline with good oscillations is interrupted by small variable decelerations. Twelve minutes before transfer to the delivery room (end of the tracing) the patient was 9 cm dilated and at 0 station. A severely depressed infant (weighing 3500 gm, placenta 600 gm) was born 15 min after transfer. The final descent in 15 min probably caused marked tightening of the cord loops wound five times around the fetal neck. Reprinted from Cibils LA: Clinical significance of fetal heart rate patterns during labor. V. Variable decelerations. *Am J Obstet Gynecol* 132:791, 1978.

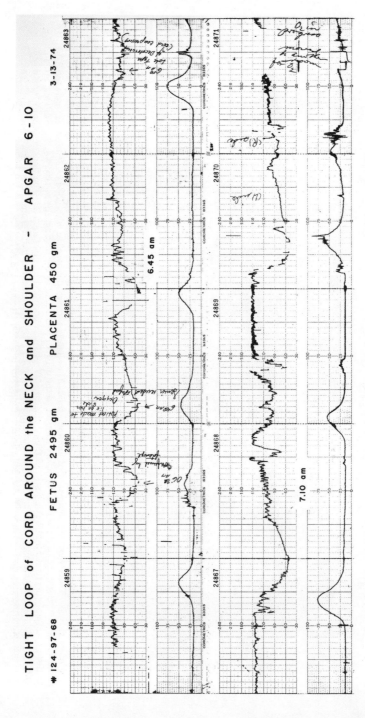

Figure 15-13 Two segments (20 min each) of direct FHR and intrauterine pressure tracings obtained from term patient in early spontaneous labor following PRM (paper speed, 3 cm/min). *(Above)* Moderate uterine activity triggering variable decelerations with prolonged slow recovery to a still oscillating baseline within normal range. *(Below)* Twenty minutes later, with contractions of low frequency, the recovery periods are more prolonged and the baseline rises steadily. Note episodes of fixed baseline and short bursts of saltatory pattern during the period of slow recovery toward a tachycardic baseline. The last deceleration did not completely recover. Emergency cesarean section produced a mildly depressed infant with meconium in the amniotic fluid. There was a tight loop of cord around neck and shoulder. Reprinted from Cibils LA: Clinical significance of fetal heart rate patterns during labor. V. Variable decelerations. *Am J Obstet Gynecol* 132:791, 1978.

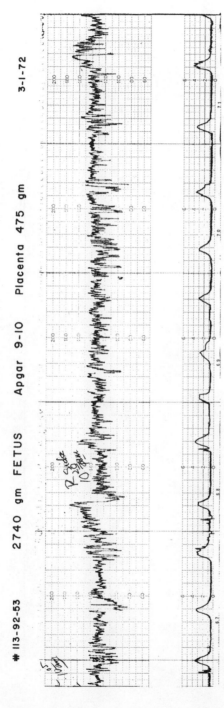

Figure 15-14 Continuous 52 min of direct FHR and intrauterine pressure recordings during enhanced labor at 37 weeks. The numerous small variable decelerations are noteworthy as well as the rapid oscillations of the baseline, interrupted in a random fashion by episodes of saltatory pattern. A normal infant with a *loose loop of cord* around the neck was delivered. Reprinted from Cibils LA: Clinical significance of fetal heart rate patterns during labor. V. Variable decelerations. *Am J Obstet Gynecol* 132:791, 1978.

356

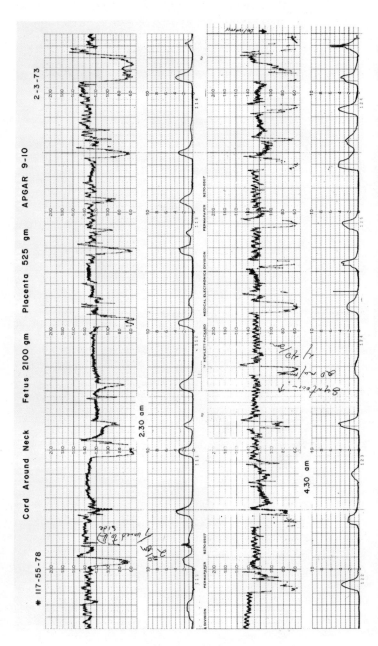

Figure 15-15 Two segments of direct FHR and uterine contraction tracings during induced labor for PRM in multipara at 36 weeks gestation. *(Above)* In mid-first stage, 50-minute tracing illustrates large variable decelerations dropping to less than 60 beats/min with quick recovery to normal baseline with rapid oscillations; some of the recovery phases seem to rebound, to come down with what appears the last part of an acceleration. *(Below)* Two hours later, the final stage of labor still with the same pattern of decelerations until the very moment of delivery (at the end of the record, small arrow). A normal fetus in good condition, with one loop of cord around the neck, was born. Reprinted from Cibils LA: Clinical significance of fetal heart rate patterns during labor. V. Variable decelerations. *Am J Obstet Gynecol* 132:791, 1978.

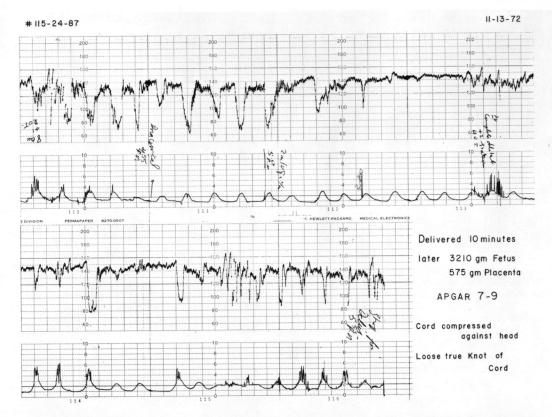

Delivered 10 minutes

later 3210 gm Fetus

575 gm Placenta

APGAR 7-9

Cord compressed
against head

Loose true Knot of
Cord

Figure 15-16   Continuous 70 min of direct FHR and intrauterine pressure tracings obtained during spontaneous labor in term primipara patient. There was meconium-stained amniotic fluid. *(Above)* At the end of first stage, very large, deep variable decelerations dropping to 65 to 70 beats/min, and lasting up to 1 min, with good recovery to a normal baseline with good oscillations. Decelerations suddenly disappear shortly after the middle of the record. *(Below)* Second stage, with some decelerations triggered by bearing down efforts, and a transient episode of saltatory pattern. At delivery the *cord was against the fetal head* and it had a *loose true knot.* Fetus and placenta were normal. Reprinted from Cibils LA: Clinical significance of fetal heart rate patterns during labor. V. Variable decelerations. *Am J Obstet Gynecol* 132:791, 1978.

decelerations, and those in which no apparent deceleration-induced alterations of baseline were observed (Figure 15-16). In spite of the benign appearance of these alterations of FHR, their effect on neonatal outcome is not negligible because there is a higher incidence of fetal depression among them when compared to cases evolving without decelerations (Figure 15-17); furthermore, they presented more baseline alterations (tachycardia, fixed and saltatory baseline) and higher neonatal deaths.

A second group of cases included those who presented in the tracings elements of what has been defined as *hypoxic components* (or late components), typically observed in late decelerations. Particularly, the slow recovery following the

deceleration (Figure 15-18) characterizes these patients who, in addition, may have other associated alterations. Among these, tachycardia—or rising baseline—and fixed baseline evolving slowly as labor progresses (Figure 15-19) are also associated with variable decelerations in cases of deteriorating fetuses. As observed in the group of late deceleration fetuses, these alterations may lead to episodes of "overlapping" decelerations or states of true bradycardia (Figure 15-20).

In other words, there is a group of cases with *variable decelerations* (as defined by the relationship of the onset of decelerations and the rising phase of the contraction) that has some of the characteristics of *late decelerations* (as defined by the recovery phase of the deceleration) and may

358

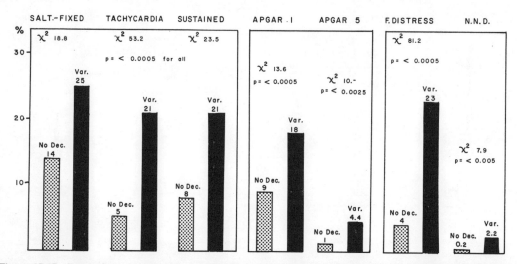

Figure 15-17 Proportion of cases with variable decelerations having FHR baseline alterations (saltatory-fixed, tachycardia), which become sustained. Neonatal outcome by Apgar scores; intrapartum clinical fetal distress, and neonatal deaths. The same incidence of abnormalities and outcome was calculated for cases without decelerations and compared statistically using the chi-square test. The exact incidences are shown on top of each bar. FHR abnormalities and poor outcome are seen in a significantly higher proportion of cases with variable deceleration. Reprinted from Cibils LA: Clinical significance of fetal heart rate patterns during labor. V. Variable decelerations. *Am J Obstet Gynecol* 132:791, 1978.

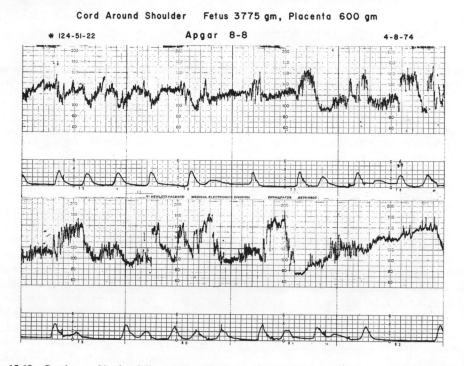

Figure 15-18 Continuous 80 min of direct FHR and intrauterine pressure tracings during enhanced labor in primipara with mild preeclampsia and PRM. The moderate variable decelerations *(top, left)* evolved into large variable decelerations (preceded by acceleration) with very *slow prolonged recovery* and some episodes of saltatory pattern. The last deceleration had a slow and prolonged recovery. The patient had a cesarean section productive of a normal infant, in good condition, with a loop of *cord around the shoulder.* Reprinted from Cibils LA: Clinical significance of fetal heart rate patterns during labor. V. Variable decelerations. *Am J Obstet Gynecol* 132:791, 1978.

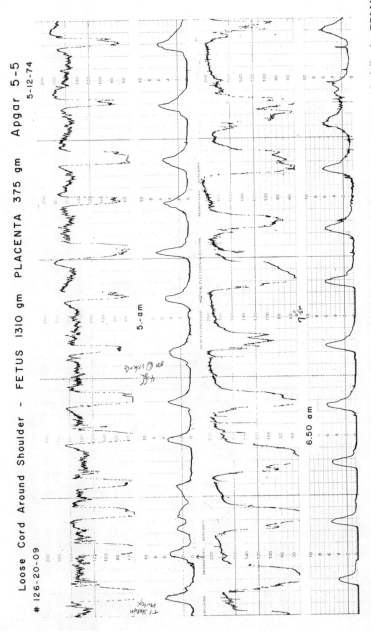

Figure 15-19 Two 50-min segments of direct FHR and intrauterine pressure tracings during premature labor at 33 weeks following PRM in primipara. *(Above)* Good uterine activity triggering *large, deep, variable decelerations* with rapid recovery to baseline with normal rapid oscillations, but rising slightly to become tachycardic; some of the decelerations appear to "blunt" accelerations. *(Below)* Recorded 70 min later, shows *deep and long lasting variable decelerations* with *slow recovery* period, hypoxic component, fixed baseline, and severe tachycardia. The total duration of the decelerations in this segment ranged from 140 to 220 sec. By emergency cesarean section, 30 min after the end of the tracing, a depressed infant with loose loop of cord around the shoulder was delivered. Reprinted from Cibils LA: Clinical significance of fetal heart rate patterns during labor. V. Variable decelerations. *Am J Obstet Gynecol* 132:791, 1978.

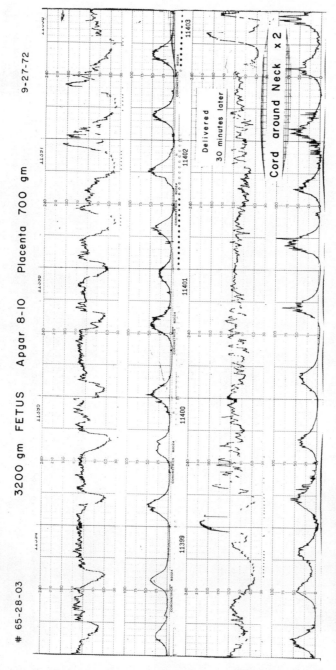

Figure 15-20 Continuous 40-min direct FHR and intrauterine pressure recording (paper speed, 3 cm/min) during induced labor for PRM in advanced first stage of primipara at term. *(Above, left)* Deep variable decelerations on a normal baseline with rapid oscillations evolving into *prolonged decelerations with slow recovery*, and at times reaching rebound tachycardia *(right)*. *(Below)* Incomplete recovery from variable decelerations. A burst of saltatory pattern interrupting a long period of moderate bradycardia preceded discontinuation of the record. A normal looking infant with two loops of cord around the neck was delivered 30 min later. Reprinted from Cibils LA: Clinical significance of fetal heart rate patterns during labor. I. Baseline patterns. *Am J Obstet Gynecol* 125:290, 1976.

have the same clinical significance as these. The comparison of the classic deceleration group with the one with hypoxic components indicates the clear deleterious effect on the fetus when the late components are observed (Figure 15-21). Close to 80% of the latter had intrapartum fetal distress and they had an exceedingly high rate of depressed fetuses. On the other hand, the associated baseline changes (saltatory and fixed baseline, tachycardia) were present in a sustained manner in over two thirds of those cases. In addition, they had a very high incidence of neonatal deaths. All these findings suggest that the *variable decelerations with late components* that induce baseline alterations present the most ominous FHR pattern, with a *high predictive value* for obtaining a depressed fetus.

MANAGEMENT

The high incidence of depressed fetuses born from labors evolving with variable decelerations attests to the potential severity of complications, which are probably preventable when the FHR tracing is carefully analyzed and followed as

labor progresses. Partial compression of the cord may induce impressive decelerations of great amplitude and duration but, with sufficient time elapsed between contractions to allow for oxygen "resupply," the fetus could maintain homeostasis and may even improve its acid–base status with the progress of labor and safely reach complete dilatation (Figures 15-22 and 15-23). When these favorable cases are recorded one may observe that the recovery phase of the deceleration is rapid, sharp, "classic," and that there are no associated baseline alterations.

On the other hand, other cases may start with the same favorable pattern and become even less impressive with the passage of time (Figure 15-24). As descent takes place or the frequency of contractions increases, the FHR pattern may show some of the elements described as late components, with acid–base status deterioration. The speed of the fetal deterioration is determined by the degree of umbilical cord occlusion taking place with each contraction, and the frequency with which contractions recur. A tight compression of the umbilical cord interferes with the blood flow almost as effectively as when clamped, and therefore the fetal oxygenation and acid–base

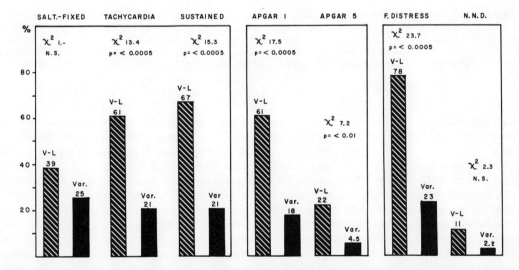

Figure 15-21 Proportion of cases with variable decelerations having FHR baseline alterations (saltatory-fixed, tachycardia) and which became sustained. Neonatal Apgar scores, intrapartum clinical fetal distress, and neonatal deaths. The same incidence of abnormalities and outcome was calculated for cases having variable decelerations with late components and compared statistically using the chi-square test. Exact incidences are shown above each bar. All *abnormalities and poor outcomes are much higher among* cases having *late components,* with the exception of saltatory-fixed and neonatal death (also higher but not significant). Reprinted from Cibils LA: Clinical significance of fetal heart rate patterns during labor. V. Variable decelerations. *Am J Obstet Gynecol* 132:791, 1978.

362

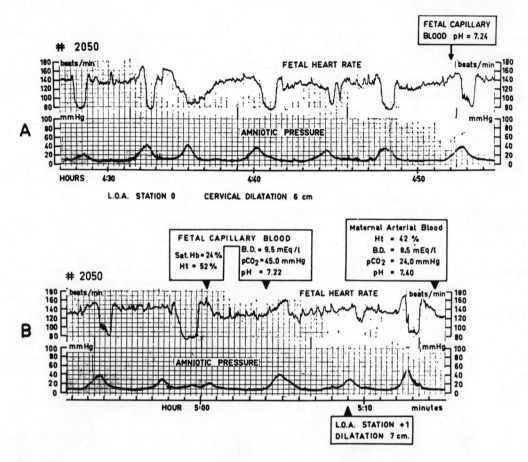

Figure 15-22 Continuous 49 min of direct FHR and intrauterine pressure tracings from advanced spontaneous first stage in multipara at term. Deep variable decelerations are triggered by contractions of moderate intensity recurring every 3.5 to 4.5 min. The fetal capillary blood pH was 7.24 *(above)* and 7.22 *(below),* while the mother's was normal. Reprinted from Caldeyro-Barcia R, et al: Fetal monitoring in labor, in Wallace HM, Gold EM, Lis EF (eds): *Maternal and Child Health Practices.* Courtesy of Charles C Thomas, Publisher, Springfield, Ill, 1973, pp 332–394.

status will deteriorate with the same rate as if subjected to complete asphyxia (see Figures 14-15 and 15-5).

When late components have been documented in the FHR tracing (Figure 15-25), the rapid production of acids during occlusion of umbilical circulation has been well documented clinically by comparing the pH difference between umbilical arteries and vein. When the frequency of contractions is high, there may not be enough time for the fetal acids to be eliminated during the short passage of blood through the placental villi, and accumulation is then inevitable.

All labors with signs of cord problems should be observed closely because changes may occur in a most unpredictable manner. The popular advice

that patients should be "turned to the left" is based on no logic whatsoever. The idea behind turning the patient is good because the aim is to move the fetus just in case the cord is compressed against limbs or shoulder, but the movement could be to a left, right, supine, or semi-Fowler's position. The most favorable position cannot be predicted because no one knows the actual position of the cord or the precise cause of the deceleration; not infrequently the less favorable position is the left lateral. Worrisome variable decelerations may suddenly disappear and evolve to a nice normal pattern (see Figure 15-16) while in other circumstances a reassuring pattern may suddenly worsen as dilatation and descent take place in advanced labor. With luck the cause may

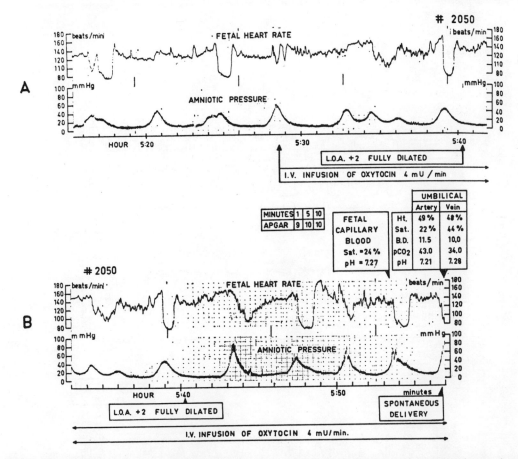

Figure 15-23 Continuation of tracings in Figure 15-22. End of first stage and oxytocin-enhanced second stage, showing the same pattern of contractions of moderate intensity, recurring every 3.5 to 4.5 min, and triggering large, deep, variable declerations. In spite of these, the fetal acid–base status improved (pH 7.27 before delivery) because of good uterine relaxation and spacing between contractions. An infant of excellent status was born. Reprinted from Caldeyro-Barcia R, et al: Fetal monitoring in labor, in Wallace HM, Gold EM, Lis EF (eds): *Maternal and Child Health Practices.* Courtesy of Charles C Thomas, Publisher, Springfield, Ill, 1973, pp 332–394.

be a relatively loose loop or loops permitting some compensatory recovery and, if delivery is rapid, the infant will be in satisfactory condition (Figure 15-26). But when the interruption of the umbilical circulation is tight, fetal deterioration may be very rapid with the delivery of a depressed infant even when one acts expeditiously (Figure 15-27).

The evolution toward fetal acidosis may follow the path of the "superacute" group (see Figure 14-16), particularly when the interruption of circulation is significant. The most clear example would be a prolapsed cord with engaging head compressing it, or a true knot in the cord, tightening with descent of the fetus (Figure 15-28). This latter situation is equivalent to complete clamping of the cord, which leads to complete anoxia within minutes; anaerobic metabolism, as the only respiratory pathway, will then cause rapid acidosis. Unless one intervenes quickly, total asphyxia is the outcome.

Even when these rapid changes are taking place in fetal acid–base balance and homeostasis, they are reflected in the FHR patterns—particularly the recovery phase of the deceleration and the associated baseline alterations. There is usually no time to take fetal scalp blood samples because of the speed with which these rare conditions develop, but a good estimation of the fetal

364

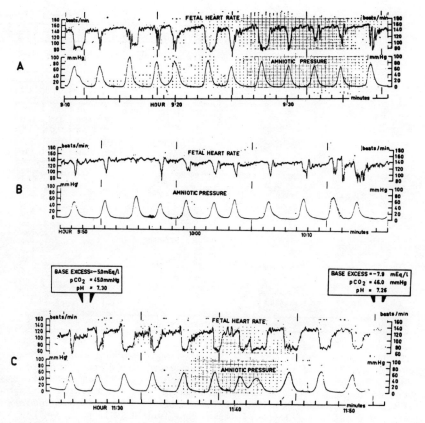

Figure 15-24 Three segments of direct FHR and intrauterine pressure tracings obtained during induced labor in term multipara. *(Above)* Deep variable declerations with good recovery to a normal baseline with rapid oscillations. *(Center)* A few minutes later, much diminished decelerations with excellent baseline characteristics. *(Below)* One hour later, large variable decelerations lasting over 2 min and *slow recovery phase* induced deteriorating fetal acid–base status (pH from 7.30 to 7.26 and rising base deficit). The progress of labor *tightened* the loop of *cord around the neck* and favored the development of FHR and acid–base status alterations quite rapidly. Reprinted from Caldeyro-Barcia R, et al: Fetal monitoring in labor, in Wallace HM, Gold EM, Lis EF (eds): *Maternal and Child Health Practices.* Courtesy of Charles C Thomas, Publisher, Springfield, Ill, 1973, pp 332–394.

condition may be made by careful analysis and interpretation of the FHR tracing.

The clinical experience, as well as the mechanical characteristics leading to them, make the *variable decelerations with late components the most severe and ominous* abnormal pattern one may observe in labor. Furthermore, because the conditions for occurrence increase as labor progresses, continuous monitoring (or frequent intermittent auscultation) should be mandatory during second stage when variable decelerations have been recorded during first stage.

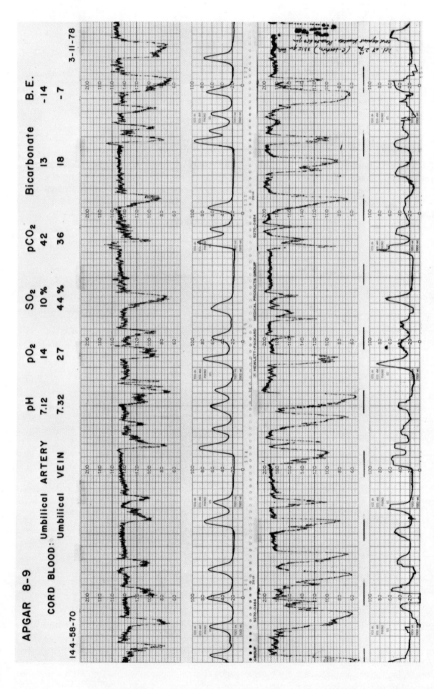

Figure 15-25 Two 50-min segments of direct FHR and uterine contraction tracings during mid-first stage of enhanced labor at term. *(Above)* Large variable decelerations dropping to 65 to 80 beats/min with fast recovery to a normal baseline with normal rapid oscillations (slight rise of baseline during those 50 min). *(Below)* Ninety minutes later, *deep variable decelerations* dropping to 55 to 80 beats/min from a fixed and tachycardic baseline of 190 beats/min; the decelerations last 60 to 180 sec. Cesarean section for fetal distress 20 min later was productive of an infant in good condition, but with large difference in the acid–base status between umbilical arteries and vein (values above). The cord was below the shoulder and compressed between the fetal shoulder and the lower segment (several contractions, in the bottom tracing, do not record the apex because of obstructed catheter).

366

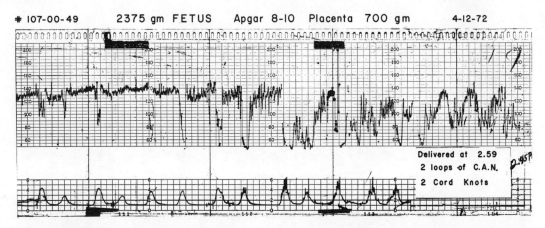

107-00-49 2375 gm FETUS Apgar 8-10 Placenta 700 gm 4-12-72

Delivered at 2.59
2 loops of C.A.N.
2 Cord Knots

Figure 15-26 Direct FHR and intrauterine pressure tracings during the last 42 min of monitoring in induced labor of patient with preeclampsia at term. Small variable decelerations *(left)* become very deep as dilatation completed, and saltatory pattern was superimposed with the decelerations until the tracing was discontinued. An infant in good condition was delivered 14 min later, and had two loops of cord around the neck and two loose true cord knots. Reprinted from Cibils LA: Clinical significance of fetal heart rate patterns during labor. II. Late decelerations. *Am J Obstet Gynecol* 123:473, 1975.

Two tights loops of Cord around the Neck   APGAR 3-7

FETUS 2325 gm   PLACENTA 675 gm

121-03-08   1-29-74

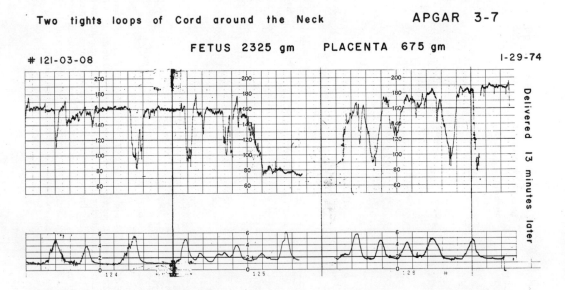

Delivered 13 minutes later

Figure 15-27 Two segments of direct FHR and intrauterine pressure tracings during early stages of premature labor following PRM. *(Left)* Progressively deepening variable decelerations on a borderline tachycardic and fixed baseline; a prolonged deceleration plateauing at about 80 beats/min prompted the transfer of the patient to the operating room (2 min not recorded). *(Right)* Rapidly rising fixed baseline and severe variable decelerations. Although the decelerations never dropped below 90 beats/min, and the delivery by emergency cesarean section was 13 min after the end of the tracing (30 min from the start of the bradycardic episode), a severely depressed infant with *two tight loops of cord around the neck* was delivered. Reprinted from Cibils LA: Clinical significance of fetal heart rate patterns during labor. V. Variable decelerations. *Am J Obstet Gynecol* 132:791, 1978.

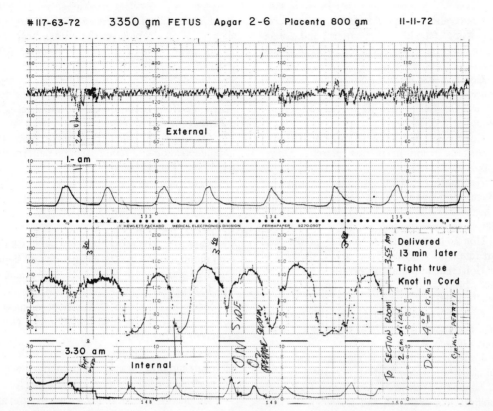

Figure 15-28 Two segments of FHR and uterine contraction tracings during early stages of induced labor at term for PRM. *(Above)* Indirect recordings of 35 min illustrate good contractility induced by 2 mU/min oxytocin, and FHR with good baseline and normal rapid oscillations. *(Below)* Direct recordings of 28 min, 2½ hours later, show *severe, deteriorating variable decelerations* with fixed and rapidly rising baseline and slow recovery (typical hypoxic pattern). By emergency cesarean section, 13 min after the end of the tracing, a severely depressed term size infant was delivered. A *tight true knot* found in the umbilical cord seems to have created this superacute fetal distress. Reprinted from Cibils LA: Clinical significance of fetal heart rate patterns during labor. II. Later decelerations. *Am J Obstet Gynecol* 123:473, 1975.

BIBLIOGRAPHY

Assali NS, Holm LW, Sehgal N: Hemodynamic changes in fetal lamb in utero in response to asphyxia, hypoxia and hypercapnia. *Circ Res* 11:423, 1962.

Barcroft J: *Researches on Prenatal Life,* chap 12. Oxford, Blackwell, 1946, pp 123–144.

Bissonnette JM: Relationship between continuous fetal heart rate patterns and Apgar score in the newborn. *Br J Obstet Gynaecol* 82:24, 1975.

Bruce SL, James, LS, Bowe TE, et al: Umbilical cord complication as a cause of perinatal morbidity and mortality. *J Perinat Med* 6:89, 1978.

Caldeyro-Barcia R, Mendez-Bauer C, Poseiro JJ, et al: Fetal monitoring in labor, in Wallace HM, Gold EM, Lis EF (eds): *Maternal and Child Health Practices,* Springfield, Ill, Thomas, 1973, pp 332–394.

Cibils LA: Clinical significance of fetal heart rate patterns during labor. I. Baseline patterns. *Am J Obstet Gynecol* 125:290, 1976.

Cibils LA: Clinical significance of fetal heart rate patterns during labor. II. Late decelerations. *Am J Obstet Gynecol* 123:473, 1975.

Cibils LA: Clinical significance of fetal heart rate patterns during labor. V. Variable decelerations. *Am J Obstet Gynecol* 132:791, 1978.

Gabert HA, Stenchever MA: The result of a five-year study of continuous fetal monitoring on an obstetric service. *Obstet Gynecol* 50:275, 1977.

Goldkrand JW, Speichinger JP: "Mixed cord compression" fetal heart rate pattern, and its relation to abnormal cord position. *Am J Obstet Gynecol* 122:144, 1975.

Goodlin RC: Fetal cardiovascular responses to distress. *Obstet Gynecol* 49:371, 1977.

Goodlin RC: Letter to the editor. *Obstet Gynecol* 51:256, 1978.

Goodlin RC, Lowe EW: A functional umbilical cord occlusion heart rate pattern. *Obstet Gynecol* 43:22, 1974.

Hammacher K, Huter KA, Bokelmann J, et al: Fetal heart frequency and perinatal conditions of the fetus and newborn. *Gynaecologia* 166:349, 1968.

Hon EH: Electronic evaluation of the fetal heart rate. *Am J Obstet Gynecol* 83:333, 1962.

Hon EH: Additional observations on "pathologic" bradycardia. *Am J Obstet Gynecol* 118:428, 1974.

Hon EH, Bradfield AH, Hess OW: The electronic evaluation of the fetal heart rate. *Am J Obstet Gynecol* 82:291, 1961.

Hon EH, Quilligan EJ: The classification of fetal heart rate. *Conn Med* 31:779, 1967.

James LS, Yeh M-N, Morishima HO, et al: Umbilical vein occlusion and transient acceleration of the fetal heart rate. *Am J Obstet Gynecol* 126:276, 1976.

Lee CY, DiLoretto PC, O'Lane JM: A study of fetal heart rate acceleration patterns. *Obstet Gynecol* 45:142, 1975.

Low JA, Boston RW, Pancham SR: The role of fetal heart rate patterns in the recognition of fetal asphyxia with metabolic acidosis. *Am J Obstet Gynecol* 109:922, 1971.

Mendez-Bauer C, Arnt IC, Gulin L, et al: Relationship between blood pH and heart rate in the human fetus during labor. *Am J Obstet Gynecol* 97:530, 1967.

Mendez-Bauer C, Poseiro JJ, Arellano G, et al: Effects of atropine on the human heart rate during labor. *Am J Obstet Gynecol* 85:1033, 1963.

Mendez-Bauer C, Ruiz-Canseco A, Andujar-Ruiz M, et al: Early decelerations of the fetal heart rate from occlusion of the umbilical cord. *J Perinat Med* 6:69, 1978.

O'Gureck JE, Roux JF, Newman MR: Neonatal depression and fetal heart rate patterns during labor. *Obstet Gynecol* 40:347, 1972.

Pardi G, Tucci E, Uderzo A, et al: Fetal electrocardiogram changes in relation to fetal heart rate patterns during labor. *Am J Obstet Gynecol* 118:243, 1974.

Paul RH, Suidan AK, Yeh SY, et al: Clinical fetal monitoring. VII. The evaluation and significance of intrapartum baseline FHR variability. *Am J Obstet Gynecol* 123:206, 1975.

Saling E, Schneider D: Biochemical supervision of the fetus during labor. *Br J Obstet Gynaecol* 74:799, 1967.

Shenker L: Clinical experience with fetal heart rate monitoring of one thousand patients in labor. *Am J Obstet Gynecol* 15:1111, 1973.

Thomas G: The aetiology, characteristics and diagnostic relevance of late deceleration patterns in routine obstetric practice. *Br J Obstet Gynaecol* 82:121, 1975.

Yeh MN, Morishima HO, Niemann WH, et al: Myocardial conduction defects in association with compression of the umbilical cord. *Am J Obstet Gynecol* 121:951, 1975.

Yeh SY, Zanini B, Petrie RH, Hon EH: Intrapartum fetal cardiac arrest. A preliminary observation. *Obstet Gynecol* 50:571, 1977.

Zilianti M, Cabello F, Estrada MA: Studies on fetal bradycardia during birth process. III. *J Perinat Med* 6:80, 1978.

CHAPTER 16
Agonal Patterns

The manifestations of fetal distress, as ascertained by FHR recording, are late decelerations, tachycardia, fixed and saltatory baseline, bradycardia, and sinusoidal pattern. This classic description applies in general to almost all cases recorded in clinical practice. However, there have been reports of fetuses dying in utero with complete absence of the most typical of all signs of fetal distress—late decelerations, a classical sign of transient significant hypoxia triggered by a contraction (Figure 16-1). Other observations have been made of fetuses subjected to prolonged periods of late decelerations (and thus distress) before objective evidence of death. The careful study of the clinical conditions of those cases, as well as of those who survived, after rapid intervention, comparable episodes of distress (as judged by the similarities of FHR tracings), indicates that there are special characteristics of the behavior of the FHR that might depend on the age of gestation of the fetus.

Several reports indicate unequal responses of fetuses to seemingly comparable stressful conditions when they are of different chronologic age. For this reason gestational age has great importance in determining the significance of FHR changes observed during distress. Thus the study of the FHR response to extreme conditions of distress preceding death (agonal) must be done by grouping observations according to fetal age: premature (or preterm), less than 36 weeks gestational age; term, between 37 and 41 weeks; and postmature (postterm), 42 weeks and beyond.

Preterm Fetuses

This span covers 10 weeks, starting with the earliest stages of viability, now about 26 weeks of gestation. Because of the large span, this group has been subdivided in two with the dividing time set arbitrarily at 32 weeks. There are numerous isolated publications of observations made a few years ago on fetuses of the youngest age group because of their borderline viability, and the usually uncontrollable developing clinical situations. The FHR alterations recorded from those fetuses may be very alarming, with all elements revealing prolonged distress (Figure 16-2). This situation notwithstanding, they are able to survive in utero for prolonged periods in spite of the adverse conditions.

The tachycardia and fixed baseline are recorded with decelerations showing hypoxic components (late and variable) for several hours, without apparent further deterioration, even when the conditions that appear to cause the distress are unchanged. The amount of oxygen supplied between contractions seems sufficient to sustain life under those precarious conditions, probably at the expense of high anaerobic metabolism. The complete suppression of umbilical blood flow precipitates a superacute state of anoxia, which may lead to a faster fetal deterioration and eventual death (Figure 16-3).

Nevertheless, even under these extreme conditions, the premature fetus demonstrates an extraordinary capacity to *withstand distress in utero*. The premature fetuses of more advanced gestational age seem to maintain their ability to survive states of marked hypoxia for long periods of time (Figure 16-4), as ascertained by the severe changes recorded in FHR tracings. The late decelerations, fixed baseline, overlapping decelerations and true bradycardias, indicators of drastic fetal homeostatic alterations, may be recorded for several hours before fetal death. Interestingly, it is exceptional for the premature fetus to pass meconium, even under conditions of terminal distress. It is not very clear at what stage of pregnancy the fetus starts to lose this characteristic quality to withstand asphyxia for such prolonged periods.

370

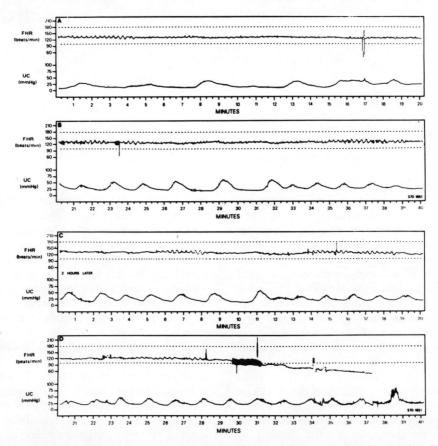

Figure 16-1 Segments of FHR and UC tracings of enhanced labor of primipara at 43 weeks gestation. Meconium-stained amniotic fluid. *(A, B)* Continuous tracings illustrate a fixed baseline of normal baseline frequency interrupted by short bursts of sinusoidal pattern. *(C, D)* Two hours later, the same pattern of FHR with uterine contractions, frequency of 2 to 2½ min. A sudden bradycardia, started in the middle of panel *D*, prompted an emergency cesarean section a few minutes after the end of the tracing. A stillborn infant weighing 4400 gm was obtained. Reprinted from Cetrulo CL, Schifrin BS: Fetal heart rate patterns preceding death in utero. *Obstet Gynecol* 48:521, 1976.

Term Fetuses

A number of publications have treated the evolution of FHR tracing from term fetuses with a fatal outcome. Characteristically, late decelerations are present throughout the stages of distress, with baseline alterations (tachycardia and fixed baseline) recorded at the same time. The controlled study of well-oxygenated fetuses subjected to states of iatrogenic hypoxia and asphyxia (Figure 16-5) has demonstrated that they also have an excellent capacity to adapt to limited oxygen availability. The intermittent supply of oxygen between contractions seems to suffice to prevent a rapid death; nevertheless these infants reach a fatal outcome in a much shorter time than their premature counterparts, although the FHR may not indicate any difference to foretell the faster death. This behavior is valid, likewise, when blood flow through the umbilical cord is completely suppressed, as seen in cases of prolapsed cord with engaged presenting part (Figures 16-6 and 16-7; compare with Figure 16-3). Another added distinguishing sign is the frequent finding of meconium-stained amniotic fluid of the term fetus in severe distress, which is probably aspirated with the gasping efforts preceding death.

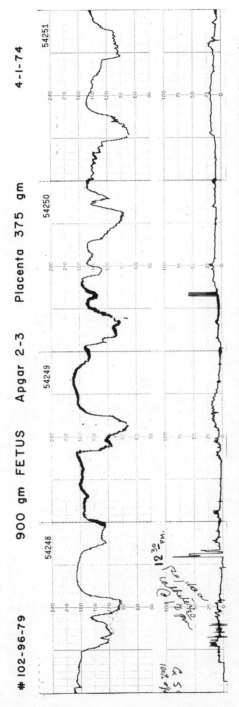

Figure 16-2 Intrauterine pressure and FHR tracings recorded for 16 min during premature labor of primipara at 27 weeks gestation. Agonal pattern recorded for over 3 hours: tachycardia, fixed baseline, and variable decelerations with late components produced by mild contractions. One hour after the end of the tracing a severely depressed premature fetus with marked acidosis (cord blood pH 7.02) was delivered. The infant died 2½ hours later. Reprinted from Cibils LA: Clinical significance of fetal heart rate patterns during labor. IV. Agonal patterns. *Am J Obstet Gynecol* 129:833, 1977.

372

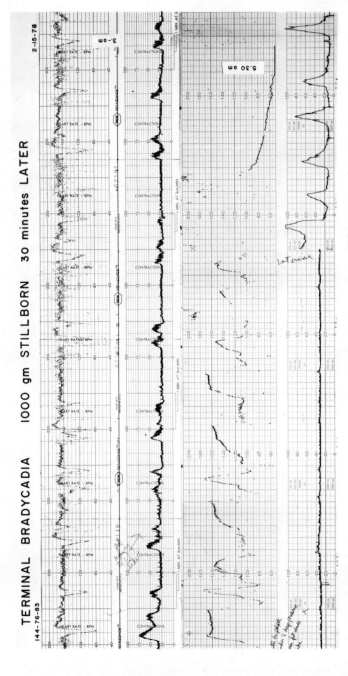

Figure 16-3 Two segments of FHR and UC recordings from obese primipara at 27 weeks gestation. Premature rupture of membranes and severe amnionitis (estimated fetal weight, 500 gm). At induction of labor, cord was prolapsed and pulsating. *(Above)* External recording of 51 min shows tachycardic baseline with variable decelerations and good recovery. *(Below)* In another monitor 90 min later, poor record of contractions but good FHR illustrates fixed baseline, variable decelerations with late components (very slow recovery) which have been recorded for over 1 hour before. Direct recording at the end documents good contractions and terminal bradycardia. A 1000 gm stillborn was delivered 30 min later.

373

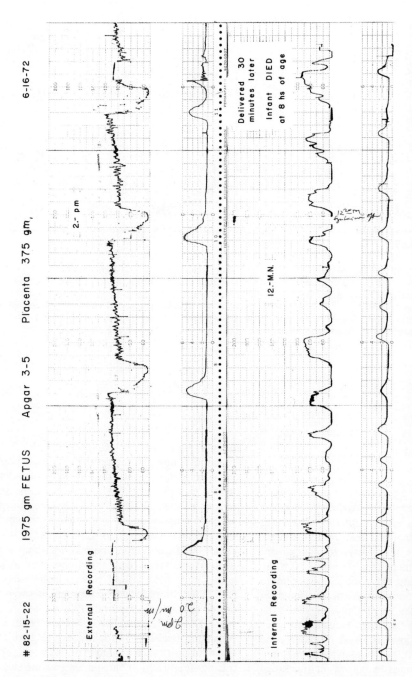

Figure 16-4 Two 50-min segments of recordings obtained from a severely hypertensive multipara at 34 weeks gestation admitted in coma for a cerebrovascular accident. *(Above)* Mild induced uterine activity with contractions every 10 min triggering severe late decelerations. *(Below)* Ten hours later, advanced first stage after induction of labor: agonal pattern with fixed baseline, overlapping late decelerations, and bradycardia. A very depressed and acidotic infant (cord blood pH 7) was born 30 min after the end of the tracing and died at 8 hours of age. Reprinted from Cibils LA: Clinical significance of fetal heart rate patterns during labor. IV. Agonal patterns. *Am J Obstet Gynecol* 129:833, 1977.

719

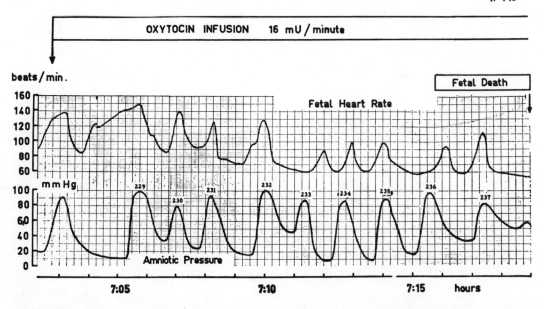

Figure 16-5 Direct FHR and UC recorded during 17 min from enhanced labor of term primipara carrying an anencephalic fetus. The number of contractions counted from the start of the recording at time 0 is shown above each contraction. The extremely strong contractions (iatrogenic hypercontracility) enhanced by 16 mU/mil oxytocin infusion (arrow) over an already high spontaneous activity produced the fixed baseline, tachycardia, overlapping late decelerations, and terminal bradycardia. The pattern persisted for over 2 hours with steady deterioration toward the agonal pattern. Fetus died during the bradycardia triggered by contraction 237. Reprinted from Caldeyro-Barcia R, et al (1963).

Postterm Fetuses

The product of a gestation chronologically 42 weeks or more is labeled *postterm,* which is not always synonymous with *postmature.* The latter have a number of anatomic features that characterize them but are not always found in cases documented to be more than 42 weeks after the last menstrual period (in patients with normal cycles). Thus, a number of postterm fetuses do not "look" what they are, because they lack the signs of intrauterine "wastage" necessary to make the diagnosis of "postmaturity." Moreover, the external, gross anatomic characteristics may not always be accompanied by equivalent functional abnormalities. Conversely, postterm fetuses without anatomic features of postmaturity may well have functional aberrations seen only in infants born after prolonged gestation. The pathophysiology of the postterm fetus is poorly understood possibly because there is no animal model in which the characteristics of the prolonged human gestation are easily reproducible without gross induced endocrine disturbances. Furthermore, close observation of human cases could significantly contribute to our knowledge about these infants, but the syndrome of prolonged gestation or "postdatism" was not appreciated in the United States for a long time and has been accepted as clinically important only in the last few years. The sporadic publication of unexplained intrapartum fetal death in labors evolving with no apparent critical pathologic disorder on FHR tracings (Figure 16-8) has stimulated a meticulous study of those cases with the finding that the majority occurred in pregnancies of 42 weeks or more (Cibils, 1977).

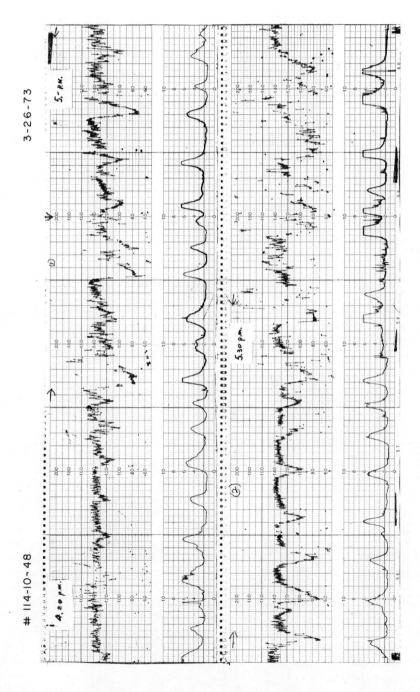

Figure 16-6 Continuous 100 min of external FHR and UC tracings from early spontaneous labor in term multipara. Obese patient, floating presenting part, breech presentation suspected. *(Above)* Minimal early decelerations. *(Below)* Evolution to variable decelerations, with slow recovery (late component) clearly seen, in spite of some interruptions at the end of the tracing. Reprinted from Cibils LA: Clinical significance of fetal heart rate patterns during labor. IV. Agonal patterns. *Am J Obstet Gynecol* 129:833, 1977.

376

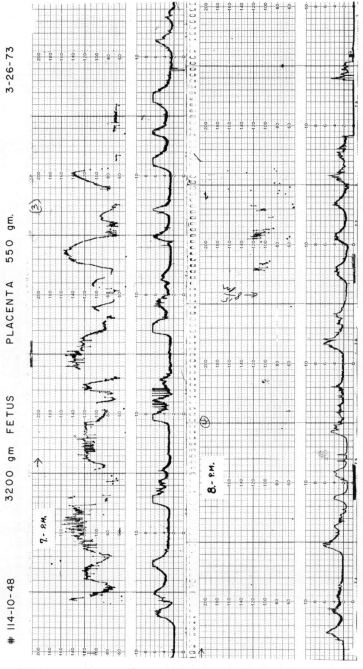

Figure 16-7 Same case as in Figure 16-6, 55 min later. Continuous 110-min recording. *(Above)* Severe variable decelerations with hypoxic component triggered particularly by the coupled contractions. When there is sufficient relaxation time between contractions (up to 5 min) there is rebound tachycardia. In spite of the external recording it is clear that the baseline is fixed. The last short recording of 65/min FHR bradycardia probably represents the moment of fetal death. *(Below)* No FHR was recorded and no FH tones heard by auscultation. Amniotomy produced meconium-stained amniotic fluid and the prolapse of a nonpulsating umbilical cord compressed by a head at 0 station. A stillborn infant was delivered 35 min after the end of the tracing. Reprinted from Cibils LA: Clinical significance of fetal heart rate patterns during labor. IV. Agonal patterns. *Am J Obstet Gynecol* 129:833, 1977.

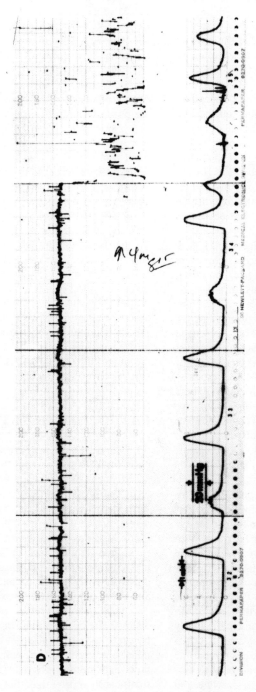

Figure 16-8 Direct FHR and UC tracings obtained from enhanced labor of *primipara at 42 weeks gestation* with meconium-stained amniotic fluid. Slow but steady progress with no other FHR alteration than moderate tachycardia and fixed baseline. Suddenly the FH tracing stopped and no FH tones could be auscultated. A stillborn 3375 gm infant was delivered within 1 hour. Reprinted from Hayashi RH, Fox ME: Unforeseen sudden intrapartum fetal death in a monitored labor. *Am J Obstet Gynecol* 122:786, 1975.

The most striking finding in the recordings of those postterm infants who seem to die intrapartum without warning is *the absence of late decelerations* (Figure 16-9), which by definition indicate episodes of hypoxia leading to severe fetal distress. One would expect that the homeostatic deterioration of the fetus terminating in death would start by hypoxia, to be followed by asphyxia, severe acidosis, and then death in a more or less protracted period of time, depending on the severity of the condition causing the hypoxia. It may well be that the cascade of alterations is the same but the FHR response is different, at least in a proportion of postterm fetuses. The other alterations of the FHR tracing seen during severe distress may or may not be present, and because of their lesser specificity as expressions of a pathologic episode, their absence is not so puzzling.

The tracing of a postterm labor may look perfectly unalarming, and the decision to interfere made on grounds unrelated to the fetal condition, but one may still be unpleasantly surprised by delivering a stillborn (Figure 16-10). Alterations of the baseline, particularly the fixed baseline, are observed in close to one-half of all prolonged gestations. Therefore in this group of patients alteration of baseline cannot be taken as a sign of distress calling for interference. Minor, inconsequential decelerations may be observed in labors of postterm pregnancies (as in all labors, see Figure 12-12), and occasionally there are decelerations that do not fit the definitions given in previous chapters. The inconspicuous tracing notwithstanding, the fetus may be in jeopardy and be born dead (Figure 16-11).

The association of a known pathologic condition with prolonged gestation does not change this unpredictable behavior of the fetus. The apparent sudden deterioration of a fetus has been observed only in this group of patients; the recording of the sinusoidal baseline pattern may precede by a very short time a fatal outcome (Figures 16-12 and 16-1). The FHR of these fetuses includes early and variable decelerations in association with baseline alterations, particularly fixed and tachycardic baseline. At the Chicago Lying-In Hospital tracings showing borderline (and apparently insignificant) bradycardia, sustained for many hours, with fixed baseline and variable decelerations have rarely been recorded. From one such case of a postterm gestation (an infant born with severe acidosis after having aspirated meconium), there was a tracing without a single late deceleration to foretell the hypoxia that must have preceded the acidosis (Figure 16-13) which ended fatally in the early neonatal period.

The risk of prolonged gestation has been emerging slowly from studies carried out in relatively small series. A review done by Vorherr (1975), from a compilation of several thousand cases, concluded that the perinatal mortality of the postterm infants is several times (5% to 7%) higher than that of term infants (1% to 2%) and that it increases as the weeks pass. Furthermore, from that review it seemed clear that the syndrome carries more than twice the risk when it occurs in primiparas as compared to multiparas. This observation has been confirmed in the series at the Chicago Lying-In Hospital (Figure 16-14), with the added ominous aspect that the majority of the fatalities did not present the classical characteristics of fetal distress until a few minutes before death, or at birth in poor condition. Moreover, the typical expression in intrauterine hypoxia, the FHR late deceleration, was conspicuously absent in all cases. This strange fact gave the impression that these infants are unable to withstand distress for any length of time; all had passed meconium in the amniotic fluid, and aspirated it before delivery.

PATHOPHYSIOLOGY

The most interesting aspect of the agonal patterns of FHR seems to be the differences established by the chronologic age of the fetuses. Preterm fetuses respond to distress with tachycardia, fixed baseline, and late deceleration *sustained for several hours* of vigorous labor before a terminal bradycardia precedes death by a few minutes. Acid–base studies have indicated that acidosis persists throughout the episode of distress and probably is the result of anaerobic metabolism and the accumulation of lactate and pyruvate.

Term fetuses present the classic signs of distress: late decelerations, tachycardia, and fixed baseline leading to acidosis and finally the terminal bradycardia. The amount of time these infants may sustain severe distress before death is significantly shorter than that for preterm fetuses, although a healthy fetus may withstand distress for a considerable period of time. Only the total suppression of blood flow through the umbilical

379

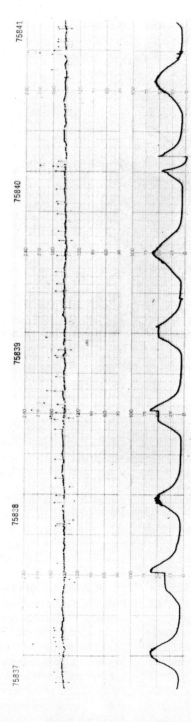

Figure 16-9 Direct FHR and UC tracings recorded for 17 min from induced labor of *primipara at 41 weeks gestation.* About 6 hours before this strip, the tracing showed variable decelerations and a short episode of bradycardia; no further alterations of the FHR tracing. Shortly after the end of this borderline tachycardic and fixed pattern the FH was no longer recorded, and the heart tones were inaudible. A 3540 gm stillborn infant was delivered 2½ hours later. Reprinted from Gaziano EP, Freeman DW: Analysis of heart rate patterns preceding fetal death. *Obstet Gynecol* 50:578, 1977.

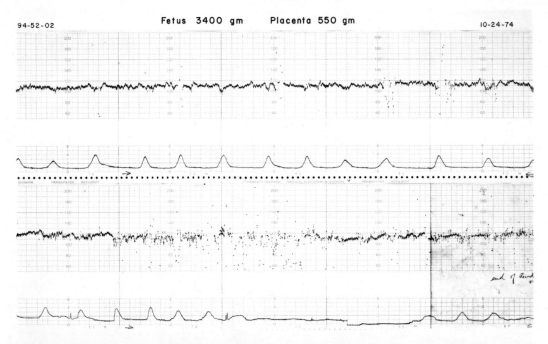

94-52-02 Fetus 3400 gm Placenta 550 gm 10-24-74

Figure 16-10 Two 50-min segments of direct FHR and UC tracings during spontaneous labor of *primipara at 41.5 weeks gestation. (Above)* Oscillating baseline, moderate bradycardia about 110 beats/min, with no decelerations triggered by contractions. *(Below)* Smaller oscillations on a still moderate bradycardic baseline 3½ hours later (recording unsatisfactory in some segments with poor FHR pickup and obstructed catheter). Because of "lack of progress" a cesarean section was performed, and 30 min after the end of the tracing a 3400 gm stillborn infant was delivered. Autopsy revealed only meconium aspiration.

cord (or complete separation of the placenta in "complete abruptio") may induce a superacute state of distress terminating in death in a short time. Even in these extreme circumstances the preterm fetuses seem to tolerate longer periods of distress than their term counterparts subjected to comparable stressful conditions (compare Figure 16-3 with Figures 16-6 and 16-7).

Postterm fetus tracings also had a fixed baseline and moderate tachycardia, as well as small early and variable decelerations but lacked the most characteristic pattern of hypoxia, the late decelerations. The absence of this symptom is important because it implies a reassuring fetal condition. In addition, the lack of late decelerations in cases of severe hypoxia and acidosis terminating in death requires an explanation of why these fetuses are set apart from all the others. Characteristically, some of these fetuses have demonstrated sinusoidal FHR shortly before death, a pattern observed almost exclusively in severely affected erythroblastotic fetuses in an

agonal state (Manseau et al, 1972). A constant sign in the agonal postterm fetus has been the presence of meconium, generally aspirated.

One can only speculate on the possible mechanisms involved in the unequal behavior of the FHR tracings among fetuses dying at different ages. Few elements are known about their physiology because there is an almost complete lack of experimental studies carried out in this particular area.

Barcroft (1946) showed, in sheep and rabbits, that the cardiovascular reflexes become operational in a sequential manner, each one appearing at an apparently set chronologic age. Observations that confirmed those studies were made later by Dawes (1969) in lamb and dog fetuses, indicating that perhaps there is a general biologic behavior applicable to the majority of fetuses, including man. There is indirect evidence that it may be so because it has been shown (Brady et al, 1962) that postmature fetuses respond in a different way from term fetuses to comparable stressful condi-

119-84-25   3650 gm FETUS   Placenta 800 gm   APGAR 0   5-15-73

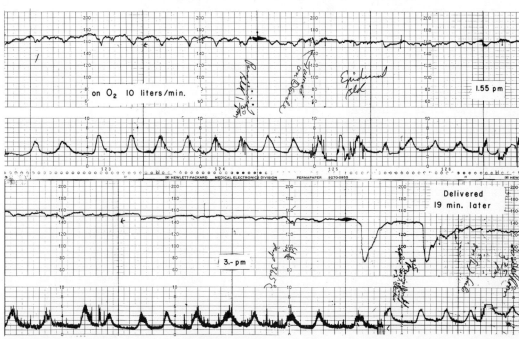

Figure 16-11 Two 50-min segments of direct FHR and external UC monitoring during spontaneous labor of *primipara at 43 weeks gestation,* with meconium-stained amniotic fluid. *(Above)* Mother receiving continuous oxygen by mask. Pattern of active labor with a fixed, tachycardic baseline and small early decelerations. Epidural anesthesia attempted and failed. *(Below)* Improvement of tachycardia 45 min later with the baseline still fixed and no more decelerations. At the end of the tracing, two large "late-like" decelerations, seemingly triggered by contractions, but with one contraction between them not affecting the FHR, were followed by the same steady pattern. Stillborn infant delivered 19 min later by low forceps under pudendal block anesthesia. Autopsy revealed stigmata of postmaturity and massive meconium aspiration. Reprinted from Cibils LA: Clinical significance of fetal heart rate patterns during labor. IV. Agonal patterns. *Am J Obstet Gynecol* 129:833, 1977

tions, behavior ascribed to differences in the development of controlling reflexes. On the other hand, the saltatory FHR pattern is almost never seen among the preterm fetuses while it is present in a high percentage at postterm; if this pattern is controlled by the nervous system, it might be that the observation of sequential development of reflexes in animals could apply to man.

The chronologic appearance of new reflexes, as the nervous system completes its anatomic and functional maturation, may not be the only critical physiologic change occurring in the fetus. In the past few years it has been observed that many enzymatic systems appear as the fetus matures, while others become less active or disappear. As an example the synthesis of lecithin in the fetal lung follows two pathways, one active from about the 22nd week, while the other appears at about

the 32nd week of pregnancy. Enzymatic systems involved in renal function or the digestive system have also been described to be absent in premature fetuses and present in normal term infants. Thus it is likely that the high capacity for anaerobic metabolism of the developing fetus may be due to an enzymatic system different from that of the predominantly aerobic term infant. The protective function of the mechanisms involved in maintaining homeostasis may be controlled by completely different enzymatic systems evolving with the growth of the fetus and depending on the age of gestation.

The interplay of chronologic maturation of enzymatic systems and operation of new reflexes may not be the sole factors that influence the different response of FHR to preterminal stresses. Anatomic relationships between the fetus and

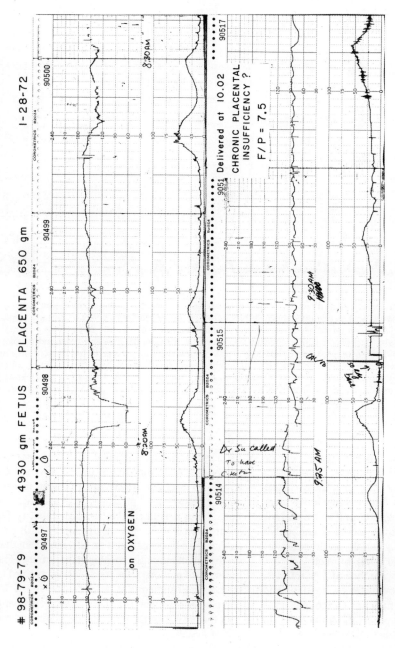

Figure 16-12 Two 16-min segments of direct FHR and UC tracings (paper speed, 3 cm/min) during spontaneous labor in multipara class B diabetic at 42 weeks gestation with advanced cervical dilatation and taking continuous oxygen by mask. *(Above)* Bigemini contractions of rather low frequency triggering a large variable deceleration with slow recovery on a fixed, tachycardic baseline. Three unimpressive small variable decelerations were triggered by subsequent contractions. *(Below)* Sudden onset of a sinusoidal pattern evolving to a progressive bradycardia, undulating around 80 beats frequency. By emergency cesarean section, 25 min after the end of the tracing, a stillborn infant was delivered weighing 4930 gm. There was, in addition, chronic placental insufficiency indicated by an F/P ratio of 7.5. Autopsy revealed postmaturity and meconium aspiration. Reprinted from Cibils LA: Clinical significance of fetal heart rate patterns during labor. IV. Agonal patterns. *Am J Obstet Gynecol* 129:833, 1977.

383

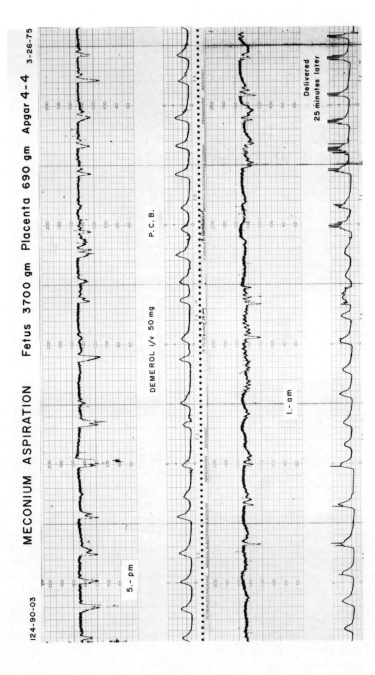

Figure 16-13 Two 50-min segments of continuous FHR and intrauterine pressure tracings during induction of labor for premature rupture of membranes in primipara at 44 weeks gestation. (*Above*) Fixed baseline, borderline tachycardia with small variable decelerations triggered by some contractions. Demerol was given, and paracervical block administered for pain. (*Below*) Seven hours later, similar pattern sustained throughout until complete dilatation. Mother given pudendal block anesthesia. By forceps rotation a very depressed and acidotic infant (cord blood pH 6.98) was delivered 25 min later. The baby had aspirated meconium, did not respond to vigorous treatment, and died at 6 hours of age. Autopsy confirmed postmaturity and meconium aspiration.

384

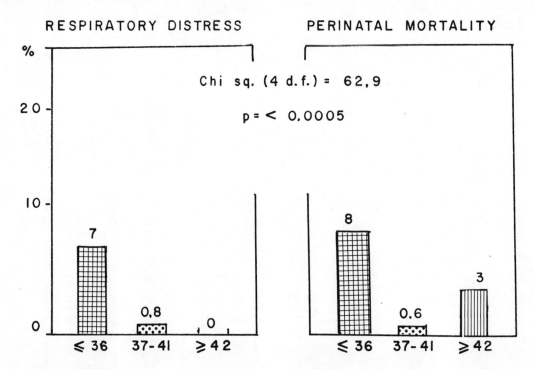

Figure 16-14 *(Left)* Incidence and comparison of neonatal morbidity (RDS), and *(right)* uncorrected perinatal mortality among perterm, term, and postterm populations at the Chicago Lying-In Hospital. Prematurity contributes heavily in both groups. Postterm infants had a very high mortality. Reprinted from Cibils LA: Clinical significance of fetal heart rate patterns during labor. I. Baseline patterns. *Am J Obstet Gynecol* 125:290, 1976.

placenta also vary. The unparallel growth of the fetus and placenta is shown by an F/P ratio of 3.2 at 28 weeks and its decline to 5.6 at term. The relatively lesser placental mass to supply the needs of a more demanding fetus must be compensated for by a faster IVS blood flow as pregnancy progresses. There are no good studies measuring the changes of blood flow with advancing gestation, but indirect evidence suggests that the circulating blood probably carries a higher oxygen tension in later pregnancy than in earlier stages (Cibils, 1967, 1974); this may be accomplished by a faster passage with less time to lose the oxygen to the fetal blood.

Other functional changes have also been observed in the placenta with the advance of gestation. Kulhanek et al (1974) have shown that placental permeability to urea (proportional to weight in early gestation) increases logarithmically, independent of weight, in late pregnancy. Functional maturation is thus unrelated to somatic growth. Finally, some observations have

indicated that the oxygen content of the postterm fetuses is lower than at term (Walker, 1958), which may lead only to potential serious hypoxia and disastrous outcome. The function of the so-called feto-placental unit also seems to be altered in prolonged gestation as the umbilical artery cortisol levels would indicate; they are significantly lower in prolonged gestations (Nwosu et al, 1975), particularly those terminated by induction of labor and/or cesarean section. If one considers the importance of adrenal steroids in adaptation to acute or chronic stress, and if these observations are accurate, it is understandable that the postterm fetus may have a response to the stress of labor different from that of the term fetus with an intact and fully functional adrenal steroid system.

In conclusion, therefore, the characteristic of the *preterm fetus* subjected to stressful situations is that it presents all the classic elements of FHR alterations seen in acute distress. It may sustain them for a *very long time* before it finally dies in severe acidosis but rarely, if ever, does it pass meconium. The *term fetus* usually presents the same signs but with a *diminished ability to withstand severe distress;* it does so for a shorter time, and generally it passes meconium shortly before the terminal bradycardia. The *postterm fetus* seems to be very fragile, if judged by the FHR characteristics. A number of them have tachycardia and fixed baseline *with meconium* in the amniotic fluid, and may be in very severe distress and acidosis *without displaying* the most notorious *sign of hypoxia, the late decerleration.* Moreover, they may very rapidly evolve toward a sinusoidal FHR pattern, a short terminal bradycardia, and death. The most puzzling feature of these cases is that they, so far, cannot predictably be singled out, and that death supervenes very rapidly before one may effectively intervene, or even when there is no apparent reason for interference.

MANAGEMENT

The observation of late decelerations is a well accepted indicator of transient fetal hypoxia and probably distress. It calls for very close observation of the evolution of that labor and readiness for intervention if associated signs of FHR alterations warrant interference (see Chapter 14). In addition to the stage of labor and possible imminent delivery, it is critical to consider FHR alterations, acid–base status, and *particularly age of gestation.* Age is extremely important because if the fetus is *preterm* the clinician may have sufficient time to observe, diagnose, and it is hoped, correct the cause of distress, or even attempt to improve the intrauterine fetal condition by controlling uterine activity and administration of oxygen to the mother. These infants will *always display late decelerations* and perhaps the other associated FHR alterations.

Term fetuses are also amenable to "intrauterine resuscitation" (see Figure 14-38) because their resistance to distress allows one time

for effective intervention. However, *postterm fetuses* have a very misleading FHR pattern: almost 50% of them have *tachycardia and fixed baseline,* alterations usually resulting from variable or late decelerations affecting the fetal homeostasis. But some of these fetuses *do not respond* on all occasions to hypoxia *with late decelerations,* a most dangerous aberration because absence of late decelerations is a reassuring sign. The management of a prolonged gestation requires close supervision of every aspect involved in labor. In particular, a *direct monitoring* system must be set up at the earliest possible time allowed by the condition of the cervix. This maneuver allows for accurate recording of FHR baseline with presence of rapid oscillations, or their absence when fixed. Moreover, the clinician may observe the amniotic fluid, which may be clear or stained with meconium. In the latter circumstance, one must attempt to obtain a sample of fetal scalp blood to evaluate acid–base status, even if the FHR is apparently reassuring. The absence of late decelerations or the sporadic recording of intermittent small ones should not serve as comfort to postpone the direct assessment of the infant (Figure 16-15). A number of authors have reported their experience with postterm or "dysmature" fetuses, born either dead or very depressed but who never presented a more alarming alteration of the FHR than tachycardia. In other circumstances one may observe strange patterns of deceleration not fitting the standard classification of early, variable, or late but still bizarre. Rapid intervention could be advised (Figure 16-16) if scalp blood sampling is not readily available in these cases. Continuous administration of oxygen to the mother cannot but help the postterm infant. Perhaps the best way to supervise the fetus would be by continuous pH monitoring, when a reliable and accessible technique is established. In the meantime, the most effective approach is the *prevention of prolonged gestation* by not allowing a pregnancy to go beyond the 41st week (288 days of amenorrhea) as the only means to avoid the death of some of these fetuses.

386

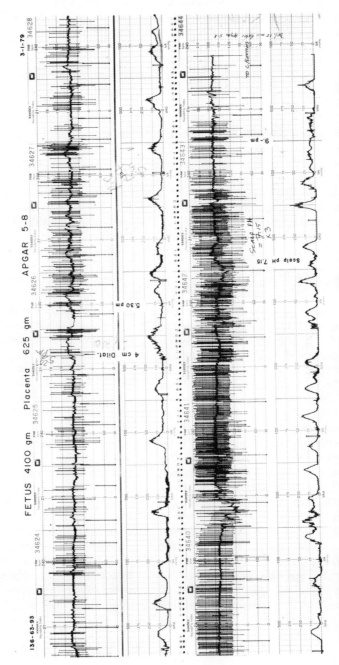

Figure 16-15 Two 60-min segments of direct FHR and UC recordings during labor of *primipara at 42 weeks gestation* induced for PRM with meconium-stained amniotic fluid. *(Above)* Moderate uterine activity with prelabor pattern. FHR with fixed baseline, and borderline tachycardia without decelerations. *(Below)* Two hours later, more satisfactory uterine activity, FHR with fixed baseline on well-established tachycardia, and three sporadic rather small late decelerations. Scalp blood pH taken where shown indicated severe acidosis for which an emergency cesarean section was performed 15 min after the end of the record. A depressed 4100 gm infant was delivered and survived.

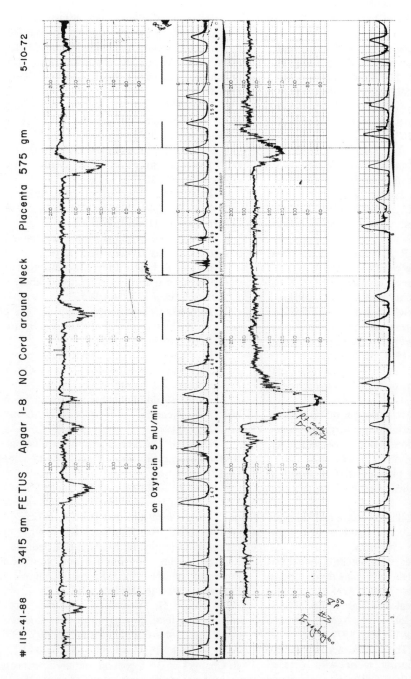

Figure 16-16 Two segments of direct FHR and intrauterine pressure changes recorded during enhanced labor of *multipara at 41.5 weeks gestation. (Above)* Good labor pattern for 50 min with severe tachycardic FHR baseline and borderline rapid oscillations. Six impressive decelerations may be seen, but three of them are not related in time to uterine contractions, the others appearing to be "late." *(Below)* Similar pattern 30 min later with the first deceleration prolonged and severe slowly recovering during a strong contraction. In spite of progress to advanced first stage, a cesarean section for fetal distress was done 45 min after the end of the tracing with the birth of a very depressed and acidotic infant (cord blood pH 7.15) who recovered satisfactorily. Reprinted from Cibils LA: Clinical significance of fetal heart rate patterns during labor. IV. Agonal patterns. *Am J Obstet Gynecol* 129:833, 1977.

388

BIBLIOGRAPHY

Assali NS, Holm LW, Sehgal N: Hemodynamic changes in fetal lamb in utero in response to asphyxia, hypoxia and hypercapnia. *Cir Res* 11:423, 1962.

Barcroft J: *Researches on Prenatal Life,* chap 12. Oxford, Blackwell, 1946, pp 123-144.

Baskett TF, Koh KS: Sinusoidal fetal heart pattern. A sign of fetal hypoxia. *Obstet Gynecol* 44:379, 1974.

Beard RW: The detection of fetal asphyxia in labor. *Pediatrics* 53:157, 1974.

Brady JP, James LS, Baker MA: Heart rate changes in the fetus and newborn during labor, delivery, and immediate neonatal period. *Am J Obstet Gynecol* 84:1, 1962.

Brady J, James LS, Baker MA: Fetal electrocardiographic studies. *Am J Obstet Gynecol* 86:785, 1963.

Caldeyro-Barcia R: Estudio de la anoxia fetal intrauterina mediante el ECG fetal y el registro continuo de la frecuencia cardiaca fetal. *II Cong Lat-Am Obstet Ginecol (Mexico)* 2:288, 1958.

Caldeyro-Barcia R, Poseiro JJ, Negreiro CE, et al: Effects of abnormal uterine contractions on a human fetus, in *Modern Problems in Pediatrics,* vol 8. Basel, Karger, 1963, pp 267-295.

Cetrulo CL, Schifrin BS: Fetal heart rate patterns preceding death in utero. *Obstet Gynecol* 48:521, 1976.

Cibils LA: Le developpement du reseau vasculaire des villosites etudie en contraste de phase au debut de la gestation. *Rev Fr Gynecol* 62:349, 1967.

Cibils LA: The placenta and newborn in hypertensive conditions. *Am J Obstet Gynecol* 118:256, 1974.

Cibils LA: Clinical significance of fetal heart rate patterns during labor. I. Baseline patters. *Am J Obstet Gynecol* 125:290, 1976.

Cibils LA: Clinical significance of fetal heart rate patterns during labor. II. Late decelerations. *Am J Obstet Gynceol* 123:473, 1975.

Cibils LA: Clinical significance of fetal heart rate patterns during labor. IV. Agonal patterns. *Am J Obstet Gynecol* 129:833, 1977.

Davidsen PCB: The significance of the fetal electrocardiogram during labor with detailed report of one case. *Acta Obstet Gynecol Scand* 50:45, 1971.

Davidsen PCB: Continuous monitoring of the fetal heart rate and uterine contractions during labor. *Acta Obstet Gynecol Scand* 50:51, 1971.

Dawes GS: Cardiovascular adjustment of the fetus during asphyxia: The aortic chemoreceptors, in *Perinatal Factors Affecting Human Development.* Washington, DC, Pan American Health Organization Scientific Publication 185, 1969, pp 199-201.

Evans TN, Koeff ST, Morley GW: Fetal effects of prolonged pregnancy. *Am J Obstet Gynecol* 85:701, 1963.

Gaziano EP, Freeman DW: Analysis of heart rate patterns preceding fetal death. *Obstet Gynecol* 50:578, 1977.

Goodlin R: Intrapartum fetal heart rate responses and plethysmographic pulse. *Am J Obstet Gynecol* 110:210, 1971.

Goodlin RC: Fetal cardiovascular responses to distress. *Obstet Gynecol* 49:371, 1977.

Hayashi RH, Fox ME: Unforeseen sudden intrapartum fetal death in a monitored labor. *Am J Obstet Gynecol* 122:786, 1975.

Hendricks CH: Patterns of fetal and placental growth: The second half of normal pregnancy. *Obstet Gynecol* 24:357, 1964.

Hon EH: The fetal heart rate patterns preceding death in utero. *Am J Obstet Gynecol* 78:47, 1959.

Hon EH: Additional observations on "pathologic" bradycardia. *Am J Obstet Gynecol* 118:428, 1974.

Hon EH, Lee ST: Electronic evaluation of the fetal heart rate. *Am J Obstet Gynecol* 87:814, 1963.

James LS, Morishima HO, Daniel SS, et al: Mechanism of late deceleration of the fetal heart rate. *Am J Obstet Gynecol* 113:578, 1972.

James LS, Rey HR, Stark RI, et al: A new approach to predicting the high-risk neonate. A scoring system for intrapartum monitoring. Presented at the 5th European Congress on Perinatal Medicine 150-155, 1976.

Klapholz H, Friedman E: The incidence of intrapartum fetal distress with advancing gestational age. *Am J Obstet Gynecol* 127:405, 1977.

Kulhanek JF, Meschia G, Makowski EL, et al: Changes in DNA content and urea permeability of the sheep placenta. *Am J Physiol* 226:1257, 1974.

Leong MKH, Murphy BEP: Cortisol levels in maternal venous and umbilical cord blood, arterial and venous serum at vaginal delivery. *Am J Obstet Gynecol* 124:471, 1976.

Manseau P, Vaquier J, Chavinie J, et al: Le rythme cardiaque foetal sinusoidal. *J Gynecol Obstet Biol Reprod (Paris)* 1:343, 1972.

Mendez-Bauer C, Monleon J, Guevara-R G, et al: Changes in fetal heart rate associated with acute intrapartum fetal distress, in *Perinatal Factors Affecting Human Development*. Washington, DC, Pan American Health Organization Scientific Publication 185, 1969, pp 178–187.

Myers RE, Mueller-Heubach E, Adamsons K: Predicatability of the state of fetal oxygenation from a quantitative analysis of the components of the late deceleration. *Am J Obstet Gynecol* 115:1083, 1973.

Nwosu U, Wallach EE, Boggs TR, et el: Possible adrenocortical insufficiency in postmature neonates. *Am J Obstet Gynecol* 122:969, 1975.

Nwosu U, Wallach EE, Boggs TR, et al: Possible role of the fetal adrenal glands in the etiology of post maturity. *Am J Obstet Gynecol* 121:366, 1975.

Pokoly TB: The role of cortisol in human parturition. *Am J Obstet Gynecol* 117:549, 1973.

Smith ID, Shearman RP: Fetal plasma steroids in relation to parturition. I. The effect of gestational age upon umbilical plasma corticosteroid levels following vaginal delivery. *J Obstet Gynaecol Br Comwlth* 81:11, 1974.

Smith ID, Shearman RP: Fetal plasma steroids in relation to parturition. II. The effect of gestational age upon umbilical plasma corticosteroids following hysterotomy and Cesarean section. *J Obstet Gynaecol Br Comwlth* 81:16, 1974.

Tushuizen PB, Stoot JE, Ubachs JM: Fetal heart rate monitoring of the dying fetus. *Am J Obstet Gynecol* 120:922, 1974.

Vapaavouri EK, Shinebourne EA, Williams RL, et al: Development of cardiovascular responses to autonomic blockade in intact fetal and neonatal lamb. *Biol Neonate* 22:177, 1973.

Vorherr H: Placental insufficiency in relation to postterm pregnancy and fetal postmaturity. *Am J Obstet Gynecol* 123:67, 1975.

Walker JJ: Prolonged pregnancy syndrome. *Am J Obstet Gynecol* 76:1231, 1958.

CHAPTER 17
Antenatal Monitoring

The clinical application of feto-maternal monitoring during labor has led, after the better understanding of the pathophysiology controlling alterations from normal patterns, to its use during the antepartum stage of gestation. The technical difficulties of obtaining good tracings for analysis in the antenatal stage contribute to uncertainties in interpretation. Recording methods are almost exclusively indirect, that is noninvasive, and therefore likely to include artifacts because observations are carried out in patients not in labor. However, a great variety of "tests" has been proposed and an even greater number of interpretations advanced to predict the condition of the fetus during the period of study as well as at the time of birth. Only tests with practical application and of recognized validity will be reviewed here.

The proportion of intrapartum deaths to perinatal mortality is relatively small, on the order of 15%; the great majority occur in the neonatal period (about 50%) or in the antepartum stage (around 35%). A high number of deaths in the antepartum stage occur in the so-called high-risk pregnancies. Thus, the importance of identifying the patients at highest risk is obvious if preventive therapeutic measures are to be applied. Several protocols have been designed with the purpose of identifying this high-risk population, which is amenable to close supervision. These schemes are more or less complicated and elaborate, encompassing medical, sociologic, economic, racial, and other factors that are weighed according to an established scale. Fortunately, only a small number of these pregnancies terminate in fetal demise, but, to prevent these, probably the majority should be tested so that the condition of the fetus and its ability to thrive in utero may be assessed. It has been estimated that in about 80% of perinatal deaths from hypoxia and asphyxia, the condition starts during gestation, whereas in only 5% does it start after delivery. The aim of the tests is to detect those cases not yet openly hypoxic but with a good chance of becoming hypoxic.

All the tests attempt to evaluate the effect of maternal pathologic conditions on the fetal well-being, which may be affected in a protracted manner so that normal growth may be retarded or arrested. On the other hand, subacute or acute conditions may interfere with adequate oxygenation of a well-grown fetus and create conditions that compromise its life in a short time. These two extremes of fetal pathology have encouraged a large number of studies over the last decade. Electronic and biochemical monitoring have been applied either in a long-term and intermittent manner or on an acute and continuous basis. This review will emphasize the electronic techniques (continuous or intermittent) with mention of the biochemical methods when they contribute to the selection of the patients to be evaluated, or when they aid in the interpretation of the tracings.

Some tests were proposed several years before being tried by other investigators and have become widely accepted only in recent times. Basically, all aim at assessing the response of the fetus to conditions indicating an acute or a chronic state of deprivation of oxygen or nutrients. The techniques employed to trigger the fetal reaction characterize the various methods to be described.

THE EXERCISE TEST

Increased oxygen consumption by the mother during physical exertion has been used by Stembera (1967) to evaluate fetal oxygen reserve and thus the potential condition of symptomatic hypoxia induced by labor contractions.

The test is based on a number of separate observations made by several investigators before the technique was devised. Morris et al (1956) demonstrated that myometrial and IVS circulation in advanced gestation are significantly lower in hypertensive than in normal patients, and that they decrease following exercise in both conditions. Moore and Myerscough (1957) corroborated that observation and further showed that in prolonged pregnancy the blood flow to the myometrium is also diminished, as ascertained by the clearance of injected radioactive sodium. Hon and Wohlgemuth (1961) observed that an exercise of 2 min, by a pregnant patient close to term, would induce a transient fetal bradycardia followed by rebound tachycardia if hypertension existed, while there were no observable changes in the FHR of normal gestations.

The test developed by Stembera consisted of recording the FHR before and after subjecting the pregnant patient to a 3-min treadmill exercise on a bicycle-like apparatus while she was supine in bed. After evaluation of the intrapartum and neonatal findings in the patients subjected to the test, he found that bradycardia following maternal exercise is frequent among distressed fetuses during labor or depressed neonates. These patients could be grouped among those who had pathologic conditions during gestation, particularly hypertension and growth-retarded fetuses. When the fetus has a borderline oxygen reserve, the increased oxygen consumption by the mother, superimposed on diminished uterine and IVS blood flow, would bring the fetal oxygen to hypoxic levels and thus trigger bradycardia. This exercise test is relatively simple and can be carried out with a bicycle or a simple two-step walking up and down for 3 min. It has not been popular in the United States, but in many European and South American countries it has had wide acceptance.

CONTRACTIONS STRESS TEST

The antepartum observation of FHR tracings recorded during a series of uterine contractions of moderate to good intensity is defined as "contractions stress test" (CST). These contractions may occur spontaneously or be triggered by the administration of an oxytocic. This test is also known by the popular misnomer "oxytocin challenge test" because of the frequent need to use oxytocin to induce the contractions.

The basic function evaluated by this test is the oxygen level in fetal blood. As extensively discussed in Chapter 14, with each uterine contraction of moderate to good intensity there is a significant decrease of blood flow to the IVS. As a corollary, there is stagnation of maternal blood, which loses its oxygen rapidly to the continuing circulating fetal blood. As the two equilibrate at low pressure, the fetus continues to consume oxygen, which must then be obtained at the expense of the so-called fetal oxygen reserve—the amount of oxygen available above the threshold of about 17–18 mm Hg, below which FHR decelerations are triggered. In other words, *the CST is a direct measure of the oxygen* reserve of the fetus and an indirect assessment of the respiratory function of the placenta.

The fetus is capable of surviving satisfactorily with such a low oxygen pressure (normal average capillary pO_2, 24 to 26 mm Hg) because a number of factors converge to facilitate maximum oxygen uptake. The high hemoglobin concentration of fetal blood, about 18 gm/100 ml, allows oxygen release more easily than adult hemoglobin, and it carries more of it at equal pressures because of its different dissociation curve. Finally, the total amount of oxygen delivered to fetal tissues at term pregnancy is very close to that of the adult because the fetal cardiac output is about twice as high per unit of body weight. The fetus is capable of withstanding the contractions of physiologic labor, under normal circumstances of IVS blood flow and maternal oxygenation, because it has a sufficient oxygen reserve to supply its needs during the approximately 40 sec that the maternal blood flow to the IVS is significantly hindered. The reserves are replenished during uterine relaxation, and the cycle repeats itself. When there is an abnormally diminished IVS blood flow, the availability of oxygen is decreased and the reserve is lower; thus the possibility of a critical transient hypoxia being triggered by a normal uterine contraction. These alterations, reviewed in Chapter 14, are called "late decelerations" and have the same pathophysiologic significance at intrapartum or antepartum stages of gestation. The test, aimed at producing labor-like contractions, is to assess this aspect of fetal physiology.

The CST as a measure of fetal well-being was first proposed independently by Pose et al (1963, 1968) and Hammacher (1966) but several years passed before its widespread application and acceptance as a clinical test. In the United States the report by Ray et al (1972) was followed fairly rapidly by a large number of publications, the majority of which suggested that this was a good method to predict fetal condition and eventual outcome. In the early stages of investigation many intrauterine fetal deaths occurred following so-called positive tests, thus substantiating the validity of a positive test to indicate fetal jeopardy. Since its introduction in 1973 as a routine test for evaluating some of the high-risk patients observed at the Chicago Lying-In Hospital, more than 800 patients have been given over 1400 tests.

Indications

A CST may be recommended whenever there is reason to suspect chronic or acute inadequate oxygen supply to the fetus. This occurs in high-risk pregnancies, and, among them, in specific syndromes where inadequate IVS blood flow constitutes one of the outstanding pathophysiologic alterations.

Hypertensive diseases of pregnancy are by definition characterized by generalized arteriolar constriction, including supply to the uteroplacental bed, and thus diminished IVS blood flow. *Chronic hypertension* is present in a high proportion of high-risk mothers and was the reason for the test in about 12% of patients seen at the Chicago Lying-In Hospital. *Preeclamptic hypertension* (subacute or "pregnancy-induced") was observed in 9% of the tested patients. The combined cases represented 21% of a highly selected population with conditions predisposing to chronic fetal oxygen deficit, antepartum fetal death, or severe intrapartum distress.

Intrauterine growth retardation of the fetus ("small for gestational age") was suspected in 23% of patients evaluated at the Chicago Lying-In Hospital. These cases had already evidence of a status of chronic placental insufficiency to supply the necessary nutrients to attain normal fetal growth. It is likely that in those patients the other vital placental function, that of respiration, may have also been impaired, creating the danger of impending asphyxia for the fetus.

Prolonged gestation, that is, pregnancy lasting more than 42 weeks after the last menses ("post-datism") has been suspected of being a condition with chronic deficiency of oxygen supply to the fetus. Furthermore, it is a syndrome with a high perinatal—particularly acute and intrapartum—mortality. Most likely hypoxia and asphyxia contribute heavily as direct causes in many of those deaths. It has been the reason for testing in 22% of the patient population at the Chicago Lying-In Hospital.

Diabetes was the indication for the test in 12% of the patients evaluated in the Chicago Lying-In Hospital series. This condition, ranging from the relatively mild class A (5%) to the progressively more severe B to F (7%), is often a cause of antepartum demise, and hypoxia is considered among the direct causes of death. In spite of a large placenta, it is believed that *relative placental insufficiency* contributes to fetal deterioration, probably initiated by the macrosomia and metabolic alterations peculiar to the disease.

The suspicion of fetal jeopardy due to *lower* than normal maternal *production of estrogens* (blood or urinary estriol) or diminished activity without any apparent pathologic disorder was the reason for testing in 10% of the Chicago Lying-In series.

History of previous fetal loss is a condition considered to increase the risk of subsequent pregnancies and was observed in 5% of the Chicago Lying-In Hospital tested population.

Miscellaneous causes, including medical complications of pregnancy and chronic drug abuse, were the reasons for conducting the test in the remainder of the population followed at the Chicago Lying-In Hospital.

Most patients with these syndromes are candidates to have the CST. Selection had been made on the basis of abnormal urinary estriol excretion and/or severity of clinical condition. The study of large, high-risk patient populations revealed that it is possible to further refine the method of selecting the candidates to be subjected to the test. Patients with an abnormal nonstress test (NST) are, in many centers, the only ones given a CST (see below, NST).

Contraindications

There are circumstances when the stimulation of uterine contractions may be contraindicated.

The suspicion, or certainty, that the patient has a *placenta previa* precludes the planned induction of uterine contractions, which may trigger or reactivate the process of bleeding that may then be difficult to control. In the case of premature *rupture of the membranes* when delivery is not yet desirable, a CST should not be given because of the probable impossibility of arresting the premature labor that may be triggered. Patients with history of *cervical incompetence,* with or without a cerclage, or with a history of repeated *premature labors* run the risk of uncontrollable premature labor if contractions are purposely stimulated.

Other means of assessing the fetal condition should be sought for the patients with these syndromes when the fetus is suspected of being in a relatively poor state.

Twin pregnancy is a relative contraindication although it is considered an absolute contraindication by some authors.

The presence of a *uterine scar* from previous cesarean section (either classic or low), myomectomy, or uteroplasty should not be contraindications to stimulate the number and quality of contractions required for a satisfactory CST. Likewise, an *overdistended* uterus of polyhydramnios should not contraindicate the test.

Technique

A quiet room with a comfortable bed is the ideal setting in which to conduct the CST. The essential elements are a *monitor* with *indirect* and *direct* recording capabilities, and an *infusion pump* capable of delivering a solution at slow and steady rates.

The patient is placed in a *supine semi-Fowler's position,* which prevents direct compression of the abdominal aorta and vena cava by the pregnant uterus. Thus there is normal unhindered circulation to the pelvic structures.

The FHR recorder — microphone, Doppler ultrasound transducer, or external ECG electrodes — is carefully placed over the area where the best signals can be obtained. Then the external tocotransducer is applied (see Chapter 4) over an area free from fetal parts. This external recording technique is used in the great majority of tests because of its easy application and its noninvasive character. However, there are circumstances when a *transabdominal catheter* may be necessary in order to record directly the intrauterine pressure changes, particularly when one is dealing with obese patients whose uteri are difficult to palpate, let alone feel the changes in consistency, and appreciate the intensity of contractions. The technique for placing the catheter is similar to that described in Chapter 4. This method carries the advantage of supplying an absolute value of the intrauterine pressure at the risk of being invasive. Maternal vital signs, especially blood pressure, should be obtained with reasonable frequency.

An intravenous catheter should be placed in one of the patient's arms and maintained open with a slow infusion of saline solution.

A control tracing of at least 30 min should be obtained before any oxytocic is administered to the patient. Relatively often, particularly in advanced gestation, spontaneous uterine contractions may be recorded, thus producing a spontaneous CST. When either no contractions are recorded or they are too infrequent and/or of low intensity, the oxytocin infusion must be started at the rate of 1 or 2 mU/min. *The aim is to trigger contractions of sufficient intensity and frequency to mimic those of early established labor.* These should be the equivalent of a 35 mm Hg intensity as a minimum, and recur at a frequency of 2½ to 3 min. If the starting oxytocin infusion does not induce the desired uterine activity after about 30 min, the rate should be doubled. This pattern should be followed until a satisfactory contractility is achieved. When late decelerations are recorded with consistency, even with low uterine activity, the oxytocin infusion must be discontinued. When the FHR is not altered by a good uterine activity maintained for about 30 min, the oxytocin is discontinued and the test considered terminated. It is good practice to maintain the monitoring until the uterine activity has returned to control values and/or the FHR has normalized after having had decelerations.

Interpretation

Although this test seems very clear cut and simple to interpret, there are in practice many circumstances when a definitive conclusion based on the available tracing cannot be reached. When presented with that dilemma one may either continue the recording until more recording is obtained or discontinue it and schedule to repeat on another date, preferably soon.

Negative The *absence of decelerations·* throughout the period of monitoring indicates that the test is negative. This suggests that at no time during the period of observation the fetus had episodes of low oxygenation with tensions below 18 mm Hg. By extension, one may conclude that the fetus is not in imminent danger of hypoxia and that, everything being equal, it may withstand labor satisfactorily. Repetition of the test should be indicated by the maternal condition or other indicators of fetal well-being. It has been established in this country, rather arbitrarily, that the CST should be repeated every week. European authors particularly do not hesitate to repeat it as often as every day in suspicious cases.

Positive The appearance of *recurrent late decelerations* triggered by either spontaneous or induced contractions indicates that the test is positive (Figure 17-1). Some authors require that 50% of the contractions produce late decelerations in order to interpret a test as positive, while others would consider results positive if only *30% of the contractions* triggered decelerations. The latter is the accepted standard at the Chicago Lying-In Hospital.

However, the amplitude of deceleration, that is the degree that FHR beats *fall* below the control

baseline, *seems to be unimportant*. Very small falls, of as little as 5 beats/min, may indicate that a fetus is in jeopardy, while larger drops may be observed in fetuses with relatively good recovery capacity. Although, in theory, the amplitude of the deceleration should be in direct relation to the degree of fall in fetal blood oxygen content, it has not been a consistent observation in clinical practice. *All amplitudes of late deceleration* should be considered equally important when observed in different patients.

In the same patient, however, there is a direct relationship between amplitude of deceleration and severity of fetal hypoxia. Decelerations of increasing amplitude suggest worsening fetal condition or, at least, more severe hypoxia during the particular contraction producing the greater decrease. When the decelerations are consistently observed with contractions of low frequency (see Figure 16-4) there is no need to enhance the con-

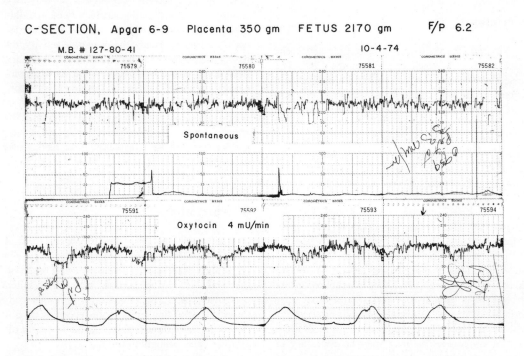

C-SECTION, Apgar 6-9   Placenta 350 gm   FETUS 2170 gm   F/P 6.2

M.B. # 127-80-41   10-4-74

Spontaneous

Oxytocin 4 mU/min

Figure 17-1 CST. Two 16-min segments of external UC and FHR tracings from hypertensive patient at 38 weeks gestation. Urinary estriol values 7 and 5 days before this recording were 8 and 7 mg/24 hours. The biparietal diameter of the fetus was 88 mm. Four days previously the patient had had a negative CST. Because the urinary estriol value fell to 4 mg/24 hours the CST was carried out. *(Above)* Control reveals no contractions. *(Below)* Steady uterine activity, triggered by 4 mU/min oxytocin, caused typical repetitive late decelerations producing a *positive CST*. In view of the clinical condition and unfavorable cervix, a cesarean section was done, and a mildly depressed, intrauterine growth-retarded infant delivered. (Paper speed, 3 cm/min.)

tractions to obtain a labor-like pattern. Nevertheless, contractions of low frequency may not trigger decelerations in a fetus with relative hypoxia because enough time elapses between contractions to allow it to build an oxygen reserve and stay above the bradycardic threshold, even through a contraction of moderate intensity. In those cases the *uterine contractility must be stimulated up to a labor-like pattern* to fully test the fetal oxygen reserve (Figure 17-2).

Oxygen administration by mask to the mother may have an important effect on the magnitude of FHR decelerations, to such an extent that potentially large decelerations are "dampened" during oxygen inhalation and become fully apparent only after oxygen is discontinued (Figures 17-2 and 17-3). The *frequency* of good contractions must not exceed the average of about 2½ min seen in active labor because *hypercontractility* (or excessive stimulation) alone is known to cause FHR alterations in normal pregnancies carrying healthy fetuses (see Figures 9-12 to 9-16, and Figure 12-25).

The intensity of the contractions must be carefully estimated by palpation when no intrauterine pressure is recorded because, as Pose has shown, a contraction of at least 35 mm Hg intensity is necessary to stress the average fetus, which may not be affected by contractions of lesser intensity (Figure 17-4). Only under extreme conditions of chronic hypoxia does a mild contraction trigger a late deceleration (see Figure 14-22).

Equivocal The recording of unusual or bizarre decelerations and late decelerations triggered by less than 30% of contractions should be interpreted as an equivocal CST. This infrequent observation creates a problem of interpretation and management not easy to solve satisfactorily. The tracing is neither clearly negative nor positive and decelerations may be of such borderline magnitude that one cannot help but accept the ill-defined label of equivocal (Figure 17-5). Tracings that cannot be properly interpreted because of interference or artifacts are not included in this category. It is seldom, if ever, impossible to stimulate the uterus to a labor-like contractility. The most likely problem in that circumstance will be the inability to record the contractions by external methods to correlate them with the FHR tracings; a transabdominal catheter is the only solution available with the added advantage of precise intrauterine pressure readings.

Unsatisfactory When the FHR cannot be recorded without too many artifacts due to excessive fetal activity, loss of signal during contractions, or electrical interference with the recording apparatus—the tracing is uninterpretable and therefore called unsatisfactory. New attempts (with a different monitor, and transducers or electrodes) should be made before the patient is discharged. Fortunately, less than 5% of all antenatal tests fall in this category. Their proportion diminishes as the experience of the person in charge of setting up the test increases.

Clinical Application

The CST has probably been, until recently, the most frequently used method to assess fetal well-being in advanced gestation due to the widespread availability of monitoring equipment and the relatively easy technique to set it up.

To take full advantage of the information, the CST should be used at the right time of gestation. It is extremely unlikely that one would have to test for fetal oxygen reserve before the 30th week of gestation because 1) the amount of placental tissue per unit of fetal weight is still high at this stage of gestation, and 2) there is very little chance that one would have to decide to terminate a pregnancy at that stage for fetal indications.

Depending on the clinical problem, the first test may be carried out at about the 35th week of gestation in diabetic patients who have good sustained estrogen levels (blood or urinary). The hypertensive patients should have the first test if the estrogen levels fall, or if there is arrest of fetal growth as ascertained by fundal examination or biparietal diameter of the head. Of course in cases of prolonged gestations the CST has to be done after the diagnosis has been made. For the patients having signs of intrauterine growth retardation one must estimate the gestational age, as accurately as possible, and indicate CSTs by the 37th week of gestation.

A *negative CST* implies that there is sufficient oxygen reserve to sustain the fetus during normal labor and, by extension, one assumes that continuation of that pregnancy for a few more days may be safe. The general clinical experience has confirmed the good predictive value of the test. The delivery of a live fetus *within 1 week* of a negative test has been shown to be predictable in 99% or more of the cases. In other words, unpredicted *intrauterine deaths* within 1 week have

396

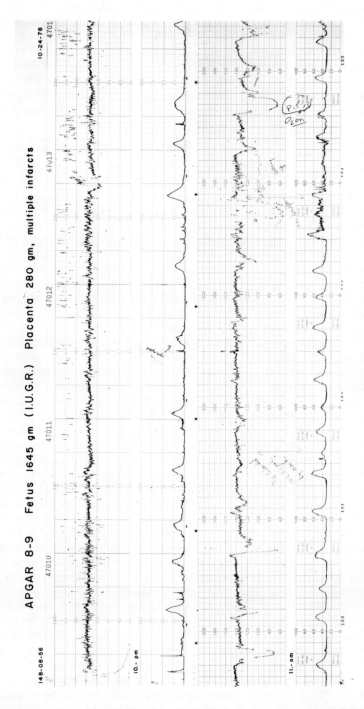

Figure 17-2 Two 60-min segments of external UC and FHR tracings at standard (1 cm/min) paper speed from preeclamptic secundipara at 34 weeks with urinary estriol excretion of 3.5 mg/24 hours. *(Above)* Mild uterine activity with contractions every 4 to 5 min and two small FHR late decelerations on a baseline of 150/min: *equivocal CST. (Below)* Increasing uterine activity, 13 hours later with contractions every 2½ to 3 min triggering frequent late decelerations, repetitive the last 25 min: *positive CST.* The clinical condition indicated a cesarean section, and a growth-retarded infant with good Apgar scores was delivered. The small placenta had several infarcts, suggesting that the F/P ratio of 5:9 may have been functionally much higher.

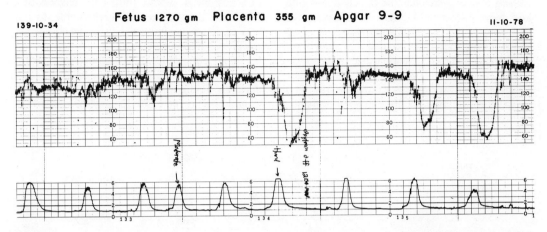

CESAREAN SECTION 40 minutes LATER   Cord pH: UV 7.31, UA 7.28

Fetus 1270 gm   Placenta 355 gm   Apgar 9-9

139-10-34   11-10-78

Figure 17-3 CST in a hypertensive multipara at 37 weeks gestation, with clinical intrauterine growth retardation. *(Left)* The mild to moderate contractions triggered only small late decelerations. *(Right)* Stronger contractions produced impressive decelerations: *positive CST*. After oxytocin was discontinued and continuous oxygen given by mask, a cesarean section produced a small infant in good condition and with normal oxygen values in the umbilical vessels.

occurred in 0.2% to 1% of the published series of negative CTS but the corrected mortality is still much lower. Intrauterine *fetal death* (or early neonatal death) without a mechanical explanation (cord accident, abruptio placentae, congenital malformations) is extremely rare following a negative CST well recorded and interpreted. In over 800 patients at the Chicago Lying-In Hospital there have been 4 cases of negative CST who died within one week: 3 had abruptio placentae, and the last one, a postmature fetus, died in utero of unexplained cause within 24 hours.

This experience agrees with the large series reported in the United States, which suggests that the incidence of true, corrected *false-negative CST* is on the order of 1/1000. Nevertheless, some short series report high incidences of up to 1/100 (Egley and Suzuki, 1977) of what must be labeled as false-negative tests.

The reassuring value of a negative CST also has been shown to indicate that intrapartum complications and neonatal "morbidity," including low Apgar scores, are on the order of only 10% to 20% in high-risk populations, much lower than observed in cases with positive or equivocal CST. Thus, it is usually recommended that the test be repeated only weekly if the first one is negative. The further analysis of FHR tracings, in addition

to decelerations, has significantly improved the prognostic value of the CST.

The predictive value of a *positive CST* has been less accurate. Nevertheless, the incidence of *intrapartum and neonatal morbidity* may complicate as many as 50% to 80% of patients having positive tests. The indirect diagnosis of low fetal oxygen reserve enables the clinician to identify the fetuses likely to have severe intrapartum hypoxia and to take the necessary steps to prevent a possible catastrophe.

The ominous significance of a positive CST is evidenced by the number of intrauterine deaths observed shortly following it when no action is taken. This fatal outcome has been evident from the first series reported by Hammacher et al (1968) and Pose et al (1969) when the clinical validity of the test was being investigated. All the authors who applied the CST to management of high-risk pregnancies have been able to confirm the ominous significance of a positive CST (see Figure 17-9). This observation has been so consistent that many investigators have recommended immediate intervention when recording a positive CST. This radical approach has been somewhat tempered by the observation that a relatively high percentage may go through labor without the need of surgical intervention.

The figures for *false-positive CSTs* vary from 25% to 70% depending on the clinical population and, more important, the criteria to classify the test. Very critical is the refinement in the analysis of the tracings now incorporated into some scoring systems designed to standardize the management. They include the study of the baseline frequency and oscillations, as well as the fetal "reactivity" or response to active movements,

With these improvements in the interpretation it is now possible to predict further the chances of a fetus to withstand labor without undue distress and to intervene immediately to avoid further fetal deterioration (Figure 17-4).

The refinements in interpretation notwithstanding, the high incidence of pathologic disorders among patients having a positive CST should remind the clinician that there is a high

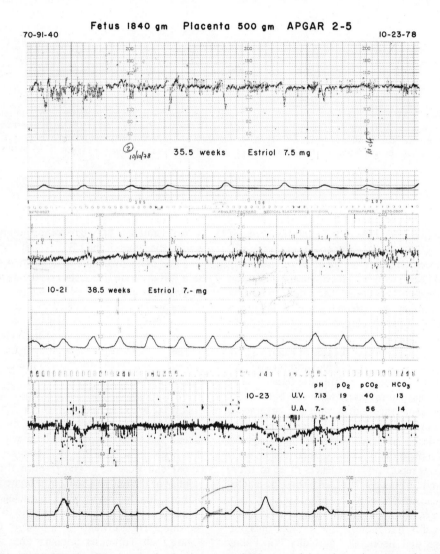

Figure 17-4 Serial CST in multipara excreting low amounts of urinary estriols and carrying a growth-retarded infant. *(Above)* At 35.5 weeks the CST was negative with a normal baseline. *(Center)* At 38.5 weeks the baseline seemed fixed but the CST was still negative. *(Below)* However, two days later, the strong contractions induced late decelerations on a fixed baseline pattern, and the smaller contractions triggered small decelerations. *Positive CST* followed by cesarean section produced a severely growth-retarded and depressed infant in state of marked asphyxia who recovered satisfactorily (cord blood values shown).

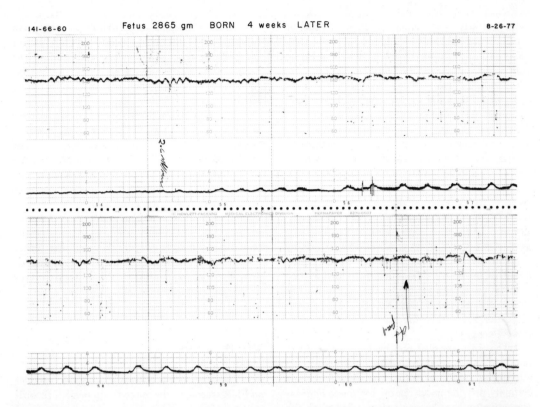

Figure 17-5 Continuous 80-min external recordings of chronic hypertensive multipara at 37 weeks gestation. *(Above)* Fixed baseline, interrupted by a transient moment of sinusoidal pattern. *(Below)* The oxytocin-induced contractions produced some barely detectable late decelerations. Neither fetal movements nor accelerations are seen: *equivocal CST*. Repeat test was scheduled for 24 hours later but *the fetus stopped moving 12 hours after the tracing*. Patient refused early induction and delivered, after spontaneous labor 4 weeks later, a macerated fetus.

number of sick fetuses in this group. A number of abnormal signs and symptoms grouped under the label of "perinatal morbidity" are detected in 75% to 92% of cases, including a perinatal mortality ranging from 12% to 18%. Clearly distressed fetuses with *intrauterine growth retardation* have been observed in about 30% to 40% of positive CSTs, and *depressed* newborns in approximately 20% to 30%. It is reasonable that one would apply a test of this kind in suspected cases to identify such a high proportion of pathologic conditions. The number of false positives seems a minor inconvenience to pay in the identification of so many severely affected fetuses.

In view of the possibility of dealing with a false-positive case, the clinician faces the dilemma of what decision to make in every case that demonstrates a positive CST. One must take into consideration the clinical picture and other tests of fetal well-being, particularly estriol values (blood or urine). The association of low estrogen value with positive CST has consistently demonstrated a severely affected fetus (see Figures 17-1, 17-2, 17-4, and 17-10). Under these circumstances one must assess the fetal viability and the amniotic fluid phospholipids (L/S ratio or phosphatidylglycerol). In many instances *active intervention* is the only choice, even when dealing with very small, borderline viable fetuses, because passive observation cannot improve the deteriorating situation of a severely compromised fetus. When one decides in favor of noninterference, the test *must be repeated as often as every day*. Some European authors repeat the test several times a day. A reassessment should be made at the completion of each new session.

On certain occasions, obvious contraction-related decelerations may be observed but they cannot clearly be classified as "late" in order to label the test as positive. These may vary—from cases having the aspect of "early" decelerations to others with an obvious "variable" pattern, as described by Mendez-Bauer et al (1978) in some antepartum tests and shown to be related to compressions of the umbilical cord. In cases of diminished amount of amniotic fluid, frequently seen in association with intrauterine growth retardation, the cord may be compressed not by being wound around the neck or limb but by its position between the fetus and the uterine walls. In cases of low oxygen reserve, the recovery leg of the deceleration will then demonstrate the characteristics of a late deceleration (see Chapter 15), suggesting that the CST is positive. The reports by Freeman and James (1975) and Baskett and Sandy (1979) of intrauterine fetal deaths following such observations demonstrate that they are at least as ominous as a typically positive CST, and perhaps more dangerous because they indicate a cord involvement.

The association of positive CST with a fixed baseline, poor fetal reactivity in response to movements, and low estrogen levels would most certainly provide good reason for *immediate intervention* (at the Chicago Lying-In Hospital, the incidence of cesarean sections has been on the order of 80% for cases with this picture). The route of delivery depends on the obstetric conditions and the characteristics of the tracing. A patient who has a ripe cervix and whose FHR baseline indicates good "reactivity" may undergo a trial of labor, while one with unripe cervix should have cesarean section. The incidence of cesarean sections ranges from 20% to 70% among the various published series in the United States—based on the interpretation of the clinicians managing the cases and therefore extremely variable. When labor is allowed to proceed, fetal scalp blood sampling must be done intermittently to assess the response of the fetus to the stress of contractions.

A positive test, with good baseline oscillations and fetal response to movements, occurs generally in cases having good estrogen value (in blood or urine). When the cervix is unripe, or the amniotic fluid phospholipid content is low, the case may be followed with daily CST and the other tests because of the reassuring significance they have as indicators of satisfactory fetal condition. A complete reassessment must be made at the end of each session.

In the Chicago Lying-In Hospital series, five fetuses died following positive CST, three antepartum when awaiting cesarean section (see Figure 17-9) and two in the early neonatal period following a vaginal delivery and a cesarean section.

The *equivocal CST* has some isolated decelerations triggered by less than 30% of all contractions. There are few of these cases in each of the published series, and when one is observed the clinician must make a decision about what action to take—either continued observation or intervention. In principle, such a test should be repeated within 24 hours but a fatal outcome may occur before that, particularly when alterations of the baseline are present (Figure 17-5). If the repeat test is still equivocal, the case should be managed as if the test were positive. When negative they should be managed as such.

NONSTRESS TEST

The antenatal nonstress test (NST) provides an FHR tracing in the antepartum period, recording baseline characteristics and accelerations following fetal movements or other stimuli such as manual palpation, sound, chemicals. It also aims at evaluating fetal condition to predict the outcome of a pregnancy.

Only recently it has been applied on a large scale even though the original observations were made more than 10 years ago by Hammacher (1968). He observed the frequency with which a *fixed baseline* ("silent") was recorded in compromised fetuses who later had either positive CSTs or even died in utero; he concluded that fixed baseline was an important sign of fetal distress and impending progressive deterioration. Only in passing did he indicate that fetal movements induce FHR accelerations and that accelerations or the lack of them may serve as an indicator of fetal well-being. Lee et al (1975) reported on a large series and concluded that when FHR accelerations followed fetal movements the CST was negative and the outcome consistently good. They went as far as suggesting that the NST should be used instead of the CST as a means for antepartum assessment of the fetus. The work of Rochard et al (1976) confirmed those observations and shortly thereafter many large and small series were published, including comparisons between NST and CST as predictors of fetal outcome.

The rationale for the test is based in the observation that fetuses in chronic distress have a fixed FHR baseline (or diminished "variability") and the interpretation that this abnormality is due to the inability of the fetal cardiovascular system to respond to sympathetic and parasympathetic stimuli, the interaction of which is responsible for the normal baseline oscillations. On the other hand, the FHR acceleration following movements (or other stimuli) is also an expression of cardiovascular response to sympathetic stimulation, and the absence of an acceleration would indicate either the inability of the cardiovascular system to respond or the lack of sympathetic stimulus. In either case it would be a sign of impaired fetal capacity to adapt to distress and thus an indication of serious fetal compromise. This sluggish cardiovascular response has been further demonstrated by the absence of tachycardia observed in the majority of affected fetuses (Kubli and Ruttgers, 1976).

The NST is indicated for any pregnancy with the possibility of a fetus in danger of intrauterine asphyxia or chronic distress. There are *no contraindications* to this test, a completely passive observation of FHR behavior.

Technique

The setting and recording methods are exactly the same as those described for the CST. Additional information must be provided by the patient, who should have a marker to trigger a signal in the tracing when she feels fetal movements, or, if this is not possible, by an observer who should do the same when palpating them. Very often the movement of the fetus triggers a deflection of the contraction-recording stylus, which thereby documents it. This pattern was originally called "reactive" by Goodlin (1972).

Interpretation

In the tracings, the following are evaluated:

1. *The baseline,* which may have the normal rapid oscillations (see Chapter 12) within the range of 5 to 20 beats. A good, precise recording, even when ob-

tained with the Doppler ultrasound transducer, will be able to pick up cases of minimal or absent oscillations. A fixed baseline ("silent," diminished beat-to-beat variability) is an ominous sign, particularly in the absence of uterine contractions, and should be interpreted as such in the overall evaluation of the tracing (Figure 17-8). In the study of fetal arousal levels by Goodlin and Schmidt (1972) this finding was considered as a "nonreactive" type of tracing. However, subsequent studies and reports by others reserved this label to FHR changes related to active fetal movements or externally applied stimuli (sounds, manipulations).

2. Recording of *at least two accelerations* of the FHR of 15 beats, as a minimum, and lasting at least 15 sec (Figure 17-6) within a period of 20 min indicates that the fetus is "reactive."

3. Complete *absence of accelerations* following fetal movements (Figure 17-7) or the *lack of any fetal activity* during two consecutive 30-min periods (Figure 17-8) characterize a "nonreactive" fetus.

Very often there is association of a fixed baseline with absence of fetal activity or poor FHR acceleration following fetal movements.

The clinical use of the NST by several investigators in the country has sparked a variety of different ways to interpret the tracings to refine the accuracy of predicting fetal condition at birth. These attempts at classification have been expressed in a number of "scoring" systems designed ostensibly to facilitate the classification of each case and with highly predictable outcomes in the hands of their proponents. However, apart from the fixed baseline and absence of acceleration following fetal movements, there is little solid additional information that one may find in a standard antepartum recording to evaluate a tracing further and facilitate the prediction with an NST only.

Other types of stimulation have been proposed if signs of fetal activity are absent. Auditory stimuli produced through a microphone placed over the maternal abdomen (Goodlin and Schmidt, 1972; Read and Miller, 1977) have been used to trigger the same type of FHR acceleration as movements; its absence would also have the

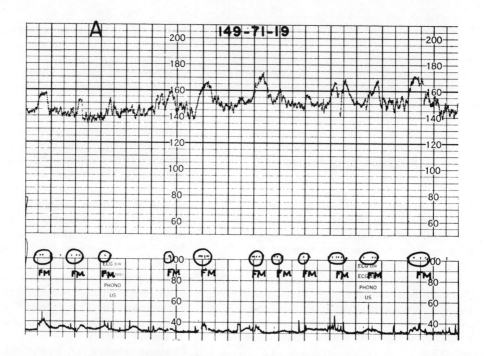

Figure 17-6 NST of primipara at 37-weeks gestation. Fetal movements (FM) indicated with a marker activated by the patient, and subsequently circled to make them stand out. Significant accelerations of FHR preceding or coinciding with the fetal movement, which often occurred in clusters. Oscillating baseline with a borderline high frequency: *reactive NST*. The patient delivered, after spontaneous labor 3 weeks later, a 3125 gm infant, Apgar 9-9.

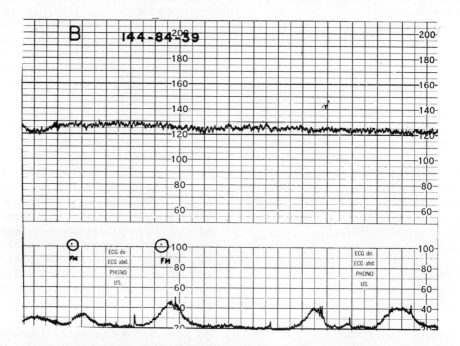

Figure 17-7 Nonreactive NST of multipara at 40 weeks gestation. Two fetal movements were recorded by the mother but there was no change observed on the FHR with almost fixed baseline and normal frequency. A CST carried out later was negative. The patient delivered, after induced labor 4 days later, a 4370 gm infant, Apgar 9-10.

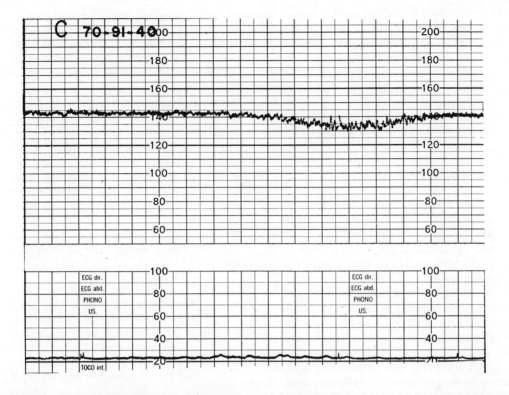

Figure 17-8 Nonreactive NST obtained on a multipara at 38.5 weeks gestation. Fixed baseline and complete absence of fetal movement. A spontaneous deceleration may be observed on the fixed baseline, and a positive CST followed (see Figure 17-4, bottom tracing). The patient was delivered by cesarean section of a 1840 gm depressed infant who recovered statisfactorily.

significance of a nonreactive fetus. Others have suggested that the fetus may be manipulated by abdominal palpation. Spellacy et al (1978), and Aladjem et al (1979) administered intravenous glucose to the mother and observed increased fetal activity in good fetuses, and unchanged activity in jeopardized fetuses. Essentially all these tests aim at assessing the integrity of the fetal neuromuscular system as an indirect indicator of possible chronic fetal distress. The nonreactive fetus would be the one affected and already in poor condition, while the reactive condition is still an acceptable situation even though this finding does not rule out a state of chronic subclinical stress.

Clinical Application

The exclusive use of the NST was proposed by Rochard et al (1976) as a means to screen large populations of high-risk patients. They rightfully claimed that it requires much less time than the CST and that, properly interpreted, could have comparable predictive value. Those authors as well as Tushuizen et al (1977) and Hammacher (1966) have shown that a significant proportion of nonreactive fetuses die in utero shortly after the test if active intervention is not undertaken.

However, the majority of clinical investigators have concluded that it is probably more advantageous to proceed with a CST in cases of a nonreactive NST. For that reason, there is no study with a substantial number of cases in which the evaluation of the fetal condition was based solely on the NST as means to decide on management. It is noteworthy to point out the extreme frequency with which one observes the *association of low estrogen* values in the mother and the presence of a *nonreactive fetus.*

COMBINED NST AND CST

The combination of NST, followed in selected cases by CST has become the method of choice to evaluate the fetal condition in a great number of high-risk pregnancy syndromes. In fact, the NST constitutes what a good control period preceding a CST should be, the only difference being that a more careful analysis of the baseline and response to movements should be done with the NST. Refinements of the test include stimulation with sound, manipulations, or increasing maternal blood glucose levels.

A *reactive NST* (see Figure 17-6) would suggest a fetus in satisfactory condition, capable of continuing in utero and perhaps of withstanding labor. The test need not be repeated more often than once per week.

A *nonreactive NST* characterized by a fixed baseline and absence of fetal movements should be followed by a CST (Figure 17-9); likewise, one characterized by fixed baseline and lack of accelerations (Figure 7-10). If the CST is negative, the usual follow-up of the patient may be conducted. In a case of positive CST the clinician must actively intervene because the association of a nonreactive NST and a positive CST (called "nonreactive responsive" by Goodlin) carries with it ominous implications. The clinical experience reported by several investigators coincides to emphasize this practice because 1) the fetus "will not tolerate labor" (see Figure 17-10) or 2) nonintervention may lead to "disastrous results" (see Figure 17-9). These findings are particularly important when one deals with fetuses in which growth has not been satisfactory, and with maternal estrogen levels (either serum or urinary) that are low.

At the Chicago Lying-In Hospital, more than 800 patients have been given simultaneous NST and CST. On the other hand, over 150 had only NST followed by CST in selected cases of "nonreactive" or "equivocal" tests, and have been in agreement with the above mentioned experience. The association of a nonreactive NST and a positive CST predicts a serious intrapartum or neonatal pathologic situation in 80% of cases, including 50% intrauterine growth-retarded fetuses. Among cases screened with NST, around 15% have a nonreactive pattern requiring a CST, which will be positive in about 35% of the patients. The unfavorable obstetric condition is reflected by a high cesarean section rate in the latter group, on the order of 65%. Furthermore, the antenatal and perinatal mortality in this group is much higher than for the cases with negative CSTs.

The clinical application of these tests is therefore, recommended in the following sequential order:

1. When the patient is deemed to require a test of fetal well-being (based on any of the indications discussed before) she should have a NST.
2. When the fetus is reactive, the patient may be retested in 1 week or sooner if the other tests deteriorate significantly.
3. If the fetus is nonreactive, a CST should be carried out. (During an NST recording session spontaneous uterine contractions may be observed thus an NST becomes a spontaneous CST.
4. If contractions are not spontaneous, they should be induced as for a CST.

Other means of stimulation may be used, if available, such as sounds, manual manipulations, or glucose administration to the mother (perhaps a meal may have the same transient mild hyperglycemic effect).

The *nonreactive* fetus may have no signs of transient hypoxia, that is, a *negative CST,* which occurs in about 65% of the cases. Under these circumstances, the case should be followed up as advised for reactive fetuses.

The *nonreactive* fetus with a positive CST constitutes about 4% to 5% of the total high-risk population and is at highest risk. Immediate intervention is advised because of impending rapid fetal deterioration (see Figures 17-9 and 17-10). About two-thirds of these patients terminate in cesarean section for fetal distress.

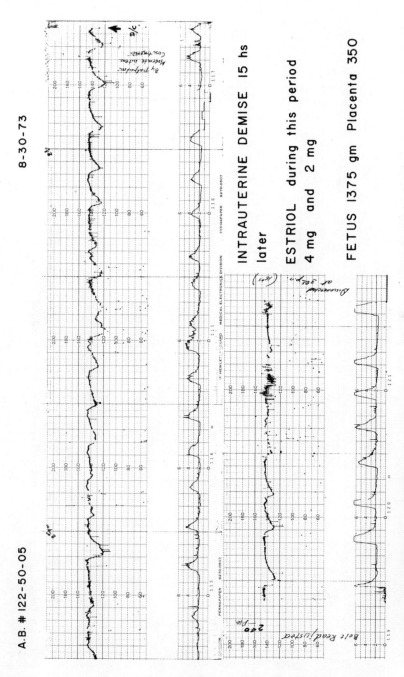

Figure 17-9 NST and CST. Continuous 75-min external UC and FHR recording in hypertensive multipara at 35 weeks gestation excreting urinary estriol 7 mg/24 hours. (*Above, left*) Some fetal movements but no accelerations of HR. Fixed baseline, *nonreactive fetus.* Repetitive late decelerations without tachycardia under oxytocin-induced contractions: *positive CST.* During the day of the test, 6-hour aliquots of urinary excretion were taken and analyzed for estriol content. Excreted equivalent to 4 and 2 mg/24 hours, the last during the night. The patient was scheduled for cesarean section the following morning, but the fetus stopped moving 15 hours after the test. Labor was induced, and a stillborn growth-retarded infant was delivered.

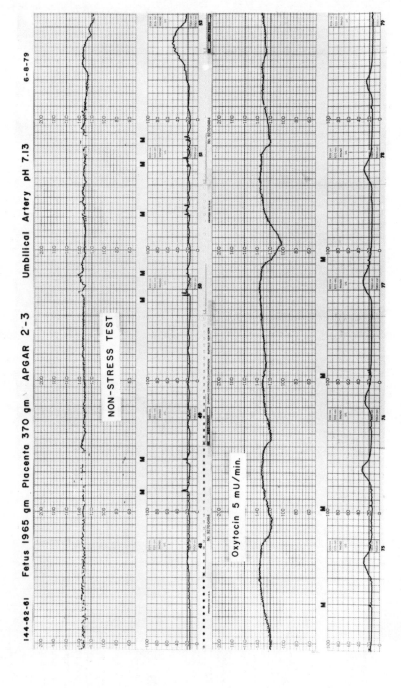

Figure 17-10 Two 16-min segments of antenatal UC and FHR tracings (paper speed, 3 cm/min) of a primipara at 37 weeks gestation with low urinary estriol excretion (5 mg/24 hours). Suspicion of intrauterine growth retardation. (*Above*) NST shows only one mild contraction at the end, but good fetal activity as indicated by deflections on the UC tracing. However, the FHR with fixed baseline had no accelerations: *nonreactive fetus.* (*Below*) Mild uterine activity 75 min later induced with oxytocin (CST) triggering repetitive late decelerations on the fixed baseline FHR, and still no accelerations with fetal movements: *positive CST.* By cesarean section performed shortly thereafter was obtained a growth-regarded, *depressed infant with marked acidosis* who recovered satisfactorily.

The *reactive* fetus with *positive CST* should be closely observed and retested within 24 hours because the borderline hypoxia, if persistent, may lead to a rapidly fatal outcome for the fetus.

The *equivocal test* (that is, a combination of either a nonreactive fetus and equivocal CST, or a *reactive fetus and equivocal CST)* presents a most puzzling problem because of the limited experience accumulated, even with the combined published reports. It probably is safest to repeat the test within 24 hours because of the unpredictable situation. As seen with the CST, the equivocal test may be followed shortly by intrauterine demise (see Figure 17-5) particularly when the baseline is fixed. However, a normal oscillating baseline or even a reactive fetus may not be completely reassuring when accompanying an equivocal CST (Figure 17-11); the likelihood of a false-negative test should always be considered as a possibility when managing these cases. The association of other abnormal findings such as growth retardation and low estrogen values should strongly influence the clinical management of those rare cases.

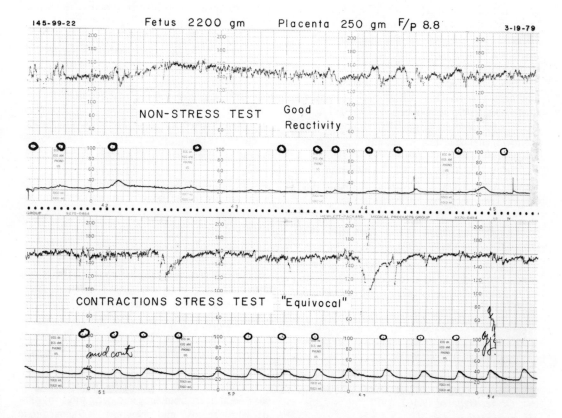

Figure 17-11 Two 40 min segments of UC and FHR tracings from a primipara at 37 weeks gestation. She had idiopathic thrombocytopenic purpura and received prednisone 120 to 40 mg/day for most of her gestation. The urinary estriol levels were about 5 to 7 mg/24 hours, and there was arrest of fundal growth with moderate growth retardation. *(Above)* NST illustrates normal baseline frequency with FHR accelerations following fetal movements, as perceived by the mother (circled points): *reactive fetus. (Below)* CST 1 hour later shows oxytocin-induced contractions that triggered only two decelerations while the fetal movements do not induce accelerations: *equivocal CST.* The patient was scheduled for induction 3 days later, stopped feeling movements 60 hours after the last tracing. The planned induction was carried out and produced a moderately growth-retarded early macerated stillborn fetus with F/P ratio of 8.8 (placental insufficiency). Autopsy revealed *severe adrenal hypoplasia.*

408

BIBLIOGRAPHY

Aladjem S, Feria A, Rest J, et al: Effect of maternal glucose load on fetal activity. *Am J Obstet Gynecol* 134:276, 1979.

Aladjem S, Feria A, Rest J, et al: Fetal heart rate responses to fetal movements. *Br J Obstet Gynaecol* 84:487, 1977.

Baskett TF, Sandy EA: The oxytocin challenge test: An ominous pattern associated with severe fetal growth retardation. *Obstet Gynecol* 54:365, 1979.

Bobitt JR: Abnormal fetal heart rate tracings, failure to intervene, and fetal death: Review of five cases reveals potential pitfalls of antepartum monitoring programs. *Am J Obstet Gynecol* 133:415, 1979.

Boyd IE, Chamberlain GVP, Fergusson ILC: The oxytocin stress test and the isoxsuprine placental transfer test in the management of suspected placental insufficiency. *J Obstet Gynaecol Br Comwlth* 81:120, 1974.

Braly P, Freeman RK: The significance of fetal heart rate reactivity with a positive oxytocin challenge test. *Obstet Gynecol* 50:689, 1977.

Cooper JM, Soffronoff EC, Bolognese RJ: Oxytocin challenge test in monitoring high-risk pregnancies. *Obstet Gynecol* 45:27, 1975.

Egley CC, Suzuki K: Intrauterine fetal demise after negative oxytocin challenge test. *Obstet Gynecol* 50:55s, 1977.

Evertson LR, Gauthier RJ, Collea J: Fetal demise following negative contraction stress tests. *Obstet Gynecol* 51:671, 1978.

Evertson LR, Gauthier RJ, Schifrin BS, et al: Antepartum fetal heart rate testing. I. Evolution of the nonstress test. *Am J Obstet Gynecol* 133:29, 1979.

Farahani G, Vasudeva K, Petrie R, et al: Oxytocin challenge test in high-risk pregnancy. *Obstet Gynecol* 47:159, 1976.

Farahami G, Fenton AN: Fetal heart rate acceleration in relation to the oxytocin challenge test. *Obstet Gynecol* 49:163, 1977.

Flood B, Lee J: Fetal death during a negative contraction stress test. *Obstet Gynecol* 52:41s, 1978.

Flynn AM, Kelly J: Evaluation of fetal well being by antepartum fetal heart monitoring. *Br Med J* 1:936, 1977.

Fox, HE, Steinbrecher M, Ripton B: Antepartum fetal heart rate and uterine activity studies. *Am J Obstet Gynecol* 126:61, 1976.

Freeman RK: The use of the oxytocin test for antepartum clinical evaluation of uteroplacental respiratory function. *Am J Obstet Gynecol* 121:481, 1975.

Freeman R, Goebelsman U, Nochimson D, et al: Evaluation of the significance of a positive oxytocin challenge test. *Obstet Gynecol* 47:8, 1976.

Freeman RK, James J: Clinical experience with the oxytocin challenge test. II. An ominous atypical pattern. *Obstet Gynecol* 46:255, 1975.

Gauthier RJ, Evertson LR, Paul RH: Antepartum fetal heart rate testing. II. Intrapartum fetal heart rate observation and newborn outcome following a positive contraction stress test. *Am J Obstet Gynecol* 133:34, 1979.

Goodlin RC, Schmidt W: Human fetal arousal levels as indicated by heart rate recordings. *Am J Obstet Gynecol* 114:613, 1972.

Goupil F, Sureau C: Rythme cardiaque fetal pendant la grossesse. *J Paris Pediatr* 118:127, 1975.

Hammacher K: Neue Methode Zur Selektiven Registrierung der fetalen Herzschlagfrequenz. *Geburtshilfe Frauenheilkd* 22:1552, 1962.

Hammacher K: The diagnosis of fetal distress with an electronic fetal heart monitor, in *Intrauterine Dangers to the Fetus*. Amsterdam, Excerpta Medica, 1967, pp 228–233.

Hammacher K: Früherkennung intrauteriner Gefahrenzustände durch Elektrophonokardiographie und Tokographie, in Elert R, Hüter KA (eds): *Die Prophylaxe frühkindlicher Hirnschäden*. Stuttgart, Thieme, 1966, p 116.

Hammacher K: The clinical significance of cardiotocography, in Huntingford PJ, Hüter KA, Saling E (eds): *Perinatal Medicine*. Stuttgart, Thieme, 1969, pp 80–93.

Hammacher K, Hüter KA, Bokelmann J, et al: Foetal heart frequency and perinatal condition of the foetus and newborn. *Gynaecologia* 166:349, 1968.

Hon EH, Wohlgemuth R: The electronic evaluation of fetal heart rate. IV. The effect of maternal exercise. *Am J Obstet Gynecol* 81:361, 1961.

Klapholz H, Burke L: Intrauterine fetal demise with a negative oxytocin challenge test. *J Reprod Med* 15:169–170, 1975.

Krebs HB, Petres RE: Clinical application of a scoring system for the evaluation of antepartum fetal heart rate monitoring. *Am J Obstet Gynecol* 130:765, 1978.

Kubli F, Boos R, Ruttgers H, et al: Antepartum fetal heart rate montioring, in *Current Status of Fetal Heart Rate Monitoring. Proc R Coll Obstet Gynaecol (Lon),* 1977, pp 29–45.

Kubli FW, Kaeser D, Hinselmann M: Diagnostic management of chronic placental insufficiancy, in Pecile A, Finzi C (eds): *The Fetal Placental Unit.* Amsterdam, Excerpta Medica, 1969.

Kubli F, Ruttgers H: Monitoring of antepartum fetal heart rate, in Tournaire M (ed): *Symposium sur la Surveillance fetale.* Paris, 1976, pp 154–163,

Lee CY, Drukker B: The non-stress test for the antepartum assessment of fetal reserve. *Am J Obstet Gynecol* 134:460, 1979.

Lee CY, DiLoreto PC, Logrand B: Fetal activity acceleration determination for evaluation of fetal reserve. *Obstet Gynecol* 48:19, 1976.

Lee CY, DiLoretto PC, O'Lane JM: A study of fetal heart rate acceleration patterns. *Obstet Gynecol* 45:142, 1975.

Lin CC, Schulman H, Saldana LR: Deceleration/contraction ratios as an index of fetal health during labor. *Obstet Gynecol* 51:666–670, 1978.

Linzey EM, Freeman RK: Antepartum fetal monitoring, in Pitkin RM, Scott JR (eds): *Yearbook of Obstetrics & Gynecology.* Chicago, Year Book, 1978, pp 85–110.

Liu DTY, Blackwell RJ, Tukel S: The relevance of antenatal and intrapartum fetal heart rate patterns to fetal outcome. *Br J Obstet Gynaecol* 85:270, 1978.

Lyons ER, Bylsma-Howell M, Shamsi S, et al: A scoring system for nonstressed antepartum fetal heart monitoring. *Am J Obstet Gynecol* 133:242, 1979.

Mendez-Bauer C, Ruiz-Canseco A, Andujar-Ruiz M, et al: Early decelerations of the fetal heart from occlusion of the umbilical cord. *J Perinat Med* 6:69, 1978.

Moore PT, Myerscough PR: Clearance rates of radiosodium from myometrium. *J Obstet Gynaecol Br Emp* 64:207, 1957.

Morris N, Osborn SB, Wright HP, et al: Effective uterine blood flow during exercise in normal and pre-eclamptic pregnancies. *Lancet* 2:481–484, 1956.

Nochimson DJ, Turbeville JS, Terry JE, et al: The nonstress test. *Obstet Gynecol* 51:491, 1978.

Pose SV, Castillo JB, Mora-Rojas EO, et al: Test of fetal tolerance to induced uterine contractions for the diagnosis of chronic distress, in *Perinatal Factors Affecting Human Development.* Washington, DC, Pan American Health Organization Scientific Publication 185, 1969, pp 96–104.

Pose SV, Castillo JB, Mora-Rojas EO, et al: Prueba de la tolerancia fetal a las contracciones uterinas inducidas. *V Cong Uruguay Ginecotocol* 1:641–646, 1969.

Pose SV, Escarcena L, Caldeyro-Barcia R: La presion parcial de oxigeno en el feto durante el parto. *IV Cong Mex Gynecol Obstet* 2:41–61, 1963.

Pose SV, Temesio P, Martino V, et al: Evaluacion de la vitalidad fetal durante el embarazo. *III Jornada Rioplatense Diabetes (Buenos Aires),* 1968.

Ray M, Freeman R, Pine S, et al: Clinical experiences with the oxytocin challenge test. *Am J Obstet Gynecol* 114:1, 1972.

Rayburn WF, Duhrling JL, Donaldson M: A study of fetal acceleration tests. *Am J Obstet Gynecol* 132:33, 1978.

Read JA, Miller FC: Fetal heart rate acceleration in response to acoustic stimulation as a measure of fetal wellbeing. *Am J Obstet Gynecol* 129:512, 1977.

Rochard F, Schifrin B, Goupil F, et al: Nonstressed fetal heart rate monitoring in the antepartum period. *Am J Obstet Gynecol* 126:699, 1976.

Schifrin B, Lapidus M, Doctor G, et al: Contraction stress test for antepartum fetal evaluation. *Obstet Gynecol* 45:433, 1975.

Schulman H, Lin CC, Saldana L, et al: Quantitative analysis in the oxytocin challenge test. *Am J Obstet Gynecol* 129:239, 1977.

Spellacy WN, Gelman SR, Abrams RM, et al: Direct observations of human fetal movements under physiologic stimulation. XXV Ann Meet Soc Gynecol Invest, Abstract 84, 1978.

410

Stembera ZK, Hodr J: The "exercise test" as an early diagnostic aid for fetal distress, in Horsky J, Stembera ZK (eds): *Intrauterine Dangers to the Fetus*. New York, Excerpta Medica, 1967, pp 349–353.

Stembera ZK, Hodr J, Brotanek B, et al: Complete early diagnosis of intrauterine fetal distress, in Horsky J, Stembera ZK (eds): *Intrauterine Dangers to the Fetus*. New York, Excerpta Medica, 1967, pp 373–376.

Trierweiler MW, Freeman RK, James J: Baseline fetal heart rate characteristics as an indicator of fetal status during the antepartum period. *Am J Obstet Gynecol* 125:618, 1976.

Tushuizen PBT, Stoot JEGM, Ubachs JMH: Clinical experience in non-stressed antepartum cardiotocography. *Am J Obstet Gynecol* 128:507, 1977.

Visser GHA, Huisjes HJ: Diagnostic value of the unstressed antepartum cardiotocogram. *Br J Obstet Gynaecol* 84:321, 1977.

Weingold AB, DeJesus TPS, O'Keiffe J: Oxytocin challenge test. *Am J Obstet Gynecol* 123:466, 1975.

CHAPTER 18
Anesthesia and Analgesia

The necessity to administer medications to the pregnant patient in advanced gestation or labor imposes on the obstetrician the need for thorough understanding of the pharmacologic effect of those drugs on the mother and the fetus in utero, and the immediate postpartum period. The response elicited by oxytocics, uterine relaxants, and other miscellaneous preparations has been reviewed in detail in Chapter 9. The substances routinely used for the *specific aim of controlling labor pains* are the subject of this chapter. However, because of their effect on the uterus, some have already been discussed in Chapter 9, to which the reader will be referred for analysis.

The discomfort produced by effective labor contractions is usually tolerable in early first stage but may require the use of analgesic (anesthetic) drugs as dilatation and descent progress. Of course the degree of pain tolerance depends on the pain threshold of the individual patient; on the other hand, cultural traditions may strongly influence pain perception or its external manifestations. Anxiety, fear, apprehension, and unfamiliar surroundings (especially for primiparas) markedly predispose to lower the pain threshold and tend to feed a vicious cycle. The number of medications or techniques advocated to diminish or control those psychogenic factors and perceived pains is countless, and more are introduced every year. There is no "ideal" drug, that is, one that is effective for the purpose given but without side effects on mother or fetus or both.

The drugs used in first stage are divided in two large groups: 1) *narcotics,* with the property of increasing pain threshold yet with minimal effect on the cardiovascular system and some upon the cortex; they act primarily on the thalamus and the reticular formation of the brain stem; 2) *ataractics and sedatives,* which do not alter the pain threshold but sedate, tranquilize, and relax the patients by their action on the hypothalamus and reticular system.

The substances used to eliminate or block pain may also be grouped in two large categories: 1) those exerting their action through the central nervous system (general anesthetics) and 2) those that block the transmission of impulses through the peripheral nerves (local anesthetics). Only the preparations utilized in daily clinical practice will be reviewed, with emphasis on their effects on mother and fetus. Their chemistry and metabolism may be reviewed in the appropriate texts of pharmacology or anesthesia and will not be discussed unless they have a direct effect on the fetal-maternal outcome.

NARCOTICS

The beneficial effect of narcotics to relieve labor pains has been known for very many years, but their use in obstetrics has been relatively limited because of the concept that they will predictably diminish uterine contractions and cause "secondary inertia." This erroneous concept has been perpetuated due, perhaps, to the excellent analgesic effect of morphine, which may induce a period of sleep and with it the impression that labor has been arrested. Moreover, several authors have postulated that some of these compounds have the wonderful specific properties to selectively "relax" the lower uterine segment and cervix, while at the same time not affecting the myometrium or the corpus. On the other hand, it has also been propounded that certain preparations have a given effect in the early stages of labor (prelabor, "latent phase") and a different action once labor is in a stage of more rapid progress (first stage, "active phase").

After the introduction of intrauterine pressure recordings, the effects of drugs on the uterus

411

have been reassessed. These observations have succeeded in clarifying numerous misconceptions. It remains now to make available to clinicians the findings observed under laboratory conditions and corroborated by other investigators in clinical settings.

Morphine

One of the oldest alkaloids used in obstetrics in its pure form, morphine is still the standard by which the analgesic properties of new compounds are evaluated. Originally thought to have uterine relaxing properties, morphine was often given when the clinician considered that "both mother and uterus needed a rest." This concept, still widely taught in modern obstetrics, has repeatedly been shown to be erroneous when the drug is injected either intramuscularly (see Figure 9-69) or intravenously (see Figures 9-70 and 9-71). The absence of any effect of morphine on the pregnant uterus in labor was first shown by Alvarez and Caldeyro-Barcia (1954) and since then corroborated by all those who studied it with the appropriate techniques. At doses of 10 to 15 mg, irrespective of the route of administration, morphine produces profound analgesia with deep respiratory movements and no alterations of maternal blood pressure or pulse rate.

The effects on the FHR are equally negligible, the baseline frequency or oscillations being unchanged. It would be an almost ideal analgesic were it not for the depressing effect on the fetal respiratory center, which seems to be greater than that produced by other synthetic narcotic preparations. The effects of morphine on the fetus have been observed to last up to 4 hours after administration to the mother. Fetuses delivered within that period of time may be significantly depressed.

Meperidine

The most widely used synthetic narcotic, meperidine (Demerol) has the majority of the effects produced by morphine with somewhat shorter duration. It has, in addition, other properties that are relevant to obstetrics. Originally believed to be "antispasmodic" it was later shown that, when given intramuscularly, meperidine has no effect on the contractions of the uterus.

However, when given intravenously, it is a potent, although transient, oxytocic, the action of which may be sufficient to trigger labor in favorable cases (Sica-Blanco et al, 1967). This oxytocic effect is dose related and depends on the concentration of the drug in the blood reaching the myometrium; small doses produce lesser and shorter responses (see Figures 9-73, 9-74, and 9-75). The effects on the maternal respiration and cardiovascular system are also similar to the response to morphine but attenuated. Patients receiving moderate to large doses of intravenous meperidine often become nauseated and vomit, with sweating and appearance of peripheral vasodilatation.

The action of meperidine on the FHR has been extensively described as markedly affecting the "beat-to-beat variability," which would diminish to almost obliteration (fixed baseline). These reports notwithstanding, in the majority of patients given the drug intravenously, the FHR pattern will be only minimally, and if so, transiently, altered (see Figures 9-73, 9-74, and 9-75) or completely unchanged with persistent, normal rapid oscillations (see Figure 12-4) throughout the remainder of labor. These observations are valid for intravenous or intramuscular doses of up to 100 mg of the drug administered alone. The simultaneous addition of other drugs (Phenergan, chlorpromazine, Valium) may affect the FHR pattern.

Pentazocine

Pentazocine (Talwin) is a potent morphine-like synthetic preparation with systemic effects similar to those of meperidine and morphine. Its effect on the myometrium is similar to that of meperidine (see Figure 9-76), that is, oxytocic when administered intravenously, capable of triggering or enhancing labor under favorable circumstances.

The FHR pattern is affected minimally, if at all by the intravenous or intramuscular administration of this substance to the mother in labor. The baseline frequency and the rapid oscillations look unchanged (Figure 18-1). It would affect the FHR pattern only if the triggered hypercontractility were to induce transient or sustained fetal hypoxia.

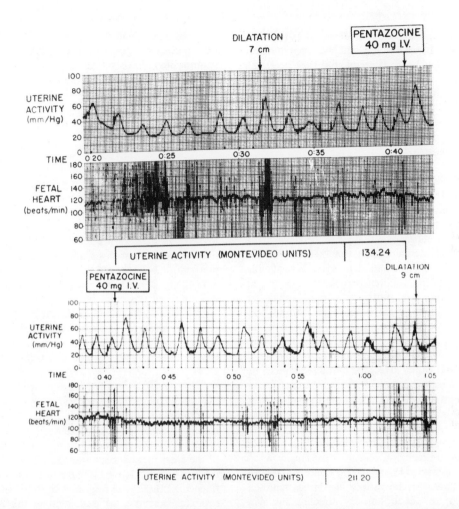

Figure 18-1 Continuous 45-min direct recordings of intrauterine pressure and FHR during advanced first stage in labor at term. Pentazocine 40 mg IV triggered a significant hypercontractility. Uterine activity increased from 134 MU to 211 MU mainly due to increased frequency of contractions. The FHR pattern was completely unchanged; the baseline continued to fluctuate around 115 to 120 beats/min with rapid oscillations in the same range. Reprinted from Filler WW, et al: Analgesia in obstetrics. *Am J Obstet Gynecol* 98:832, 1967.

Fentanyl

One of the newer synthetic analgesics, fentanyl (Sublimaze) per unit of weight is about 100 times more potent than meperidine. Very commonly used as a preanesthetic drug or a sedative to supplement local anesthesia, it affects the pregnant uterus in a manner very similar to meperidine when given intravenously (see Figure 11-6). Likewise, the effect on the FHR does not significantly affect either baseline frequency or rapid oscillations.

This drug has important potential implications for obstetrics because in combination with

the ataractic droperidol it is part of the popular preparation Innovar. This combination does not neutralize the effect of fentanyl on the myometrium and it still has minimal action on the FHR pattern.

ATARACTICS AND SEDATIVES

The extensive use of sedatives and tranquilizers during labor imposes the need to understand their effects on the uterus and the fetus when administered alone or in combination with analgesic preparations. It seems apparent that they tend to relieve the patient's apprehension; on the other hand, it seems that they potentiate the effect of analgesics, thereby allowing the use of lower amounts of these drugs to control labor pains.

Chlorpromazine

The first ataractic used in clinical medicine, and still frequently used, chlorpromazine (Thorazine) is usually administered in single doses of 25 to 50 mg or in combination with other ataractics and/or narcotics. When given alone it has no effect on the uterine activity (see Figure 9-77). The effect on maternal blood pressure is negligible, particularly in normotensive patients; in hypertensive subjects and, particularly, preeclamptic patients it may induce a moderate fall in both systolic and diastolic pressures, perhaps by influencing the sympathetic nerve action. In combination with meperidine and promethazine, it does significantly affect the blood pressure of the patients (see Figure 9-78). This combination has been used in the management of preeclampsia and eclampsia in many European and South American hospitals. The effect on the FHR may be the direct consequence of the degree of fall in blood pressure: when blood pressure drops below a safe level, diminished IVS blood flow and fetal distress will follow with the various alterations representative of this condition. By affecting the sympathetic nervous system, this combination of drugs may induce fetal tachycardia and diminution of the rapid oscillations (tendency to fixed baseline).

Promethazine

A "back-up" ataractic, promethazine (Phenergan) is an excellent sedative with neither the intrinsic analgesic action nor the potentiating effect of simultaneously administered narcotics. It has no effect on uterine activity or FHR patterns. This absence of significant action is not altered by the simultaneous administration with meperidine using either the intramuscular (Figure 18-2) or intravenous route (Figure 18-3). These observations are at variance with some reports, which indicate that the rapid oscillations of the FHR baseline are diminished or obliterated.

The other phenothiazines also used in obstetrics, promazine (Sparine) and prochlorperazine (Compazine), have similar negligible effects on uterine activity and FHR patterns.

Diazepam

The most widely used sedative in medicine, diazepam (Valium) was thought to have no effect on the fetus after extensive studies undertaken in Europe. However, following the close observation of the newborn infants in modern neonatal units it has been reported that diazepam has a prolonged, albeit barely noticeable, effect on the neuromuscular system of the newborn when the mother in labor received the drug in doses greater than 10 mg. Some investigators have reported that it diminished the rapid oscillations (or "beat-to-beat variability") of the baseline. It has been our consistent observation that diazepam alone has a negligible effect on the parameters of the FHR tracing usually analyzed by the clinicians (Figure 18-4).

The association of diazepam with narcotic substances, particularly meperidine, is often used to attempt to sedate anxious patients who are having severe labor pains. This combination may affect the FHR pattern predictably. In about 50% of the cases it produces a transient diminution of the baseline oscillations (Figure 18-5) without influencing other reflex responses of the FHR. The neonatal outcome, as evaluated by the Apgar score, is not affected by this drug; when there is fetal depression it is generally possible to single out the condition that provoked the distress.

Magnesium Sulfate

This salt has long been used in obstetrics for its anticonvulsant properties as part of the classic Stroganoff method to treat eclampsia. After a period of disfavor it was reintroduced in the United States by Pritchard and Zuspan as an important therapeutic tool in the management of preeclampsia and eclampsia. It is now recommended as the single drug of choice to prevent convulsions in those conditions.

Originally thought to act exclusively through its effect on the neuromuscular plate, it has been more recently shown (Borgers and Gücer, 1978) that it has a significant effect on the cortex. This

415

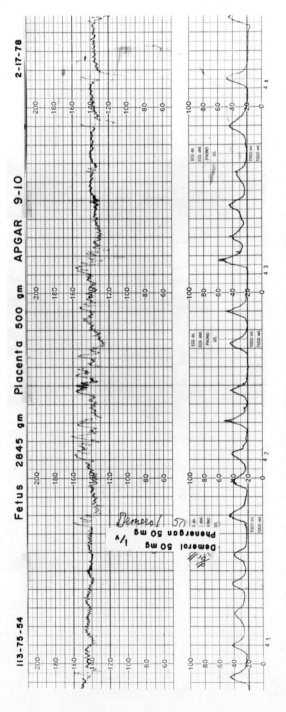

Figure 18-2 Direct UC and FHR tracings from enhanced labor of multipara at term. Promethazine 50 mg IM and meperidine 50 mg IM-IV induced no change in FHR baseline frequency or rapid oscillations. Transient increase in contractility following the small intravenous dose of meperidine. An infant in good condition was delivered 90 min later.

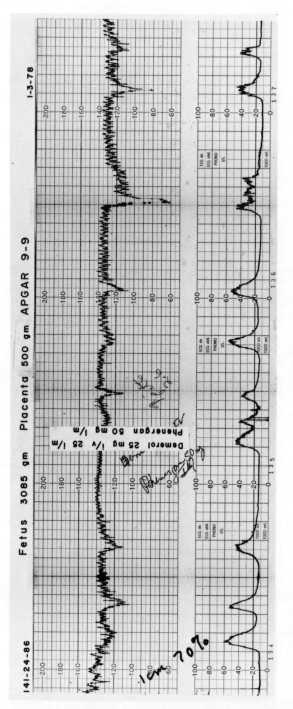

Figure 18-3 Direct UC and FHR tracings from secundipara in spontaneous labor. Administration of promethazine 50 mg and meperidine 50 mg IV, where indicated, did not diminish the rapid oscillations of the baseline. In fact, there is a transient period of 6 min with bursts of saltatory pattern. An infant in excellent condition was delivered 40 min later.

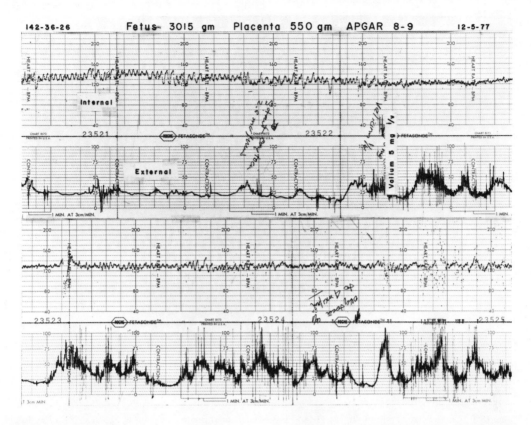

Figure 18-4 Continuous 36 min of direct FHR and external UC tracings from early enhanced labor of preeclamptic primipara at term. Rapid oscillations of the FHR baseline are diminished for about 10 min just preceding and following the intravenous administration of 5 mg diazepam. No change in baseline frequency.

relatively recent observation has been instrumental in explaining the *sedative action* of magnesium sulfate observed by the clinicians when it is administered in significant doses to usually anxious young preeclamptic patients. In fact, magnesium sulfate is an *excellent anticonvulsant,* when given in sufficient amounts, and effective blood levels are maintained. The uterine effects and method of administration have been discussed in Chapters 9 and 11. There is almost unanimous agreement that it does not affect the contractility pattern at therapeutic doses of 7 to 8 mEq/liter (8 to 10 mg/100) blood levels. The current teaching is that the FHR is significantly affected by the administration of magnesium sulfate to the mother: the "beat-to-beat variability" is obliterated to the point of fixed baseline. In fact, the administration of *prolonged infusions of this salt does not affect the FHR pattern:* the rapid oscillations of the baseline are maintained as well as the known

changes produced by other factors (Figure 18-6). Likewise, large "loading" doses of magnesium sulfate given to patients with severe preeclampsia and marked hyperreflexia do not significantly affect the FHR baseline pattern (Figure 18-7). The prolonged administration of maintenance doses, after the patient has been "loaded," do not change the pattern of FHR tracing (see Figure 18-47).

The significant magnesium blood levels reached by the fetus (usually equilibrated with those of the mother) do not seem to induce any depression at birth, as judged by the Apgar score or the acid–base status of the infant.

Antihypertensive drugs commonly used to control dangerous hypertension do not affect the FHR unless the blood pressure drops below safe levels because of transient overdose or the superimposed effect of vasodilating medications. When magnesium sulfate is given too rapidly, transient vasodilatation occurs (see Figures 9-79

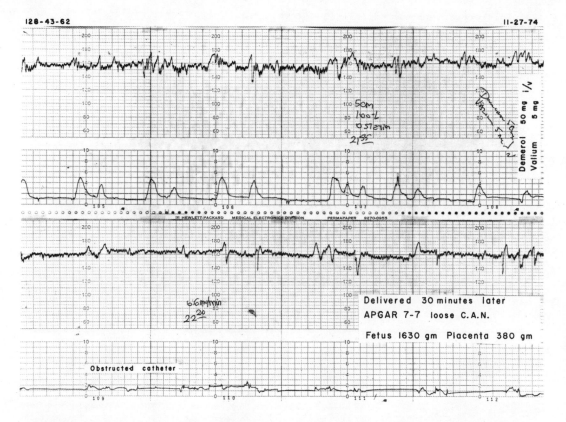

Figure 18-5 Continuous 80 min of direct UC and FHR recordings of premature labor at 32 weeks gestation. Rapid oscillations of the tachycardic baseline are diminished after diazepam 5 mg IV and meperidine 50 mg IV. However the accelerations of FHR recorded simultaneously with the contractions continue unchanged. *(Below)* Intrauterine catheter obstructed throughout recording. A small infant in good condition was delivered 30 min after end of the recording.

and 9-80), and the FHR may be momentarily altered (Figure 18-7) as it would during any other episode of hypotension.

ANESTHETICS

Among the extraordinary number of preparations with the property of blocking pain, some exert their action by their effect on the central nervous system while others act by blocking the painful impulses without affecting consciousness. The first group are the general anesthetics, and the second group produce either local or regional anesthesia. The intimate mechanism of action will not be discussed here (the interested reader is referred to the texts of pharmacology or anesthesiology). Their effects on the

uterus, vital signs of the mother, and the FHR are the specific aim of this chapter.

General Anesthetics

These substances have the potential of blocking the perception of sensation at various levels, depending on the amount of medication received and the strength of the stimulus applied. The majority of them are administered by mask, mixed with oxygen, or by the intravenous route generally in combination with other drugs.

Volatile substances *Trichloroethylene* A liquid that evaporates at low temperature, trichloroethylene (Trilene) has been used as an analgesic during first stage and rarely as anesthetic in second stage. It is administered in a mixture of

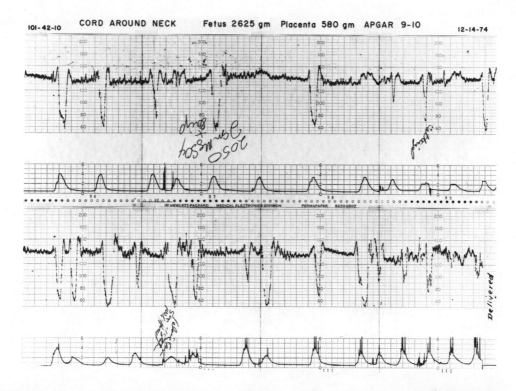

Figure 18-6 Two 40-min segments of direct UC and FHR recordings from induced labor of preeclamptic secundipara at term. *(Above)* FHR baseline frequency is normal with good rapid oscillations interrupted by large variable decelerations. Administration of 2 gm magnesium sulfate IV followed by maintenance infusion did not alter the FHR pattern. *(Below)* After 100 more min of continuous infusion, normal baseline oscillations and the large variable decelerations were still maintained. At the end of the tracing a slightly growth-retarded infant was born in excellent condition with one loop of cord around the neck.

0.4 to 0.6 vol% and is relatively slowly absorbed when administered by vaporizer. It has an acceptable analgesic effect at blood concentration of 5 to 6 mg/100 ml. When given continuously, trichloroethylene has a moderate effect on the uterine activity by its action on the frequency of the contractions—somewhat diminished, but with intensity unaffected (Figure 18-8). However, no change of the FHR has been observed with this drug administered at either analgesic or anesthetic levels. When given in the usual interrupted fashion it does not affect uterine contractility.

Ether The classic general anesthetic "par excellence" as uterine relaxant, ether, was for a long time the single effective medication to induce safely and predictably, in a sustained manner, the relaxation of the uterus in advanced labor, at second stage or postpartum when intrauterine manipulation was indicated. It influences both the intensity and frequency of uterine contractions, but its effect is clearly observed, and is of clinical usefulness only at the third anesthetic stage, that is, at the surgical plane of anesthesia. To reach that point, the anesthetic must be administered for several minutes at the appropriate concentration of 5 to 8 vol%. In general, a minimum of 10 min will elapse between the moment the anesthesia is started and a satisfactory relaxation is obtained with blood levels of 50 to 60 mg/100 ml (Figure 18-9). It is therefore impossible to induce with it very rapid relaxation, as may be necessary in certain clinical situations—a critical fact to remember when intrauterine manipulations are contemplated. Ether has no direct effect on the FHR.

Nitrous oxide A very popular analgesic-anesthetic in obstetrics, nitrous oxide has long been considered to have no direct effect upon the

420

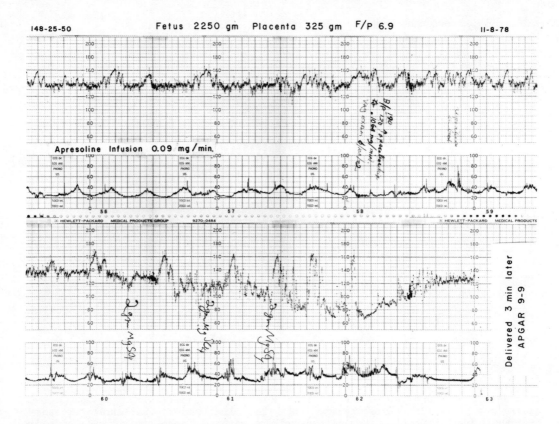

Figure 18-7 Continuous 75-min direct UC and FHR recordings of advanced first stage of multipara at term in spontaneous labor. Neurofibromatosis with severe hypertension of 190/120 mm Hg, patient receiving continuous infusion of hydralazine, 0.09 mg/min. *(Above)* Normal baseline frequency and rapid oscillations interrupted by accelerations related to fetal movements. Because of hyperreflexia the patient was given 6 gm magnesium sulfate IV over 11 min. Some bradycardia coincides with the transient *relative* maternal hypotension induced by too rapid magnesium sulfate administration. However, the baseline oscillations remain unchanged, or even slightly exaggerated, as do the accelerations of the fetal heart. A growth-retarded infant in excellent condition was born 3 min after the end of the tracing. Evidence of placental insufficiency with an F/P ratio of 6.9.

myometrium. This concept is based on observations made during its administration as an analgesic in labor, in an intermittent fashion, during each contraction and discontinuing it during uterine relaxation. Given in this manner, at the 50% mixture with oxygen, it has negligible analgesic effect and no action on the uterine activity at a blood level of 25 to 30 mg/100 ml. However, when administered in a continuous way it diminishes the uterine activity when reaching analgesic planes (40 to 50 mg/100 ml blood levels). When nitrous oxide is given to obtain anesthesia one should expect to see a *clear uterine relaxant effect* within 5 min of its continuous administration (Figure 18-10). The intensity of the contractions is primarily affected as the frequency

is usually unaltered. The recovery of preanesthetic pattern of uterine activity is also rapid, being reached within 5 min of discontinuing the gas mixture. This not-too-well-known effect of nitrous oxide may be the cause of preventable bleeding when it is used to maintain anesthesia in cesarean sections after "crash induction" and removal of the fetus. Likewise, it may be indirectly responsible for significant blood loss when used as anesthetic to complete second trimester abortions or perform first trimester abortions. Fortunately, its rapid elimination facilitates the hemostatic action of the recovered uterine contractions.

Nitrous oxide has no direct effect on the FHR patterns when used as analgesic during labor or in superficial anesthetic planes.

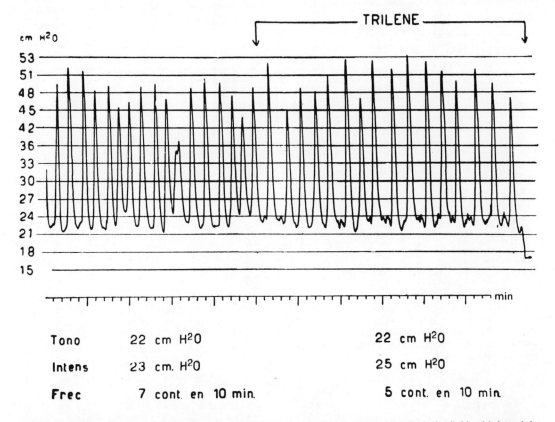

Figure 18-8 Intrauterine pressure tracing of term spontaneous labor following amniotic fluid withdrawal in polyhydramnios. (Note scale in cm H_2O and very slow paper speed.) Continuous administration of trichloroethylene is followed by mild reduction in frequency of contractions without change in intensity. Reprinted from Alvarez and Caldeyro-Barcia (1954).

Methoxyflurane This potent volatile anesthetic from the group of halogenated preparations was introduced to clinical medicine in relatively recent times and has demonstrated a remarkable effect on the pregnant myometrium. Used at very low concentration in a mixture with oxygen (0.5% to 1.5%) it induces deep anesthesia within a few minutes. Its action on the uterus is characterized by *diminution of both the intensity and frequency of contractions* within 2 min of starting the administration of the mixture at 1% (Figures 18-11 and 18-12), and its uterine relaxant effect is in direct proportion to the blood concentration of the drug. At over 2 mg/100 ml concentration, reached very rapidly, uterine contractions are diminished in intensity and frequency, and with levels of over 5 mg/100 ml one may obtain almost complete relaxation of the uterus. The recovery of uterine contractility is also relatively

fast and follows the clearance of the drug from the bloodstream, which takes longer than the induction time. As much as 15 min after discontinuing methoxyflurane (Penthrane) one may still measure it in the blood and observe incompletely recovered uterine activity. No effect has been observed on FHR, provided the cardiovascular changes do not interfere with effective IVS blood supply.

The effect of methoxyflurane on the blood pressure and pulse rate are marked and should be clearly understood when this anesthetic is to be used. At blood concentrations of slightly over 2 mg/100 ml the systolic and diastolic pressures fall and the pulse rate rises. When the blood concentration reaches 5 mg/100 ml the blood pressure may reach dangerously low values; this effect seems to be the direct consequence of a marked vasodilatation triggered by the anesthetic. The

422

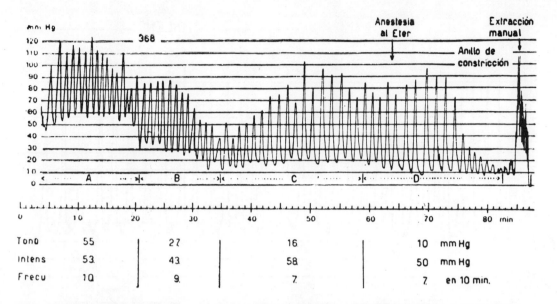

Tono	55		27		16		10	mm Hg
Intens	53		43		58		50	mm Hg
Frecu	10		9		7		7	en 10 min.

Figure 18-9 Intrauterine pressure recording of third stage obtained by catheterization of the umbilical vein, the placenta serving as intrauterine balloon. Patient received ergometrine postpartum but the placenta was not expelled. Extremely high tonus and frequency induced by the medication. Ether anesthesia started (arrow), and after 12 min the contractions relaxed and permitted an easy manual extraction of the placenta. Reprinted from Alvarez and Caldeyro-Barcia (1954).

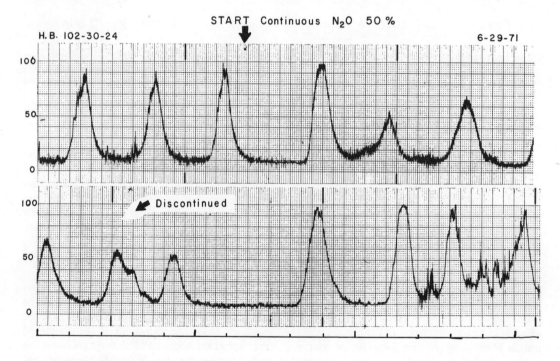

Figure 18-10 Continuous 32-min intrauterine pressure recording of enhanced labor of multipara at term. Strong contractions diminish in intensity 4 min after continuous nitrous oxide at 50% concentration was started (arrow, *above*). The contractions recurred with normal frequency but with significantly lesser intensity. The contraction occurring 6 min after discontinuing the anesthetic *(below)* was the first one where the preanesthesia strength was regained. A transiently increased frequency and tonus may be appreciated by the end of the recording.

423

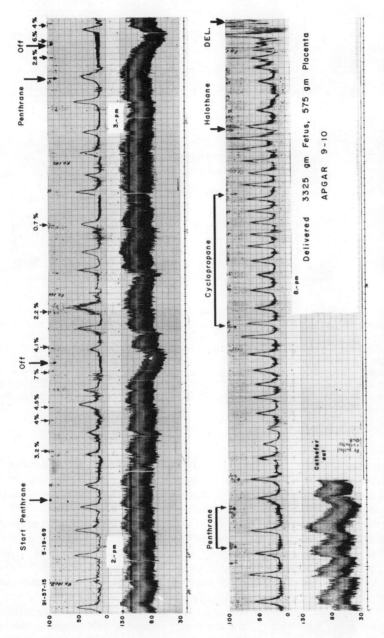

Figure 18-11 Two segments of direct UC and intraarterial (femoral) pressure recordings in spontaneous labor of multipara at term. (UC and blood pressure scales in mm Hg at left; paper speed, 6 mm/min, the small marks at the bottom indicating 1 min.) *(Above)* Methoxyflurane given in early labor (between large arrows), and the arterial blood concentration serially followed (small arrows). Blood levels of 2 and 3 mg/100 ml are rapidly reached with a significant diminution of intensity and frequency of contractions. With levels above 4.5 mg/100 ml there is marked hypotension in addition to profound uterine relaxation; the recovery of both is rapid after discontinuing the anesthetic. *(Below)* Four hours later, a brief administration of methoxyflurane (arterial catheter being lost). Farther on, the continuous administration of cyclopropane with an apparent increased uterine contractility in spite of good anesthetic level. After 10 min of interruption halothane was given and the uterine contractility dropped dramatically within 2 min. With mother under light halothane anesthesia, a fetus in excellent condition was delivered.

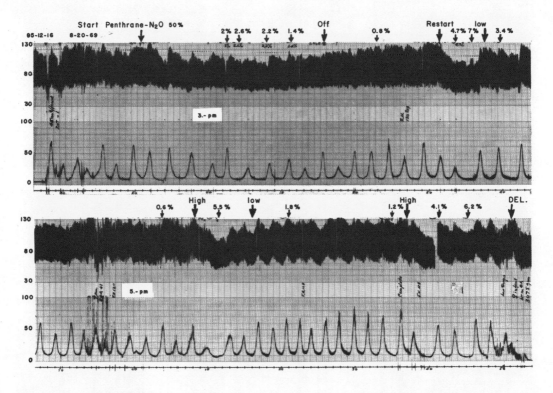

Figure 18-12 Two 68-min segments of direct UC and intraarterial (femoral) pressures obtained in middle and late first stage of enhanced labor at term. (Recording scales are in mm Hg at left, and the time in minutes.) A mixture of methoxyflurane 0.5% and nitrous oxide–oxygen 50% was started (arrow), and 6 min later uterine activity was noticeably diminished. However, the blood pressure started to fall by the third minute. Decreased uterine activity was maintained with methoxyflurane blood levels of around 2 mg/100 ml (small arrows). After the drugs were discontinued, recovery seemed fairly complete with blood levels of 0.8 mg/100 ml. Resumption of the gas mixture at higher flow had an almost immediate effect, and blood level reached 7 mg/100 ml at 4.5 min with sharp fall in blood pressure. The same response was elicited over 1 hour later in advanced first stage and second stage. A mildly depressed infant who did well was delivered by low forceps.

recovery from the hypotension is rapid and reasonably good blood pressures may be observed at blood concentrations of 2 mg/100 ml, still with low uterine activity maintained.

The association of methoxyflurane and nitrous oxide appears to have the added effect of these two anesthetics (Figure 18-12) diminishing uterine contractility with Penthrane concentrations of 1 to 2 mg/100 ml. Dramatic diminution of uterine contractility may be observed with blood levels below 7 mg/100 ml. The cardiovascular changes of the mother are as significant as with methoxyflurane given alone. Penthrane anesthesia will "break through" the strong effect of oxytocin and even ergotrate.

The newborn is not dramatically affected by this anesthetic even though there is rapid passage into the fetal circulation. Apgar scores are usually good, and fetal blood levels of the anesthetic equal to those in the mother. Likewise, fetal acid–base status is not deleteriously influenced by this substance (Ivankovic et al, 1971).

Halothane A volatile anesthetic popular for some time, halothane (Fluothane) is now relatively infrequently used because of some sporadic cases of severe hepatic problems following its administration. However, it is an excellent uterine relaxant with a very rapid action on both intensity and frequency of contractions when used in a mixture of about 1% with oxygen to obtain blood levels on the order of 10 mg/100 ml. The relaxant action on the myometrium may be seen within 2 min of starting the administration (Figure 18-11). The effect on the fetus is negligible, either on FHR pattern or neonatal condition evaluated by Apgar score and acid–base state. When rapid uterine relaxation is needed, Fluothane is an excellent preparation to use because the effect may be obtained even when the uterus has recently been stimulated with oxytocin or ergotrate. Elimination is also very rapid, the blood levels dropping dramatically while the uterine activity recovers quickly.

Fluothane has a very clear hypotensive and tachycardic effect at blood concentrations producing anesthesia. These effects are caused by peripheral vasodilatation; nevertheless, the recovery is also rapid after discontinuing the anesthetic.

Enflurane One of the newest anesthetics available for use in obstetrics, enflurane (Ethrane) has the same general characteristics as its related compound Fluothane and is also similar to Penthrane. It is a volatile agent that has a short period of induction with rapid general effect when given at concentrations of 0.5 to 1.5 vol% with oxygen.

With this amount in a non-rebreathing system it reaches the effective level of 12 mg/100 ml within 2 min. With this or higher concentrations in blood it produces a marked depression of uterine contractions (Figure 18-13), which will occur even when the uterus has been stimulated with either oxytocin or ergotrate. It is an excellent compound to use when rapid uterine relaxation is needed for intrauterine manipulations. As with the other volatile anesthetics, enflurane does not seem to affect the FHR pattern at the time of induction.

Cyclopropane This substance is considered to be the most potent gas anesthetic for clinical use; its advantage is rapid, easy induction. The two main problems inherent in its use are that it is explosive, and that it produces cardiac arrhythmias, particularly extrasystoles. Thus its use in obstetrics has been somewhat restricted in the last few years. Nevertheless, because it is one of the few volatile anesthetics with short induction

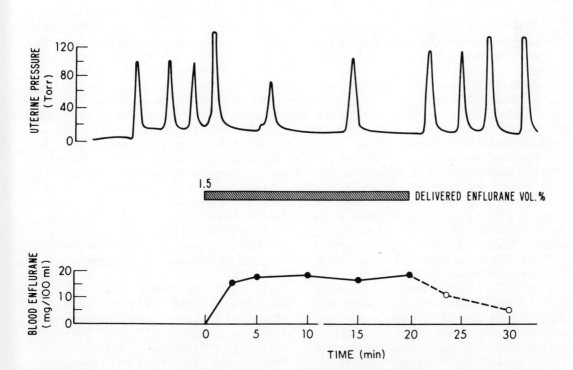

Figure 18-13 Postpartum intrauterine pressure recorded by means of a microballoon inserted after third stage. The rhythmic activity is rapidly diminished when enflurane 2% was given and the blood level exceeded 14 mg/100 ml. Uterine contractility recovered rapidly after discontinuing the anesthetic with rapid fall in its blood levels. Reprinted from Marx GF, et al: Postpartum uterine pressure under halothane or enflurane anesthesia. *Obstet Gynecol* 51:695, 1978.

time and minimal or no effect on uterine contractility there is still room for this preparation in modern obstetrics.

At mixture concentrations with oxygen of 5% to 10%, it rapidly reaches blood levels of 5 to 8 mg/100 ml—sufficient to produce good anesthesia without significant change in uterine contractility (see Figure 18-11). At moderate anesthetic levels one may see the suggestion of a mild increase in frequency of contractions, perhaps the uterine response to endogenous release of norepinephrine, which is known to be triggered by these levels of cyclopropane. It is therefore a good, rapid anesthetic but *inappropriate when one needs uterine relaxation.*

No significant changes in FHR pattern may be observed under standard conditions; likewise, superficial anesthesia causes minimal neonatal depression while prolonged anesthesia has been observed to correlate with significant fetal asphyxia and low Apgar scores.

Intravenous Substances

The anesthetic medications routinely used by the intravenous route do not have clinical use as analgesics but their effects are relevant to the obstetrician because they are used as general anesthetics for both vaginal delivery and cesarean section. Because these preparations are generally used in combination or rapid sequence they will be discussed as components of the so-called balanced method of anesthestia.

Balanced anesthesia The concept of balanced anesthesia implies that different medications are given simultaneously or in rapid succession to take advantage of their pharmacologic effect on specific target organs or systems at the minimum possible effective dose. To be properly applied, balanced anesthesia requires complete understanding of the pharmacologic actions of the various drugs used and skillful use of such knowledge. Each agent is used with the specific aim of controlling one aspect of anesthesia: anxiety, pain relief, paralysis of striated muscles. For cesarean section, the induction of the anesthesia, after premedications, generally entails the use of a muscle relaxant and a barbiturate of rapid action.

Thiopental As all barbiturates, thiopental (Pentothal) is a poor analgesic that exerts its effect at the cortical level as a hypnotic. It does not interfere with the conduction of stimuli from the periphery and therefore, to induce anesthesia, the cortex must be significantly depressed. It does not produce muscle relaxation; for this reason it is used in association with the so-called skeletal muscle relaxants.

When thiopental is given intravenously at the standard dose of 200 to 300 mg to the patient in advanced gestation or in labor, uterine activity does not seem to be significantly affected by it. The frequency as well as the intensity of contractions are unaltered (Figure 18-14) even though the patient may have entered into a satisfactory anesthetic plane. Likewise, the FHR is not significantly affected by such doses of the barbiturate. The neonates are usually born with very good Apgar scores, an indication of very limited depressant action of Pentothal at moderate doses.

Succinylcholine One of the most frequently used skeletal muscle relaxants, succinylcholine prevents repolarization of the cells after "firing" and thus exerts its relaxing action. This effect is sought, as part of balanced anesthesia, to facilitate a surgical procedure. A dose of 1 to 1.5 mg/kg injected rapidly by the intravenous route produces paralysis of striated muscles facilitating intubation of the patients. This enables the anesthesiologist to administer oxygen and other volatile anesthetics to sustain the short superficial anesthesia obtained by the preceding injection of thiopental.

The effects on the pregnant uterus have been studied only in passing because usually the uterus is emptied within minutes of the induction. The few observations carried out with intrauterine catheters suggest that succinylcholine, at the doses usually employed to start general anesthesia, triggers a moderate state of hypercontractility, mainly at the expense of frequency and tonus (Felton and Goddard, 1966). In vitro studies indicate that myometrium exposed to high doses of the drug may diminish its contractility while that exposed to lighter concentrations is stimulated (Iuppa et al, 1971).

This interesting finding corroborates the clinical observation of stimulation seen during induction of anesthesia. Even though modest, nevertheless, uterine activity is clearly increased (Figure 18-15) at the expense of a higher frequency of contractions. Close observation of patterns of uterine activity reveal an increased frequency of contractions following the induction of general anesthesia even in cases of moderately irregular contractility (Figure 18-16). In either case, the

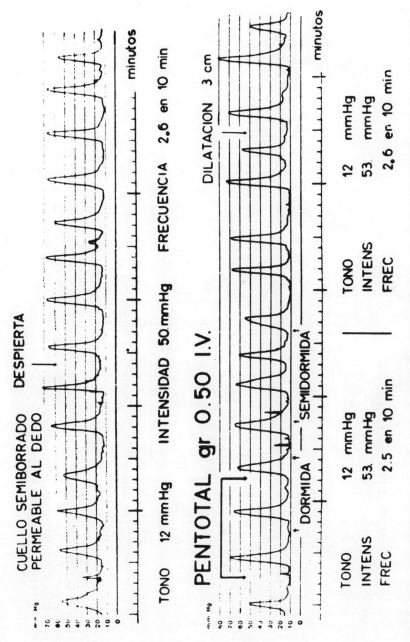

Figure 18-14 Continuous 100 min of intrauterine recording of spontaneous late prelabor in term pregnancy. *(Above)* Uterine activity with the patient awake. *(Below)* Thiopental 500 mg (arrows) given intravenously followed by anesthetic sleep. Analysis of uterine contractility indicated no apparent change following anesthetic. Reprinted from Alvarez and Caldeyro-Barcia (1954).

428

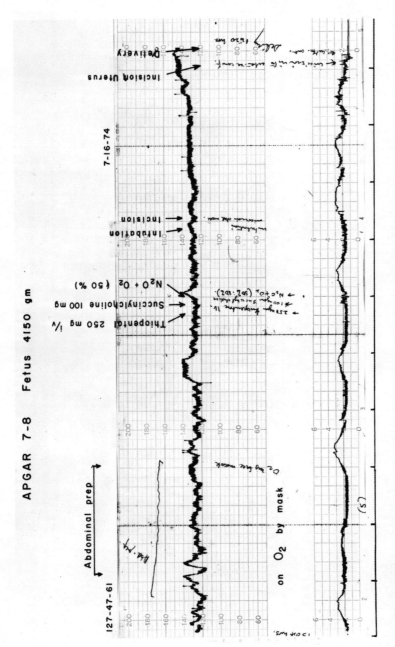

Figure 18-15 Direct intrauterine pressure and FHR recordings just before and during a cesarean section for relative cephalopelvic disproportion. (Paper speed, 3 cm/min.) Uterine contractility seems to have increased following the administration of "balanced" anesthesia (arrows). In spite of N₂O content of the method, the frequency of contractions increased from 5 to 8/10 min before a 4150 gm infant was delivered in good condition (Apgar 7-8).

effect of succinylcholine on the FHR is negligible: the patterns preceding anesthesia will continue unchanged until the fetus is removed from the uterus. When there are decelerations triggered either by hypoxia or cord problems they will still recur as before (Figure 18-16).

The effect of balanced anesthesia on the neonate seems not to alter its homeostasis because Apgar scores and acid–base status are not significantly different from the average populations delivered under local or no anesthesia.

Conduction Anesthesia

The blockade, at the level of the spinal cord, of the painful stimuli triggered by uterine contractions and the delivery of the infant stands out among the important contributions of modern anesthesiology to improve the care of the laboring patient. The techniques to obtain the blockade vary: intrathecal injection of local anesthetics, or administration in the epidural space, either caudal or lumbar. In either case, there is complete sensory blockade below the level of injection. There is also partial motor blockade ("weakening of muscles") with the extradural techniques, and complete muscular paralysis with the intrathecal method.

Simultaneously with the blockade of the sensory (posterior) roots there is blocking of the sympathetic nerves and thus important alterations of the peripheral vascular system controlled by them. Because a large part of the vascular tree can be affected by this anesthesia technique, it is of utmost importance to be sure of the normal status of the

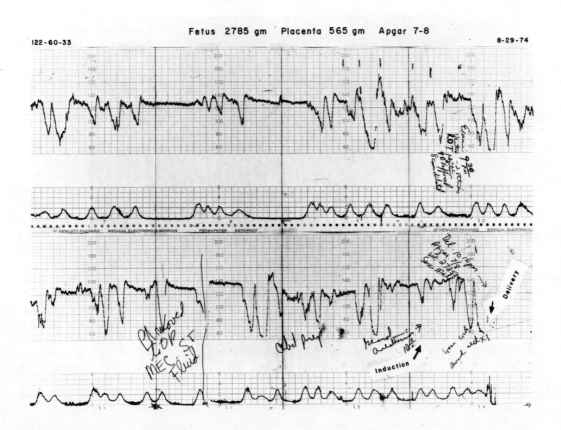

Figure 18-16 Continuous 80-min direct UC and FHR recordings of advanced labor of patient at term. Meconium-stained amniotic fluid and FHR decelerations interpreted as fetal distress. The somewhat irregular pattern of uterine contractility triggered variable decelerations. *(Below)* After transfer to the operating room, the "balanced" anesthesia (given at arrow) seemed to induce increased contractility, particularly frequency and tonus, breaking the pattern maintained before anesthesia. An infant in good condition with a loop of cord around the neck was extracted.

cardiovascular system of the patient and her blood volume before giving conduction anesthesia. Indirectly, by affecting the IVS blood flow, these techniques of pain relief may alter the fetal well-being rapidly and dramatically.

On the other hand, blocking of the motor (anterior) roots will produce complete muscular paralysis and relaxation of striated muscles below the level of the blockade. Depending on the technique used, the block may preferentially affect the sensory roots with only moderate effect upon the motor roots (extradural methods), or affect equally both groups of roots and produce a "functional section" of the spinal cord (intrathecal method).

The agents used to produce conduction anesthesia are known by the generic name of local anesthetics. Those used in clinical work are synthetic substances that affect the transmission of nerve impulses. (For detailed information on mechanism of action, physicochemical properties, metabolism, and techniques of administration the reader is referred to the specialized texts on pharmacology and anesthesia.) The intimate mechanism of action is unknown; the membrane potential of the nerve fibers is unaltered, and it is speculated that sodium transport through the nerve membrane may be involved in the mechanism of blocking the impulses. The duration of action and toxicity of these substances is variable as it is their potency per unit of weight. All have a completely reversible action and are administered as water-soluble, more or less acid salts.

Spinal Anesthesia

This method has been used extensively in obstetrics after its introduction in 1900, and one of its variants—the "saddle block" technique—was probably at one time the most widely used type of anesthesia for the relief of spontaneous and/or operative delivery pains. In spite of this widespread utilization there was and still is controversy with regard to its effects on uterine contractility and the progress of labor, when it is given before full dilatation.

With accurate monitoring of uterine contractions, it is possible to document that the pattern preceding the block does not usually change after the anesthesia has been achieved (Figure 18-17). These results may in general be expected, regard-

less of the level of anesthesia obtained; in other words, *a successful spinal block neither depresses nor increases the preceding uterine activity*. An exception to this general principle has been observed in cases of painful, irregular, or incoordinated activity in first stage: as soon as the pain is relieved the contractility pattern takes the aspect of a perfectly normal uterine activity (Figure 18-18). In spite of the complete sensory, motor, and sympathetic blockade the uterine contractility pattern continues to appear as it would without anesthesia with regard to its changes; according to the position of the patient—usually more regular and with higher frequency when supine, and stronger with less frequent contractions when in the lateral position (Figures 18-19, 18-20, 18-21).

The cardiovascular system of the patient is of course significantly affected by the sympathetic block. There is a tendency to a moderate degree of systolic and diastolic hypotension due to the peripheral pooling of blood. With adequate circulating blood there is good compensation and minimal systemic repercussions. The blood pressure and pulse rate continue to fluctuate in response to the contractions. Likewise, the cerebrospinal fluid pressure parallels the blood pressure and intrathoracic pressure changes (Figures 18-19 and 18-20), indicating the homogeneity and continuity of the internal fluid system.

These observations are valid for the majority of patients, regardless of the level of anesthesia and block obtained. This is, in general, true for the well-hydrated and compensated patients. This is also true for *the effects of spinal anesthesia on the FHR pattern: usually no changes* over the preexisting pattern. Changes occur only when significant hypotension at the level of the iliac vessels contributes to diminished IVS blood flow. This syndrome may be observed when the patient has apparent good systemic pressure from the reading taken only on the brachial artery, and it may coexist with hypotension below the bifurcation of the aorta. The clinical result in these cases will be evidence of fetal distress manifested as late decelerations (Figure 18-21). Observations of this type are particularly dangerous for the fetus when the spinal anesthesia is either unexpected (accidental) or at very high level. Even then, rapid intervention should prevent fetal deterioration and facilitate the delivery of a nondepressed fetus with good Apgar scores.

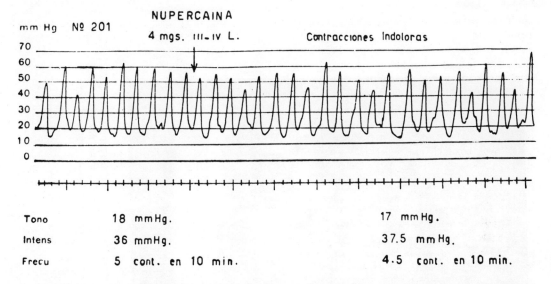

Figure 18-17 Direct UC recording during spontaneous labor at term. Strong uterine contractions did not change in pattern after the intrathecal administration of 4 mg dibucaine between L3-4. Analysis of contractility *(bottom)* documents lack of change. Reprinted from Alvarez and Caldeyro-Barcia (1954).

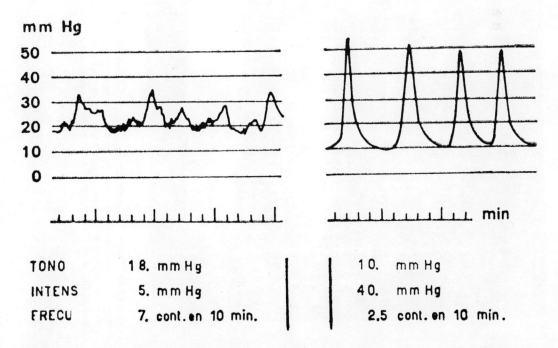

Figure 18-18 Two segments of direct UC tracings of early labor at term. *(Left)* Irregular pattern, incoordinated and with high tonus (hypertonic inertia). *(Right)* Normal contractility after successful spinal anesthesia. Analysis of the recording at the bottom. Reprinted from Alvarez and Caldeyro-Barcia (1954).

432

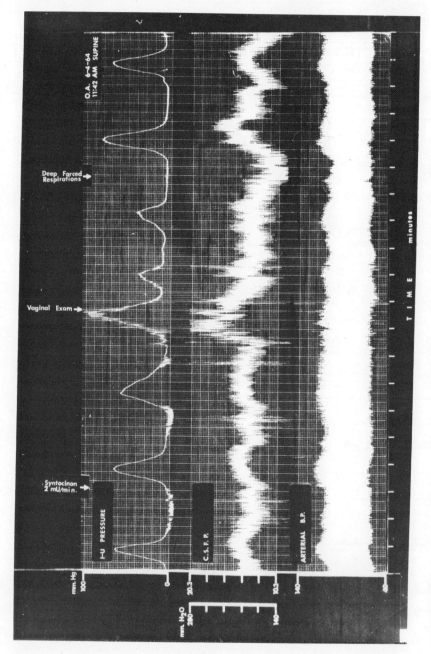

Figure 18-19 Direct UC, intrathecal, and intraarterial (femoral) pressures recorded during spontaneous labor at term. The patient received continuous spinal anesthesia, and the uterine contractility demonstrated the same pattern as before anesthesia. The blood pressure was steady but slightly lower than preanesthetic readings. CSF pressure changes were not influenced by the spinal block. Reprinted from Hopkins EL, et al: Cerebrospinal fluid pressure in labor. *Am J Obstet Gynecol* 93:907, 1965.

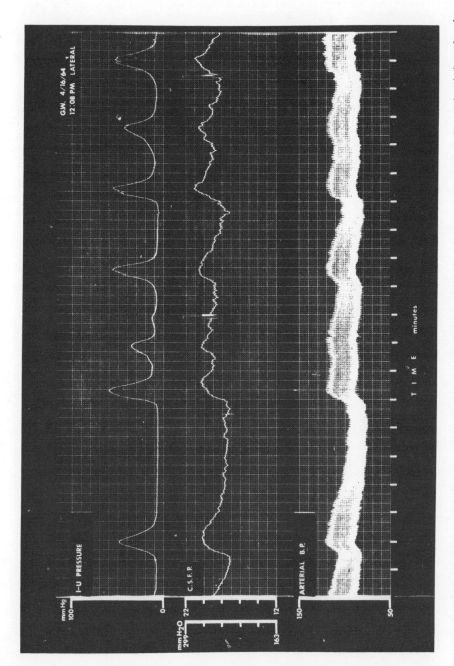

Figure 18-20 Direct UC, intrathecal, and intrarterial (femoral) pressures recorded during term enhanced labor. The patient in lateral position, under continuous spinal anesthesia, labors with a normal contractility pattern that responds readily to position changes. The blood pressure and CSF pressure demonstrate the normal hemodynamic changes produced by contractions. Reprinted from Hopkins EL, et al: Cerebrospinal fluid pressure in labor. *Am J Obstet Gynecol* 93:907, 1965.

434

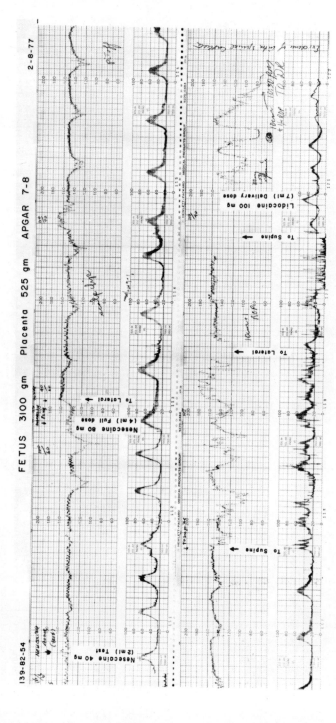

Figure 18-21 Continuous 115-min direct UC and FHR recordings during enhanced labor at term. *(Top)* Epidural anesthesia test dose (chloroprocaine 40 mg) was given (arrow) and 15 min later FHR decelerations were recorded. Full dose of 80 mg was given, rapidly followed by hypotension and good anesthesia to T-9. Patient turned to lateral position and so maintained for 47 min. The uterine contractility and brachial blood pressure were minimally affected while the FHR continued to demonstrate moderate decelerations. *(Bottom)* Supine position for 15 min induced more severe FHR decelerations and saltatory pattern corrected by returning the patient to lateral position. Delivery dose of 100 mg mepivacaine brought above severe worsening of FHR decelerations and total anesthesia to T-2. Oxygen by mask, lateral position, and forceps delivery helped to obtain a fetus in good condition. It was possible to *aspirate spinal fluid* through the catheter indicating that the *last dose was intrathecal.* (Possible secondary perforation of dura mater.)

Caudal Anesthesia

The use of the peridural space to inject an anesthetic substance was first suggested in the early part of the century. Soon thereafter European obstetricians applied it as means to relieve labor and delivery pains using the sacral canal—the terminal part of the vertebral canal—occupied by nerve roots and very loose adipose and areolar tissue as the site of injection. This sacral canal is anatomically a semiclosed system, the "leaky" areas being the foramina partially filled by nerve roots. The anesthetic injected into this space therefore literally bathes the nerve roots it contains and thereby exerts its blocking action. Because these roots are the "cauda equina" the technique is known as caudal anesthesia.

The popularity of caudal anesthesia in obstetrics followed the report by Edwards and Hingson (1942) who advocated its use after evaluating its safety and efficacy. The technique of a single dose is used for late first stage and second stage, whereas the continuous technique is usually started in mid-first stage with repeated doses as needed. In spite of the general agreement that it is an effective method of anesthesia, there is not such agreement with regard to its effects on uterine activity, the progress of labor, and the cardiovascular system. The majority of the publications on these aspects are based on purely clinical reports and have contradictory conclusions, while the few studies conducted with accurate monitoring techniques agree on results. Among the possible causes for very strongly held different opinions may be the effect of added epinephrine as an adjuvant with the intention of prolonging the anesthetic action (Rucker, 1925). On the other hand, the method of calculating first- and/or second-stage effects is basically prone to subjective influences and thus the results strongly weighed by the investiagor's preexisting ideas.

Oxytocin-*induced uterine contractility is usually not affected by* the administration of caudal anesthesia. Neither the pattern of contractions (Figures 18-22 and 18-23) nor the calculated uterine activity is significantly changed: only the normal cyclic fluctuations of uterine activity are observed (Figure 18-24) as seen in induced labors progressing without anesthesia. Likewise, *uterine contractility of spontaneous labor does not seem to be significantly affected* by caudal anesthesia (Figures 18-25 and 18-26). The contractility patterns and the calculated uterine activity are not changed after the anesthesia is administered (Figure 18-24).

The *efficiency of uterine contractions* to dilate the cervix, evaluated *by calculating the uterine work* required to produce, under stable conditions, a given amount of cervical dilatation ("partial uterine work") does not change in about 70% of spontaneous or induced labors; it could be expected to increase in 25%, and to decrease in 5% (Figure 18-27). The "total uterine work" required to dilate the cervix in first stage conducted under caudal anesthesia should be expected to be within the normal range, depending on the parity, variety of position, and state of membranes (see Chapter 5 and Figures 5-38 through 5-42) because the efficiency of the contractions is not significantly altered.

Only the addition of epinephrine to the anesthetic solution will predictably influence the contractility by decreasing it temporarily.

Caudal anesthesia predictably triggers mild degrees of *fall in systolic and diastolic blood pressures* preceding the relief of pain. The average anticipated drop in blood pressure is on the order of 15 to 20 mm Hg for both systolic and diastolic pressures (Figure 18-22). It appears within 10 or 12 minutes after the total dose has been given, with the pulse rate following in mirror image the fluctuations in blood pressure (Figure 18-23). Perhaps because of pressure exerted by the uterus over the aorta and vena cava the blood pressure changes are more clearly manifested with the patient in supine position. When the blood pressure falls significantly it may be easily corrected by two maneuvers: either elevating the patient's legs up to 90 degrees (Figure 18-25) or turning the patient to a right or left lateral position (Figure 18-23). These falls in blood pressure do not appear to be related to the level of anesthesia obtained; they are rather influenced by the patient's circulating blood volume and the lability of her cardiovascular system. Preeclamptic patients are much more labile and prone to severe hypotension than normotensive pregnant patients. In cases of acute hypotension it is much better to change the position of the patient to correct hypotension than to administer vasoactive substances, which are usually ineffective (Figure 18-26). Vasoactive substances may, in addition, worsen the fetal effect of hypotension by increasing the uterine contractility, a common characteristic of such drugs: the more frequent contractions will further interfere with the already compromised IVS blood

436

flow brought about by the hypotension. The result would be more prolonged fetal hypoxia in spite of a transiently reassuring improvement in blood pressure.

The FHR is not directly affected by this method of conduction anesthesia. It may indirectly change in cases of significant maternal hypotension that would induce hypoxia and late decelerations. The amount of anesthetic drug transferred to the fetus is not sufficient to affect the patterns of the commonly evaluated elements of FHR.

Epidural (Lumbar) Anesthesia

The injection of the anesthetic solution into the peridural space, in the region corresponding to the thoracic and/or lumbar segments of the

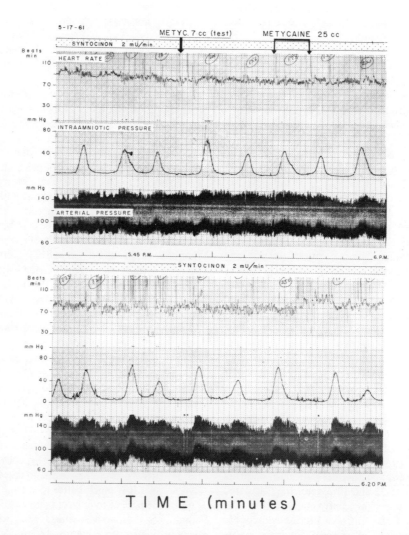

Figure 18-22 Continuous 40-min recordings of maternal heart rate, direct UC, and intraarterial (femoral) pressure recordings in first stage of *induced labor* (oxytocin dose, dotted area) in primipara with intact membranes in supine position. The administration of piperocaine test (100 mg) and full dose (375 mg) did not affect the uterine contractility pattern. The blood pressure demonstrated a small fall and clear fluctuations with the contractions, while heart rate followed the arterial pressure changes in mirror image. There were no appreciable changes in FHR. Reprinted from Cibils LA, Spackman TJ: Caudal analgesia in first stage of labor: Effect on uterine activity and the cardiovascular system. *Am J Obstet Gynecol* 84:1042, 1962.

spine, is commonly known as epidural anesthesia and is to be distinguished from caudal block. The medication bathes preferentially the nerve roots traversing the posterior aspect of the space, that is the sensory roots emerging from the spinal cord, and only to a lesser degree the motor roots emerging from the anterior aspect of the cord.

The clinical use of epidural block, first established in general surgery in the mid-1920s, gained its place in obstetrics much later, after Bromage (1954) reported its many advantages with observations made on a solid scientific basis. At the present time it is probably the method most frequently used (other than the local procedures)

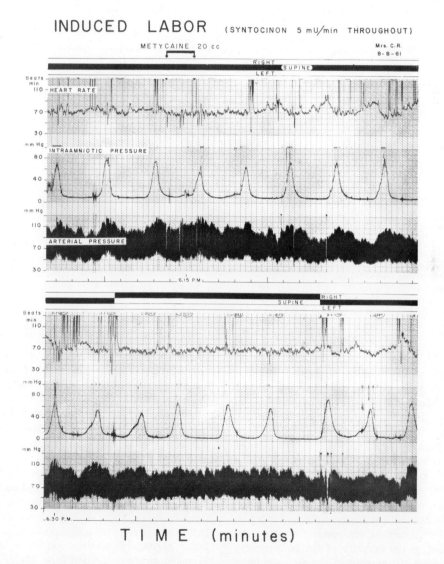

Figure 18-23 Continuous 46-min recordings of maternal heart rate, direct UC, and intraarterial (femoral) pressure in mid-first stage of *induced labor* in multipara at term. (Patient's position indicated by horizontal black bar, above tracings.) The administration of a full dose (300 mg) of piperocaine, (arrows) did not induce any change in uterine contractility. The blood pressure had a small fall starting 4 min after the anesthetic injection and reached maximum effect 8 min later. *(Below)* Turning of the patient to her right stabilized the blood pressure in a good range and corrected the fluctuations of blood pressure and pulse rate. No changes in FHR were appreciated clinically. Reprinted from Cibils LA, Spackman TJ: Caudal analgesia in first stage of labor: Effect on uterine activity and the cardiovascular system. *Am J Obstet Gynecol* 84:1042, 1962.

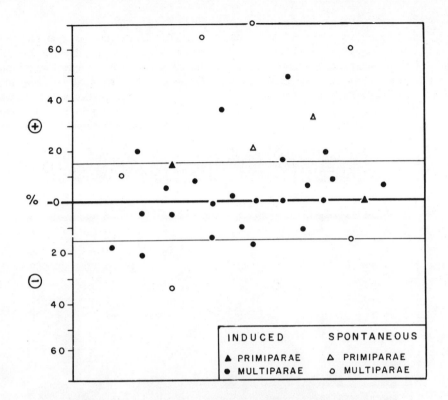

Figure 18-24 Maximum percentage variations of uterine activity calculated after effective caudal anesthesia. The preinjection average was taken as 100% and the two thin lines at 15% indicated the range of normal spontaneous fluctuations of unmedicated labors. Clearly the majority of cases fell within the normal expected values, regardless of parity or type of labor. Reprinted from Cibils LA, Spackman JF: Caudal analgesia in first stage of labor: Effect on uterine activity and the cardiovascular system. *Am J Obstet Gynecol* 84:1042, 1962.

for relief of pain during labor and delivery. Nevertheless, some controversial points still remain regarding the effects of epidural block on uterine contractility, the fetal well-being, and the maternal cardiovascular system. However, there is significant agreement among those studies conducted with accurate means of observation, which are thus free from the pitfalls of subjective interpretations.

The *uterine contractility is usually decreased when the anesthetic is given with added epinephrine.* The diminished contractility is due to a diminution in the intensity of the contractions, the frequency remaining almost unaltered (Figures 18-28 and 18-33). The calculated uterine activity tends to fall in the majority of cases when epinephrine is given with the anesthetic (Figure 18-29). This diminution in uterine activity is usually in proportion to the total amount of epinephrine given (compare Figures 18-28, 18-33,

and 18-34). The rationale behind this pharmacologic manipulation (adding epinephrine) aims at preventing excessive vasodilatation and to give "cardiovascular support" to the laboring patient. When *plain anesthetic solution* is given uterine contractility may increase, decrease, or *remain unchanged* (Figure 18-30). The *calculated uterine activity continues* the normal fluctuations observed in unmedicated labors and therefore it may appear as increased, decreased, or *unchanged* (Figure 18-31). These fluctuations of uterine activity and the effect of added epinephrine may be better appreciated when a number of cases are averaged and compared (Figure 18-32); the depressant effect of epinephrine is then more clearly observed.

In fact, the uterine relaxing action observed when epinephrine is added to the anesthetic solution is perfectly predictable and understandable when one remembers that epinephrine given in ad-

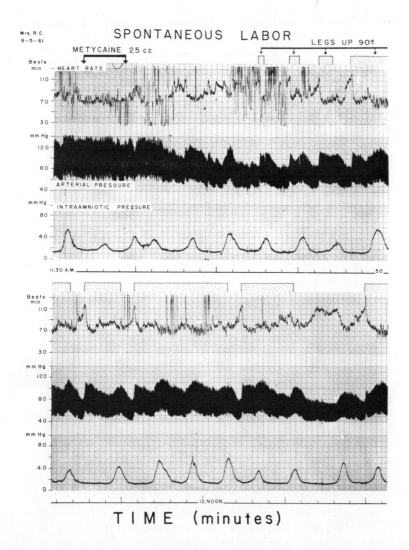

Figure 18-25 Continuous 41-min recordings of maternal heart rate, direct UC, and intraarterial (femoral) pressure during *spontaneous labor* of multipara at term in mid-first stage with intact membranes and in supine position. *(Above, left)* Administration of a full dose of piperocaine (375 mg) (arrows) was followed within 4 min by a significant fall in systolic and diastolic blood pressures. *(Above, right)* This fall is instantly attenuated by raising the legs 90 degrees and is sustained as long as legs are maintained in that position. *(Below)* As soon as the legs are brought down the blood pressure falls to much lower levels. Uterine activity had only the normal fluctuations in pattern. No FHR changes were observed. Reprinted from Cibils LA, Spackman TJ: Caudal analgesia in first stage of labor: Effect on uterine activity and the cardiovascular system. *Am J Obstet Gynecol* 84:1042, 1962.

vanced gestation exerts a predominantly β-mimetic effect (see Chapter 9, Figures 9-43, 9-44, 9-46, 9-47, and 9-48) on the uterine contractility. Furthermore it is clearly why small amounts of epinephrine may not have the same effect as larger doses. The absorption of what amounts to a large single dose of epinephrine rapidly takes

place by the very rich paravertebral venous plexus occupying the peridural space, and has an effect comparable, to a certain extent, to an intravenous injection of the β-adrenergic substance.

The effect of lumbar epidural block on the *cardiovascular system* is, in a way, similar to what has been described for caudal anesthesia but on a

440

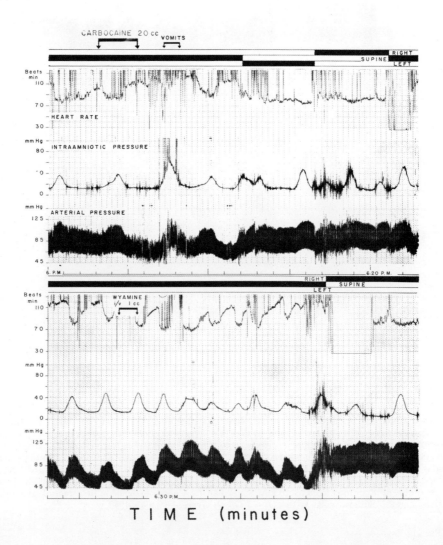

T I M E (minutes)

Figure 18-26 Continuous 46-min recordings of maternal heart rate, direct UC, and intraarterial (femoral) pressure during *spontaneous labor* of multipara at term with intact membranes in mid-first stage. (Patient position indicated by the black horizontal bars above tracings.) Full dose of mepivacaine (200 mg) was rapidly followed by hypotension corrected by turning the patient to her left and right (to allow for good even anesthesia). Back to supine *(top right and bottom)*, the patient had severe hypotension not corrected by the intravenous injection of 15 mg mephentermine sulfate (arrows) which induced only a very transient and partial improvement. The blood pressure returned to normal only after the patient was turned to her right. During all this time the pulse rate followed in mirror image the dramatic changes in blood pressure. The uterine contractility increased after the patient was turned to supine position and received mephentermine; it diminished after she was put on her side. There was clinical evidence of FHR alterations during the period of severe maternal hypotension. Reprinted from Cibils LA, Spackman TJ: Caudal anesthesia in first stage of labor: Effect on uterine activity and the cardiovascular system. *Am J Obstet Gynecol* 84:1042, 1962.

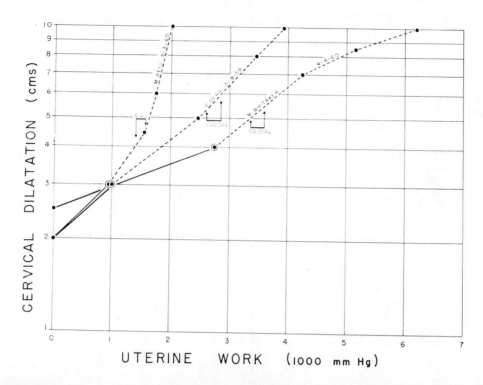

Figure 18-27 The slope of cervical dilatation plotted on semilog paper against the uterine work of three representative patients given caudal anesthesia at the moment indicated for each. The single points represent pelvic examinations and the double circles the moment of amniotomy. The straight line in the middle case is characteristic of the majority (70%) of normal labors; the one on the left, increased efficiency (25%), and the one on the right decreased efficiency (5%) of contractions to dilate the cervix following caudal anesthesia. Reprinted from Cibils LA, Spackman TJ: Caudal anesthesia in first stage of labor: Effect on uterine activity and the cardiovascular system. *Am J Obstet Gynecol* 84:1042, 1962.

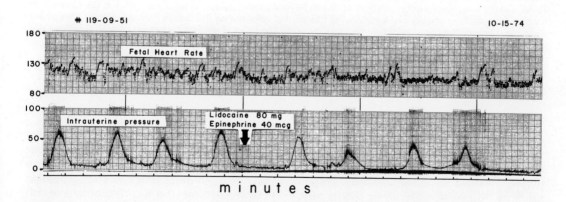

Figure 18-28 Direct FHR and UC recordings of *induced labor* in multipara at term in mid-first stage. The administration of *80 mg lidocaine with 40 μg epinephrine,* as full epidural dose, was followed by a clearly diminished uterine contractility mainly due to decreased intensity of contractions. There was no appreciable effect on the FHR, and the accelerations continued to recur regularly. From Matadial L, Cibils LA: The effect of epidural anesthesia on uterine activity and blood pressure. *Am J Obstet Gynecol* 125:846, 1976.

442

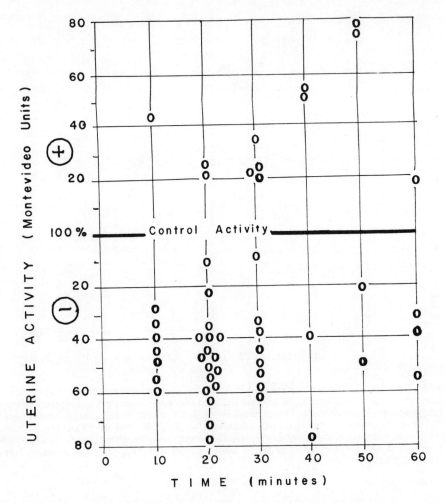

Figure 18-29 Maximum relative changes in uterine activity, from preanesthetic baseline, in a group of patients following epidural block carried out *with epinephrine added to lidocaine.* The preinjection activity was taken as 100%, and the subsequent values calculated at 10-min intervals; the maximum change was plotted at the corresponding time. The majority of cases had a relative fall (the normal spontaneous fluctuation is on the order of 15% above and below control). Reprinted from Matadial L, Cibils LA: The effect of epidural anesthesia on uterine activity and blood pressure. *Am J Obstet Gynecol* 125:846, 1976.

more limited scale. The majority of cases respond with *minimal hypotension* and slight *compensatory tachycardia* if there are changes at all (Figure 18-33). Less often one may observe *significant hypotension* developing shortly after the total dose has been given (Figure 18-34) with a corresponding tachycardia. This hypotension may well be the result of the added effect of sympathetic block on the vena cava and aortic compression, creating below the promontory a more

significant hypotension than one may realize when checking the brachial blood pressure (see Figure 18-30). The best maneuver to correct this problem is to turn the patient to a lateral position (it is irrelevant whether it is right or left) so that the blood pressure and pulse rate will stabilize in a normal range (Figure 18-34). The overall expected fall in blood pressure averages 10 mm Hg systolic and 5 mm Hg diastolic, and about 15 beats/min rise in pulse rate.

443

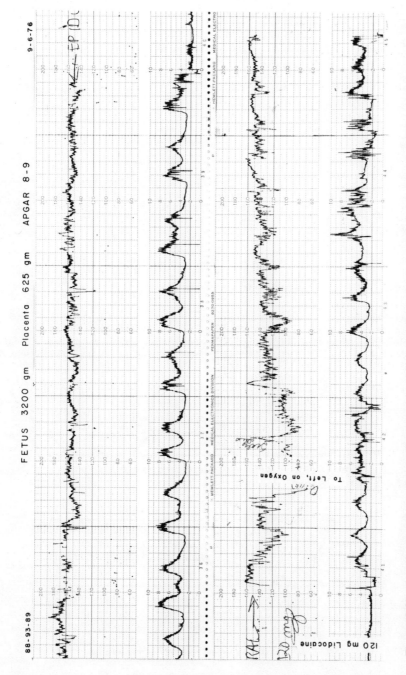

Figure 18-30 Continuous 100-min direct FHR and external UC recordings of multipara at term in advanced first stage of spontaneous labor. *(Below, left)* The full dose of epidural anesthesia, 120 mg lidocaine, triggered FHR decelerations corrected after turning the patient to her side and giving her oxygen. There was minimal brachial hypotension. Note that uterine activity remained unchanged and that dilatation progressed normally. A fetus in good condition was delivered 14 min after the end of the tracing.

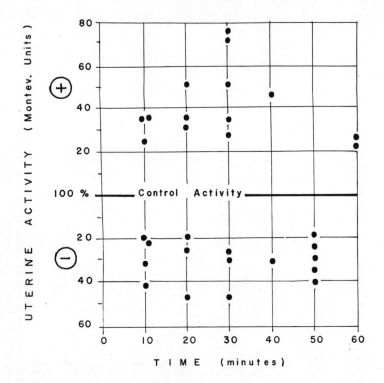

Figure 18-31 Maximum relative changes from preanesthetic baseline uterine activity in a group of patients, following epidural anesthesia obtained with *plain lidocaine*. (Calculations as in Figure 18-29.) The cases are equally distributed above and below the control values, suggesting that the cause of change may be independent of anesthesia. Reprinted from Matadial L, Cibils LA: The effect of epidural anesthesia on uterine activity and blood pressure. *Am J Obstet Gynecol* 125:846, 1976.

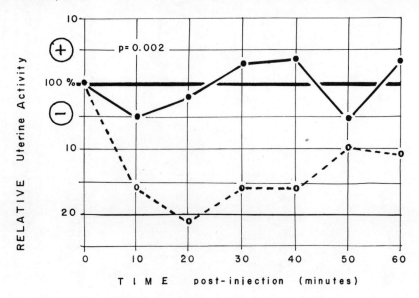

Figure 18-32 Mean values of uterine activity in two groups of patients following successful epidural anesthesia obtained with plain lidocaine (solid line) and epinephrine added to lidocaine (broken line). Activity was calculated at 10-min intervals and separately averaged for each group. The two curves are significantly different, the respective fluctuations being part of spontaneous variations of normal contractility. Reprinted from Matadial L, Cibils LA: The effect of epidural anesthesia on uterine activity and blood pressure. *Am J Obstet Gynecol* 125:846, 1976.

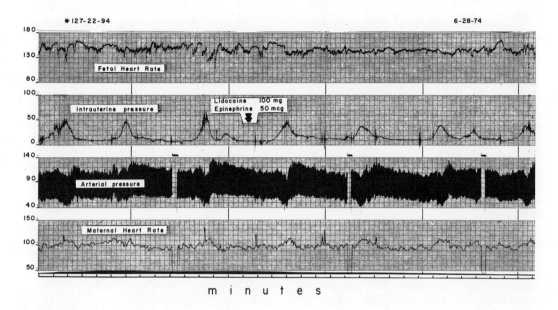

Figure 18-33 Direct FHR, UC, intraarterial (femoral) pressure, and maternal heart rate recordings during oxytoxin-enhanced labor in patient at term, supine position. The epinephrine-added full dose of lidocaine was followed by a decrease in uterine contractility due to diminished intensity of contractions. No changes in blood pressure or maternal heart rate. FHR continued to oscillate without significant changes. Reprinted from Matadial L, Cibils LA: The effect of epidural anesthesia on uterine activity and blood pressure. *Am J Obstet Gynecol* 125:846, 1976.

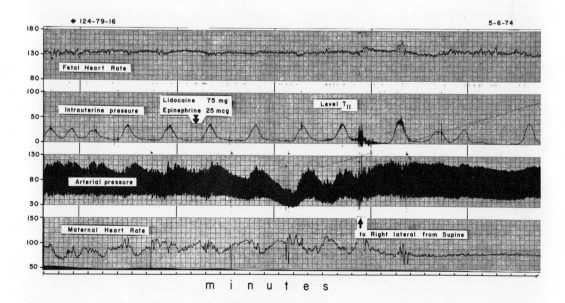

Figure 18-34 Direct FHR, UC, intraarterial (femoral) blood pressure, and maternal heart rate recordings during term spontaneous labor at 4 cm dilatation. The dose of epidural anesthesia (lidocaine 75 mg with epinephrine 25 μg) was followed promptly by a severe fall in blood pressure corrected after turning the patient to her side. The pulse rate followed in mirror image the blood pressure changes and stabilized when the patient adopted the lateral position (blood pressure dropped in spite of "cardiovascular support" of epinephrine). Good anesthesia level was obtained. Note minimal effect on uterine contractility and the expected change following the adoption of lateral position. No changes in FHR observed during the transient hypotension. Reprinted from Matadial L, Cibils LA: The effect of epidural anesthesia on uterine activity and blood pressure. *Am J Obstet Gynecol* 125:846, 1976.

The best known technical difficulty in administering lumbar epidural anesthesia is accidental perforation of the dura mater, obvious by the flow of cerebrospinal fluid. However, a less well-known, and potentially dangerous, complication is *secondary perforation of the dura* after the patient has received more than one dose of medication with good results with the expected pattern of analgesia and partial motor paralysis. This rate problem has been observed after successful caudal and lumbar epidural blocks in about 1 of every 6000 to 20,000 cases; there is no satisfactory explanation apart from the suggestion that the catheter may secondarily "erode" the dura mater and penetrate the intrathecal space. However, one may produce a massive spinal block when repeating the dose, with potential hypotension and secondary fetal compromise (see Figure 18-21). Needless to say, serious problems of severe hypotension and/or respiratory insufficiency may arise as consequence of this accident.

More rarely one may observe untoward cardiovascular effects of epidural anesthesia, particularly when the anesthetic has added epinephrine solutions. In certain instances of hypersensitive vascular system the patients may respond with *severe hypertension,* perhaps due to the rapid absorption of epinephrine (Figure 18-35). In those cases it is absolutely essential to make the differential diagnosis from intravascular injection which may give a relatively similar picture.

The *effects of epidural anesthesia on FHR* have been variably reported as increased, decreased, to have late decelerations, or not affected. Many clinical reports were reviews of material studied retrospectively and/or without precise recording methods. When the information is obtained in a prospective manner and with refined monitoring techniques one must reach the conclusion that *epidural anesthesia itself does not affect the FHR patterns* (Figures 18-28, 18-33, 18-34, 18-36). Some authors assumed that when

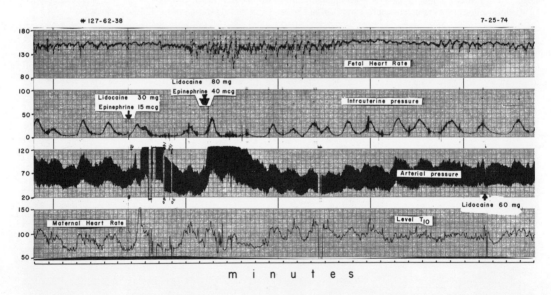

Figure 18-35 Direct FHR, UC, intraarterial pressure (femoral), and maternal heart rate recordings during term spontaneous labor in young primipara, 4 cm dilated. The test dose of 30 mg lidocaine and 15 μg epinephrine for epidural anesthesia triggered a sharp bout of hypertension and bradycardia with diminished uterine activity (blood pressure scale was adjusted to pick up maximum values). Full dose given 5 min later was immediately followed by a higher and more prolonged bout of hyperstension (with severe headaches), and also diminished uterine contractility. As the hypertension subsided, a significant hypotension with tachycardia was established. The uterine contractility rebounded with polysystoly. The FHR had a transient period of saltatory pattern and mild tachycardia. On the extreme right is shown the level of anesthesia (T-10) and that the repeat injection of plain lidocaine did not produce cardiovascular changes. The good level and absence of CNS reaction ruled out intravascular injection. Reprinted from Matadial L, Cibils LA: The effect of epidural anesthesia on uterine activity and blood pressure. *Am J Obstet Gynecol* 125:846, 1976.

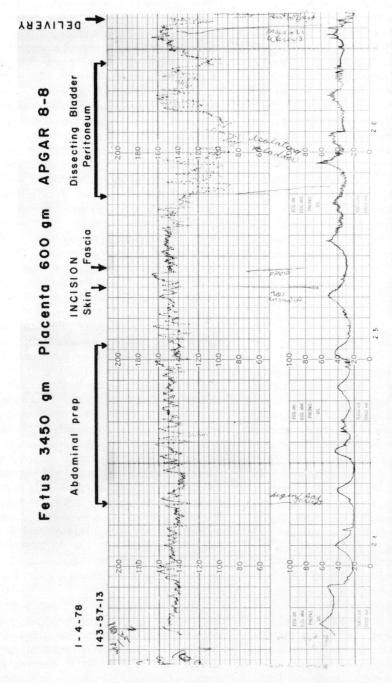

Figure 18-36 Direct UC and FHR tracings during preparation for, and performance of, extraperitoneal cesarean section for "relative cephalopelvic disproportion," carried out with patient under continuous epidural anesthesia. The FHR pattern maintained a good baseline frequency and oscillations. Fetal response to head compression (during separation of bladder and lower segment peritoneum) were not altered, showing the expected bradycardia. An infant in good condition was delivered.

alterations of the FHR were seen they were due to the toxic effect of the anesthetic reabsorbed from the peridural space and transferred to the fetus. But very small amounts of those substances have been measured in the fetal blood—usually much less than 2 $\mu g/ml$ of the local anesthetic. Others considered that the "inevitably high incidence of FHR alterations" was due to the high incidence of significant maternal hypotension. However, the few episodes of hypotension are easily correctable, and the FHR alterations, representing transient fetal hypoxia, are also amenable to prompt recovery by the same maneuvers (Figure 18-30). In the rare circumstances of observing other systemic side effects the FHR presents the alterations seen in fetal distress (saltatory pattern, tachycardia) and the subsequent recovery patterns (see Figure 18-35) when corrective measures are taken.

For pain relief during first stage or for operative deliveries of normal patients epidural block offers minimal interference with the maternal cardiovascular system and absence of deleterious effects on uterine activity and FHR patterns (Figure 18-36).

LOCAL ANESTHESIA

The perineural infiltration of a peripheral nerve, small branches or their endings, or a nervous plexus with a substance to obtain analgesia-anesthesia is defined as local anesthesia. In obstetrics there are several areas where the injection can be made depending on the moment of labor when the pain relief is sought. In some cases there are several ways to reach the nerves intended for blocking. Those blocks more frequently used are: local abdominal (for cesarean section), local perineal, pudendal, and paracervical blocks.

The maternal and fetal repercussions of *abdominal, perineal,* and *pudendal blocks* should be negligible under normal circumstances. Maternal systemic reaction (convulsion) with fetal compromise may occur following either the intravascular injection of the anesthetic or the administration of an excessive amount, which may lead to intoxication and fetal deterioration from placental transfer of the anesthetic. These complications are strictly preventable if the physician pays the required attention to technical details and knows the anatomy.

Paracervical block The infiltration of the lateral fornices of the vagina in the region of the hypogastric plexus and ganglia (plexus of Frankenhäuser) to block labor pains was first applied in Europe in the late 1920s. It was not until Rosenfeld (1954) published his first short series that it was introduced in the United States. Others published their experiences, thus contributing to the slow but steady increase in popularity and acceptance of this method of pain relief. With the increase in number of publications came, inevitably, the realization that there are potential fetal hazards inherent in this particular technique of anesthesia. A great amount of work on animals and humans has been carried out to clarify the mechanisms involved in the untoward fetal response occasionally seen after paracervical block (PCB). There are a number of hypotheses entertained by those investigators who worked on this problem, but at the present time there is no unanimous agreement on why the fetus may be unfavorably affected in some cases. Nevertheless, PCB is used extensively because it offers several advantages: excellent pain relief during the advanced stages of dilatation, administration by the obstetrician, and unlike conduction anesthesia methods, minimal maternal supervision after administration.

The *systemic maternal effects* are related mainly to the degree of pain relief obtained and the repercussion of pain on the cardiovascular system. Unrelieved pain probably triggers the release of endogenous catecholamines which, in turn, influence the blood pressure and pulse rate. Painless contractions would have a systemic effect on the cardiovascular system only as they directly influence the hemodynamics of circulation. The alterations triggered by pains are suppressed but reappear when the anesthetic effects pass and the sensation of pain returns. Among those cardiovascular effects, moderate degrees of hypertension and rapid oscillations of the blood pressure are obliterated by a good paracervical block (see Figure 7-19). At the same time, the fluctuations in pulse rate that follow the blood pressure changes are clearly affected when there is good pain relief (Figure 18-37).

There is no unanimous agreement with regard to the *effects of PCB on uterine contractility.* In some cases one may observe decreased contractility (Figure 18-38) while in others this may appear increased (Figure 18-41). However, in the majority of cases the *uterine contractility does not seem affected,* and when the activity is calculated no changes are observed from the preinjection values. Likewise, the efficiency of the contrac-

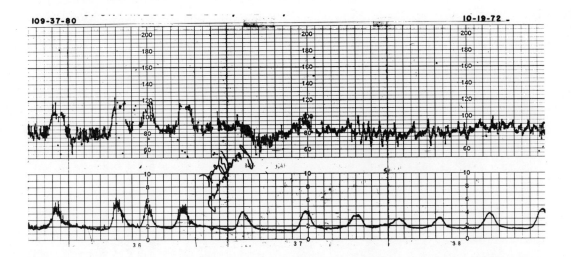

Figure 18-37 Direct intrauterine pressure recordings and maternal heart rate obtained through scalp electrode applied to a dead fetus. Active first stage of labor with painful contractions. Paracervical block anesthesia produced rapid relief without alteration of uterine contractility. The maternal heart rate pattern changed in that the accelerations observed with each painful contraction disappeared when anesthesia was obtained.

tions to dilate the cervix, assessed by the uterine work required for continuous steady progress, does not change after the administration of PCB.

Alterations of the FHR have been observed by almost all clinicians who have used PCB or studied its effects upon the fetus. The majority of observers have reported *bradycardias* occurring in variable proportion, ranging from 2% to 56%. There are numerous factors affecting the fetal response to PCB and the severity of the alterations observed. For some, they are so severe that they contraindicate its use in obstetrics while others advise against its use only in cases of high-risk gestation—perhaps because in almost all large clinical series there are intrapartum or neonatal deaths, and some are attributed to the PCB. However, in the majority of those deaths one may clearly find other factors that may have contributed to the fetal death.

The *alterations of the FHR* always occur within 8 min after the anesthetic injection, and often within 2 to 3 min, that is very rapidly. The changes in FHR range from minimal alterations to very severe bradycardias. The most frequently observed are transient bradycardias with or without superimposed baseline alterations (Figure 18-38) followed by rapid recovery. The mild episodes of bradycardia may also have superimposed decelerations, particularly during the

recovery periods (Figure 18-39). These may be followed by episodes of "rebound" tachycardia (Figure 18-40), which may last a relatively long time before returning to preinjection levels and, at the same time, manifest baseline changes indicative of alterations of fetal homeostasis (Figure 18-41). Often one may observe decelerations superimposed on the bradycardia and, on the period of recovery, to the tachycardia and fixed baseline (Figure 18-42). The less frequently described saltatory pattern is often present as part of the alterations of FHR following PCB. They may appear superimposed on periods of bradycardia (Figure 18-43) and followed by rebound tachycardia and fixed baseline, or may alternate with decelerations and even short periods of bradycardia, the pattern lasting for a prolonged period of time (Figure 18-44). Severe episodes of bradycardia and slow recovery are relatively infrequent, but they have a frightening appearance (Figure 18-45) with all the characteristics of altered fetal homeostasis. Recovery may be so slow that in spite of sufficient time elapsed between PCB and delivery the infant may be born before apparent complete recovery as suggested by the FHR pattern (Figure 18-46).

The overall incidence of FHR alterations (not only bradycardia, as reported by many) was 28% in the high-risk monitoring unit of the Chicago

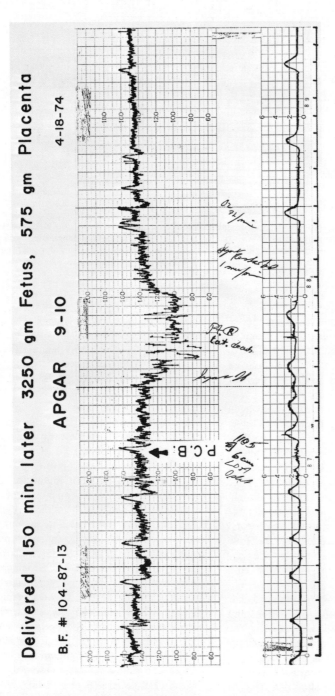

Figure 18-38 Direct FHR and UC recordings during enhanced labor of primipara at term, 6 cm dilatation. Within 4 min of PCB the FHR showed a transient bradycardia with superimposed saltatory pattern lasting about 4 min. The recovery was rapid followed by some diminution in the range of baseline oscillations. There is a clearly *decreased uterine activity* following a short polysystoly of two contractions and patient's turning to lateral. An infant in excellent condition was born 150 min later. Reprinted from Cibils LA, Santonja-Lucas JJ: Clinical significance of fetal heart rate patterns during labor. III. Effect of paracervical block anesthesia. *Am J Obstet Gynecol* 130:73, 1978.

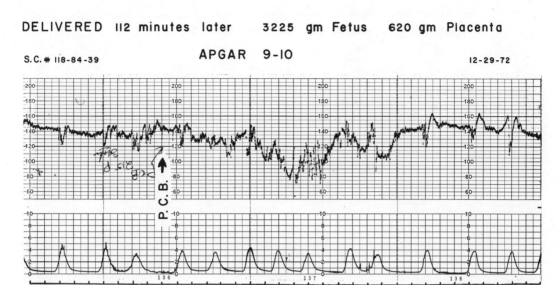

DELIVERED 112 minutes later   3225 gm Fetus   620 gm Placenta

S.C. # 118-84-39   APGAR 9-10   12-29-72

Figure 18-39 Direct FHR and UC recording advanced first stage of enhanced labor of term primipara. Within 6 min of PCB a *bradycardia* started with *superimposed saltatory pattern and late decelerations.* The latter continued to recur during the recovery phase completed 18 min after anesthesia. An infant in excellent condition was born 112 min later. Reprinted from Cibils LA, Santonja-Lucas JJ: Clinical significance of fetal heart rate patterns during labor. III. Effect of paracervical block anesthesia. *Am J Obstet Gynecol* 130:73, 1978.

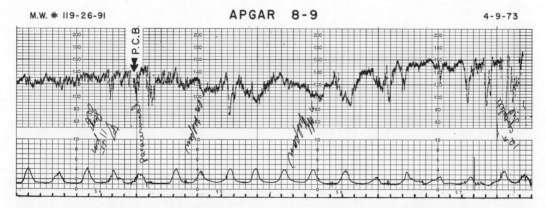

DELIVERED 54 minutes later 1900 gm Fetus, 360 gm Placenta

M.W. # 119-26-91   APGAR 8-9   4-9-73

Figure 18-40 Direct FHR and UC recordings from advanced first stage of premature labor in dichorionic twin gestation. A *moderate bradycardia* with *superimposed late decelerations* developed 5 min after PCB. Decelerations persisted during the period of recovery. *Rebound tachycardia* and tendency to fixed baseline were also present. No change in uterine contractility. A premature infant in good condition was delivered 21 min after the end of the record. Reprinted from Cibils LA, Santonja-Lucas JJ: Clinical significance of fetal heart rate patterns during labor. III. Effect of paracervical block anesthesia. *Am J Obstet Gynecol* 130:73, 1978.

452

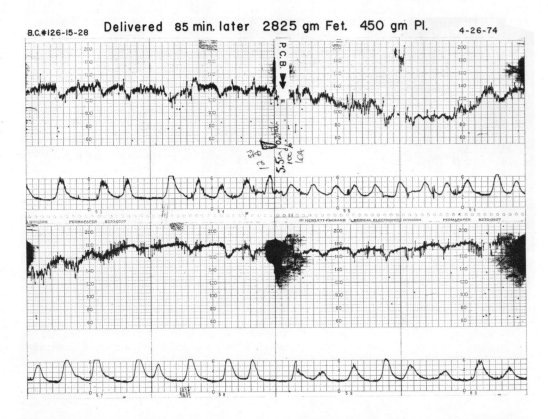

Figure 18-41 Continuous 80-min direct UC and FHR recordings during mid-first stage of spontaneous labor in primipara at term. Following PCB, a transient period of *increased uterine activity*. The normal baseline frequency with rapid oscillations and some early decelerations evolve within 3 min of anesthesia to an episode of *bradycardia* lasting 12 min followed by a significant *rebound tachycardia, fixed baseline, and small late decelerations* sustained until the end of the tracing. An infant with Apgar scores 8 and 10 was delivered 25 min later. Reprinted from Cibils LA, Santonja-Lucas JJ: Clinical significance of fetal heart rate patterns during labor. III. Effect of paracervical block anesthesia. *Am J Obstet Gynecol* 130:73, 1978.

Lying-In Hospital until some adjustments of technique were made. Since then the incidence has been significantly lower.

Numerous clinical conditions and technical details have been considered as *predisposing or determining factors to trigger FHR alterations*. Those patients who received *repeat PCB* have a significantly higher incidence of FHR changes; however, when the total number of injections is considered, the incidence is much the same as in the patients who received single injections. As in these patients, the changes are of the same type, on some occasions of moderate degree and on others of severe intensity (Figure 18-47). Of course when one overlooks some technical recom-

mendations (to reinject only after at least 40 min have passed since the previous injection) the chances of triggering severe FHR alterations are increased with the repeat dose (Figure 18-48).

Despite the potentially increased fetal hazard of repeat PCB, neonatal outcome is similar in both groups of patients. One should anticipate that Apgar scores of ≤ 6 at 1 and 5 minutes will be very similar: 14% and 16%, and 2% and 3% respectively in the Chicago Lying-In Hospital series, indirect evidence that the repeated injections do not seem to increase the chances of fetal depression. With routine use of PCB, one must expect that a greater number of primiparas will require repeat injections because they require longer

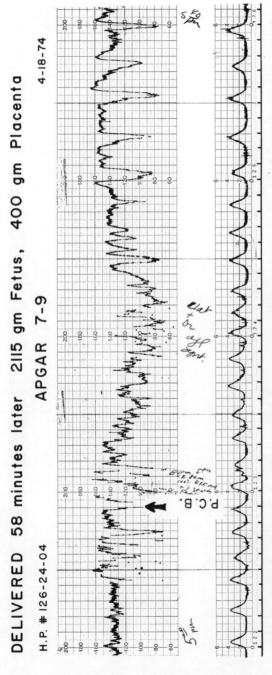

Figure 18-42 Direct UC and FHR recordings obtained from primipara in premature induced labor (PRM) and advanced first stage. Moderate hypercontractility precedes PCB, which is followed, within 4 min, by bradycardia, saltatory pattern, and superimposed decelerations. The recovery after 11 min is followed by rebound tachycardia, large decelerations lasting about 50 sec, and diminished baseline oscillations. An infant in good condition was born 26 min after the end of tracing. Reprinted from Cibils LA, Santonja-Lucas JJ: Clinical significance of fetal heart rate patterns during labor. III. Effect of paracervical block anesthesia. *Am J Obstet Gynecol* 130:73, 1978.

454

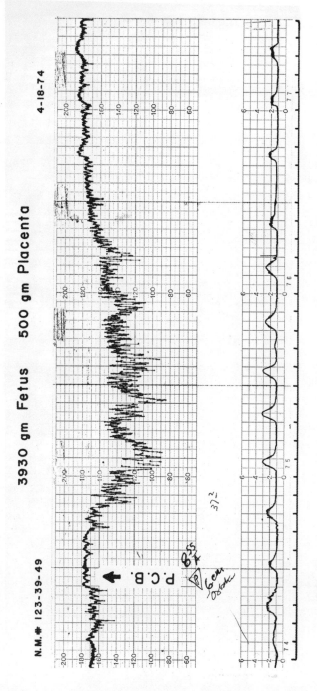

Figure 18-43 Direct UC and FHR tracings obtained from mid-first stage in enhanced labor of primipara with prolonged gestation (42 weeks). On a preexisting tachycardia, PCB triggered, within 4 min, a period of prolonged bradycardia with superimposed late decelerations and persistent saltatory pattern. This continued through part of the slow recovery ending in still higher tachycardia and fixed baseline. An infant in good condition was born 1 hour after the end of the tracing. The F/P ratio of 7.85 indicates chronic placental insufficiency. Reprinted from Cibils LA, Santonja-Lucas JJ: Clinical significance of fetal heart rate patterns during labor. III. Effect of paracervical block anesthesia. *Am J Obstet Gynecol* 130:73, 1978.

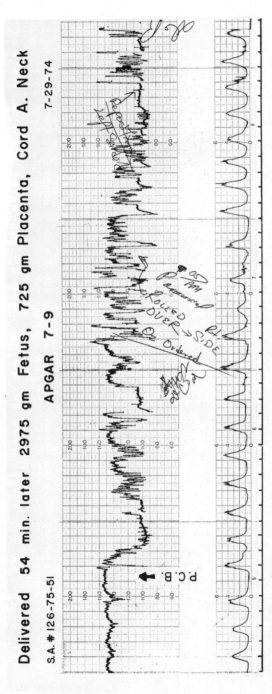

Figure 18-44 Direct UC and FHR tracings of advanced first stage induced labor of preeclamptic patient at term. Within 2 min of PCB there was a significant bradycardia followed by a pattern of alternating saltatory pattern, decelerations, and bradycardia; all these were still present 35 min after anesthesia when the record was discontinued. Delivery 16 min later produced an infant in good condition with one loop of cord around the neck. Reprinted from Cibils LA, Santonja-Lucas JJ: Clinical significance of fetal heart rate patterns during labor. III. Effect of paracervical block anesthesia. *Am J Obstet Gynecol* 130:73, 1978.

456

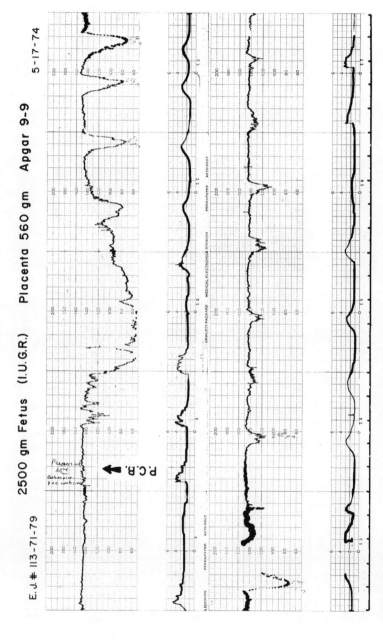

Figure 18-45 Continuous 50 min direct UC and FHR recordings of spontaneous labor at term in a patient who had low urinary estrogen level. (Paper speed, 2 cm/min, twice the standard recording speed.) A *fixed baseline* preceded the PCB, given with only 140 mg mepivacaine, and which within 4 min triggered *a severe and prolonged bradycardia.* The recovery was slow and marked by *severe late decelerations,* still present but somewhat diminished at the end of the recording. No change in uterine contractility. A growth-retarded infant in good condition was delivered 20 min after the end of tracing. Reprinted from Cibils LA, Santonja-Lucas JJ: Clinical significance of fetal heart rate patterns during labor. III. Effect of paracervical block anesthesia. *Am J Obstet Gynecol* 130:73, 1978.

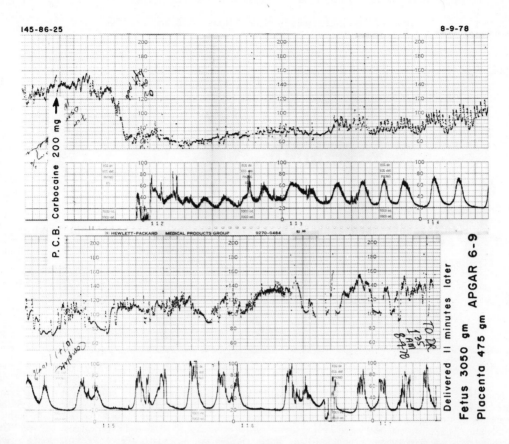

Figure 18-46 Continuous 64-min direct UC and FHR recording of advanced first and second stage of primipara at term in spontaneous labor. PCB given with 200 mg mepivacaine triggered within 4 min a *prolonged severe bradycardia* with superimposed saltatory pattern *(above, right)* in spite of continuous oxygen administration with patient in left lateral position. *(Below, left)* After completion of dilatation the FHR still continued in the bradycardic frequency with superimposed late decelerations marring the extremely slow recovery. It appears to be a significant hypercontractility coinciding with the onset of bradycardia but since there is no preceding tracing it is not possible to affirm that it was triggered by the anesthetic. A moderately depressed infant was delivered 11 min after the end of tracing.

labors to complete dilatation. On the other hand, FHR alterations recorded after one PCB do not necessarily indicate that the subsequent doses will similarly affect the fetus (Figure 18-49).

It is frequently pointed out that *maternal hypertension* should be a contraindication to the use of PCB; however in the Chicago Lying-In Hospital series there was exactly the same incidence of FHR alterations among the normotensive population (27%) as among the patients with increased blood pressure (28%). A given type of specific alteration may occur more often depending on the preexisting baseline pattern or frequency, but these do not indicate predisposition to alterations.

The *total dose* and the *concentration* of the drug used as anesthetic appear to influence the FHR response to PCB; the higher either one of them, the more chances of alterations. Likewise, the *addition of epinephrine to the anesthetic* solution markedly increases the likelihood of significant FHR alterations. This is so predictable that the use of epinephrine should be discouraged with the solution used for PCB.

Other factors have been incriminated as predisposing, like preeclampsia, fetal distress, primiparity, diabetes, but there is no convincing evidence that they are significant.

The repercussions of the FHR alterations following the anesthesia seem to be negligible with

458

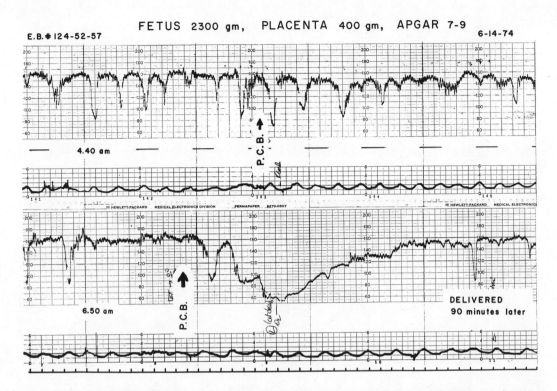

FETUS 2300 gm, PLACENTA 400 gm, APGAR 7-9

E.B.#124-52-57   6-14-74

Figure 18-47 Two 45-min segments of direct UC and FHR recordings of preeclamptic primipara at term in spontaneous labor, carrying twins. Uterine contractions are of low intensity due to the overdistension of the uterus. At the beginning of the tracing there are variable FHR decelerations on a borderline tachycardic baseline with normal oscillations. The *patient had been receiving magnesium sulfate intravenously* to control hyperreflexia. *(Above)* PCB triggered *three late decelerations* without baseline changes. *(Below)* Two hours later a repeat PCB triggered a *severe and prolonged bradycardia with fixed baseline* followed by a slow recovery. This twin was delivered in good condition 1 hour after the end of the tracing. Reprinted from Cibils LA, Santonja-Lucas JJ: Clinical significance of fetal heart rate patterns during labor. III. Effect of paracervical block anesthesia. *Am J Obstet Gynecol* 130:73, 1978.

regard to *fetal outcome:* there is no difference in the incidence of depressed infants between those who had alterations and those who did not have FHR changes. Interestingly, *there is a negative correlation between anesthesia to delivery time and Apgar scores.* In other words, the shorter the elapsed time from PCB to delivery, the higher the Apgar score. This fact disputes the standard advice given in textbooks and monographs that delivery should be postponed for at least 30 min or more after post-PCB alterations of the FHR, to allow for recovery of normal heart function and fetal homeostasis. That recommendation is further disputed because infants delivered within 20 min of PCB administration have the same incidence of neonatal depression as those delivered beyond that span of time: approximately 15% in-

cidence of Apgar scores of 6 or less for both groups of patients. Vigorous infants are delivered even when apparently still recovering from an episode of bradycardia (Figure 18-50).

Several hypotheses attempt to explain the mechanism whereby PCB alters the FHR patterns: uterine hypercontractility, anesthetic intoxication, and uterine artery spasm.

The uterine hypercontractility hypothesis postulates that the anesthetic administration triggers an increased uterine activity and/or tonus that would interfere with blood flow to cause hypoxia with alterations of FHR. This very sensible theory is at variance with the facts: only exceptionally have hypercontractility (polysystoly and/or hypertonus) been documented, even by those authors who support this mechanism of

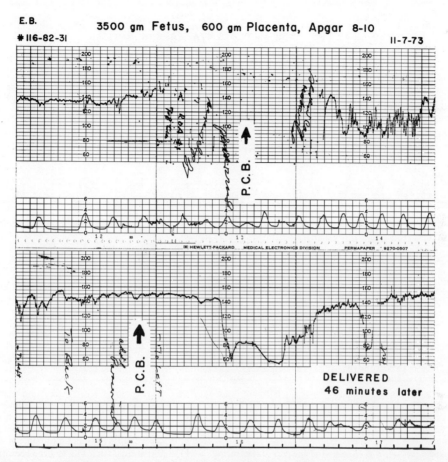

Figure 18-48 Continuous 60-min direct UC and FHR recordings during enhanced labor of primipara at term in advanced first stage (7.5 cm dilatation). *(Above)* First PCB was followed 5 min later by an episode of moderate bradycardia with superimposed saltatory pattern from which it recovered rapidly. *(Below)* A second PCB was given only *22 min after the first one* and was followed within 6 min by a severe and *prolonged bradycardia* with slow recovery without rebound. An infant in good condition was delivered 46 min after the end of the recording. Reprinted from Cibils LA, Santonja-Lucas JJ: Clinical significance of fetal heart rate patterns during labor. III. Effect of paracervical block anesthesia. *Am J Obstet Gynecol* 130:73, 1978.

action. As a matter of fact, even the use of β-mimetic substances to depress uterine contractility have not been sufficient to prevent or correct FHR alterations produced by PCB (Santonja and Bonilla, 1974).

The *anesthetic intoxication* hypothesis suggests that the drug is absorbed and transferred to the fetus with "production of sudden cardiovascular insufficiency through a direct effect on the fetal heart and/or CNS leading to tissue hypoxia. . . . Acidosis is mainly metabolic, and therefore it cannot originate from an acute placental insufficiency" (Teramo, 1969). This hypothesis has been extensively investigated by

several authors, but a number of important inconsistencies remain, without explanation, between the clinical observations and the pharmacology and toxicology of local anesthetics.

1. The FHR alterations *start within 8 min* after PCB (often within 2 to 3 min whereas the highest *maternal and fetal blood levels* are seen at about 20 min. At this moment the toxic effects should be maximum, but FHR alterations have already returned to normal or are well on their way to normalization in the majority of cases.

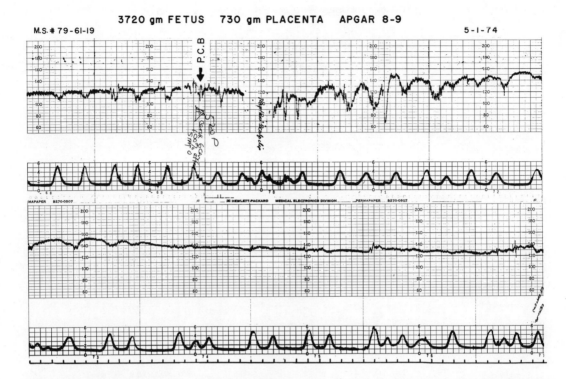

Figure 18-49 Continuous 92-min direct UC and FHR recordings of term spontaneous labor of primipara, 6 cm dilatation. Minimal early FHR decelerations before PCB, which was followed, within 5 min, by a moderate bradycardia, late decelerations, and rebound tachycardia with fixed baseline. The slow recovery was completed only 60 min after the anesthesia and strongly resembles the recoveries observed after hypercontractility-induced hypoxia. The patient received a *second PCB* 15 min after the end of the tracing. No FHR alterations. An infant in good condition was delivered 55 min later. Reprinted from Cibils LA, Santonja-Lucas JJ: Clinical significance of fetal heart rate patterns during labor. III. Effect of paracervical block anesthesia. *Am J Obstet Gynecol* 130:73, 1978.

2. The *tolerance and toxicity studies* in animals and human fetuses (after large intravenous injections to the mother) indicate that the blood concentrations needed to trigger cardiovascular changes or CNS symptoms are much higher than the values recorded in clinical observations (usually 2 μg/ml or less; rarely 3 μg/ml or above). The accidental intoxication by large intrafetal injections documented that 8 μg/ml does not produce tachycardia or vascular collapse (Finster et al, 1965). Likewise, the massive planned injection of local anesthetic to a fetus does not induce bradycardia (Freeman et al, 1972) which occurs only with further intoxication and as a terminal phenomenon.

3. The *fetal ECG changes* recorded during post-PCB bradycardias have no QRS abnormalities and only P wave changes. The *fetuses receiving toxic doses of local anesthetic* have prolonged P-R intervals and *widened QRS complex but without bradycardia.* These findings suggest that post-PCB bradycardia is not the cardiac response to anesthetic intoxication.

4. The clinical observations of fetuses born in excellent condition shortly after an episode of severe bradycardia (Figure 18-51) or during the period that should be maximum intoxication (Figure 18-52) further suggest that a mechanism other than direct intoxication may be responsible for the FHR alterations.

DELIVERED   20 minutes later   2975 gm Fetus, 450 gm Placenta

G.K.# 95-53-54   Apgar   9-10   7-17-72

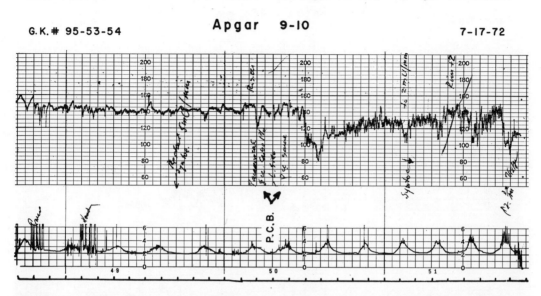

Figure 18-50   Last 32 min of direct UC and FHR tracingss of enhanced labor of multipara at term. Mepivacaine 150 mg was given for PCB and within 2 min an episode of *moderate but sustained bradycardia* with increased baseline oscillations was observed. No complete recovery had occurred when the record was discontinued, and an infant in excellent condition was born 5 min after this, and 20 min after anesthesia. Reprinted from Cibils LA, Santonja-Lucas JJ: Clinical significance of fetal heart rate patterns during labor. III. Effect of paracervical block anesthesia. *Am J Obstet Gynecol* 130:73, 1978.

To be acceptable, a hypothesis must reconcile all the clinical observations with known principles of physiology and pharmacology. The uterine artery spasm hypothesis (Cibils, 1976) appears to answer the majority of the questions.

The *uterine artery spasm hypothesis* postulates that the first link in the chain of events that follows the PCB anesthesia that triggers FHR alterations is a spastic response of the uterine arteries exposed to a high concentration of the anesthetic substances — potent oxytocics that also strongly stimulate the smooth muscle of the uterine arteries at concentrations many times lower than those used in clinical practice for nerve blocking (Figure 18-53). This contractile response is dose-dependent, the strongest and most prolonged effect seen with the larger and more concentrated doses. The spasm would cause severe curtailment of IVS blood flow and consequently diminished oxygen supply to the fetus and hypoxia.

As discussed previously, late decelerations and bradycardia are only different degrees of response to episodes of hypoxia triggered by uterine contractions. The recovery patterns following them are usually rebound tachycardia and fixed baseline. Saltatory patterns are also often seen in situations of transient fetal hypoxia and distress.

Animal studies conducted by Greiss and associates (1976) corroborated these in vitro observations. They demonstrated that local anesthetics infused into the uterine arteries markedly decreased uterine blood flow independent of the effects on uterine contractility. This response is also dose-dependent, and at equiactive concentrations bupivacaine (Marcaine) has a much stronger and prolonged effect than mepivacaine or lidocaine.

The standard concentration of 1% solutions would make a concentration of 10,000 μg/ml at the site of injection, but due to dilution in interstitial fluid the actual concentration must be lower at the periphery of the infiltrate. However, this would be many times higher than the in vitro concentrations producing strong, sharp, contractile responses in uterine artery specimens. The

462

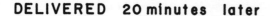
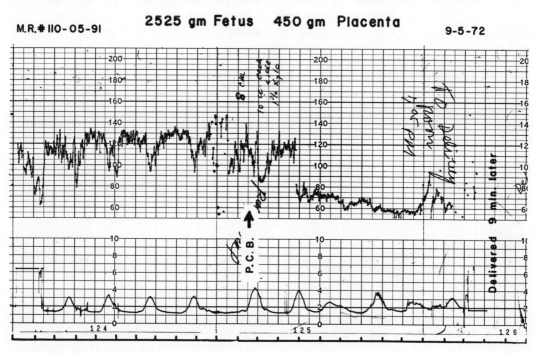

Figure 18-51   Last 22 min of direct UC and FHR tracings of enhanced labor of multipara at term. Lidocaine, 200 mg, given for PCB triggered within 3 min a prolonged bradycardia without recovery until the recording was discontinued. Nine minutes later (20 min after anesthesia) an infant in good condition was delivered. Reprinted from Cibils LA, Santonja-Lucas JJ: Clinical significance of fetal heart rate patterns during labor. III. Effect of paracervical block anesthesia. *Am J Obstet Gynecol* 130:73, 1978.

duration of the spasm and recovery time must be related to the drug concentration and to the distance from the artery at which the injection is made. The hypoxic episode may be moderately benign (Figure 18-37) or trigger severe FHR changes (Figures 18-45, 18-46) — additional indirect evidence of the variation in degree of vascular spasm or its duration.

The comparison of the FHR alterations triggered by hypercontractility with those following PCB further illustrates the similarities between them. Compare Figure 18-54 with Figures 9-12 and 12-25. The quickly triggered bradycardia, the late decelerations, the rebound tachycardia, fixed baseline, and slow recovery are all indistinguishable in both situations. The ideal observation would be if both types of episodes could be observed in the same patient. If the FHR altera-

tions are similar, one may safely postulate that indeed the two circumstances are due to the same mechanism; such an example may be seen in Figure 18-55.

Only one question remains to be answered if the uterine artery spasm hypothesis is the most likely mechanism involved in FHR alterations following PCB. Why is it that only less than one-third of all cases manifest these changes? Probably because of a combination of several factors: the uterine arteries are exposed to different degrees of drug concentrations depending on the variable depths of the injection. This situation would explain, in different cases, the unequal severity of vasospasm, which is dose-dependent. On the other hand, in sheep (Assali et al, 1962) and rhesus monkeys (Myers, 1972) it has been shown that it is necessary to diminish the IVS

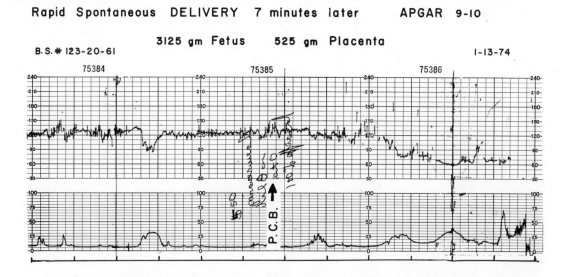

Figure 18-52 Last 12 min of direct UC and FHR tracings (paper speed, 3 cm/min) of enhanced labor of multipara at term. Within 3 min of PCB the fetus developed severe bradycardia, *and delivery occurred during the episode of bradycardia* 1 min after the end of the tracing. Infant was in excellent condition. Reprinted from Cibils LA, Santonja-Lucas JJ: Clinical significance of fetal heart rate patterns during labor. III. Effect of paracervical block anesthesia. *Am J Obstet Gynecol* 130:73, 1978.

blood flow by at least 50% in fetuses in good condition to induce bradycardia or symptomatic fetal hypoxia.

This wide range of "fetal reserve" would explain why FHR alterations are not seen more often while moderate arterial spasms may be very frequently induced. It is then clear that post-PCB alterations of the FHR are expressions of transient or moderately sustained hypoxia due to decreased IVS blood flow. This mechanism would also explain why the fetuses born during, or shortly after, episodes of severe bradycardia (see Figures 18-51, 18-52) are in such excellent condition. Thus, the recommendation that delivery be postponed in those cases for at least 30 min to allow for "fetal detoxification and recovery" is not warranted. When FHR alterations are observed there is no need to hasten labor or delivery. It is a self limiting episode that subsides relatively rapidly. Probably the administration of oxygen to the mother is the only potentially effective thing to do, and this helps in a very limited way.

From the foregoing it seems that the clinical manifestation of uterine artery spasm should be preventable, providing some technical points are carefully observed.

There should be no need to ban the use of PCB. The anesthetic drug should be used at concentrations no higher than 1%, in moderate volume and without added epinephrine. Bupivacaine, which at the standard concentration has a very strong and prolonged effect on the uterine vascular tree, should be avoided. The most critical point is that the injection site must be rather superficial (Figure 18-56), made at a reasonable distance from the uterine artery pedicles. If the procedure is done in this manner, the nervous plexus will still be infiltrated but the arteries would not be exposed to high concentrations of the drug.

If these steps are taken there is no reason to withhold this excellent method of pain relief from high-risk patients in general or hypertensive patients in particular.

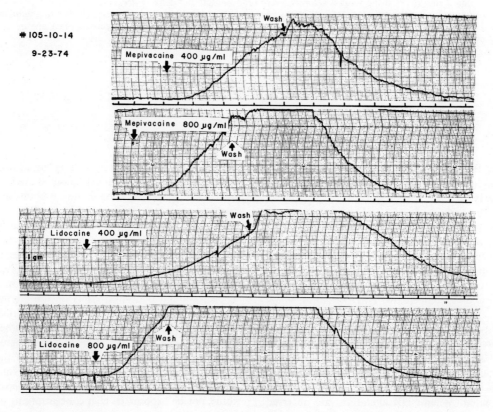

Figure 18-53 In vitro response to local anesthetics of radial uterine artery strips obtained from term pregnancy during cesarean hysterectomy. Note the steeper rise of the contraction wave with higher concentrations of both drugs, as well as the more prolonged time taken for relaxation after they have been washed out of the bath and rinsed with fresh Krebs' solution. (Time scale in min in the abscissa, and five thick lines in ordinates = 1 gm tension. The arrows indicate the addition of the anesthesia to the bath and its final concentration.) Reprinted from Cibils LA: Response of human uterine arteries to local anesthetics. *Am J Obstet Gynecol* 126:202, 1976.

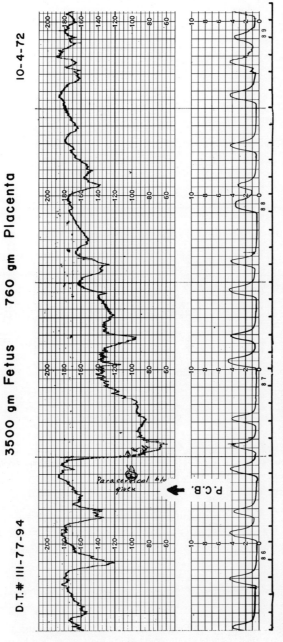

Figure 18-54 Direct UC and FHR tracings of advanced enhanced labor of multipara at term with meconium-stained amniotic fluid. Uterine contractility is normal. FHR illustrates tachycardia and late decelerations before PCB, which was followed within 2 min by severe prolonged bradycardia, slow recovery with late decelerations, fixed baseline, and tachycardia. A mildly depressed infant was delivered 20 min after the end of the tracing. Reprinted from Cibils LA, Santonja-Lucas JJ: Clinical significance of fetal heart rate patterns during labor. III. Effect of paracervical block anesthesia. *Am J Obstet Gynecol* 130:73, 1978.

466

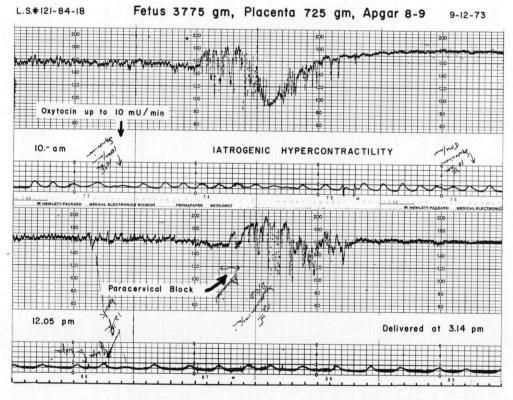

Figure 18-55 Two 40-min segments of direct UC and FHR tracings obtained during enhanced labor of primipara at term with meconium-stained amniotic fluid. *(Above)* Hypercontractility (polysystoly and hypertonus) following increase of oxytocin infusion to 10 mU/min, which triggered a marked saltatory pattern and bradycardia followed by rebound tachycardia and fixed baseline. *(Below)* A similar episode with less bradycardia was recorded 2 hours later during normal uterine contractility maintained with 1 mU/min oxytocin and within 2 min after PCB. An infant in good condition was born 3 hours later. Reprinted from Cibils LA, Santonja-Lucas JJ: Clinical significance of fetal heart rate patterns during labor. III. Effect of paracervical block anesthesia. *Am J Obstet Gynecol* 130:73, 1978.

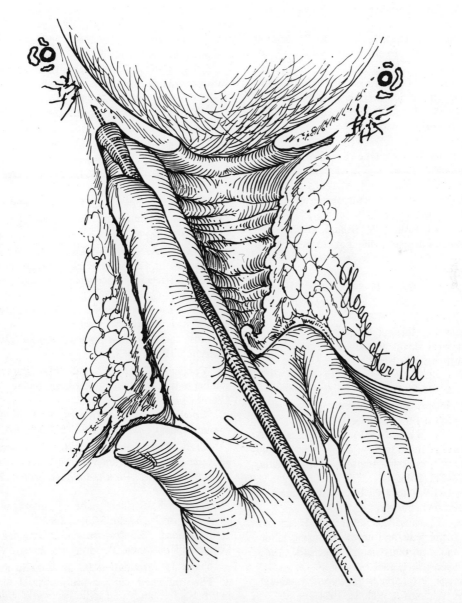

Figure 18-56 Technique of injection to obtain a safe paracervical block anesthesia. The injection must be done between 3 and 4 and 8 and 9 o'clock positions with the needle entering only superficially and the *guide not pushing* through the fornix. The anesthetic should diffuse and reach the nervous plexus, while the uterine arteries should be exposed to only minimal amounts. Modified from Davis JE, et al: The combined paracervical-pudenal block anesthesia for labor and delivery. *Am J Obstet Gynecol* 89:366, 1964.

BIBLIOGRAPHY

Akamatsu TJ, Ueland K, Der Yuen D, et al: Maternal cardiovascular dynamics. VII. Cesarean section under epidural anesthesia with epinephrine. *Obstet Gynecol* 43:616, 1974.

Althabe O, Schwarcz RL, Pose SV, et al: Effects on fetal heart and fetal pO_2 of oxygen administration to the mother. *Am J Obstet Gynecol* 98:858, 1967.

Alvarado A, Bazan T, Peredo C: Continuous paracervical block. *Am J Obstet Gynecol* 97:367, 1967.

Alvarez H, Caldeyro-Barcia R: Fisiopatologia de la contraccion uterina y sus aplicaciones en clinica obstetrica. *II Cong Lat-Am Obstet Ginecol (Brasil)* 1:1, 1954.

Alver EC, White CW, Weiss JB, et al: An effect of succinylcholine on the uterus. *Am J Obstet Gynecol* 83:795, 1962.

Asling JH, Shnider SM, Margolis AJ, et al: Paracervical block anesthesia in obstetrics. II. *Am J Obstet Gynecol* 107:626, 1970.

Assali NS, Holm LW, Sehgal N: Hemodynamic changes in fetal lamb in utero in response to asphyxia, hypoxia and hypercapnia. *Circ Res* 11:423, 1962.

Beazley JM, Taylor G, Reynolds F: Placental transfer of bupivacaine after paracervical block. *Obstet Gynecol* 39:2, 1972.

Bloom SL, Horswill CW, Curet LB: Effects of paracervical blocks on the fetus during labor: A prospective study with the use of direct fetal monitoring. *Am J Obstet Gynecol* 114:218, 1972.

Bonica JJ: *Principles and Practice of Obstetric Analgesia and Anesthesia,* Philadelphia, Davis, 1972.

Bonica JJ, Kennedy WF, Ward RJ, et al: A comparison of the effects of high subarachnoid and epidural anesthesia. *Acta Anaesthesiol Scand [Suppl]* 23:429, 1966.

Borgers LF, Gücer G: Effect of magnesium on epileptic foci. *Epilepsia* 19:81, 1978.

Brady JP, James LS, Baker MA: Heart rate changes in the fetus and newborn during labor, delivery and immediate neonatal period. *Am J Obstet Gynecol* 84:1, 1962.

Bromage PR: *Spinal Epidural Analgesia.* Baltimore, Williams & Wilkins, 1954.

Bromage PR: Physiology and pharmacology of epidural analgesia. *Anesthesiology* 28:592, 1967.

Bromage PR: Continuous lumbar epidural analgesia for obstetrics. *Can Med Assoc J* 85:1136, 1961.

Bromage PR, Robson JG: Concentrations of lignocaine in the blood after intravenous, intramuscular, epidural and endotracheal administration. *Anaesthesia* 16:461, 1961.

Caldeyro-Barcia R, Mendez-Bauer C, Poseiro J, et al: Fetal monitoring in labor, in Wallace HM, Gold EM, Lis EF (eds): *Maternal and Child Health Practices.* Springfield, Ill, Thomas, 1973, pp 332–394.

Cibils LA: Clinical significance of fetal heart rate patterns during labor. I. Baseline patterns. *Am J Obstet Gynecol* 125:290, 1976.

Cibils LA: Clinical significance of fetal heart rate patterns during labor. II. Late decelerations. *Am J Obstet Gynecol* 123:473, 1975.

Cibils: LA: Response of human uterine arteries to local anesthetics. *Am J Obstet Gynecol* 126:202, 1976.

Cibils LA: Clinical significance of fetal heart rate patterns during labor. IV. Agonal patterns. *Am J Obstet Gynecol* 129:833, 1977.

Cibils LA, Santonja-Lucas JJ: Clinical significance of fetal heart rate patterns during labor. III. Effect of paracervical block anesthesia. *Am J Obstet Gynecol* 130:73, 1978.

Cibils LA, Spackman TJ: Caudal analgesia in first stage of labor: Effect on uterine activity and the cardiovascular system. *Am J Obstet Gynecol* 84:1042, 1962.

Cooper K, Gilroy KJ, Hurry DJ: Paracervical nerve block in labor using bupivacaine. *Br J Obstet Gynaecol* 75:863, 1968.

Cowles GT: Experiences with lumbar epidural block. *Obstet Gynecol* 26:734, 1965.

Craft JB, Epstein BS, Coakley CS: Effect of lidocaine with epinephrine versus lidocaine (plain) on induced labor. *Anesth Analg (Cleve)* 51:243, 1972.

Crawford JS: The place of halothane in obstetrics. *Br J Anaesth* 34:386, 1962.

Crawford JS: *Principles and Practice of Obstetrics Anesthesia.* London, Blackwell, 1978.

Davis JE, Frudenfeld JC, Frudenfeld K, et al: The combined paracervical-pudendal block anesthesia for labor and delivery. *Am J Obstet Gynecol* 89:366, 1964.

DeMot E, Muller G, Irrmann M, et al: The role played by uterine hypertonia in the fetal risk associated with paracervical block. *Proc 2nd Eur Cong Perinatal Med,* London, 1970, p 26.

DeVoe SJ, DeVoe K, Rigsby WC, et al: Effect of meperidine on uterine contractility. *Am J Obstet Gynecol* 105:1004, 1969.

Edwards WB, Hingson RA: Continuous caudal anesthesia in obstetrics. *Am J Surg* 57:459, 1942.

Evans JA, Chastain GM, Phillips JM: The use of local anesthetic agents in obstetrics. *South Med J* 62:519, 1969.

Felton DJC, Goddard BA: The effect of suxamethonium chloride on uterine activity. *Lancet* 1:852, 1966.

Fernandez R, Gomez-Rogers C: Single-dose caudal anesthesia. *Am J Obstet Gynecol* 98:847, 1967.

Filler WW, Hall WC, Filler NW: Analgesia in obstetrics. *Am J Obstet Gynecol* 98:832, 1967.

Finster M, Poppers PJ, Sinclair JC, et al: Accidental intoxication of the fetus with local anesthetic drug during caudal anesthesia. *Am J Obstet Gynecol* 92:922, 1965.

Foldes FF, Molloy R, McNall PG: Comparison of toxicity of intravenously given local anesthetics in man. *JAMA* 172:1493, 1960.

Freeman DW, Bellville TP, Barno A: Paracervical block anesthesia in labor. *Obstet Gynecol* 8:270, 1956.

Freeman RK, Gutierrez N, Ray ML, et al: Fetal cardiac response to paracervical block anesthesia. I. *Am J Obstet Gynecol* 113:583, 1972.

Friedman EA, Sachtleben MR: Caudal anesthesia. The factors that influence its effect on labor. *Obstet Gynecol* 13:442, 1959.

Gabert HA, Stenchever MA: Electronic fetal monitoring in association with paracervical blocks. *Am J Obstet Gynecol* 116:1143, 1973.

Gomez DF: Paracervical block in obstetrics. *Lancet* 1:1163, 1969.

Gordon HR: Fetal bradycardia after paracervical block. *N Engl J Med* 279:910, 1968.

Greiss FC, Still JG, Anderson SG: Effects of local anesthetic agents on the uterine vasculatures and myometrium. *Am J Obstet Gynecol* 124:889, 1976.

Grimes DA, Cates W: Deaths from paracervical anesthesia used for first-trimester abortions. *N Engl J Med* 295:1397, 1976.

Gunther RE, Bauman J: Obstetric caudal anesthesia. *Anesthesiology* 31:5, 1969.

Hamilton LA, Gottschalk W: Paracervical block: Advantages and disadvantages. *Clin Obstet Gynecol* 17:199, 1974.

Hehre FW, Moyes AZ, Senfield RM, et al: Continuous lumbar epidural anesthesia in obstetrics. II. *Anesth Analg* 44:89, 1965.

Hendricks CH: The hemodynamics of a uterine contraction. *Am J Obstet Gynecol* 76:969, 1958.

Hingson RA, Cull WA: Conduction anesthesia and analgesia for obstetrics. *Clin Obstet Gynecol* 4:87, 1961.

Hollmen A, Korhonen J, Ojala A: Bupivacaine in paracervical block. Plasma levels and changes in maternal and fetal acid-base balance. *Br J Anaesth* 41:603, 1969.

Hon EH: Additional observations on "pathologic" bradycardia. *Am J Obstet Gynecol* 118:428, 1974.

Hopkins EL, Hendricks CH, Cibils LA: Cerebrospinal fluid pressure in labor. *Am J Obstet Gynecol* 93:907, 1965.

Hyman MD, Shnider SM: Maternal and neonatal blood concentrations of bupivacaine associated with obstetrical conduction anesthesia. *Anesthesiology* 34:81, 1971.

Ivankovic AD, Elam JO, Huffman J: Effect of maternal hypercarbia on the newborn infant. *Am J Obstet Gynecol* 107:939, 1970.

Ivankovic AD, Elam JO, Huffman J: Methoxyflurane anesthesia for cesarean section. *J Reprod Med* 6:105, 1971.

Iuppa JB, Smith GA, Colella JJ, et al: Succinylcholine effect on human myometrial activity. *Obstet Gynecol* 37:591, 1971.

James LS, Gordon HR, Finster M: Fetal mepivacaine toxicity not established. *N Engl J Med* 278:1072, 1968.

James LS, Morishima HO, Daniel SS, et al: Mechanism of late deceleration of the fetal heart rate. *Am J Obstet Gynecol* 113:578, 1972.

Jung H, Kopecky P, Klock FK: Die fetale Gefahrdung durch die "Parazervikalblockaden." *Geburtshilfe Frauenheilkd* 29:519, 1969.

Kobak AJ, Sadove MS: Combined paracervical and pudendal nerve blocks—A simple form of transvaginal regional anesthesia. *Am J Obstet Gynecol* 81:72, 1961.

Koback AJ, Sadove MS, Mazeros WT: Anatomic studies of transvaginal regional anesthesia. *Obstet Gynecol* 19:302, 1962.

Lehew WL: Paracervical block in obstetrics. *Am J Obstet Gynecol* 113:1079, 1972.

Liston WA, Adjepon-Yamoah KK, Scott DB: Fetal and maternal lignocaine levels after paracervical block. *Br J Anaesth* 45:750, 1973.

Lowe HJ: Flame ionization detection of volatile organic anesthetics in blood, gases and tissues. *Anesthesiology* 25:808, 1964.

Lowensohn RI, Paul RH, Fales S, et al: Intrapartum epidural anesthesia. *Obstet Gynecol* 44:388, 1974.

Martin K, Rathgen GH, Schwethelm R, et al: Mepivacain (Scandicain) Blutspiegel-Untersuchungen nach parazervikalen block. *Geburtshilfe Frauenheilkd* 29:711, 1969.

Marx GF, Kim YI, Lin CC, et al: Postpartum uterine pressure under halothane or enflurane anesthesia. *Obstet Gynecol* 51:695, 1978.

Matadial L, Cibils LA: The effect of epidural anesthesia on uterine activity and blood pressure. *Am J Obstet Gynecol* 125:846, 1976.

Moir DD: Anesthesia for cesarean section. *Br J Anaesth* 42:136, 1970.

Moore DC, Bridenbaugh LD, Bagdi PA, et al: Accumulation of mepivacaine hydrochloride during caudal block. *Anesthesiology* 29:585, 1968.

Morishima HO, Daniel SS, Finster M, et al: Transmission of mepivacaine hydrochloride across the human placenta. *Anesthesiology* 27:147, 1966.

Morishima HO, Gutsche BG, Stark RI, et al: Relationship of fetal bradycardia to maternal administration of lidocaine in sheep. *Am J Obstet Gynecol* 134:289, 1979.

Morishima HO, Heymann MA, Rudolph AM, et al: Toxicity of lidocaine in the fetal and newborn lamb and its relationship to asphyxia. *Am J Obstet Gynecol* 112:72, 1972.

Morishima HO, Heymann MA, Rudolph AM, et al: Transfer of lidocaine across the sheep placenta to the fetus. *Am J Obstet Gynecol* 122:581, 1975.

Murphy PJ, Wright JD, Fitzgerald TB: Assessment of paracervical nerve block anesthesia during labor. *Br Med J* 1:526, 1970.

Myers RE: Two patterns of perinatal brain damage and their conditions of occurrence. *Am J Obstet Gynecol* 112:246, 1972.

Noriega-Guerra L, Rodriguez de la Fuente F, Arevalo N, et al: Efecto de la bupivacaina sobre la contractilidad uterina. *Ginecol Obstet Mex* 27:639, 1970.

Nyirjesy I, Hawks BL, Hebert JE, et al: Hazards of the use of paracervical block anesthesia in obstetrics. *Am J Obstet Gynecol* 87:231, 1963.

Paul RH, Freeman RK: Fetal cardiac response to paracervical block anesthesia. II. *Am J Obstet Gynecol* 113:592, 1972.

Petrie RH, Paul WL, Miller FC, et al: Placental transfer of lidocaine following paracervical block. *Am J Obstet Gynecol* 120:791, 1974.

Pose SV, Cibils LA, Zuspan FP: Effect of *l*-epinephrine on uterine contractility and cardiovascular system. *Am J Obstet Gynecol* 84:297, 1962.

Riffel HD, Nochimson DJ, Paul RH, et al: Effects of meperidine and promethazine during labor. *Obstet Gynecol* 42:738, 1973.

Ritmiller LF, Rippman ET: Caudal analgesia in obstetrics: Report of thirteen years' experience. *Obstet Gynecol* 9:25, 1957.

Rosefsky JB, Petersiel ME: Perinatal deaths associated with mepivacaine paracervical-block anesthesia in labor. *N Engl J Med* 278:530, 1968.

Rosenfeld S: Paracervical anesthesia for the relief of labor pains. *Am J Obstet Gynecol* 50:527, 1945.

Rucker JP: The action of adrenalin on the pregnant human uterus. *South Med J* 18:412, 1925.

Rucker JP: The use of Novocain in obstetrics. *Am J Obstet Gynecol* 9:35, 1925.

Santonja-Lucas JJ, Bonilla-Musoles F: Anestesia paracervical en obstetricia: Efectos sobre la dinamica uterina y frecuencia cardiaca fetal. *Rev Esp Obstet Gynecol* 33:87, 1974.

Shnider SM: Serum cholinesterase activity during pregnancy, labor and the puerperium. *Anesthesiology* 26:335, 1965.

Shnider SM, Asling JH, Holl JW, et al: Paracervical block in obstetrics. I. Fetal complications and neonatal morbidity. *Am J Obstet Gynecol* 107:619, 1970.

Shnider SM, Asling JH, Margolis AJ, et al: High fetal blood levels of mepivacaine and fetal bradycardia. *N Engl J Med.* 279:947, 1968.

Shnider SM, Gildea J: Paracervical block anesthesia in obstetrics. III. Choice of drug. *Am J Obstet Gynecol* 116:320, 1973.

Shnider SM, Way EL: The kinetics of transfer of lidocaine across the human placenta. *Anesthesiology* 29:944, 1968.

Shnider SM, Way EL: Plasma levels of lidocaine in mother and newborn following obstetrical conduction anesthesia. *Anesthesiology* 29:951, 1968.

Sica-Blanco Y, Rozada H, Remedio MR: Effect of meperidine on uterine contractility during pregnancy and pre-labor. *Am J Obstet Gynecol* 97:1096, 1967.

Sinclair JC, Fox HA, Lentz JF, et al: Intoxication of the fetus by a local anesthetic. *N Engl J Med* 273:1173, 1965.

Steffenson JL, Shnider SM, DeLorimier AA: Transarterial diffusion of mepivacaine. *Anesthesiology* 32:459, 1970.

Steinhaus JE: Local anesthetic toxicity: A pharmacological re-evaluation. *Anesthesiology* 18:275, 1957.

Sunshine I, Fike WW: Value of thin layer chromatography in two fatal cases of intoxication due to lidocaine and mepivacaine. *N Engl J Med* 271:487, 1964.

Tafeen CH, Freedman HL, Harris H: Combined continued paracervical and continuous pudendal nerve block anesthesia in labor. *Am J Obstet Gynecol* 100:55, 1968.

Taw RL: Paracervical-pudendal block (discussion). *Am J Obstet Gynecol* 89:375, 1964.

Teramo K: Studies on foetal acid–base values after paracervical blockade during labor. *Acta Obstet Gynecol Scand* (suppl 3)48:80, 1969.

Teramo K: Fetal acid–base balance and heart rate during labour with bupivacaine paracervical anesthesia. *Br J Obstet Gynaecol* 76:881, 1969.

Teramo K: Effects of obstetrical paracervical blockade on the fetus. *Acta Obstet Gynecol Scand* (suppl 16)50:6, 1971.

Teramo K, Benowitz N, Heymann MA, et al: Effects of lidocaine on heart rate, blood pressure, and electrocardiogram in fetal sheep. *Am J Obstet Gynecol* 118:935, 1974.

Teramo K, Rajamaki A: Foetal and maternal plasma levels of mepivacaine and fetal acid–base balance and heart rate after paracervical block during labour. *Br J Anaesth* 43:300, 1971.

Teramo K, Widholm O: Studies of the effects of anesthetics on the fetus. I. The effect of paracervical block with mepivacaine upon fetal acid–base values. *Acta Obstet Gynecol Scand* (suppl 2)46:3, 1967.

Thiery M, Vroman S: Paracervical block analgesia during labor. *Am J Obstet Gynecol* 113:988, 1972.

Thomas J, Climie CR, Mather LE: The maternal plasma levels and placental transfer of bupivacaine following epidural analgesia. *Br J Anaesth* 41:1035, 1969.

Tyack AJ, Parsons RJ, Millar DR, et al: Uterine activity and plasma bupivacaine levels after caudal epidural analgesia. *J Obstet Gynaecol Br Comwlth* 80:896, 1973.

Van Liere EJ, Bell WE, Mazzocco TR, et al: Mechanism of action of nitrous oxide, ether, and chloroform on the uterus. *Am J Obstet Gynecol* 90:811, 1964.

Vasicka A, Hutchinson TT, Eng M, et al: Spinal and epidural anesthesia, fetal and uterine response to acute hypo- and hypertension. *Am J Obstet Gynecol* 90:800, 1964.

Vasicka A, Kretchmer H: Effect of conduction and inhalation anesthesia on uterine contractions. *Am J Obstet Gynecol* 82:600, 1961.

Vasicka A, Robertazzi R, Raji M, et al: Fetal bradycardia after paracervical block. *Obstet Gynecol* 38:500, 1971.

Ward GH, Anz UE, McCarthy AM: Sustained contractions of the gravid uterus during spinal anesthesia. *Am J Obstet Gynecol* 64:406, 1952.

Wingate MB, Wingate L, Iffy L, et al: The effect of epidural analgesia upon fetal and neonatal status. *Am J Obstet Gynecol* 119:1101, 1974.

Yeh SY, Paul RH, Cordero L, et al: A study of diazepam during labor. *Obstet Gynecol* 43:363, 1974.

Zourlas PA, Kumar D: An objective evaluation of paracervical block on human uterine contractility. *Am J Obstet Gynecol* 91:217, 1965.

CHAPTER 19
Complications and Advantages

The continuous recording of the various pathophysiologic phenomena evolving during labor and delivery implies a number of manipulations and the use of equipment (see Chapter 4) that may predispose to complications (physical or psychological) while contributing to the benefit of the patients being monitored.

The most important of the complications have been briefly mentioned. They will be described in more detail here, with emphasis on means of preventing them. Furthermore, the possible benefits and inconveniences to the patient will be discussed.

COMPLICATIONS

Circumstances that affect the physical well-being of mother and fetus as direct consequences of intrapartum electronic monitoring may, for practical purposes, be considered to be the result of direct or internal monitoring exclusively. The invasive transvaginal intrauterine catheter and the fetal scalp subcutaneous electrode are the most extensively used methods of direct monitoring. Other modes of recording are so seldom used by so few that this discussion will center only on the problems created by the transvaginal catheter and fetal scalp subcutaneous electrode.

Maternal

Traumatic Careless manipulation at introducing the internal catheter may produce moderate to severe complications that may or may not be recognized at the time they occur. The first to be reported was the *perforation of the lower segment* by the catheter guide (Haverkamp and Bowes, 1972) with subsequent development of a parauterine abscess requiring drainage. *Unrecognized perforations* have been found at the time of cesarean sections. The *perforation into the broad ligament* without untoward effects has been documented by injection of contrast medium through the obstructed catheter (Figure 19-1). From the few published observations it is difficult to assess the overall incidence of this accident; the problem of an accurate estimate is further compounded by the possible "silent" perforations unrecognized by the operators. They occur as a consequence of faulty technique: the insertion of the guide much beyond the tip of the examining fingers applied between cervix and presenting part. The observance of the proper technique (see Figure 4-26) should completely prevent this potentially serious problem. In the Chicago Lying-In Hospital series of more than 7000 cases of direct monitoring there has been no recognized case of uterine perforation.

It is obvious that the consequences of this type of perforation may be very serious: laceration of a large vessel may cause either a severe hemorrhage or the formation of a hematoma of unpredictable size. Furthermore, the latter may become infected with all the consequences of a large abscess.

Another mechanical accident produced by faulty technique at introduction of the catheter is *perforation of placental vessels*. In general, it is manifested by minimal external bleeding or staining of the amniotic fluid; more significant is the progressive fetal tachycardia without apparent good reason, but actually due to progressive fetal anemia. When fetal distress is not rapidly recognized and treated the infant may be lost (Trudinger and Pryse-Davies, 1978). The diagnosis of fetal distress with prompt intervention may produce an anemic infant who would require neonatal transfusion. The laceration of a large placental vessel (Figure 19-2) explains the rapid blood loss somewhat dampened by the partial plugging effect of the threaded-in catheter.

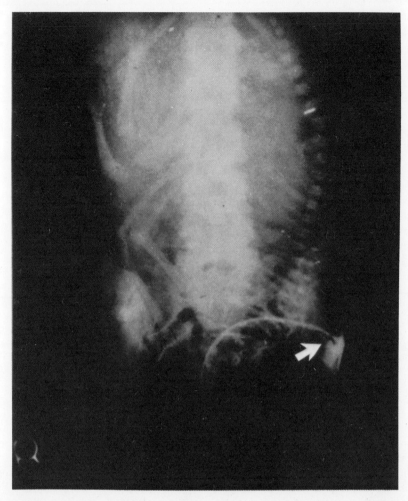

Figure 19-1 Radiography of lower abdomen of patient in labor. Intrauterine catheter not recording contractions. Transcatheter injection of Hypaque reveals accumulation in the left broad ligament (arrow). Reprinted from Chan WH, et al: Intrapartum fetal monitoring. *Obstet Gynecol* 41:7, 1973.

The *entanglement of the catheter with the umbilical cord* has been reported even though it is extemely rare (Trudinger and Pryse-Davies, 1978). It requires that the catheter be more pliable than that usually available, and that too much of it be introduced. The presence of variable type decelerations, totally unrelated to contractions, seems to be the symptom that should alert the clinician.

Another potential accident, not yet reported, is the partial separation of the placenta when the guide is introduced too far and acts as a

bougie—also due to inappropriate technique.

When the catheter is inserted transabdominally, one may observe all the traumatic complications reported for amniocentesis. In particular, the transplacental insertion of the needle and the possible laceration of a vessel on the fetal side should now be avoidable when localization of the placenta is possible by means of ultrasound imaging. The lesion of an umbilical artery has occurred without effect on fetal outcome; however, if the lacerated vessel is the umbilical vein the exsanguination of the fetus may be rapid. The

474

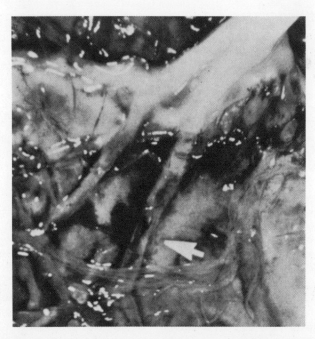

Figure 19-2   Fetal side of placenta showing perforation of an important venous branch (arrow) produced by the intrauterine catheter. Rapidly developing fetal anemia is the logical consequence. Reprinted from Nuttal ID: Perforation of a placental fetal vessel by an intrauterine pressure catheter. *Br J Obstet Gynaecol* 85:573, 1978.

spasm of the artery may prevent massive bleeding, whereas the vein has no adequate walls to actively participate in the process of hemostasis.

Infection   The potential infection of the amniotic cavity by the insertion of a transvaginal catheter should always be in the mind of the obstetrician contemplating direct monitoring. It is now known that the "normal" vaginal flora contains a variety of strains of potentially pathogenic aerobes and anaerobes. If a sufficient number of them are carried to the amniotic cavity it is conceivable that a clinical infection may supervene. The contamination of the cavity is a certainty a few hours after labor with ruptured membranes even in nonmonitored labors. (For the effect of internal monitoring on postpartum infection, see Advantages and Hazards.)

The use of transabdominal catheters does not predispose to intrauterine infections when appropriate aseptic technique is observed. Recordings of up to 3 days have evolved without the slightest sign of infection.

Fetal

Traumatic   Because the recording electrode must be implanted in the fetal subcutaneous tissue, traumatic accidents may occur. This possibility has become more evident with the generalized use of the spiral electrode, which may be (and generally is) applied blindly. This step has been an improvement in the ease of application, compared to the necessity of exposing the scalp through an amnioscope when the clip was the electrode in use. The convenience of blind insertion of the spiral electrode predisposes to the possibility of its implantation on a nonrecommended area—particularly when the presenting part is high or abnormal. Application on the *eyelid,* in case of face presentation, has been observed (Thomas and Blackwell, 1975). Likewise, in a case of breech presentation the electrode was applied on the *vulvar fourchette with subsequent rectal laceration* (Pugh and Weiss, 1976). The insertion of the electrode directly over a fontanelle allows the possibility of lacerating the underlying large venous sinuses, and, when too deep, the penetration *through the dura mater and into the CSF space;* the relatively prolonged drainage of CSF subsequent to this trauma has been reported (Goodlin and Harrod, 1973). The *laceration of arterioles* with persistent "spurting" bleeding causing anemia and requiring suture has been reported (Scanlon and Walkley, 1972). On the other hand, the mistaken placement of the electrode on the cervix may expose the pointed tip to the passing fetus at the time of delivery and produce significant lacerations. One such case with a *laceration affecting the cheek, trunk, and thigh* was reported (Atlas and Serr, 1976).

An unknown coagulation defect of the fetus may be a very serious cause of bleeding, particularly when fetal scalp blood sampling is used as a complement to electronic monitoring. Fortunately these cases are extremely rare.

The transabdominal insertion of the needle to set the intrauterine catheter may also wound the fetus, if the necessary care is not taken. Scratches and small punctures have been observed following amniocentesis aimed at obtaining amniotic fluid for various purposes, and the same may occur when the puncture is done to pass a catheter.

The prophylaxis of these complications requires strict adherence to the principle of meticulous technique. Among the several thousand cases monitored at the Chicago Lying-In Hospital no traumatic complications related to electrode application have been observed. Likewise, no traumatic fetal lesions have been found following the transabdominal insertion of catheters when this technique was required.

Infection The vagina, normally populated by potentially pathogenic aerobic and anaerobic bacteria, constitutes a possible source of infection following the subcutaneous implantation of a needle on the fetal presenting part. Although the number of reported infections is relatively low, nevertheless it represents a potential serious complication that may or may not be completely preventable. In large series it has been estimated that *fetal scalp abscesses occur* in about 4 to 9 per 1000 cases (Cordero and Hon, 1971; Plavidal and Werch, 1976; Yasunaga, 1976; Feder et al, 1976). However, others have osbserved a much higher incidence, 4% to 5% (Winkel et al 1976; Okada et

al, 1977) when conducting meticulous observations of fetal scalps.

Etiology Relatively large numbers of so-called sterile or aseptic abscesses were observed shortly after internal monitoring was introduced; nevertheless, recent, more elaborate methods of culture have yielded consistent positive multibacterial cultures. Among the more frequently found are *Staphylococcus epidermidis; Streptococcus* A, viridans, β-hemolytic); *Peptostreptococcus; Peptococcus; Escherichia coli;* and *Bacteroides. S. epidermidis* has been found consistently in over 40% of cases, while the others have been found in lower proportions.

The majority of these abscesses are seen when the infant is about 4 days of age, the "incubation" period ranging from 2 to 10 days. The lesions tend to be relatively small in size, averaging 1 to 3 cm, and are *usually superficial.*

In rare cases the infection may extend in depth to reach under the occipitofrontal aponeurosis and produce *subgaleal abscesses* (Goodman et al, 1977), which of course may be severe and extend very rapidly. The deep penetration of the infection may also affect the subjacent bone to produce a limited *osteomyelitis* (Yasunaga, 1976; Plavidal and Werch, 1976). Delay in treating this complication may lead to a more severe form of bone infection with partial destruction (Figure 19-3).

The subcutaneous localization of the infection does not preclude a severe clinical picture. When the offending organism is a highly pathogenic anaerobe one might have *crepitation and gas formation* detectable by x-ray (Turbeville et al, 1976). In this circumstance the outcome may be fatal.

Even when the infection responds to aggressive treatment there may be significant local *necrosis with loss of tissue* (Figure 19-4) which imposes the necessity of grafting for a complete recovery.

Septicemias due to gonococcus (Thadepalli et al, 1976), and/or associated with streptococcus (Plavidal and Werch, 1977) have been reported and required prolonged treatment before full recovery could be obtained.

Treatment The treatment of choice is drainage and local care as soon as a collection is detectable. In the majority of cases this simple procedure, without the use of systemic antibiotics

476

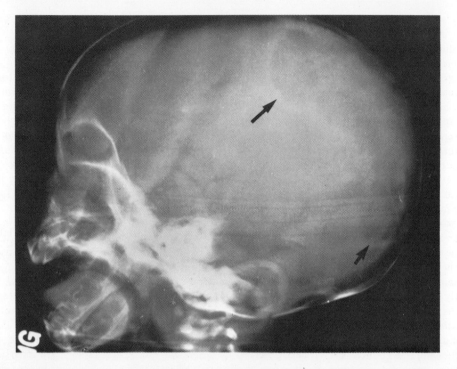

Figure 19-3 Lateral radiography of newborn skull with severe scalp infection. The large area of bone destruction (arrows) extending from the parietal to the occipital was produced by *Staphylococcus epidermidis*. Drainage and debridement facilitated eventual but delayed healing. Reprinted from Overturf GD, Balfour G: Osteomyelitis and sepsis: Severe complications of fetal monitoring. *Pediatrics* 55:244, 1975. Copyright American Academy of Pediatrics, 1975.

has been sufficient to obtain complete healing. However, when the extent or depth of the infection is significant, generous debridement and large doses of systemic antibiotics may be necessary to control the infection.

Predisposing factors With a relatively low incidence, these infections seem sometimes to be the consequence of factors present in clusters in selected cases. In some series the factor seems to have been determined by the *model of the subcutaneous electrode* (Winkel et al, 1976). Another presumed incriminating factor has been *prematurity* (Okada et al, 1977). Plavidal and Werch (1976) found that in 48% of the abscesses they observed, there was *premature rupture of the membranes,* in 39% of them for more than 24 hours. This finding notwithstanding, the duration of monitoring seems to contribute only peripherally as a determining factor: the range of 2 to 21 hours has been reported in the larger series; this extremely wide range indicates that it does not seem to be an important contributing cause.

A circumstance probably directly responsible for the infection is the type of *vaginal flora* present in the mother. In several cases the same strain of bacteria was found present in the scalp abscesses of gonococcal infections and *β-hemolytic Streptococcus.*

A large caput succedaneum or a cephalohematoma are definitely points of call for an infection. In fact, one reported case of osteomyelitis (Figure 19-3) developed in a newborn having a cephalohematoma. In these circumstances, one might consider the possibility of a secondary infection, perhaps unrelated to the monitoring. Yasunaga (1976) ascribed a number of the cases he observed to *deficient sterilization techniques* that clustered around a given period. Changes in procedure seemed to have been enough to prevent this complication.

In the series of more than 7000 cases at the Chicago Lying-In Hosital about 20 abscesses, none severe, have been observed. No deep infections have, so far, been found. Almost 50% of

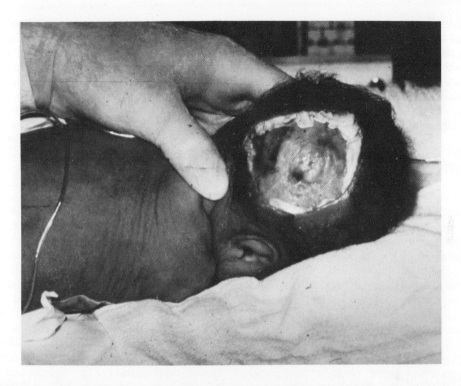

Figure 19-4   Large slough of fetal scalp following a postdirect monitoring abscess (β-hemolytic streptococcus group A). It required prolonged antibiotic therapy and skin grafting. Reprinted from Feder HM, et al: Scalp abscess secondary to fetal scalp electrode. *J Pediatr* 89:808, 1976. Courtesy H.M. Feder.

them occurred during a short period of time when the treatment of the small wound was not carried out with the attention and technique established in the protocol. Enforcement of the technical steps eradicated the "minor epidemic."

Prophylaxis   A survey of factors associated with monitoring accidents suggests that *some are preventable* if appropriate care is taken to use proper sterilization techniques and standard fine stainless steel electrodes; to insert the needle (transabdominal tap) without forcing and away from placenta and fetal parts; and to insert the catheter guide up to the tip of the operator's fingers (never beyond). When the operator is in doubt as regards the presenting part and the precise anatomic site selected for implantation, he should not proceed. Gentle manipulation is absolutely mandatory in all circumstances.

Other circumstances may contribute to accidents that are less predictable or preventable. The fact that a patient has premature rupture of membranes often dictates the need of induction and monitoring, which tends to occur often among preterm pregnancies. The presence of a vaginal infection should be a strong contraindication to the use of transvaginal direct monitoring, unless other methods are not applicable and monitoring is absolutely essential.

The presence of a large caput succedaneum or a cephalohematoma should temper the enthusiasm for the implantation of an electrode. Also, the electrode *should never be applied over a suture or fontanelle.*

Probably the most important step in preventing a scalp infection (other than using properly sterilized material) is *meticulous treatment of the small wound immediately after delivery.* After completion of cleaning the airway and execution of the eye treatment (Credé's method) for prophylaxis of ophthalmia neonatorum, attention should be turned to the scalp. After inspection and localization, the wound must be thoroughly cleansed with an antiseptic detergent and a broad-spectrum antibiotic cream applied locally. Very hairy infants should be shaved to facilitate cleansing and follow-up of the wound. If caput succedaneum or cephalohematoma are found under the scalp where the electrode has been inserted, closer observation should be exerted to detect early infection and treat it vigorously. In these cases more prolonged follow-up is advisable because of the possibility of delayed infection.

ADVANTAGES AND HAZARDS

Continuous feto-maternal monitoring was for more than a decade strictly a research tool, but in the past 10 years it has acquired widespread clinical application. Unfortunately its rapid acceptance as adjuvant in the conduction and supervision of labor has not been accompanied by the necessary in-depth education of all those in charge of interpreting the tracings and managing the cases. Along with many advantages and benefits, some hazards have been observed (those affecting the fetus more directly have already been reviewed) and these hazards may have a detrimental effect on the outcome of some pregnancies. Strong emotional attitudes by those espousing opposing viewpoints have not helped in carrying out an objective evaluation of the rightful place of this new tool in the practice of obstetrics.

Disadvantages

Because monitoring has been considered as "interference" with the spontaneous "natural" process of labor, some refuse to use it except under extreme circumstances. This concept applies not only to the invasive internal techniques but to the external noninvasive methods as well, and the areas presumably affecting the patients involve psychological and physical aspects of their well-being.

Psychological The first reaction of the pregnant patient to electronic monitoring of her labor cannot be indifferent. The need to apply and/or introduce the gadgets used to pick up the signals to be recorded may create a feeling of either fear or reassurance, depending on her knowledge regarding the instrumentation and its aim. A well-informed patient may respond with a calm reaction and cooperation to the manipulations required to establish a good recording, while a fearful or inadequately prepared patient may be

extremely apprehensive and manifest even distrust at what she is about to undergo.

This negative attitude is not attenuated by the stimulus of a vociferous campaign propounding that monitoring "dehumanizes" the process of labor and delivery and the relationship between the patient and those charged with the responsibility of assisting her in that process. This concept is, in part, supported by the relative immobilization required of the patient after the recording devices have been applied, particularly the "external" methods. The immobilization is most noticeable in the early stages of dilatation when many patients have the desire to move about in bed or even walk around in the labor room. In the more advanced stages of dilatation they are more willing to remain in bed, and this becomes a necessity for those who request anesthesia to relieve their labor pains. Internal methods allow for only slightly more mobility in bed, and in addition are less bothersome physically, but this advantage is countered by the more uncomfortable manipulations necessary for their application.

The patient's fear or apprehension may alter the normal evaluation of an otherwise potentially normal labor. The release of catecholamines, especially norepinephrine, must affect the progress of labor because they have a direct effect on uterine contractility. This reaction may affect the patient's blood pressure in those cases where there is increased vascular reactivity to these amines (preeclampsia, hypertension). By influencing the uterine contractility and maternal blood pressure, the release of norepinephrine may, in extreme cases, affect the well-being of the fetus by interfering with IVS blood flow.

It seems evident that for an improperly informed patient, or one indoctrinated against electronic monitoring, this technique may induce such an important psychological burden as to lose all its potential advantages and in fact be detrimental to her labor and delivery.

Physical *Cesarean sections* One of the most important objections made against the use of electronic intrapartum monitoring by its detractors is that one consistently sees a significant increase in the proportion of cases terminating in cesarean section. Clearly this is a more traumatic way of delivery than the vaginal route and carries with it a significant risk of serious complication. To document this point of view, this group often quotes the consistent and impressive rise in cesarean section rates across the country coincidental with the introduction of widespread use of electronic monitoring. The average overall less than 10% section rate observed 10 years ago has risen to an impressive 25% to 30% in some hospitals, and in general to approximately 20% in the majority of them. This increase is usually ascribed exclusively to the use of electronic monitoring (implying intrapartum fetal distress), disregarding all the other clinical conditions in which the more liberal use of cesarean section has successfully (perhaps not always justifiably) been advocated and with great acceptance: all breech presentations, premature labor with very small fetuses, rupture of membranes for more than 24 hours, therapeutic termination of pregnancy with unripe cervices, so-called borderline cephalopelvic dysproportions or "lack of progress." Very few randomized studies have been conducted to evaluate this problem. The most frequently quoted is that of Haverkamp et al (1976) in which the monitored group had a 16.5% section rate compared to 6.8% for the unmonitored. However, Renou et al (1976) found no difference in their cesarean section rate in a parallel controlled study. Other authors have found that, in fact, the incidence of cesarean sections for *fetal distress* actually fell from 9.5% to 6% (Edington et al, 1975) and even 4% after electronic monitoring was widely applied in their hospitals (Shenker et al, 1975) while, at the same time, the primary section rate increased because of other factors. It appears that *experience in interpretation of the tracings is critical to avoid unnecessary cesarean sections*. Another group of investigators (Tipton and Lewis, 1975) found no increase in their cesarean section rate in consecutive years in spite of a marked rise in the use of continuous intrapartum monitoring as an adjuvant in the management of their cases.

The uncritical evaluation of the increased incidence of cesarean sections coinciding with the generalized use of continuous intrapartum monitoring observed in the past few years would suggest a direct connection. However, the more detailed assessment of other possible broadened indications for cesarean section in reasonably large and comparable series would indicate that the more liberal indications may be responsible for the observed increase. In fact, when properly interpreted by experienced individuals, electronic monitoring tracings should avoid unnecessary cesarean sections. By the same token, the analysis of recordings by inadequately trained individuals will logically increase the number of cesarean sections by "overcalling" some FHR alterations. *The need for experience and caution when evaluating an electronic monitoring record cannot be overemphasized.*

In the clinical material of the Chicago Lying-In Hospital (3200 to 3500 deliveries a year) the proportion of continuously monitored cases has steadily risen from 15% (1970) to more than 90% (1979), while the overall incidence of cesarean sections has fluctuated between 10% and 12%. The primary section rate remained within the range of 6% and 8%, with the year 1979 being 7%. The liberalization of indications has contributed to a small increase, while the incidence of cases operated for fetal distress have remained very stable.

Infection The manipulations involved in setting up "direct" monitoring carry with them the potential for infection; in particular the need to rupture membranes should be recognized as a most important possible drawback of the technique. The remainder of this discussion will refer exclusively to cases monitored by direct techniques because there is no danger of intrauterine contamination with indirect methods.

It has been repeatedly claimed by the critics who oppose continuous monitoring that it is responsible for an inordinate number of intrapartum and postpartum infections. However, no differences in puerperal infection rates have been observed when comparing monitored and unmonitored patients (Wiechetek et al, 1974). Curiously, Haverkamp et al (1976) found a significantly higher puerperal infection rate among the "monitored" cases even though their control cases were equally manipulated and monitored but the tracings disregarded for management. In a large series of vaginal deliveries Ledger (1978) reported a low incidence, 3%, of puerperal infections (Figure 19-5) among the cases with internal monitoring; furthermore, the duration of monitoring did not seem to influence the incidence of puerperal infection. And, the "fever index" was shown to be comparable in two infected populations of monitored and unmonitored patients with the conclusion that "internal monitoring alone is not a significant clinical factor in the development of infection in a high risk obstetric population."

The more intense investigations carried out to evaluate the possible effect of internal monitoring on postpartum infections have been on the

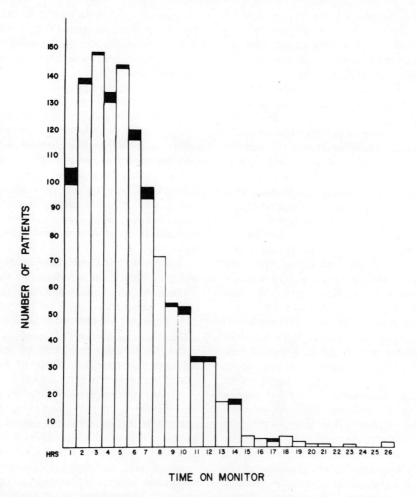

Figure 19-5 Series of patients who delivered vaginally following internal monitoring. The length of time with the monitor applied is shown in the abscissa, and the numer of patients monitored for each hour in the ordinates. Open bars indicate the number of patients with normal puerperium (1159 cases), and the black bars (on top) indicate the number of those who had puerperal infection (33 cases). Reprinted from Ledger WJ: Complication associated with invasive monitoring. *Semin Perinatol* 2:187, 1978. By permission.

group of patients undergoing *cesarean sections*. The overall incidence of "infectious morbidity" following this operation has consistently been astonishingly high, ranging from 35% to 50%. The breakdown into various groups indicates that perhaps labor before monitoring could be considered a strong causative factor facilitating a higher incidence of infections (Hagen, 1975; Gassner and Ledger, 1976). Several studies have been conducted to evaluate these and other possible variables; the general assessment indicates that duration of monitoring before cesarean section does not influence the rate of postoperative infec-

tions (Figure 19-6). On the other hand, labor before the operation significantly increases the postoperative "fever index," which is still further increased when the membranes have been ruptured for some time (Figure 19-7). This factor seems to be independent of the time the monitoring lasted before the cesarean section, but there is a clear positive correlation between duration of ruptured membranes and propensity to postoperative pelvic infection (Figure 19-8).

The combination of ruptured membranes and labor constitutes a definite risk for postoperative infection regardless of method of

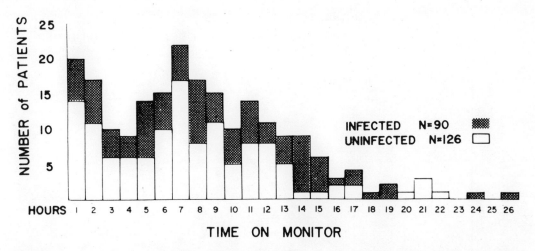

Figure 19-6 Series of patients who had a cesarean section following internal monitoring. Tabulation as in Figure 19-6 shows a much higher infection rate. Reprinted from Ledger WJ: Complication associated with invasive monitoring. *Semin Perinatol* 2:187, 1978. By permission.

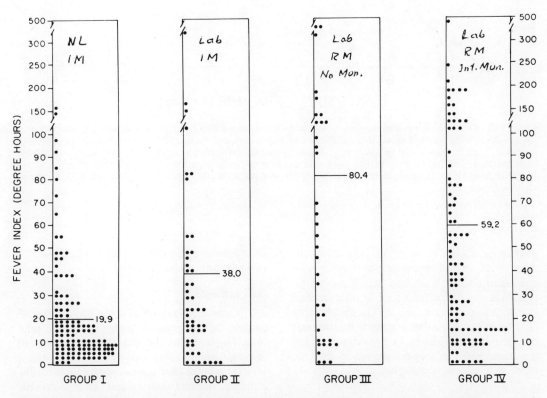

Figure 19-7 Postoperative "fever index" in four groups of patients who underwent cesarean section (each dot represents a patient). Group I with intact membranes and not in labor. Group II with intact membranes and with labor preceding the operation. Group III in labor with ruptured membranes and no internal monitoring. Group IV in labor with ruptured membranes and internal monitoring before the operation. There is no difference between the averages of Group III and IV. Reprinted from Gibbs RS, et al: Internal fetal monitoring and maternal infection following cesarean section. *Obstet Gynecol* 48:653, 1976.

482

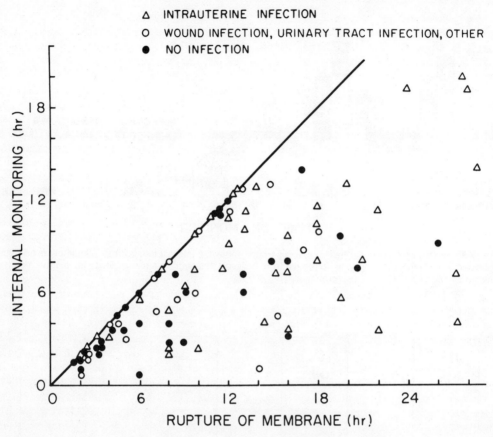

△ INTRAUTERINE INFECTION

○ WOUND INFECTION, URINARY TRACT INFECTION, OTHER

● NO INFECTION

Figure 19-8 Duration of ruptured membranes and internal monitoring in a group of patients who had cesarean section. Each point is placed to indicate the duration of both parameters, and the type of symbol represents the puerperal evolution. The distribution of points does not incriminate internal monitoring as a risk factor independent of rupture of membranes. The points over the line show that in those cases the duration of both parameters is the same. Reprinted from Gibbs RS, et al: Internal fetal monitoring and maternal infection following cesarean section. *Obstet Gynecol* 48:653, 1976.

monitoring (Gibbs et al, 1976). Moreover, the number of vaginal examinations further contributes to possible infections, which are not increased in severity or frequency by prior internal monitoring (Gibbs et al, 1978). Endometrial cultures in postoperative infections demonstrate the same bacterial strains in nonmonitored and monitored patients; they are present in amniotic fluid, decidua, and membranes.

In conclusion, it seems that continuous direct monitoring does not predispose to postpartum and postoperative infections. The factors that facilitate infection seem to be labor, time elapsed

since amniotomy, number of pelvic examinations, and preexisting vaginal flora.

Advantages

It stands to reason that the continuous recording of intrapartum pathophysiologic data *should be beneficial* and make an improvement in perinatal results obtained without monitoring. This theoretical (and logical) statement notwithstanding, the fact remains that, to be accepted, such a postulate needs scientific demonstration. There are numerous difficulties intrinsic in a retrospective evaluation of clinical data, even accumulated at the same institution and by the same group of investigators. The changing variables include some circumstances already mentioned, to which one must add the improvements in prenatal diagnosis, neonatal care (assisted respiration, electrolyte balance, new antibiotics, parenteral feeding, continuous monitoring of vital signs) and diagnostic methods (ultrasound, computerized tomography) which have contributed to a marked improvement in neonatal survival. The problems are compounded by the strong emotions of those involved in the controversy (physicians and lay people). In spite of this fact one may still attempt an objective evaluation of the published reports and draw *tentative conclusions* regarding the possible benefits of continuous monitoring.

Psychological For the well-informed and receptive patient, continuous monitoring of her labor constitutes an important reassuring element. A positive attitude cannot but help in its successful conduction and outcome. This acceptance and the awareness of the contribution the procedure makes in the management of her labor are of particular importance in the group of high-risk gestations. The recordings allow the repeated review of the various elements that influence maternal and fetal well-being and that are the basis for changes or adjustments of the therapeutic procedures employed to manage those labors. The graphic documentation should help the physician to convey to the patient the reasons, when the need arrives, for planning or taking certain unexpected therapeutic steps.

Physical *Uterine contractility* Adequate evaluation of the contractility pattern during labor can be done only by continuous recording of the contractions. In fact, for a precise assessment of all the important elements of the contractions, *"internal" or direct recordings* are the only ones giving the necessary information. The policy at the Chicago Lying-In Hospital, since the section of Fetal-Maternal Medicine was established in 1969, is that whenever the use of drugs, with their potential effect on uterine contractility is contemplated, continuous monitoring is carried out. Only with the continuous tracing of contractions can the clinician make objective decisions with regard to the changes in dose of medications or the administration of new ones. It is probably safe to state that even those strongly opposed to continuous monitoring recognize the need for this procedure when there is need to induce or enhance a labor. Likewise, an accurate diagnosis of dysfunctional labor or relative cephalopelvic disproportion can be made only

when one has available the information about the pattern and the intensity of contractions, the latter possible only with the output of the internal monitoring recordings.

Neonatal status The condition of the fetus at birth has been one of the elements evaluated by the majority of observers in assessing the fetal condition: the Apgar score and the acid–base balance of the newborn. Ideally, both should be in the normal range if one attempts to practice effective prophylaxis. However, the detractors of monitoring usually criticize the "uselessness" of the procedure because the incidence of depressed infants is only slightly higher among those monitored and diagnosed to have intrapartum distress; presumably an indicated intervention producing a nondepressed infant is a "false positive" case and thus unnecessary interference. In fact, the delivery of a good infant following FHR alterations that indicate impending or developing problems should be considered a therapeutic success rather than labeled as a false alarm. Under ideal circumstances, the delivery of a depressed infant who demonstrated FHR alterations during labor should be interpreted perhaps as failure to intervene or delay in taking therapeutic steps. These considerations are made with the awareness that low Apgar scores do not always indicate fetal acidosis. Conversely, only in states of severe acidosis is there good correlation with low Apgar scores; a high proportion of fetuses with moderate acidosis have good Apgar scores.

The outcome of monitored compared to unmonitored labors gives consistently better Apgar scores according to several large series collected in centers where there is sufficient experience to interpret the tracings (Shenker et al, 1975; Lee and Baggish, 1976; Gabert and Stenchever, 1977; Amato, 1977). These findings would, indirectly, suggest that warnings of impending fetal deterioration, detected in the tracings, probably helped to establish corrective steps or to decide on successful interference before the fetus could undergo homeostatic alterations.

When fetal acid–base status has been studied in similar patient populations, it has been observed that the unmonitored fetuses have lower pH and less oxygen in the umbilical artery (Renou et al, 1976). Nevertheless, Haverkamp et al (1976) were unable to detect any difference between two comparable patient populations and their outcomes. The judicious interpretation of continuous intrapartum monitoring by experienced physicians

484

should contribute to better overall newborn condition than observed in unmonitored populations, as the large clinical studies indicate.

Perinatal morbidity and mortality Fetal mortality during labor and in the neonatal period is usually reviewed to evaluate the quality of intrapartum care (It is recognized that mortality constitutes an extreme indication of such care). Furthermore, other factors heavily influence perinatal mortality. A somewhat better indicator should be neonatal morbidity, and still better the long-term assessment of the physical and mental condition of the infants studied. Nevertheless, only perinatal results are available for review, with very few exceptions of prospective longitudinal studies.

Immediate and *short-term neonatal morbidity* has been studied by Renou et al (1976) in two randomized groups of high-risk patients, and their findings seem to indicate that continuous monitoring, properly interpreted, should help in preventing damage in a number of neonates (Figure 19-9). Other authors have found that

intrapartum fetal distress and homeostatic imbalance are particularly damaging to premature fetuses and suggest that among these infants the early warning of impending distress indicated by monitoring should diminish the incidence of depressed neonates and handicapped infants.

The overall perinatal mortality in the United States was on the order of 25 per 1000 in the 1960s and fell to about 15 per thousand in the late 1970s. It is generally accepted that this improvement has been the result of several factors: better prenatal care, a more aggressive management of obstetric complications, the application of new concepts in the management of premature infants, and for some the use of continuous intrapartum monitoring. This last point has been the subject of much controversy charged with emotion. The position of those who believe that continuous monitoring improves perinatal survival has been substantiated by reports involving control groups from several institutions, although these studies have not been done on matched populations. Paul and Hon

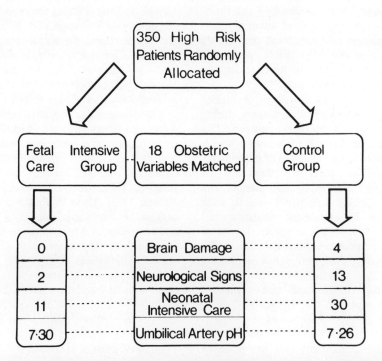

Figure 19-9 Diagram showing the results of a controlled study carried out on a group of high-risk pregnancies. One half (175) had continuous monitoring and scalp blood analysis while the controls (175) had routine periodic checks of vital signs. The number of cases for each parameter studied is shown. All differences are significant. Reprinted from Wood C: Fetal scalp sampling: Its place in management. *Semin Perinatol* 2:169, 1978. By permission.

(1974) observed lower mortality (11 per 1000) among a group of high-risk patients than in a low-risk population (21 per 1000).

Likewise, Shenker et al (1975) observed a marked fall in perinatal mortality, from 17 to 9 per 1000 after the routine use of continuous monitoring. Tipton and Lewis (1975) observed in 2 years a fall from 10 to 3 per 1000 in intrapartum and neonatal deaths; Edington et al (1975) from 15.5 to 4.5 per 1000. Lee and Baggish in 3 years reported a fall in perinatal mortality from 24 to 15 per 1000; Hochuli et al (1976) in 10 years from 10.4 to 4.7 per 1000.

In a 2-year period, in two populations cared for in the same hospital and at the same time, Amato (1977) observed a 23 per 1000 mortality in the unmonitored group and only 3 per 1000 in the monitored patients. All these authors indicate that continuous monitoring probably contributed significantly to the better outcomes.

Neutra et al (1978) reviewed a large collaborative material and concluded that monitoring seems to be effective in improving perinatal mortality only in high-risk populations, while in low-risk groups the potential benefit was not noticeable.

The most impressive findings have been observed in the prevention of intrapartum deaths (Figure 19-10). Shenker et al (1975) have not observed an intrapartum death among the monitored patients, and 1.2 per 1000 among the unmonitored. Edington et al (1975) observed a

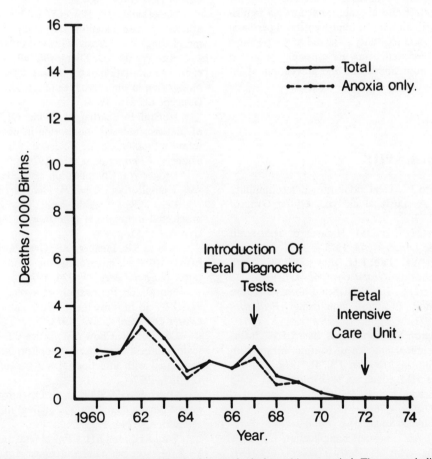

Figure 19-10 Incidence of intrapartum fetal deaths for anoxia during a 14-year period. The arrows indicate years when procedures that presumably would influence the outcome were introduced. No intrapartum deaths (excluding malformation) were recorded after continuous monitoring was established as routine. Reprinted from Wood C: Fetal scalp sampling: Its place in management. *Semin Perinatol* 2:169, 1978. By permission.

dramatic fall from 4.5 to 0.5 per 1000 after continuous monitoring was routinely applied. Likewise, Lee and Baggish (1976) observed a difference from 3.7 to 0.3 per 1000 intrapartum deaths between unmonitored and monitored patients. In comparable groups of patients Amato (1977) found 0.5 per 1000 intrapartum deaths among monitored patients and 4 per 1000 in unmonitored.

It seems undeniable that intensive observation and continuous recording of pathophysiologic data during labor contributes to identify cases of preventable intrapartum death.

In conclusion, the objective review of the available clinical data suggests that continuous intrapartum monitoring, *applied with the appropriate technique and interpreted by adequately trained individuals,* does not significantly predispose to fetal or maternal morbidity. On the other hand, it appears that it has made a significant contribution to the improvement of perinatal morbidity and mortality observed in the past few years. These statements are especially valid for high-risk populations and the prevention of intrapartum deaths.

BIBLIOGRAPHY

Amato JC: Fetal monitoring in a community hospital: A statistical analysis. *Obstet Gynecol* 50:269, 1977.

Atlas M, Serr DM: Hazards of fetal scalp electrodes. *Lancet* 1:648, 1976.

Chan WH, Paul RH, Toews J: Intrapartum fetal monitoring. *Obstet Gynecol* 41:7, 1973.

Cordero L, Hon EH: Scalp abscess: A rare complication of fetal monitoring. *Pediatrics* 78:533, 1971.

Edington PT, Sibanda J, Beard RW: Influence on clinical practice of routine intrapartum fetal monitoring. *Br Med J* 3:341, 1975.

Feder HM, MacLean WC, Moxon R: Scalp abscess secondary to fetal scalp electrode. *J Pediatr* 89:808, 1976.

Fernandez-Rocha L, Oullette R: Fetal bleeding: An unusual complication of fetal monitoring. *Am J Obstet Gynecol* 125:1153, 1976.

Gabert HA, Stenchever MA: The results of a five-year study of continuous fetal monitoring on an obstetric service. *Obstet Gynecol* 50:275, 1977.

Gassner CB, Ledger WJ: The relationship of hospital-acquired maternal infection to intrapartum monitoring techniques. *Am J Obstet Gynecol* 126:33, 1976.

Gibbs RS, Jones PM, Wilder CJY: Internal fetal monitoring and maternal infection following cesarean section. *Obstet Gynecol* 52:193, 1978.

Gibbs RS, Listwa HM, Read JA: The effect of internal fetal monitoring on maternal infection following cesarean section. *Obstet Gynecol* 48:653, 1976.

Goodlin RC, Harrod JR: Complications of fetal spiral electrodes. *Lancet* 1:559, 1973.

Goodman SJ, Cahan L, Chow AW: Subgaleal abscess. A preventable complication of scalp trauma. *West J Med* 127:169, 1977.

Hagen D: Maternal febrile morbidity associated with fetal monitoring and cesarean section. *Obstet Gynecol* 46:260, 1975.

Haverkamp AD, Bowes WA: Uterine perforation: A complication of continuous fetal monitoring. *Am J Obstet Gynecol* 110:667, 1972.

Haverkamp AD, Thompson HE, McFee JG, et al: The evaluation of continuous fetal heart rate monitoring in high-risk pregnancy. *Am J Obstet Gynecol* 125:310, 1976.

Hochuli E, Eberhard J, Dubler O: The effect of modern intensive monitoring in obstetrics on infant mortality and the incidence of hypoxia and acidosis. *J Perinat Med* 4:78, 1976.

Ledger WJ: Complication associated with invasive monitoring. *Semin Perinatol* 2:187, 1978.

Lee WK, Baggish MS: The effect of unselected intrapartum fetal monitoring. *Obstet Gynecol* 47:516, 1976.

Neutra RR, Fienberg SE, Greenland S, et al: Effect of fetal monitoring on neonatal death rates. *N Engl J Med* 299:324, 1978.

Nuttal ID: Perforation of a placental fetal vessel by an intrauterine pressure catheter. *Br J Obstet Gynaecol* 85:573, 1978.

Okada DM, Chow AW, Bruce VT: Neonatal scalp abscess and fetal monitoring: Factors associated with infection. *Am J Obstet Gynecol* 129:185, 1977.

Overturf GD, Balfour G: Osteomyelitis and sepsis: Severe complications of fetal monitoring. *Pediatrics* 55:244, 1975.

Paul RH, Hon EH: Clinical fetal monitoring. V. Effect on perinatal outcome. *Am J Obstet Gynecol* 118:529, 1974.

Plavidal FJ, Werch A: Fetal scalp abscess secondary to intrauterine monitoring. *Am J Obstet Gynecol* 125:65, 1976.

Plavidal FJ, Werch A: Gonococcal scalp abscess: A case report. *Am J Obstet Gynecol* 127:437, 1977.

Pugh C, Weiss DB: Hazards of fetal scalp electrodes. *Lancet* 1:803, 1976.

Renou P, Chang A, Anderson A, Wood C: Controlled trial of fetal intensive care. *Am J Obstet Gynecol* 126:470, 1976.

Scanlon JW, Walkley EI: Neonatal blood loss as a complication of fetal monitoring. *Pediatrics* 50:934, 1972.

Shenker L, Post RC, Seiler JS: Routine electronic monitoring of fetal heart rate and uterine activity during labor. *Obstet Gynecol* 46:185, 1975.

Thadepalli H, Rambhatla K, Maidman JE, et al: Gonococcal sepsis secondary to fetal monitoring. *Am J Obstet Gynecol* 126:510, 1976.

Thomas G, Blackwell RJ: A hazard associated with the use of spiral fetal scalp electrodes. *Am J Obstet Gynecol* 121:1118, 1975.

Tipton RH, Lewis BW: Induction of labour and perinatal mortality. *Br Med J* 1:391, 1975.

Trudinger BJ, Pryse-Davies J: Fetal hazards of the intrauterine catheter: Five case reports. *Br J Obstet Gynaecol* 85:567, 1978.

Turbeville DF, Heath RE, Bowen FW, et al: Complications of fetal scalp electrodes: A case report. *Am J Obstet Gynecol* 122:530, 1976.

Tutera G, Newman RL: Fetal monitoring: Its effect on the perinatal mortality and cesarean section rates and its complications. *Am J Obstet Gynecol* 122:750, 1975,

Wiechetek WJ, Horiguchi T, Dillon T: Puerperal morbidity and internal fetal monitoring. *Am J Obstet Gynecol* 119:230, 1974.

Winkel CA, Snyder DL, Schlaerth JB: Scalp abscess: A complication of the spiral fetal electrode. *Am J Obstet Gynecol* 126:720, 1976.

Wood C: Fetal scalp sampling: Its place in management. *Semin Perinatol* 2:169, 1978.

Yasunaga S: Complications of fetal monitoring: Scalp abscess and osteomyelitis. *IMJ* 150:41, 1976.

492